UPDATE

I

THE
HEART

UPDATE

I

THE
HEART

Editor

J. Willis Hurst, M.D.

Professor of Medicine (Cardiology)
Chairman, Department of Medicine
Emory University School of Medicine
Atlanta, Georgia

McGraw-Hill Book Company

New York St. Louis San Francisco Auckland Bogotá Düsseldorf
Johannesburg London Madrid Mexico Montreal New Delhi
Panama Paris São Paulo Singapore Sydney Tokyo Toronto

UPDATE I: THE HEART

ISBN 0-07-031490-x

1 2 3 4 5 6 7 8 9 0 MUMU 7 8 3 2 1 0 9

This book was set in Times Roman by Precision Typographers Inc.
The editors were J. Dereck Jeffers,
Richard S. Laufer, and Henry C. De Leo;
the designer was Elliot Epstein;
the production supervisor was Jeanne Selzam.
The Murray Printing Company was printer and binder.

NOTICE

Medicine is an ever-changing science. As new research and clinical experience broaden our knowledge, changes in treatment and drug therapy are required. The editors and the publisher of this work have made every effort to ensure that the drug dosage schedules herein are accurate and in accord with the standards accepted at the time of publication. Readers are advised, however, to check the product information sheet included in the package of each drug they plan to administer to be certain that changes have not been made in the recommended dose or in the contraindications for administration. This recommendation is of particular importance in regard to new or infrequently used drugs.

Contents

Preface   ix

The contribution of Allan Burns   1
J. Willis Hurst, M.D.

Limitations of symptoms in the recognition of coronary atherosclerotic heart disease   3
John S. Douglas, Jr., M.D., and J. Willis Hurst, M.D.

The diagnostic capabilities and limitations of the electrocardiogram   13
Mark E. Silverman, M.D., and Barry D. Silverman, M.D.

The value and limitations of echocardiography   47
Joel M. Felner, M.D.

The use and misuse of digoxin blood levels   75
Thomas W. Smith, M.D., Gregory D. Curfman, M.D., and Laurence H. Green, M.D.

Advances in cardiac pathology   83
Bernadine H. Bulkley, M.D.

From Harvey to coronary bypass surgery: An exercise in logic and scientific analysis   115
J. Willis Hurst, M.D., and Spencer B. King III, M.D.

Coronary bypass surgery at Emory University Clinic: Service organization, surgical technique and selected surgical results   139
Charles R. Hatcher, Jr., M.D.

Myocardial infarction with normal coronary arteries   147
Albert E. Raizner, M.D., and Robert A. Chahine, M.D.

Vasodilator therapy of congestive heart failure   167
James F. Spann, M.D., and J. Willis Hurst, M.D.

Cardiovascular manifestations of sickle-cell anemia   185
Joseph E. Hardison, M.D., and C. Milford Rogers, M.D.

The heart in protein-calorie undernutrition   191
Steven B. Heymsfield, M.D., and Donald O. Nutter, M.D.

Heart disease in the elderly (geriatric cardiology)   211
R. Joe Noble, M.D., and Donald A. Rothbaum, M.D.

Exercise and the heart   235
Donald O. Nutter, M.D.

Alcohol and the heart   259
Timothy J. Regan, M.D., and Philip O. Ettinger, M.D.

Surgical treatment of Wolff-Parkinson-White syndrome   275
Will C. Sealy, M.D., Edward L. C. Pritchett, M.D., Jackie Kasell, and
John J. Gallagher, M.D.

Antiplatelet medication and cardiovascular disease   291
Sidney F. Stein, M.D., and Bruce L. Evatt, M.D.

Arrhythmias related to abnormal repolarization   305
Paul F. Walter, M.D.

Cardiovascular Nuclear Medicine   239
H. William Strauss, M.D., Kenneth A. McKusick, M.D., and Gerald M. Pohost, M.D.

Preface

I began the preparation for the first edition of THE HEART in 1962 and the first edition was published in 1966. The fourth edition was published in 1978. The objective of *The Heart* has always been to present in one or two volumes a complete treatise on the heart and blood vessels with the patient and the practicing physician as the focal point. Since the field is vast, it is necessary to use every method of editing in order to limit the size of the book(s). Accordingly, the allocation of space to a discussion of new advances that have not been tested by practicing physicians must be limited. For example, only a few pages were allocated to radionuclide imaging of the heart in the fourth edition. Similarly, the space allocated to a relatively small but important subject must be limited. For example, arrhythmias related to abnormal repolarization of the myocardium were not discussed in great detail in the fourth edition of the book, whereas a great deal is known about the subject. Finally, it has been necessary to limit the number of illustrations and references in *The Heart* in order to conserve space. This always concerns good teachers and good writers since such restraints may blunt their ability to express themselves as freely as they would like to do.

Toward the end of the preface of the fourth edition of *The Heart*, I wrote:

> Now that the fourth edition of *The Heart* is completed, the fifth edition is underway. The gestation period will be 3 or 4 years. The product of this gestation, the fifth edition, will be different from the first, second, third, and fourth editions. This is true because new information is being generated at such a rapid pace. I and the other authors who contribute to the book will evolve new ideas as new data dictate we should.

Since publication of the fourth edition the rapidly expanding body of knowledge has compelled me to search for an additional medium of communication. At times, just after a new edition of *The Heart* has been published, a new concept or a new procedure has come to my attention. Since the book is on a 4-year cycle, the new concept or procedure could not be presented for 4 years. Although this has never been a major problem, developments are coming at an ever-increasing pace, and it seems appropriate now to develop a method of assuring readers of *The Heart* that they will be apprised of every significant advance in the subject in the shortest possible period of time.

If one reflects carefully on this, one is led to the idea of periodic updates. I am eternally grateful for the worldwide acceptance *The Heart* has enjoyed (it has been translated into Spanish, Portuguese, Italian, and Japanese), and its objective will not be changed. It will remain a complete treatise on the heart and blood vessels contained in one or two volumes and, as always, will be written with the patient and the practicing physician in mind. The Updates will be used to fulfill the needs stated above. Accordingly, four to six will be created to appear between editions of *The Heart*. Some of them will have no particular theme and will be journallike, containing a number of articles on a variety of subjects, while others will be thematic minibooks and will contain a number of articles on the same subject. The reader should see the continuity of the Updates and their umbilical attachment to the mother of them all, *The Heart*. The material presented in detail in the Updates will then be "summarized" in the subsequent edition of *The Heart*.

This, then, is the first of the Updates. It is of the journal nature. There is no particular theme expressed in it. Two articles deal with medical history. This fascinating aspect of our heritage not only brings enjoyment to us all but is essential to one who desires to be a logical thinker and needs to know if current thought is an appropriate extension of the beliefs of our predecessors. Regrettably, the limitation of space will not permit most textbooks to include such vital information. The discussion of radionuclide imaging of the heart presented in this Update is quite long compared to the few pages allocated to the subject in the fourth edition of *The Heart*. Although the field is still developing, it seems appropriate to give a progress report on this important subject since the procedure is being used by an ever increasing number of institutions. On the other hand, there are four articles that deal with old subjects such as the use of the patient's history, the electrocardiogram, the echocardiogram and blood level of digoxin. The thrust of these articles is different from the usual discussion, however, since the authors emphasize the *limitations* of the methods of examination as well as the value of the methods. Finally, a number of articles, including arrhythmias related to abnormal repolarization, are presented in greater detail than space permitted in *The Heart*. These subjects were chosen by me by simply asking—

x

if I had unlimited space in *The Heart* what would I add?

The Heart and its daughters, the Updates, will, I hope, assure the reader that he or she has access to all of the important information regarding the cardiovascular system. *The Heart* was conceived in 1962 and delivered in 1966. It then developed and matured through four editions and now—not surprisingly—it plans to have daughters.

I wish to thank Carol Miller in my office. She keeps order, translates and types my own unique brand of shorthand, detects and corrects errors, and does so with a smile. I also wish to thank my publisher McGraw-Hill for its interest in these Updates. The very talented Dereck Jeffers and Rich Laufer deserve my special thanks.

J. Willis Hurst

UPDATE

I

THE HEART

The Contribution of Allan Burns [1,2]

J. WILLIS HURST, M.D. *

The third edition of Sir William Osler's *The Principles and Practice of Medicine* was published in 1899.[3] He listed four theories of angina pectoris. They are reprinted here in order to mark the views at the turn of the century and to place Allan Burns in the spotlight of history.[4]

Theories of Angina Pectoris.— (1) That it is a neuralgia of the cardiac nerves. In the true form the agonizing cramp-like character of the pain, the suddenness of the onset, and the associated features, are unlike any neuralgic affection. The pain, however, is undoubtedly in the cardiac plexus and radiates to the adjacent nerves. It is interesting to note, in connection with the almost constant sclerosis of the coronary arteries in angina, that Thoma has found marked sclerosis of the temporal artery in migraine and Dana has met with local thickening of the arteries in some cases of neuralgia. (2) Heberden believes that it was a cramp of the heart-muscle itself. Cramp of certain muscular territories would better explain the attack. (3) That it is due to the extreme tension of the ventricular walls, in consequence of an acute dilatation associated, in the majority of cases, with affection of the coronary arteries. Traube, who supported this view, held that the agonizing pain resulted from the great stretching and tension of the nerves in the muscular substance. A modified form of this view is that there is a spasm of the coronary arteries with great increase of the intracardiac pressure.

(4) The theory of Allan Burns, revived by Potain and others, [is] that the condition is one of transient ischaemia of the heart-muscle in consequence of disease, or spasm, of the coronary arteries. The condition known as intermittent claudication illustrates what may take place. In (man and in the horse), in consequence of thrombosis of the abdominal aorta or iliacs, transient paraplegia and spasm may follow exertion. The collateral circulation, ample when the limbs are at rest, is insufficient after the muscles are actively used, and a state of relative ischaemia is included with loss of power, which disappears in a short time. This "intermittent claudication" theory has been applied to explain the angina paroxysm. A heart the coronary arteries of which are sclerotic or calcified, is in an analogous state, and any extra exertion is likely to be followed by a relative ischaemia and spasm. In Allan Burns's work on The Heart (1809) the theory is discussed at length, but he does not think that spasm is a necessary accompaniment of the ischaemia.

* From the Department of Medicine, Emory University School of Medicine, Atlanta.

In fatal cases of angina the coronary arteries are almost invariably diseased either in their main divisions, or there is chronic endarteritis with great narrowing of the orifices at the root of the aorta. Experimentally, occlusion of the coronary arteries produces slowing of the heart's action, gradual dilatation, and death within a very few minutes. Cohnheim has shown that in the dog ligation of one of the large coronary branches produces within a minute a condition of arrhythmia, and within two minutes the heart ceases in diastole. These experiments, however, do not throw much light upon the etiology of angina pectoris. Extreme sclerosis of the coronary arteries is common, and a large majority of the cases present no symptoms of angina. Even in the cases of sudden death due to blocking of an artery, particularly the anterior branch of the coronary artery, there is usually no great pain either before or during the attack.[4]

Some years ago, while reading Osler, I discovered Allan Burns. When I read Burns' work I became embarrassed and felt I owed him an apology. The contributions of Heberden, Hunter, Parry, and Jenner were well known to me, but I had not known of Burns' remarkable contributions.

Allan Burns was a genius. He belongs, along with Laennec, to a small group of exceptional people who were able to make breathtaking contributions to medicine at a very young age. (Laennec and Burns were born in the same year. Laennec died at the age of 45 and Burns died at the age of 31). Burns broke with the convention of the day and "did it his way." He was born September 18, 1781, in Glasgow, Scotland. His father was a minister. Burns began studying medicine at age 14. The reasons for discontinuing his formal schooling are not known, but it is likely that his creative mind was restricted by the rigid thought of his instructors.

Burns was an original thinker and investigator. When he was 16 years of age he became the laboratory assistant to his brother, Dr. John Burns, who was destined to have a "checkered career" but who emerged as a prominent surgeon in Glasgow. Allan Burns was the "director of the dissecting rooms" and must have been one of the first physician's assistants.

He was obsessed by a desire to understand the human body. He became a skilled dissector. He kept accurate records. He observed the patients of his brother and others. He began to write scientific papers on anatomy and clinical problems when he was 21 years of age.

Empress Catherine of Russia heard of the young genius Burns. She enticed him to go to St. Petersburg as director and surgeon of a new hospital. Burns was 23 years old at the time. He remained there for about 6 months and returned to Glasgow.

Upon his return he discovered that his brother had been charged with body snatching and for this reason could not continue his lectures on anatomy. Accordingly, Allan Burns gave the lectures. He propelled Glasgow into medical prominence, and during the year 1814 there were 800 studies in anatomy.

Burns championed anatomy and learned pathology. He thought physiologically. He "attended" patients with his brother, who was professor of surgery at the university. (British law allowed his brother to continue to practice even though he had been accused of body snatching.) Burns also performed a great deal of surgery even though he held no degree in medicine or surgery. He was, however, a member of the Royal College of Surgeons, London, and a lecturer on anatomy and surgery in Glasgow. Burns wrote two books, and each displays the brilliance of the young genius. The first book, *The Most Frequent and Important Diseases of the Heart,* was published in 1809 when Burns was 28 years old. His second book, *Observations on the Surgical Anatomy of the Heart and Neck,* was published in 1811.

Burns died of a ruptured appendix when he was 31 years old (1813).

Herrick was intrigued by Burns and his writing. Herrick wrote:

The coronary artery theory of angina pectoris and his experiment with ligatures, his clear statement of the back pressure theory of dilatation and hypertrophy, whether from valvular obstruction or leakage, and his discussion of ante-mortem thrombi, aortic aneurysm, the falciform ligament, postmortem digestion, and the ligation of the thyroid arteries for goitre, are all notable contributions.[5]

This short dissertation on Allan Burns has been presented for several reasons. It is always interesting to observe a creative thinker in action. Burns was clearly a genius and had made his mark in medicine by the time he was 16 years old. His thinking had a cutting edge that few men possess, and his writing was simple, clear, and accurate (see the quotation from Burns in Ref. 6, Chap. 11).[6] The question is, had others listened to Burns' magnificent pathophysiologic explanation of angina pectoris, would our management of coronary atherosclerotic heart disease be different today? Burns, at age 28 (in 1809), knew that coronary artery obstruction produced myocardial ischemia and that this, in turn, produced angina pectoris and death. He postulated that coronary artery spasm might play a role in some patients. Many of us have only recently understood these "truths."

REFERENCES

1 Burns, A.: "Observations on Some of the Most Frequent and Important Diseases of the Heart," with an introduction by D. W. Richards, M.D., published under the auspices of the Library of The New York Academy of Medicine, Hafner Publishing Company, Inc., New York, 1964.

2 Bing, R. J.: Coronary Circulation and Cardiac Metabolism, in A. P. Fishman and D. W. Richards (eds.), "Circulation of the Blood Men and Ideas," Oxford University Press, New York, 1964, p. 199.

3 Osler, W.: "The Principles and Practice of Medicine," 3d ed., D. Appleton and Company, New York, 1899, p. 1150.

4 Osler, W.: Angina Pectoris, in W. Osler (ed.), "The Principles and Practice of Medicine," D. Appleton and Company, New York, 1899, pp. 762–763.

5 Herrick, J. B.: Allan Burns: 1781–1813: Anatomist, Surgeon, and Cardiologist, *Bull. Soc. Med. Hist.,* 4:457, 1935.

6 Burns, A.: "Observations on Some of the Most Frequent and Important Diseases of the Heart; on Aneurism of the Thoracic Aorta; on Preternatural Pulsation in the Epigastric Region: and on the Unusual Origin and Distribution of Some of the Large Arteries of the Human Body," printed by James Muirhead for Thomas Bryce and Co., Medical Booksellers, London, 1809.

Limitations of Symptoms in the Recognition of Coronary Atherosclerotic Heart Disease[*]

JOHN S. DOUGLAS, JR., M.D. and J. WILLIS HURST, M.D.

Discomfort in the chest, whether actually painful or not, is usually due to a relatively innocent or a potentially grave disorder. Unfortunately there is no parallelism between the severity of the distress and the gravity of its cause.

TINSLEY RANDOLPH HARRISON, M.D. (1900–1978) and T. JOSEPH REEVES, M.D.[1]

INTRODUCTION

The masterful description of effort-related angina pectoris by the English physician William Heberden over 200 years ago[2] has not been improved upon. The interpretation of chest discomfort remains to this day the most important method of recognizing coronary atherosclerotic heart disease. There are, however, many reasons for failure to recognize coronary artery disease from its symptomatic expressions. A minority of affected patients have the classical symptoms described by Heberden, and even these symptoms are not specific indicators of disease. Symptoms tend to occur late in the course of the disease. Autopsy studies of presumably healthy soldiers killed in action suggest that the majority of individuals with significant coronary atherosclerosis are asymptomatic.[3,4] When symptoms do develop, even to a mild degree, most patients have stenosis of two or more coronary arteries.[5–7] Symptoms characteristically wax and wane. It is reported that angina pectoris disappears in 25 percent of patients on follow-up.[8] When sudden death occurs as the first manifestation of the disease, pathologic examination usually indicates advanced and obviously long-standing coronary atherosclerosis.[9] The apparently healthy individual who develops ischemic changes during treadmill testing commonly has multivessel coronary obstruction.[10] The lack of parallelism between the severity of symptoms and anatomic disease is distressing. Furthermore, it has been observed that myocardial infarction is unrecognized in 12 percent[11] and unaccompanied by chest pain in up to 25 percent of patients.[12]

Early pathologic studies confirmed the presence of severe coronary atherosclerosis in virtually all patients with angina pectoris.[13–15] Angiographic studies of the coronary arteries, available during the past decade, have afforded the opportunity to study patients with chest pain during life and reveal that many who were thought to have coronary artery disease do not.[7,16,17] These studies and subsequent clinical experience indicate that chest discomfort can be misinterpreted even by the most experienced practitioners. The predictive value of the history has been shown to be better in some types of chest pain than in others[7,16,17] and diminishes as the prevalence of disease declines in a population (Bayes' rule).[18,19] The following comments briefly detail some of the factors important to the development and interpretation of symptoms resulting from coronary atherosclerosis. Insight into the reliability and limitation of symptoms as indicators of coronary atherosclerosis is a prerequisite for the optimal management of individuals with chest discomfort or other clinical parameters suggesting coronary artery disease.

FACTORS INFLUENCING THE VALUE OF THE HISTORY

In order for the physician to recognize coronary atherosclerotic heart disease by its symptomatic expressions, a chain of circumstances must exist. Sufficient coronary stenosis must be present to produce myocardial ischemia at activity levels encountered by the patient. Metabolic changes of ischemia and stimulation of afferent cardiac nerves by as yet undefined mechanisms[20] must occur. The patient must be alert enough to perceive any uncomfortable sensations and to communicate them accurately to the physician. These sensations experienced by the patient must have characteristics unique to the ischemic myocardium in order for them to be differentiated from other causes of chest discomfort. The physician must collect all useful information with regard to symptoms and make correct judgments as to the importance of these symptoms. If any link in the chain is absent, an incorrect diagnosis is likely to be made. If other causes of chest pain are present in addition to myocardial ischemia or if other pains have some features of myocardial ischemia, the stage is set for misdiagnosis.

[*] From the Departments of Medicine and Radiology, Emory University School of Medicine, Atlanta.

Factors such as the patient's emotional state may influence the history given. Fear may prevent thoughtful recounting of subtle chest tightness or pressure. Denial may thwart all attempts at exploring the history. Symptoms may be minimized by the stoic or embellished by those who seek secondary gain. If there are major economic considerations in the balance, the pressure upon the patient to conceal the truth may be overwhelming. Master clinicians have emphasized the difficult but key role of the physician in gently extracting all pertinent information regarding the patient's symptoms.[21-24] Harrison and Reeves state, "Of the many arts of clinical medicine, that of questioning the patient so that he, like Othello 'will a round unvarnished tale deliver', requires the largest measure of tact, skill, experience and wisdom."[1]

It is clear that symptoms do not mean disease. Symptoms are simply temporary disturbances of function which may be independent of structural pathologic change. Attempts to make anatomic diagnoses from symptoms are always subject to error. Skilled physicians know the range of error when they use symptoms to diagnose disease.

THE RELATIONSHIPS OF CORONARY STENOSIS, CORONARY FLOW, AND MYOCARDIAL ISCHEMIA

Myocardial ischemia is defined as a condition of oxygen deprivation secondary to reduced perfusion.[25,26] In coronary atherosclerotic heart disease, coronary artery stenosis is the usual cause of reduced coronary blood flow and the unfavorable oxygen supply/demand ratio which results in myocardial ischemia. In experimental studies, the resting flow rate in a coronary artery remains normal until the coronary stenosis exceeds 85 percent.[27] Lesser degrees of stenosis are compensated for by reduction in arteriolar resistance distal to the stenosis which is probably mediated by a local increase in adenosine[28] or prostaglandin F.[29] When the coronary peripheral vascular bed is fully dilated and coronary flow approaches maximal levels, a 35 percent reduction in coronary artery diameter (equivalent to a 60 percent cross-sectional area stenosis) reduces flow.[27] Under such conditions, flow decreases continuously with increasing coronary artery stenosis.[30] In a study of stenosed human coronary arterial segments removed at autopsy, Logan showed that resistance at 90 percent cross-sectional stenosis is fourfold to fivefold greater than that at 80 percent stenosis and that when stenosis exceeds 90 percent, resistance increased extremely rapidly.[31] Less than 80 percent stenosis caused small changes in resistance.

Studying patients during coronary bypass surgery, Smith reported that coronary arteries with a diameter reduction of less than 80 percent had pressure gradients of less than 20 mm Hg and normal coronary blood flow, while those with over 80 percent stenosis had reduced flow and higher gradients.[32] Massie and coworkers[33] and Horwitz and associates[34] showed that 70 percent cross-sectional stenosis limits flow during exercise. These experimental data are consistent with the clinical observations that anginal symptoms seldom occur with less than 50 percent cross-sectional stenosis and are often present with greater than 75 percent stenosis and that angina at rest is frequently associated with over 90 percent stenosis. The relationship between resistance and cross-sectional area also demonstrates that in far-advanced stenosis, slight progression can produce significant hemodynamic changes.

Ischemia is a result of the interactions of determinants of myocardial oxygen consumption, coronary flow, and the degree to which collateral channels compensate for the deficit. Although many patients experience emergence of angina at a myocardial workload that is relatively fixed,[35,36] variations in angina threshold may be accounted for by (1) a failure of the initial sympathetic increase in coronary tone with exercise to be overcome by local vasodilator mechanisms (explaining "walk-through" angina);[20] (2) reflex changes in coronary vascular resistance resulting from physical stimuli;[37] and (3) poorly understood mechanisms by which psychologic stimuli appear to induce angina independent of myocardial work.[38,39]

A significant number of patients have been reported and are seen daily in clinical practice who have typical histories of angina pectoris but normal coronary arteriograms.[40-42] The majority of these patients are female and have been shown to have normal coronary blood flow and myocardial oxygen extraction. Some produce lactate during stress. Fortunately, the outlook for these patients is quite good.[41] The mechanisms in this syndrome are unclear. A significant proportion, however, appear to have underlying psychologic problems.[43] Myocardial infarction in the presence of normal coronary arteriograms is an uncommon "accident" of the coronary circulation and is most likely thrombotic or thromboembolic.[44] Fortunately, the prognosis in these patients is also good.[45,46]

LIMITATIONS OF SYMPTOMS AS INDICATORS OF MYOCARDIAL ISCHEMIA

In the time course of progression of coronary atherosclerosis from insignificant plaque to the clinical manifestations of angina pectoris and myocardial infarction, there is ample evidence that myocardial ischemia occurs that is both asymptomatic and deadly.[47–49] Laboratory studies indicate that a moderately reduced coronary blood flow sufficient for resting metabolic needs is well tolerated, but subsequent increases in myocardial work are accompanied by mechanical, metabolic, and electrophysiologic markers of myocardial ischemia. Alteration of cardiac mechanics is the first readily detectable change and is closely associated with abnormalities of regional metabolism resulting in lactate formation.[50,51] These changes consistently precede ST-segment alterations over the ischemic zone.[51,52] Changes in global left ventricular performance are recorded when a large mass of myocardium is affected. In patients with coronary artery disease subjected to stress in the form of atrial pacing, hand-grip tests, or catecholamine infusion, alterations in regional left ventricular contraction, lactate production, and ST-segment shifts accompanying myocardial ischemia regularly occur prior to the onset or in the absence of symptoms.[53,54] Similar observations are made daily in the cardiac catheterization laboratory, where patients with coronary artery disease undergoing arteriographic studies are noted to have spontaneous and stress-induced myocardial ischemia, recognized by ST-segment shifts and alterations in left ventricular compliance, that is totally asymptomatic or followed shortly thereafter with typical ischemic pain. Patients with unstable angina who are free of pain at the time of ventriculography have been shown to have large areas of left ventricular dyskinesia which can be reversed by nitroglycerin therapy or revascularization surgery.[55,56] During coronary care unit monitoring of patients with unstable angina, ST-segment shifts are noted in the absence of symptoms, and the occasional patient with a critical balance between myocardial oxygen supply and demand may receive nitrate therapy aimed at correcting ST-segment abnormalities which occur prior to the onset of angina. On the treadmill, ST-segment shifts are commonly noted in patients with severe coronary stenosis prior to the onset of any symptoms. Recently myocardial imaging with radionuclides has been used in patients with transient myocardial ischemia, revealing perfusion defects in such patients at times when ST-segment shifts have occurred but prior to the onset of symptoms.[57] Some studies suggest that the scintigraphic technique is more sensitive in the detection of myocardial ischemia than either symptoms or standard electrocardiographic maximal stress testing.[58] In patients with severe coronary stenosis, left ventricular failure during exercise has been noted as reflected by precipitous decreases in systemic blood pressure prior to the onset of pain or ST-segment changes.[59] This mechanism of "ischemic paralysis" accounts for the common complaints of fatigue experienced by many patients as the sole indicator of serious underlying coronary stenosis and can produce acute left ventricular failure with pulmonary edema or shock without complaints of chest discomfort. In association with myocardial ischemia, patients may experience dyspnea as a result of acute elevations in pulmonary venous pressure, early interstitial pulmonary edema, and alterations in pulmonary compliance.[60] The above laboratory and clinical observations indicate that a hierarchy of recognizable manifestations of myocardial ischemia exists and suggest that the *presence of symptoms* is a relatively insensitive indicator which is usually associated with severe myocardial ischemia.

SYMPTOMS AS INDICATORS OF MYOCARDIAL INFARCTION

In a classical paper which presents the earliest complete clinical description of acute myocardial infarction, Herrick noted that clinical manifestations of acute infarction may be variable and complex.[61] An intense and protracted bout of angina pectoris may be simulated or discomfort in the abdomen accompanied by nausea may point to a serious abdominal accident. Patients with little or no pain were discussed. Early pathologic studies reported that approximately 40 percent of patients with "coronary thrombosis" had no history of chest pain.[62,63] However, Paul Dudley White commented that in his experience with 56 cases of acute myocardial infarction proved at autopsy, only 4 percent of patients had no chest pain.[22] Paul Wood similarly noted that less than 5 percent of patients he observed with acute infarction were free of chest discomfort.[24] In a study of acute myocardial infarction in a community, Kinlen found that 12.5 percent of patients had predominating symptoms other than chest pain and noted that an unusual degree of fatigue was a common symptom in patients without chest pain.[64] In a recent report of the symptoms of 102 patients with acute infarction, Uretsky noted that 76 patients had chest or arm pain, 14 had dyspnea, and the remaining 12 had abdominal symptoms, fatigue, nausea, or syncope.[12] Patients with atypical symptoms were older, had a lower prevalence of preceding angina (4 percent versus 37 percent), and had a higher morbidity and mortality associated with the infarction.

Symptoms in unhospitalized patients, perhaps with smaller infarctions, may appear less frequently. In the Framingham study the prevalence of unrecognized or silent myocardial infarction was 12 percent,[11] and in the Western Collaborative Group Study, it was 30 percent.[65] Roberts, in reporting the pathologic findings of 27 patients with isolated angina pectoris, none of whom had had a myocardial infarction, recorded that 52 percent had small myocardial scars judged to be the result of small, presumably silent, myocardial infarctions.[66] In a recent pathologic study of 47 patients with stable and unstable angina, Gutherie reported that 60 percent had histories of prior myocardial infarction and that 77 percent had myocardial scars, and he postulated that the remaining 17 percent had sustained silent myocardial infarctions.[15]

That myocardial infarction can occur and escape recognition is clear. The frequency with which this occurs in the general population remains unknown. Clinical and epidemiologic studies suggest that 10 to 20 percent of nonfatal myocardial infarctions which could be potentially recognized and confirmed clinically are silent. Smaller infarctions that are not easily documented clinically are apparently more common.

SYMPTOMS AS A PREDICTOR OF SUDDEN DEATH

Sudden and unexpected death occurs annually in hundreds of thousands of individuals in this country with symptomatically silent coronary disease. The mechanism is usually ventricular fibrillation as a result of myocardial ischemia or necrosis. The majority of these patients have multivessel coronary disease and would be candidates for coronary bypass surgery if they could be identified.[48] Liberthsome, in reporting 300 sudden deaths in the community, noted that one-half occurred with no warning, with collapse and death within 1 min, and on arrival of rescue squads, ventricular fibrillation was present in 72 percent.[9] Of 220 autopsies performed, 94 percent revealed severe stenosis of at least one coronary artery, and in 86 percent, two coronary arteries were involved. One-half of these patients had had no prior history of angina, chest pain, or myocardial infarction. Thirty-nine percent evolved electrocardiographic (ECG) changes of acute myocardial infarction and 34 percent had ECG changes of myocardial ischemia. Kannel indicates that one-half of all deaths resulting from coronary atherosclerotic heart disease are sudden and that 60 percent of middle-aged men dying suddenly had no prior evidence of coronary disease.[67] Weaver reported 64 patients with coronary disease resuscitated from sudden death, and in 28 percent ventricular fibrillation was the first manifestation of disease.[48] The majority of these patients were candidates for coronary bypass surgery. Myerburg, in a study of 1,348 sudden deaths resulting from coronary atherosclerosis, reported that sudden death was the first and only manifestation of disease in 41 percent.[68] It is apparent that within the population at large, a significant reservoir of patients exist with pre-

symptomatic lethal myocardial ischemia which is, in most cases, amenable to treatment.

CLINICAL SYMPTOMS AS PREDICTORS OF CORONARY ARTERY STENOSIS

Pathologic Studies

Early pathologic studies indicated that virtually all patients with angina pectoris had severe coronary atherosclerosis and that the remainder had some form of heart disease.[13,14,69-71] It was also noted that some patients with severe atherosclerotic occlusion of the coronary arteries remained asymptomatic, and compensation by collateral channels was hypothesized.[14,69] Zoll made a comprehensive comparison between the occurrence of angina pectoris and autopsy findings in 848 cases and noted that the incidence of angina was 5 percent when coronary stenosis was present but was 52 percent in those with occlusion of a coronary artery.[14] When one major coronary artery was occluded, angina pectoris was present in 60 percent of cases, and when two or more major coronary arteries were occluded, the incidence of angina was about 85 percent. Gutherie[15] and Roberts,[66] reporting on the pathologic findings of a total of 74 patients characterized as having stable or unstable angina, noted that the degree of stenosis in patients with stable and unstable angina pectoris was similar. An average of three of four major coronary arteries had greater than 75 percent cross-sectional stenosis; 1 patient had single-vessel disease. Roberts performed approximately 60 histologic sections of coronary arteries in each of 27 patients and all contained atherosclerotic plaques.

The majority of autopsy studies contain a large proportion of patients dying of coronary disease and are therefore not representative of this disease in the general population. In a study of American servicemen aged 18 to 46 killed during the Korean war, Enos reported that 77 percent had some coronary atherosclerosis and 15 percent had severe disease.[3] Comparable autopsy studies from the Vietnam conflict have been reported in which 45 percent of men had some and 5 percent had severe coronary atherosclerosis.[4] These studies suggest that the majority of persons in the general population with significant coronary atherosclerosis have no symptoms suggestive of heart disease.

Angiographic Studies

Proudfit reported the first large study correlating clinical symptoms and findings at coronary arteriography.[16] This was a retrospective study in which diagnoses were made by reviewing the patient's clinical record without knowledge of the results of coronary arteriography. The clinical findings were then compared with the presence or absence of coronary artery stenosis. The highest correlation of symptoms with coronary stenosis occurred in patients judged to have effort-related angina pectoris, 94 percent of whom had significant coronary artery stenosis (Table 1). Any departure of the history from one of effort-related angina resulted in a lower incidence of coronary artery stenosis. The clinical subgroup in which the lowest incidence of coronary stenosis occurred was that of atypical angina, a category for patients in whom there were "unusual or inconstant features in the history" but some characteristics and precipitating factors of angina pectoris. In this group of patients, 65 percent had significant coronary stenosis. Of patients who had had effort-related angina and who developed angina pectoris at rest, 87 percent had significant coronary artery stenosis.

The patient with rest pain alone or prolonged pain presents a difficult clinical problem because of the high likelihood that either life-threatening or inconsequential disease is present. Of the patients in these clinical subgroups, 21 percent had no significant coronary artery stenosis. In these patients, the need for a diagnostic coronary arteriogram is readily apparent. In a relatively small group of patients thought to be normal, only 4 percent had coronary artery stenosis. Two factors contribute to this unusually high correlation between clinical findings and the coronary arteriogram: (1) the use of a "probably normal" designation in which a 19 percent incidence of coronary stenosis was observed, and (2) the presence in the study group of 114 women under the age of 50, of whom a high proportion (75 percent) had no significant coronary disease.

At the Emory University Hospital, 1,308 males and 490 females with chest pain were studied prospectively.[7] After interviewing the patient and prior to the coronary arteriogram, each patient was assigned to one of several subgroups of angina pectoris or classified as normal (Table 1). Clinical judgments were compared with the results of coronary arteriography. The findings in males were remarkably similar to those of Proudfit. The highest correlation between clinical symptoms and coronary stenosis occurred in patients with effort angina. However, no category of atypical angina was utilized in the Emory study. Patients with effort-related chest pain with some atypical features were placed in the effort angina category if they were thought to have coronary disease and into the normal group if not. In the Proudfit study, such a patient would probably have been classified as having atypical angina. This resulted in a slightly lower correlation of 90 percent, as compared to 94 percent in the Proudfit study, which used a more clear-cut definition of effort-related angina. Of patients classified as having recent

TABLE 1
Correlation of clinical symptoms with findings at coronary arteriography

Patients	Cleveland Clinic[16] (786 males, 214 females)	Emory University[7] (1308 males)	Cleveland Clinic[17] (1000 females, < 50 years)	Emory University[7] (490 females)
Clinical assessment	Percentage of patients with CAD*	Percentage of patients with CAD*	Percentage of patients with CAD†	Percentage of patients with CAD*
Initial onset angina	—	81	—	73
Effort-related angina	94	90	48	57
Stable, mild	—	87	—	60
Stable, disabling	—	90	—	60
Progressive	—	91	—	54
Effort- and rest-related angina	87	89	51	74
Rest-related angina only	79	—	—	—
Prolonged pain	78	86	59	77
Atypical angina	65	—	26	—
Probably normal	19	—	10	—
Normal	4	32	1	18
All angina subsets	82‡	87‡	42‡	70‡
All normal subjects	15	32	9	18
All patients	63	75	24	44

* Equal to or greater than 50 percent cross-sectional stenosis.

† Equal to or greater than 50 percent lumen diameter reduction.

‡ Predictive value of a positive history.

onset angina (a designation not used in the Proudfit study), 19 percent had no significant coronary artery stenosis. The proportion of patients having coronary stenosis in the groups with effort-related angina plus rest pain and in patients with prolonged pain was similar to that in the Proudfit study. The sensitivity [true positives/(true positives + false negatives)] of the history was 0.92 in the Proudfit study and 0.93 in the Emory males. Simply stated, this indicates that 93 percent of males with coronary stenosis were classified as having ischemic pain. Extrapolation of this data to the general population is hazardous, however. Patients in these studies had chest pain and a very high incidence of coronary artery disease. In the general population, the incidence of coronary artery disease is unknown but much lower than that in the study groups. In addition, many individuals in the general population with coronary artery disease have no symptoms.

In comparing symptoms with coronary arteriography in women, studies at the Cleveland Clinic[17] and at Emory Hospital[7] failed to reproduce the high correlation observed in males between effort-related angina and coronary stenosis. Only 50 percent of women with effort-related angina had coronary stenosis. The clinical implications of these data are significant and point to a need for diagnostic coronary arteriography when symptoms suggest angina pectoris in women, even if the symptoms are classical. A much better correlation was observed in women who were thought to be "normal," of whom only 1 percent had coronary stenosis, or "probably normal," of whom 10 percent had coronary stenosis in the Cleveland Clinic study. In the study of women at Emory, 18 percent who were thought to be normal had coronary artery stenosis. The very poor correlation between anginal symptoms and anatomy observed in women and the differences between the Cleveland Clinic and the Emory data are almost totally explained by the differences in the prevalence of disease in the study groups and by consideration of Bayes' rule.

Bayes' rule states that the predictive value of a test (in this case the analysis of symptoms) decreases as the prevalence of disease diminishes in a population. This is illustrated in Table 1, where the predictive value or occurrence rate of coronary disease in patients with angina falls from 87 percent in the Emory males to 42 percent in the Cleveland Clinic young females as the prevalence of disease in the study groups diminishes from 75 percent in males to 24 percent in young females. This relationship between the predictive value of a test and the prevalence of disease in the population accounts for many of the striking differences noted between the four study groups. This major influence of Bayes' rule can be demonstrated by using the sensitivity (0.92) and specificity (0.67) of

Proudfit's group in col. 1 (Table 1) and calculating expected occurrence rates of coronary disease for patients judged to have angina in the other three study groups with their different prevalences of disease. For patient populations with coronary disease prevalences of 75, 24, and 44 percent, the calculated occurrence rate of coronary stenosis in patients with angina (the predictive value of a positive test) is 89, 46, and 69 percent, respectively, showing that the major differences in ability to predict coronary stenosis in the groups relates to the prevalence of disease. In a study of 239 women under the age of 45 who had a coronary disease prevalence of 48 percent, Waters reported that 68 percent of women judged to have coronary disease on the basis of symptoms had significant coronary stenosis.[72] The calculated predictive value of the history was 70 percent using the same sensitivity and specificity from Proudfit's study as above. The difficulty in recognizing coronary artery disease in women arises as a result of the lower prevalence of disease in women. When the prevalence of disease is higher, for instance in the older Emory women, the value of the history in predicting coronary stenosis is greater.

In Proudfit's study, 85 percent of patients thought to be normal were normal (15 percent had disease), while in the group of Emory males, 68 percent judged to be normal were, in fact, free of stenosis (32 percent had disease). The differences are totally explained by a lower prevalence of normals (higher prevalence of disease) in the Emory males, and this can be shown again by calculating the expected occurrence rate of normal anatomy in a population with 25 percent normals using the sensitivity and specificity of Proudfit's study. The calculated occurrence rate of normal anatomy in patients judged to be normal on the basis of symptoms in such a population is 68 percent (32 percent with disease), and this was the exact observed result in the Emory males.

These data illustrate that the prevalence of disease in a population in question must be a prime consideration in judging the value of a positive test result whether it is a clinical assessment or a more objective evaluation. If the prevalence of disease is quite low, the positive result will have less import because of the greater opportunity for false positive occurrences.

Table 2 reports the distribution of coronary stenosis in groups of men based on symptoms. Perhaps the most surprising observation is the lack of differences in severity of disease. Only in initial onset angina, where a relatively low incidence of left main coronary stenosis was observed, did appreciable differences in coronary anatomy occur. Patients with mild, disabling, and progressive effort-related angina had virtually the same incidence of 75 percent coronary stenosis, one-vessel, two-vessel, three-vessel, and left main disease. It is apparent, however, that

TABLE 2
Clinical symptoms and coronary artery stenosis at coronary arteriography in 1,308 males at the Emory University Hospital[7]

Clinical assessment	Patients (no.)	Patients grouped by extent of disease (%)					
		None*	Mild†	1V‡	2V‡	3V‡	Left main§
Initial onset angina	159	19	8	22	22	22	4
Effort-related angina	338	10	3	22	24	29	11
Stable, mild	100	13	5	21	22	28	11
Stable, disabling	105	10	3	25	22	28	13
Progressive	133	9	2	20	29	31	9
Effort- and rest-related angina	394	11	3	22	27	27	13
Prolonged pain	156	14	5	21	30	20	10
Normal	261	68	9	14	4	3	1

* Normal or less than 50 percent cross-sectional stenosis of a coronary artery.

† Greater than 50 percent but less than 75 percent cross-sectional stenosis, except the left main coronary artery.

‡ Greater than or equal to 75 percent cross-sectional stenosis of one, two, or three coronary arteries.

§ Greater than or equal to 50 percent cross-sectional stenosis of the left main coronary artery.

the extent of distal disease, the number of sites of stenosis, and the degree of stenosis exceeding 75 percent may differ. In patients thought to be normal, the incidence of severe disease was low, with 4 percent having left main or three-vessel disease. As stated in the above discussion of Bayes' rule, extrapolation of these data is valid only when dealing with a population with the disease prevalence of 75 percent.

The correlation between *severity* of symptoms and *severity* of disease was higher in women than in men (Table 3). None of the women with mild stable angina had three-vessel or left main disease, as compared to women with disabling and progressive effort-related angina, of whom 10 and 24 percent, respectively, had three-vessel or left main disease. Of patients with effort-related angina plus rest pain, 34 percent had three-

vessel or left main stenosis. The reason for this difference between the sexes is not apparent. Possible factors may include a more liberal use of treadmill tests in males, the result being a selection of more males with mild symptoms but positive treadmill test results. Any tendency for males to minimize symptoms and thereby achieve an anginal description inferring less difficulty than actually experienced would contribute to the differences which were observed.

CONCLUSION

The challenge of coronary atherosclerotic heart disease is identification of affected individuals prior to

TABLE 3
Clinical symptoms and coronary artery stenosis at coronary arteriography in 490 females at the Emory University Hospital[7]

Clinical assessment	Patients (no.)	Patients grouped by extent of disease (%)					
		None*	Mild†	1V‡	2V‡	3V‡	Left main§
Initial onset angina	22	27	0	33	36	4	0
Effort-related angina	77	43	5	22	18	6	6
Stable, mild	18	54	8	23	15	0	0
Stable, disabling	35	40	7	23	20	3	7
Progressive	24	46	0	17	13	12	12
Effort- and rest-related angina	112	26	4	19	17	30	4
Prolonged pain	37	23	6	14	37	14	6
Normal	242	82	6	6	4	1	1

* Normal or less than 50 percent cross-sectional stenosis of a coronary artery.

† Greater than 50 percent but less than 75 percent cross-sectional stenosis, except left main coronary artery.

‡ Greater than or equal to 75 percent cross-sectional stenosis of one, two, or three coronary arteries.

§ Greater than or equal to 50 percent cross-sectional stenosis of the left main coronary artery.

morbid events so that modern therapeutic measures may be applied. The high percentage of individuals whose initial manifestation is sudden death brings this problem into focus. Current clinical tools are inadequate, and the following approaches are needed: (1) A method for identifying patients with myocardial ischemia prior to the development of symptoms. Treadmill testing is inadequate because of the number of false positive results. An approach to this problem has been conceptualized.[73] (2) An aggressive approach to the identification of coronary risk even in mildly symptomatic patients appears warranted. Coronary arteriography is the most direct diagnostic approach. (3) In patients with chest pain, consideration of Bayes' rule will aid in interpretation of these symptoms and the need for objective documentation of coronary status.

REFERENCES

1 Harrison, T. R., and Reeves, T. J.: "Principles and Problems of Ischemic Heart Disease," Year Book Medical Publishers, Inc., Chicago, 1968, pp. 197 and 57.

2 Heberden, W.: Some Account of a Disorder of the Breast, *Med. Trans. R. Coll. Physicians,* 2:59, 1772.

3 Enos, W. F., Holmes, R. H., and Beyer, J.: Coronary Disease among United States Soldiers Killed in Action in Korea: Preliminary Report, *J.A.M.A.,* 152:1090, 1953.

4 McNamara, J. J., Molot, M. A., Stremple, J. F., et al.: Coronary Artery Disease in Combat Casualties in Vietnam, *J.A.M.A.,* 216:1185, 1971.

5 Fuster, V., Frye, R. L., Connolly, D. C., et al.: Arteriographic Patterns Early in the Onset of Coronary Syndromes, *Br. Heart J.,* 37:1250, 1975.

6 Walsh, W., Rickards, A. F., and Balcon, R.: Coronary Arteriographic Study of Mild Angina, *Br. Heart J.,* 37:752, 1975.

7 Douglas, J. S., Jr., and King, S. B., III.: Limitations of the History in the Diagnosis of Obstructive Coronary Atherosclerotic Disease, submitted for publication.

8 Burggraf, G. W., and Parker, W. D.: Prognosis in Coronary Artery Disease: Angiographic, Hemodynamic, and Clinical Factors, *Circulation,* 51:146, 1975.

9 Liberthson, R. R., Nagel, E. L., Hirschman, J. C., et al.: Pathophysiologic Observations in Prehospital Ventricular Fibrillation and Sudden Cardiac Death, *Circulation,* 49:790, 1974.

10 Erikssen, J., Enge, I., Forfang, K., et al.: False Positive Diagnostic Tests and Coronary Angiographic Findings in 105 Presumably Healthy Males, *Circulation,* 54:371, 1976.

11 Margolis, J. R., Kannel, W. B., Feinleib, M., et al.: Clinical Features of Unrecognized Myocardial Infarction—Silent and Symptomatic, *Am. J. Cardiol.,* 32:1, 1973.

12 Uretsky, B. F., Farquhar, D. S., Berezin, A. F., et al.: Symptomatic Myocardial Infarction without Chest Pain: Prevalence and Clinical Course, *Am. J. Cardiol.,* 40:498, 1977.

13 Blumgart, H. L., Schlesinger, M. J., and Davis, D.: Studies on the Relationship of the Clinical Manifestations of Angina Pectoris, Coronary Thrombosis, and Myocardial Infarction to the Pathologic Findings, *Am. Heart J.,* 19:1, 1940.

14 Zoll, P. M., Wessler, S., and Blumgart, H. L.: Angina Pectoris: Clinical and Pathologic Correlations, *Am. J. Med.,* 11:331, 1951.

15 Gutherie, R. B., Vlodauer, Z., Nicoloff, D. M., et al.: Pathology of Stable and Unstable Angina Pectoris, *Circulation,* 51:1059, 1975.

16 Proudfit, W. L., Shirey, E. K., and Sones, F. M., Jr.: Selective Cine Coronary Arteriography: Correlation with Clinical Findings in 1000 Patients, *Circulation,* 33:901, 1966.

17 Welch, C. C., Proudfit, W. C., and Sheldon, W. C.: Coronary Arteriographic Findings in 1000 Women under Age 50, *Am. J. Cardiol.,* 35:211, 1975.

18 Lusted, L. B.: "Introduction to Medical Decision Making," Charles C Thomas, Publisher, Springfield, Ill. 1968.

19 Jelliffe, R. W.: Quantitative Aspects of Clinical Judgment, *Am. J. Med.,* 55:431, 1973.

20 Schlant, R. C.: "Altered Cardiovascular Physiology of Coronary Atherosclerotic Heart Disease," in J. W. Hurst (ed.) "The Heart," 4th ed., McGraw-Hill Book Company, New York, 1978, p. 1134.

21 Osler, W.: "Lecture on Angina Pectoris and Allied States, Lecture One," D. Appleton and Company, Inc., New York, 1897.

22 White, P. D.: "Heart Disease," 4th ed., The Macmillan Company, New York, 1951, Chaps. 3 and 21.

23 Levine, S. A.: "Clinical Heart Disease," 5th ed., W. B. Saunders Co., Philadelphia, 1958, Chap. 6.

24 Wood, P.: "Disease of the Heart and Circulation," J. B. Lippincott Company, Philadelphia, 1956.

25 Hillis, L. D., and Braunwald, E.: Myocardial Ischemia (first of three parts), *N. Engl. J. Med.,* 296:971, 1977.

26 Neely, Jr., and Morgan, H. E.: Relationship between Carbohydrate and Lipid Metabolism and the Energy Balance of Heart Muscle, *Annu. Rev. Physiol.,* 36:413, 1974.

27 Gould, K. L., Lipscomb, K., and Hamilton, G. W.: Physiologic Basis for Assessing Critical Coronary Stenosis. Instantaneous Flow Response and Regional Distribution During Coronary Hyperemia as Measures of Coronary Flow Reserve, *Am. J. Cardiol.,* 33:87, 1974.

28 Fox, A. X., Reed, G. E., Glassman, E., et al.: Release

of Adenosine from Human Hearts during Angina Induced by Rapid Atrial Pacing, *J. Clin. Invest.*, 53:1447, 1974.

29 Berger, H. J., Zaret, B. L., Speroff, L., et al.: Cardiac Prostaglandin Release during Myocardial Ischemia Induced by Atrial Pacing in Patients with Coronary Artery Disease, *Am. J. Cardiol.*, 39:481, 1977.

30 Lipscomb, K., and Gould, K. L.: Mechanism of the Effect of Coronary Artery Stenosis on Coronary Flow in the Dog, *Am. Heart J.*, 89:50, 1975.

31 Logan, S. E., Tyberg, J. V., Parmley, W. W., et al.: A Hemodynamic Basis for the Stress Test: The Relationship between Coronary Perfusion Pressure, Flow, and Percent Stenosis in Human Coronary Arteries, *Clin. Res.*, 22:147A, 1974.

32 Smith, S. C., Gorlin, R., Herman, M. U., et al.: Myocardial Blood Flow in Man: Effects of Coronary Collateral Circulation and Coronary Artery Bypass Surgery, *J. Clin. Invest.*, 51:2556, 1972.

33 Massie, B., Morady, F., Botvinick, E., et al.: Quantitative Assessment of Coronary Stenosis: Correlation with Coronary Flow, *Circulation*, 51, 52 (suppl. 2):26, 1975.

34 Horwitz, L. D., Curry, G. C., Parkey, R. W., et al.: Differentiation of Physiologically Significant Coronary Artery Lesions by Coronary Blood Flow Measurements during Isoproterenol Infusion, *Circulation*, 49:55, 1974.

35 Ronghgarden, J. W.: Circulatory Changes Associated with Spontaneous Angina Pectoris, *Am. J. Med.*, 41:947, 1966.

36 Robinson, B. F.: Relation of Heart Rate and Systolic Blood Pressure to the Onset of Pain in Angina Pectoris, *Circulation*, 35:1073, 1967.

37 Mudge, G. H., Jr., Grossman, W., Mills, R. M., et al.: Reflex Increase in Coronary Vascular Resistance in Patients with Ischemic Heart Disease, *N. Engl. J. Med*, 295:1333, 1976.

38 Levine, S. A.: Some Notes concerning Angina Pectoris, *J.A.M.A.*, 1838, 1959. (Editorial.)

39 Lown, B.: Verbal Conditioning of Angina Pectoris during Exercise Testing, *Am. J. Cardiol.*, 40:630, 1977.

40 Kemp, H. G., Jr., Vokonas, P. S., Cohn, P. F., and Gorlin, R.: The Anginal Syndrome Associated with Normal Coronary Arteriograms: Report on a Six Year Experience, *Am. J. Med.*, 54:735, 1973.

41 Bemiller, C. R., Pepine, C. J., and Rogers, A. K.: Long-term Observations in Patients with Angina and Normal Coronary Arteriograms, *Circulation*, 47:36, 1977.

42 Kemp, H. G., Jr., Elliott, W. C., and Gorlin, R.: The Anginal Syndrome with Normal Coronary Arteriography, *Trans. Assoc. Am. Physicians*, 80:59, 1967.

43 McLaurin, L. P., Raft, D., Tate, S., et al.: Chest Pain with Normal Coronaries—a Psychosomatic Illness? *Circulation*, 51, 52 (suppl. 3):174, 1977.

44 Arnett, E. N., and Roberts, W. C.: Acute Myocardial Infarction and Angiographically Normal Coronary Arteries: An Unproven Combination, *Circulation*, 53:395, 1976.

45 Khan, A. H., and Haywood, L. J.: Myocardial Infarction in Nine Patients with Radiographically Patent Coronary Arteries, *N. Engl. J. Med.*, 291:427, 1974.

46 Rosenblatt, A., and Selzer, A.: Nature and Clinical Features of Myocardial Infarction with Normal Coronary Arteriogram, *Circulation*, 55:578, 1977.

47 Kuller, L. H., Perper, J. A., and Cooper, M. C.: Sudden and Unexpected Death Due to Atherosclerotic Heart Disease, in M. F. Oliver (ed.), "Modern Trends in Cardiology," 3d ed., Butterworth & Co. (Publishers), Ltd., London, 1975, p. 292.

48 Weaver, W. D., Lorch, G. S., Alvarez, H. A., et al.: Angiographic Findings and Prognostic Indicators in Patients Resuscitated from Sudden Cardiac Death, *Circulation*, 54:855, 1976.

49 Julian, D.: Sudden Death, in L. McDonald, J. Goodwin, and L. Resnekov (eds.), "Very Early Recognition of Coronary Heart Disease," Excerpta Medica, Amsterdam-Oxford, 1978.

50 Lekven, J., Mjos, O. D., and Kjekshus, J. K.: Compensatory Mechanisms during Graded Myocardial Ischemia, *Am. J. Cardiol.*, 31:467, 1973.

51 Waters, D. D., Daluz, P., Wyatt, H. L., et al.: Early Changes in Regional and Global Left Ventricular Function Induced by Graded Reductions in Regional Coronary Perfusion, *Am. J. Cardiol.*, 39:537, 1977.

52 Sheuer, J., and Brachfeld, N.: Coronary Insufficiency: Relations between Hemodynamic, Electrical, and Biochemical Parameters, *Circ. Res.*, 18:178, 1966.

53 Parker, J. O., Chiong, M. A., and West, R. O.: Sequential Alterations in Myocardial Lactate Metabolism, S-T Segments, and Left Ventricular Function during Angina Induced by Atrial Pacing, *Circulation* 40:113, 1969.

54 Cohen, L. S., Elliott, W. C., Klein, M. D., et al.: Coronary Heart Disease: Clinical, Cinearteriographic, and Metabolic Correlations, *Am. J. Cardiol.*, 17:153, 1966.

55 Helfant, R. H., Pine, R., Meister, S. G., et al.: Nitroglycerin to Unmask Reversible Asynergy: Correlation with Post Coronary Bypass Ventriculography, *Circulation*, 50:108, 1974.

56 Bryson, A. L., Aycock, A. C., Flamm, M. D., et al.: Changes in Regional Ventricular Contraction of the Arteriosclerotic Heart Following Nitroglycerin Administration—Surgical Correlation, *Circulation*, 50 (suppl. 3):44, 1974.

57 Maser, A., Parodi, O., Severi, S., et al.: Transient Transmural Reduction of Myocardial Blood Flow, Demonstrated by Thallium-201 Scintigraphy, as a Cause of Variant Angina, *Circulation*, 54:280, 1976.

58 Berman, D. S., Salel, A. F., Denardo, G. L., et al.: Non Invasive Detection of Regional Myocardial Ischemia Using Rubidium-81 and the Scintillation Camera. Com-

parison with Stress Electrocardiography in Patients with Arteriographically Documented Coronary Stenosis, *Circulation,* 52:619, 1975.

59 Thomson, P. D., and Kelemen, M. H.: Hypotension Accompanying the Onset of Exertional Angina. A Sign of Severe Compromise of Left Ventricular Blood Supply, *Circulation,* 52:28, 1975.

60 Pepine, C. J., and Winer, L.: Relationship of Anginal Syndromes to Lung Mechanics during Myocardial Ischemia, *Circulation,* 46:863, 1972.

61 Herrick, J. B.: Clinical Features of Sudden Obstruction of the Coronary Arteries, *J.A.M.A.,* 59:2015, 1912.

62 Davis, N. S.: Coronary Thrombosis without Pain: Its Incidence and Pathology, *J.A.M.A.,* 98:1806, 1932.

63 Gorham, L. W., and Martin, S. J.: Coronary Artery Occlusion with and without Pain, *Arch. Intern. Med.,* 112:821, 1938.

64 Kinlen, L. J.: Incidence and Presentation of Myocardial Infarction in an English Community, *Br. Heart J.,* 35:616, 1973.

65 Rosenman, R. H., Friedman, M., Jenkins, C. D., et al.: Clinically Unrecognized Myocardial Infarction in the Western Collaborative Group Study, *Am. J. Cardiol.,* 19:776, 1967.

66 Roberts, W. C.: The Coronary Arteries and Left Ventricle in Clinically Isolated Angina Pectoris: A Necropsy Analysis, *Circulation,* 54:388, 1976.

67 Kannel, W. B., Doyle, J. T., McNamara, P. M., et al.: Precursors of Sudden Coronary Death. Factors Related to the Incidence of Sudden Death, *Circulation,* 51:606, 1975.

68 Myerburg, R. J., and Davis, J. H.: The Medical Ecology of Public Safety: I. Sudden Death Due to Coronary Heart Disease, *Am. Heart J.,* 68:586, 1964.

69 Schlesinger, M. J.: An Injection plus Dissection Study of Coronary Artery Occlusions and Anastomosis, *Am. Heart J.,* 15:528, 1938.

70 Lenegre, J. and Himbert, J.: Critical Study of the Relationship between Angina Pectoris and Coronary Atherosclerosis, *Am. Heart J.,* 58:539, 1959.

71 Vlodaver, Z., Neufeld, H. N., and Edwards, J. E.: Pathology of Angina Pectoris, *Circulation,* 46:1048, 1972.

72 Waters, D. D., Halphen, C., Theroux, P., et al.: Coronary Artery Disease in Young Women: Clinical and Angiographic Features and Correlation with Risk Factors, *Am. J. Cardiol.,* 42:41, 1978.

73 Swan, J.: Implications of Regional Cardiac Mechanical Function in Myocardial Ischemia and Infarction—a Strategy for Presymptomatic Detection, in L. McDonald, J. Goodwin, and L. Resnekov (eds.), "Very Early Recognition of Coronary Heart Disease," Excerpta Medica, Amsterdam-Oxford, 1978.

The Diagnostic Capabilities and Limitations of the Electrocardiogram*

MARK E. SILVERMAN, M.D., and BARRY D. SILVERMAN, M.D.

It is a sound diagnostic principle to lean toward the interpretation of normality when the indications of abnormality are questionable. To paraphrase the American legal rule of thumb, 'The patient is innocent of disease until proven guilty.

ERNST SIMONSON[1]

INTRODUCTION

The electrocardiogram (ECG) is an imperfect diagnostic method used in diagnosing and screening for the presence of acute or residual cardiac disease or arrhythmia. Since the first clinical application by Einthoven in 1906, the ECG has been highly esteemed by physicians and often accorded a diagnostic precision that is not always warranted. In this review we will try to place the resting and exercise ECG in a perspective that emphasizes its capabilities as well as its limitations as a diagnostic method.

General Considerations

In the daily practice of interpreting electrocardiograms, scant attention is given to a number of known constitutional, physiologic, and technical influences that can substantially affect the ECG.[1]

Constitutional variables include age, sex, body weight, body height, chest configuration, anatomic position of the heart, and race. Age is the single most important biologic factor, causing a significant decrease in the R and S wave amplitudes and a shift to the left of the QRS axis.[2,3] The P-R interval lengthens, while the QRS interval remains the same. Most, if not all, of these changes parallel the increasing incidence of heart disease with age, variously estimated to be present in 10 to 49 percent of the geriatric population. Other factors associated with aging, such as emphysema, kyphotic chest configuration, greater motion of the heart, and changed conductivity through chest wall and mediastinal tissues have also been implicated.[1]

Until age 60, women have smaller amplitude R, S, and T waves, particularly in the precordial leads.[4-6] There is a higher incidence of decreased or absent initial anterior QRS forces; the QRS, P-R, and

Q-T intervals are shorter; and the J point and ST segment are more superiorly-posteriorly directed than in men.[6] These electrocardiographic differences in women have been attributed to a different chest configuration, smaller heart size, higher content of body fat, breast tissue under the electrode, and lower hemoglobin levels and metabolic rate.[1] Older women with osteoporosis often have a pronounced collapse of their chest, bringing the heart closer to the chest wall, enhancing R wave amplitude, and producing a misleading appearance of cardiomegaly on chest x-ray.

An increase in body weight over normal is associated with a shift in the QRS axis leftward to a horizontal position and a decrease in R and T amplitude.[1] A lower than normal body weight is associated with a more vertical axis. The changes related to body weight are greatest in the 40 to 59 age range and may be caused by the gain in weight with age in Americans. Interestingly, a study correlating electrocardiographic and constitutional variables in an adult Japanese population showed body weight and height to be a stronger influence than age on the ECG.[7] Postulated mechanisms for the effect of body weight on the ECG are positional factors, chest configuration, tissue conductivity, and body fat content.[1]

The electrical position of the heart will play a role in determining the QRS and T wave amplitudes in the frontal and horizontal planes and the location of the precordial transition zone. Although various constitutional factors, including age, body weight, and chest configuration, may contribute to the orientation of the electrical position, recent studies have shown that the frontal plane QRS axis is primarily determined by the anatomic position of the heart.[8] Different values for the normal ECG are apparently present in different races.[1] This has been studied in blacks, who have been noted to have a shorter QRS interval, larger QRS amplitude, and a more posterior T vector than a white population.[4]

Physiologic variables include alterations in systemic blood pressure, intracardiac pressures, hematocrit values, heart size, electrolytes, body temperature, exercise conditioning, hyperventilation, emotions, high altitude, recent meal, and smoking.[1,9] Many of these physiologic variables exert their influence on the ECG only when they plunge or rise rapidly to abnormal levels.

* From the Departments of Medicine, Emory University School of Medicine and Piedmont Hospital and Northside Hospital, Atlanta, Georgia.

13

Technical considerations include position of precordial leads relative to anatomic position of the heart, width of the sternum, fidelity of the ECG machine, conducting medium used under electrodes, observer variability, error of measurement, base-line variation, and normal day-to-day variation.[1] These technical problems are a source of great concern, for they potentially contribute a significant variability to each tracing. The relation of the traditional precordial leads to the anatomic position of the heart will obviously vary considerably, depending on the chest configuration. Electrocardiographic machines vary in their proficiency in responding faithfully to small deflections or to rapid rates of deflection.[10] Diagnostic Q waves that are apparent when recorded on one machine may be slurred into the R wave by another machine. ST-segment depression in the precordial leads may reflect a problem with frequency response and not ischemia. Corroded or unkempt electrodes, the incorrect use of alcohol rather than saline pads, and imperfect contact of the electrode with the skin may affect voltage.[1]

Disagreement in the interpretation of the same ECG among experienced observers is common.[1] The discrepancies can be quite significant, averaging about 30 percent.[11] The same observer may offer a different opinion on the same ECG on repeat interpretation. Different observers often disagree on the measurements of intervals and amplitudes. This error of measurement adds to the difficulties of human interpretation of the ECG.

The computer has been called upon to improve the diagnostic accuracy of interpretation.[11–13] The computer is superior to human interpretation in measurements of intervals, amplitudes, and axis; is more consistent in its application of criteria; has reduced technical errors in recording, mounting, and reporting; and provides a cost saving when applied to large populations. There remain problems with interpreting arrhythmias and certain types of abnormalities, comparing old and current tracings, reading technically poor tracings, and incorporating clinical information into the final interpretation. Nevertheless, computer interpretation with physician over-read has current approval and promises added precision and improved criteria of interpretation.

A day-to-day variation of the normal ECG has been documented.[14] Even when scrupulous attention is given to placing chest leads in the identical position by marking the chest, there is a substantial fluctuation in the QRS and T amplitude and QRS axis. This is most marked for small deflections such as Q waves and R wave amplitude. Time measurements are only minimally affected. The variation is exaggerated when technicians are not using lead placement markers. These day-to-day changes explain, at least in part, why an ECG will easily meet criteria for left ventricular hypertrophy (LVH) on one day but not on the next or be diagnostic of inferior infarction on one occasion but show small initial R waves in the inferior leads on another.

Confirmation of Electrocardiographic Criteria

Electrocardiographic criteria are only as reliable as the standard against which they are verified. Standards have changed, however, as new techniques have become available. Early studies used clinical criteria of "disorders capable of producing strain on the left or right side of the heart," chest pain thought to result from angina pectoris, and chest x-ray evidence of cardiac chamber enlargement for comparison.[15] Each of these approaches is seriously flawed since none is subject to precise measurement and pathologic authentication. For example, as many as 20 percent of patients who have chest discomfort confidently diagnosed as angina pectoris have been found to have normal coronary arteries. Yet many of our current standards have been predicated on these precarious clinical criteria. At first glance, autopsy confirmation would seem to be the desirable standard. Autopsy information, although of great importance, suffers several limitations.[1] It cannot reveal the physiologic influences, such as intraluminal pressure, heart rate, and blood pressure, that may influence the ECG in the living individual. Nor is the tension and thickness of the postmortem myocardial wall the same as that in a living individual. Autopsy technique differs greatly from study to study—the septum may or may not be included as part of the left heart, the epicardial fat may or may not be removed, the measurements of thickness may be taken in different places. Since the autopsy population is highly selected for advanced disease, autopsy data are highly skewed information and endow the ECG with an exaggerated precision.[1]

Newer diagnostic techniques, such as intracardiac pressures and electrophysiologic measurements, angiography, echocardiography, radioisotopic scans, myocardial biopsy, and a more sophisticated understanding of epidemiologic approaches, statistical methods, and computer science have provided a better definition of normal values and enhanced electrocardiographic correlations.

Statistical Considerations

The contribution of any diagnostic test is highly dependent on its ability to discover a high percentage of the patients with the disorder while excluding those without it. This is commonly expressed in terms of sensitivity, specificity, and predictive accuracy.[1,16,17] An understanding of these terms is essential in order to appreciate the capabilities and limitations of the resting ECG.

The *sensitivity* of a test is defined as the probability of a positive result for a disease if all the patients have the disease. This may be restated as

$$\text{Sensitivity } (\%) \ = \ \frac{TP}{TP + FN} \times 100$$

where TP = true positives (number of patients abnormal for the condition being tested which meet the criterion)

FN = false negatives (number of patients abnormal for the condition being tested which do not meet the criterion)

Therefore, a test which correctly detects all the patients with the disease has a sensitivity of 100 percent.

The *specificity* of a test is defined as the probability of a negative result for a disease if none of the patients have the disease. This may be restated as

$$\text{Specificity} = \frac{TN}{TN + FP} \times 100$$

where TN = true negatives (number of patients without the condition being tested which do not meet the criterion)

FP = false positives (number of patients without the condition being tested which do meet the criterion)

Therefore, a test with a specificity of 100 percent detects only the patients with the disease.

The *predictive accuracy* is the percentage of positive results that are truly positive, or

$$\text{Predictive accuracy} = \frac{TP}{TP + FP} \times 100$$

where TP = true positives (number of patients abnormal for the condition being tested which meet the criterion)

FP = false positives (number of patients without the condition being tested which do meet the criterion)

The value of a test is highly dependent on the prevalence of the disease in the study population. The number of false positive results increases as the prevalence of the disease decreases and the predictive accuracy is correspondingly lower. Bayes' theorem incorporates the prevalence of the disease in the study population into the analysis and allows the clinician to predict more accurately the chance of disease being present given a positive or negative test.[18]

These considerations are nicely illustrated by the following example adapted from Redwood, Borer, and Epstein:[19]

Assume that the ECG criteria for left ventricular hypertrophy has both a specificity and a sensitivity of 95 percent and that 1000 patients are tested from a population in which 90 percent have LVH. Since the test has a sensitivity of 95 percent, then 855 (900 × 95 percent) would be true positives. If the specificity is 95 percent, 5 of the 100 patients without LVH will be false positives. Since a total of 855 of the 860 patients actually have LVH, there is a predictive accuracy of 99.4 percent. If, however, the prevalence of LVH in the 1000 patients is only 2 percent, then 20 patients would have LVH and 980 would not. This time 19 of 20 will be true positives and 49 of 980 will be false positives. The predictive accuracy, based on 19 true positives out of 68 with a positive test result, is now only 28 percent. In actuality, the sensitivity for commonly used precordial plane criteria for LVH is about 55.0 percent and the specificity is around 89 percent. Again, assuming a population of 1000 patients and a prevalence of 2 percent, a predictive accuracy of only 9.3 percent is obtainable. Redwood, Borer, and Epstein used this approach to stress the very limited diagnostic value of the exercise test in screening an asymptomatic population.

The accuracy of electrocardiographic criteria, particularly the differentiation between normal and abnormal, has been extensively studied by Simonson.[1,20] In his many articles, which are fundamental to understanding the limitations of the ECG, he stresses the following problems:

1 Inadequate sample size: Because of the significant effect of constitutional factors—age, sex, race, weight, chest configuration—and unknown factors, a large sample is necessary to arrive at meaningful conclusions. Simonson estimates a minimal sample size of 1000 men and women and a desirable sample size of 1800 is necessary to determine normal limits for various subgroups. This figure contrasts with the sample size of 100 to 200 used in many studies.

2 Composition of the sample: An ideal sample would be truly representative of the average, healthy population. This requires fastidious screening to eliminate any disorder that may conceivably influence the ECG. Common pitfalls include the use of hospitalized patients, patients who have died with "normal" hearts, or a group preselected in some way, such as medical students, people who answer an ad to have a free ECG, etc. This concern has plagued many studies and is a major reason why the results of one study cannot be compared with or added to those of another study.

3 Adequate statistical evaluation: Studies that compile values for a "normal population" and use the extreme values as the limits of normal include many false normals. This error increases as the sample enlarges. This was the method, however, used by many early studies that are now the basis for current criteria. A more acceptable method for achieving a statistically sound boundary of normal is to determine percentile distribution and establish a cutoff point at both ends of the normal distribution. A frequently used cutoff is 2.5 percent at each end so that 95 percent of the normal population is included in the limits. This approach still strands 2.5 percent of the normal subjects below and 2.5 percent above the normal limits. Multivariate analysis, aided by a computer, greatly strengthens the validity of this approach.

Specific Diagnostic Considerations

ATRIAL ABNORMALITY

Normal The normal, sinus-initiated P wave is a composite of two forces: an initial inferior, anterior, and leftward force caused by right atrial depolarization and a later left atrial contribution directed inferiorly, leftward, and posteriorly.[18a,18b,21,22] Right atrial activation time occurs from 20 to 45 ms, and left atrial depolarization is from 30 to 90 ms. The resultant normal P vector is oriented near +60° in the frontal plane, registering best in lead II, and is slightly anterior, often producing a biphasic configuration in lead V_1. The normal P wave amplitude is less than 2.5 mm, and the duration does not exceed 0.10 s.

Correlations Many studies have been aimed at correlating P wave alterations with left or right atrial weight at autopsy; with atrial dimension by echocardioangiogram, chest x-ray, or surgery; with direct or indirect atrial pressure; and with diseases that are known to impose a burden upon the left or right atrium.[23–31] Although these studies have shown some degree of correlation of P wave alterations with each of these anatomic, physiologic, or clinical measurements, the frequent occurrence of a normal P wave in the presence of a definitely enlarged or hypertrophied atrium remained difficult to explain.[32] Most importantly, the abnormal P wave is sometimes present only intermittently. Recent studies have shown an excellent correlation of P wave alterations with interatrial electrical conduction defects.[33] Since changes in atrial pressure, volume, and wall structure could all alter atrial conduction velocity or conceivably cause a shift in the atrial conduction pathway, a harmonious explanation can be provided that relates all the influences on the atrium to electrical conduction.

Right atrial abnormality A right atrial abnormality (RAA) shifts the P vector anteriorly and increases its magnitude without prolonging the P wave. Previously, a diagnosis of "P pulmonale" was made when tall, peaked, relatively narrow P waves ≥ 2.5 mm and less than 0.11 s were inscribed in lead II or V_1. Although it is true that this pattern is frequently seen with chronic lung disease, cor pulmonale, and diseases afflicting the pulmonic and tricuspid valves, a similar P wave can also be present in diseases known to affect the left atrium. Chou and Helm have labelled this "pseudo P pulmonale" and have pointed out that the pattern of RAA is not very specific in favoring the

right atrium over the left.[34] For this reason the use of the term "P pulmonale" is now discouraged in favor of "right atrial enlargement" or "right atrial abnormality."[35]

Left atrial abnormality A left atrial abnormality (LAA) produces a posterior shift of the P vector in the horizontal plane and a prolonged P wave duration. The following have been proposed as useful diagnostic criteria for LAA:

1 P terminal force in $V_1 \geq - 0.04$ mm/s (calculated as the product of the depth in millimeters and duration in sections of the terminal negative deflection of the P wave in lead V_1 and referred to as the Morris index).[25]

2 P wave in Lead II > 2.5 mm in amplitude and/or ≥ 0.12 s in duration.[21]

3 Notching of the P wave in any lead with the peaks separated by more than 0.04 s.[28]

4 P wave duration: A P wave duration/PR segment ratio exceeding 1.6 (PR segment measured from end of P wave to the onset of the QRS, known as the Macruz index).[26]

A number of studies have compared these criteria to left atrial size or weight, left atrial pressure, or diseases that affect the left side of the heart such as hypertension, cardiomyopathy, and aortic and mitral valve disease. The Morris index, which utilizes the P terminal force in lead V_1 (PTF-V_1) has generally been found to be the most sensitive and specific measurement, particularly for left atrial dimension and an interatrial conduction defect.[25,28] A P wave duration ≥ 0.12 s is the second most useful measurement. Notching of the P wave is not helpful, since it is often present normally and may or may not be demonstrable, depending upon the technical quality of the ECG machine.[28] The ratio of P wave duration to PR segment (Macruz index) is of limited usefulness, since it is less sensitive and less specific than other criteria and cannot be applied when the patient is receiving digitalis. All the criteria suffer a high yield of false negative and false positive diagnoses, a problem that is improved when several criteria are met. The following is the result of one study of 100 patients that compared the

Criteria	% Sensitivity	% False pos.	% False neg.
P wave ≥ 0.12 s (lead II)	62	33	5
Notching (any lead)	64	24	12
P terminal force (V_1)	77	12	11
P/PR ratio (lead II)	50	50	0

ECG criteria for LAA with left atrial echo dimension greater than 4.0 cm:[28]*

Correlations between P wave morphology and specific disease entities have also been made.[36–39] An abnormal PTF-V_1 has proved to be a sensitive finding in acute pulmonary edema, being present acutely in 76 percent and 91 percent of patients in two different studies.[39,40] The P wave abnormality was often transient and disappeared with clinical improvement. Similar findings were also reported in patients with acute myocardial infarction and an elevated left ventricular filling pressure.[41] A LAA is a common occurrence in patients with hypertension and may supply the earliest clue to hypertensive heart disease.[37] In mitral stenosis, one study found a sensitivity of PTF-V_1 of 68 percent and a Macruz index of 76 percent.[27] Notching was present in 52 percent, and a P duration ≥ 0.12 was present in 69 percent. These findings did not correlate well with atrial size at surgery and were sometimes visible with normal atrial size. For this reason, and for other reasons stated earlier showing the P wave morphology to correlate best with interatrial conduction defects, the term "P mitrale" is in disrepute in favor of "left atrial abnormality."[35]

Left ventricular hypertrophy Left ventricular hypertrophy (LVH) produces the following electrocardiographic alterations:[18a,18b,21,22]

1 Increased magnitude of the mean left ventricular vector

2 Shift in the mean left ventricular vector superiorly, posteriorly, and to the left

3 ST-T vector opposite the mean QRS vector

4 Left atrial involvement

5 Prolonged left ventricular activation time

These effects of LVH have led to criteria that are often applied to the analysis of the electrocardiogram.

These criteria have been critically examined by Romhilt and associates, who provide the following correlations:[42]†

A Limb lead criteria	Sensitivity	Specificity
RI + SIII > 25 mm	10.6%	100%
RaV_L > 7.5 mm	22.5%	96.5%
RaV_L > 11 mm	10.6%	100%
RaV_F > 20 mm	1.3%	99.5%

B Precordial lead criteria	Sensitivity	Specificity
SV_1 + RV_5 or RV_6 > 35 mm	42.5%	95%
SV_1 or V_2 + RV_5 or RV_6 > 35 mm	55.6%	88.5%
SV_1 + RV_5 or RV_6 > 30 mm	55.6%	89.5%
Greatest R + greatest S > 45 mm	45%	93%
RV_5 or RV_6 > 26 mm	25%	98.5%

Supportive criteria
Ventricular activation time ≥ 0.05 s in V_5 or V_6
ST-T opposite the QRS (patient not on digitalis)
LAD: $-30°$

C Left atrial involvement (see below)

D **Point score system of Romhilt and Estes**‡[43]

Sensitivity	Specificity
54%	97%

1 Amplitude   3 points
Any of the following:
  a Largest R or S wave in the limb leads ≥ 20 mm
  b S wave in V_1 or $V_2 \geq 30$ mm
  c R wave in V_5 or $V_6 \geq 30$ mm

2 ST-T-segment changes (typical pattern of left ventricular strain with the ST-T segment vector shifted in direction opposite to the mean QRS vector)
  Without digitalis   3 points
  With digitalis   1 point

3 Left atrial involvement   3 points
  Terminal negativity of the P wave in V_1 is 1 mm or more in depth with a duration of 0.04 s or more

4 Left axis deviation: $-30°$ or more   2 points

5 QRS duration ≥ 0.09 s   1 point

6 Intrinsicoid deflection in $V_{5,6} = 0.05$ s   1 point

Correlations[16,42–56] Using the above criteria, an autopsy-proven diagnosis of LVH can be made by the ECG less than 60 percent of the time. The limb lead criteria are much less sensitive, though more specific, than the precordial lead criteria. The point score system devised by Romhilt and Estes seems to offer the most satisfactory approach but still leaves a 46 percent incidence of false negative results. Although it is tempting to improve the disappointing sensitivity by lowering the voltage criteria, this manipulation inevitably produces an unacceptably large number of false positive results.

There are many reasons why the correlation between the electrocardiogram and the cardiac anatomy is poor.[1] The differentiation between a normal heart and a hypertrophied heart at autopsy is imprecise. Total heart weight or chamber weight is dependent upon dissection techniques that vary considerably from one study to the next. The number of "normal" hearts for various age groups and body sizes is very limited, particularly since death from infectious illness has declined. Most studies that use heart weight criteria depend on the 1942 study by Zeek in which heart

---

* Used by permission of the authors and *The Southern Medical Journal*.

† Used by permission of the authors and by the American Heart Association, Inc.

‡ LVH, 5 points; probable LVH, 4 points.

weight is correlated with body length. Unfortunately, the correlation was relatively weak. Measurement of wall thickness at autopsy is virtually useless because of a postmortem loss of muscle tone and controversy as to the proper point of measurement. There is no correlation of heart weight or left ventricular thickness with QRS voltage over the range of normal heart weights.[46,57] The QRS amplitude seems to increase mainly when heart size increases over the original value. Normal factors of age, sex, race, body build, and skin and fat thickness are important in determining QRS amplitude.[1,58] Age in particular is a consideration, since voltage may be very high in men under age 30 with $SV_2 + RV_5$ reaching 65 mm in normal teenage boys and $SV_1 + RV_5$ or RV_6 exceeding 40 in the 20 to 25 age range.[59]

Alterations in QRS voltage may also be produced by other pathologic changes. Patients with long-standing LVH and congestive heart failure commonly develop right ventricular hypertrophy (RVH).[46,60,61] The increased rightward and anterior forces of RVH subtract from the posteriorly directed forces of LVH, producing a false negative electrocardiogram for LVH. Acute cardiac enlargement, possibly through an ill-defined effect of the intracavitary blood pool, decreases QRS amplitude.[59] This may explain the lower QRS voltage found in congestive heart failure when compared to the compensated heart. The electrocardiogram is more sensitive in diagnosing the presence of LVH when the heart is chronically large (50 to 60 percent precordial lead sensitivity) as compared to smaller hearts (30 to 40 percent sensitivity) at autopsy.[42] Since ventricular hypertrophy may be a response to a number of diseases which produce varying effects of preload and afterload, the resultant heart size, configuration, and degree of left and right ventricular hypertrophy may differ. The ECG may therefore be more sensitive to ventricular hypertrophy in one disease than in another. Myocardial fibrosis, myocardial infarction(s), left bundle branch block, left anterior hemiblock, and electrolytes also alter QRS amplitude, so that a diagnosis of LVH is more difficult and often impossible.[56,61,62] Extracardiac effects of lung or mediastinal disease, left mastectomy, anasarca, pleural or pericardial effusion, and obesity are additional concerns.

Because of these numerous difficulties, newer techniques have been applied to the measurement of ventricular hypertrophy. Simonson et al., in an extensive review comparing the diagnostic accuracy of the vectorcardiogram (VCG) and ECG, found the ECG to be a superior method of diagnosing LVH.[63] The echocardiogram has been most helpful, particularly in ruling out hypertrophy in children with very large QRS voltage.[50] Significant correlations have been found between derived echo measurements of left ventricular

mass and the thickness of the interventricular septum but not necessarily with the thickness of the posterior left ventricle. Echocardiographic techniques offer the opportunity to correlate the ECG with the living heart and should eventually provide newer, more accurate criteria for the diagnosis of ventricular hypertrophy.[48–52]

Right ventricular hypertrophy Right ventricular hypertrophy (RVH) produces the following electrocardiographic alterations:[18a,18b,21,22,64]

1 The right ventricular vector is increased in magnitude.

2 There is a displacement of the QRS vector anteriorly, to the right, and either superiorly or inferiorly. Uncommonly the vector may be oriented to the right, posteriorly, and either inferiorly or superiorly. A clockwise rotation of the transverse loop is characteristic of more severe RVH.

3 The ST-T vector may be displaced to the left, posteriorly, and either superiorly or inferiorly. The magnitude of the ST or T vector is usually small and may not be noticeable unless an advanced degree of RVH is present.

4 Right atrial involvement may be seen.

5 A prolonged right ventricular activation time is often present.

The following criteria have been developed and critically analyzed in several studies:[56,65]

A	Precordial lead criteria	Sensitivity	Specificity
	R/S ratio $V_1 \geq 1$	6%	98%
	qR in V_1	5%	99%
	$RV_1 \geq 7$ mm	2%	99%
	R/S ratio $V_6 \leq 1$	16%	93%
	Deep SV_1, V_2, or V_3	*	*
	Dip in the normally rising R/S curve between any pair of pretransitional leads	28%	76%

* Not available.

B	Limb lead criteria	Sensitivity	Specificity
	Right axis deviation $\geq 110°$	12–19%	96%
	SI, II, III pattern	24%	87%
	$RaV_R \geq 5$ mm	0%	100%

Additional findings
Ventricular activation time ≥ 0.035 s in V_1.
T inversion right precordial leads.
ST depression right precordial leads.
Shortening and notching of SV_1.
QRS may be normal or slightly prolonged.
A right ventricular conduction delay producing an R′ may occur.
Small r and deep S may be seen in $V_{5,6}$.

Correlations The criteria listed above enjoy a high specificity for adults but provide a very low degree of sensitivity. Roman, Massie, and Walsh, after applying multiple older proposed criteria for RVH to a large autopsy series, concluded that the most useful criteria were a right axis deviation (RAD) greater than +110°, an R/S amplitude ratio in $V_1 > 1$, and an R/S amplitude ratio in $V_6 \leq 1$.[69] These three criteria used together diagnosed RVH correctly in 87.2 percent of the hearts, with a false positive incidence of 38 percent. In a more recent autopsy study, Flowers and Horan found the following criteria to be helpful:[16,70]*

Criteria	Sensitivity	Specificity
SV_5 or $V_6 \geq 7$ mm	26%	90%
Rv_1 and SV_5 or $V_6 > 10.5$ mm	18%	94%
Rv_5 or $V_6 > 5$ mm	13%	87%
R/S V_5 or $V_6 \leq 1$	16%	93%
SI, II, III	24%	87%
SI, QIII	25%	87%
SV_5 & V_6	58%	53%
Dip in R/S ratio	28%	76%

The difficulty in recognizing hypertrophy of the right ventricle stems from the normal marked predominance of left ventricular forces in the adult. The normal right ventricle is only 3 mm or so in thickness and contributes very little to the formation of the QRS unless a right bundle branch block is present. Scott estimates that the right ventricular wall may double in thickness and still not generate enough voltage to wrench the left ventricular forces anteriorly and to the right. Therefore, RVH is very difficult, if not impossible, to recognize in its early stages. This is particularly true in the older population with acquired RVH, since the mean QRS axis is already horizontal and RAD, one of the most helpful clues to RVH, is found in only a minority of patients. In addition, the degree of acquired RVH seldom exceeds the thickness of the left ventricle. In contrast, in congenital heart disease the mean QRS begins and remains rightward and the RVH may outstrip the left ventricle. Numerous studies have confirmed that RVH is easier to recognize in congenital heart disease such as pulmonic stenosis and Eisenmenger's physiology as compared with acquired RVH from mitral stenosis or left-sided heart failure.[67,71] Other factors, such as duration of the disease, left or right ventricular or pulmonary artery pressures, anatomic position of the heart, and presence of LVH in the acquired group, are also important. False negative results also occur because of LVH, left or right bundle branch block, and anteroseptal myocardial infarction. A false positive diagnosis of RVH may be made in patients with normal hearts, right bundle branch block, posterior myocardial infarction, left posterior hemiblock, type A Wolff-Parkinson-White Syndrome, chronic lung disease, dextrocardia or acquired ana-

tomic shifts of the heart, and rarely isolated cases of LVH.[56,72]

Other techniques of measuring for RVH, besides a careful physical examination, are not particularly helpful, including the echocardiogram and vectorcardiogram.

Chronic obstructive lung disease Chronic obstructive lung disease (COLD)[18a,18b,21,22] may produce the following electrocardiographic effects:[73-78]

1 Posteriorly displaced mean QRS vector with a marked counterclockwise rotation of the transverse loop. The terminal forces may be rightward and superior.

2 Rightward shift of the mean QRS vector in the frontal plane.

3 Decreased magnitude of ventricular forces.

4 Enlarged P vector which is oriented between +75° and +90° in the frontal plane.

5 Minimal effect on the normal ST or T vector.

The following criteria relate to these effects and are applied to the diagnosis of COLD:

1 The mean QRS axis is shifted to the right and is equal to or exceeds +90° in the frontal plane. An apparent left axis can be present a minority of the time.

2 Low voltage equal to or less than 5 mm in the frontal plane is often seen.

3 A small *r* wave is found in the right precordial leads.

4 There is a shift in the transition zone so that the R wave does not exceed the S wave until V_5 or V_6.

5 The P wave is tall, peaked, or notched and equals or exceeds 2.5 mm in one or more inferior leads (usually II). A tall upright P wave in V_1 is an uncommon sign. The P wave is often isoelectric in lead I.

6 An SI,II,III pattern can be found and an S wave may be present in the left precordial leads.

7 Signs of RVH may appear in lead V_1 with severe COLD.

Correlations[73-79] Many studies indicate that the ECG is quite inadequate in recognizing mild to moderate lung disease. As the lung disease progresses, ECG alterations occur that reflect the vertical position of the heart, the effect of the lower diaphragm on cardiac position, and the presence of hyperinflated lungs. Lung functions were studied in 103 patients who met one or more of the ECG criteria for COLD in a study by Kamper et al.[78] A sensitivity of 88.7 percent was found, with a specificity of only 31.7 percent. The high number of false positive results could be improved when a combination of criteria was required. A P vector $\geq 80°$ was the most sensitive criteria. An SI, II, III pattern was fairly specific for severe COLD, prob-

---

* Used by permission of the authors and the F. A. Davis Company.

ably representing the presence of RVH. False positive results were seen with pleural effusion, hypertension, and congenital, rheumatic, and coronary heart disease. There was a good correlation between the severity of the lung disease and the ECG criteria. A study by Littman of a male population at a Veterans Administration Hospital revealed similar findings.[73] Virtually all the patients with clinical, symptomatic lung disease had recognizable ECG alterations. The P wave changes provided a sensitive, early clue. RVH could be diagnosed by the ECG in 5 to 8 percent of patients but was almost always present at autopsy.

Acute alterations of pulmonary artery pressure and of chamber size in the right side of the heart may be witnessed on the ECG according to Ferrer.[79] The most sensitive findings are T wave inversion or flattening in the right precordial leads and a 30° shift of the mean QRS axis to the right of the previous axis. Less commonly, transient ST depression in leads II, III and aV_F and right ventricular conduction delays occur. A variability of the P wave has been noted by others. These abnormalities are reversible with improvement in pulmonary artery pressures.

The dilemma of separating the effects of COLD from the additional changes resulting from RVH has not been resolved.[80] RVH, a very late finding in COLD, could be diagnosed accurately in only 16 to 30 percent of patients with cor pulmonale resulting from COLD. This may be partly related to the coexistance of LVH, which is present in as many as 90 percent of autopsies of patients with COLD.[77] Scott, as well as Phillips and Burch, feels that RVH can be recognized when RAD > +110°, right ventricular conduction delays, and classic V_1 criteria are present in addition to the usual changes due to COLD.[74,75]

Pulmonary embolus[18a,18b,21,22] Since the normal electrocardiogram is preponderantly determined by left ventricular forces, acute stresses on the right side of the heart have little or no effect unless the strain is fairly intense.[81] Studies have shown that ECG changes do not often occur until 50 percent or more of the pulmonary vasculature is obstructed.[81,82] Even with massive obstruction, the previously normal right ventricle is unable to generate a mean pulmonary arterial pressure (PAP) much greater than 40 mm Hg. Patients with normal ECGs usually have a mean PAP below 30mm Hg, whereas patients with a mean PAP above 30 mm Hg usually, but not always, have an abnormal ECG.[82]

Massive and submassive pulmonary embolization, however, may alter the ECG in the following manner:

1 Mean QRS vector is shifted to the right or to the left.

2 Initial QRS vector is shifted superiorly, posteriorly, and to the left.

3 Terminal QRS vector is shifted superiorly, posteriorly, and to the right.

4 QRS vector in the horizontal plane is shifted posteriorly.

5 ST-T wave changes.

6 P vector is shifted rightward and the magnitude of the vector is increased.

7 Transient atrial or ventricular arrhythmias.

These effects of pulmonary embolus may be manifest by classical or nonspecific changes,[83] including:

1 SI, QIII, TIII (McGinn and White pattern)

2 Right axis deviation

3 SI,II,III

4 Right ventricular conduction defect

5 Right atrial abnormality

6 Shift of transition zone to the left (V_4)

7 ST-segment elevation or depression in right precordial leads

8 T wave inversion in right precordial leads

9 Pseudoinfarction patterns—Q waves with or without ST-T changes in inferior and anteroseptal areas

These changes have been attributed to acute dilatation of the right side of the heart and to the secondary effects produced by hypoxemia, hemodynamic changes, and coronary blood flow.

Correlations Table 1, collected from the Urokinase-Pulmonary Embolism Trial (UPET study), lists the changes that were seen on the ECG and frequency of occurrence in 90 patients with massive or submassive pulmonary embolism.[83,84] By design, the patients in this trial had symptoms suggesting pulmonary embolus in the preceding 5 days, and pulmonary arteriography confirmed an obstruction or filling defect in at least one segmental pulmonary artery. Massive pulmonary embolization was designated by similar findings in two or more lobar pulmonary arteries or their equivalent in other vessels. This major study, as well as virtually all other similar studies, are, by necessity, highly selective for symptomatic patients who might be expected to have significant embolization and electrocardiograhic alterations. Presumably, patients with lesser degrees of pulmonary embolization, which are more difficult to diagnose, would exhibit an even higher incidence of normal ECGs. In addition, the UPET study and other studies attempted to distinguish patients with normal hearts from those with

TABLE 1
Electrocardiographic manifestations*: Patients without prior cardiac or pulmonary disease

Electrocardiogram	50 Points, massive pulmonary embolism,† percent	40 Points, submassive pulmonary embolism, percent	90 Points, massive or submassive pulmonary embolism, percent
Normal electrocardiogram	6	23	13
Rhythm disturbances			
Premature atrial beats	2	3	2
Premature ventricular beats	4	3	3
Atrio-ventricular conduction disturbances			
First degree AV block	0	3	1
P pulmonale	6	5	6
QRS abnormalities			
Right axis deviation	8	5	7
Left axis deviation	4	10	7
Clockwise rotation (V_5)	10	3	7
Incomplete right bundle branch block	8	3	6
Complete right bundle branch block	8	10	9
Right ventricular hypertrophy	6	5	6
S_1,S_2,S_3 Pattern	6	8	7
$S_1,Q-3,T-3$ Pattern	18	5	12
Pseudoinfarction	16	5	11
Low voltage (frontal plane)	8	3	6
Primary RST segment and T wave abnormalities			
RST segment depression (not reciprocal)	28	23	26
RST segment elevation (not reciprocal)	18	13	16
T wave inversion	46	38	42

*Some patients had more than one abnormality.

† The prevalence of none of the various electrocardiographic abnormalities differed significantly between patients with massive or submassive pulmonary embolism (chi square greater than 0.05).

SOURCE: The Urokinase-Pulmonary Embolism Trial.[84]

preexisting heart disease in whom ST-T changes or infarction patterns might be a consequence of prior disease and not necessarily right-sided heart strain.

The UPET study shows that ST depression or T wave inversion or both are the most common abnormalities. One or more classical changes of acute cor pulmonale, such as SI, QIII, TIII; right ventricular conduction delay; peaked P waves; and right axis deviation were present in 31 percent of 78 patients with massive embolization. A normal ECG was found in 23 percent of patients with submassive pulmonary embolism as well as in 6 percent with a massive embolus. By 5 days the majority of the QRS changes had disappeared, while T wave inversion persisted in 51 percent at 2 weeks. This study and others observed that left axis deviation is as common or more common than a rightward shift and that atrial fibrillation or flutter is rare unless prior heart disease is present. Previous studies have also emphasized the low degree of ECG sensitivity and specificity for pulmonary embolus.

McIntyre et al., in a study of 20 patients with 13 to 68 percent embolic obstruction by angiography, concluded that the ECG was of no positive value in 80 percent, was nonspecific but consistent with or suggestive of the diagnosis in 15 percent, and was diagnostic in only 5 percent.[82] They felt that the only role of the ECG was in distinguishing acute myocardial infarction from massive pulmonary embolism. Spodick, in an editorial, noted that right-sided heart strain patterns are seen in roughly 15 to 40 percent of patients and that a normal or unchanged ECG is common, particularly in mild degrees of embolism.[81] Smith and Ray, however, found that slurring of the ascending limb of the S wave in right precordial leads and regression of the R/S ratio between two successive precordial leads was a sensitive sign of early right ventricular enlargement, being present in 58 percent of 127 patients with acute pulmonary embolism.[85] These changes were transient and usually abated in 30 min to 48 h.

CORONARY ARTERY DISEASE

Myocardial infarction The electrocardiographic diagnosis of an acute myocardial infarction depends upon one or more of the following observations:[18a,18b,21,22]

1 A partial or total subtraction of the normal forces generated by a segment of the myocardium. This loss enhances opposing forces, and as a consequence the mean initial (0.04 s) vector points away from the site of the infarction. Abnormally wide and deep Q waves are therefore recorded in leads that provide information from the infarcted area.

2 A "current of injury" emanates from the area of infarction, resulting in ST-segment deviation from the isoelectric line on the surface ECG. Either ST-segment elevation or depression can be seen, depending upon the anatomic location and the leads subserving the injured area.

3 T wave abnormalities occur. Acutely a transient T vector, larger than normal, is directed toward the fresh infarction. Later the T vector rotates away from the area.

The age of the infarction is judged by the stage of the ST-T evolution as compared to the usual course of an infarction. The following terms are applied: acute—less than 3 days; recent—less than 1 month; old—more than 3 months, and age undetermined—unspecified.[35]

These well-known QRS-ST-T changes are further classified by assuming that a correlation exists between the ECG leads and the underlying cardiac anatomy. The accepted correlations are:[35]

Site	ECG leads
Septal	V_1, V_2
Anteroseptal	V_1-V_4
Anterior	V_3, V_4
Anterolateral	I, a V_L, V_3-V_6
Extensive anterior	I, V_1-V_6
Apical	II, III, AV_F, V_3, V_4
Inferior	II, III, aV_F
Inferolateral	II, III, aV_F, aV_L, $V_{5,6}$
Posterior	V_1, V_2 (wide, tall R)
Posterolateral	I, aV_L, V_1, V_6

An infarction is also defined from the ECG by estimating if the involved tissue is confined to the subendocardium or the subepicardium or is a full thickness "transmural" injury. The ST vector points away from an injured subendocardial area and toward a subepicardial injury. Therefore, ST-segment depression is seen with anterior or inferior subendocardial injury, and ST-segment elevation is seen with anterior or inferior subepicardial injury. An alteration in the initial portion of the QRS is the hallmark of a transmural

infarction. Nontransmural infarction, a newer term, describes ST-T changes without accompanying QRS modification.

Pathologic correlations By definition, an abnormal Q wave extends 0.04 s in duration and reaches a certain depth, often stated as 25 percent of the following R wave (if present) in leads I, III, aV_F, and V_2-V_6 and 15 percent in aV_L. In practice, a width slightly exceeding 0.03 s is often applied.

In the 1930s the concept of a myocardial dead zone permitting an intracavitary potential to be viewed via an inert electrical window was conceived, and a Q wave was considered to be synonymous with a transmural infarction. Current information has dispelled this notion. With ischemia, Q waves may appear and quickly vanish.[86] Q waves may also come or go immediately following coronary bypass surgery.[87,88] Their appearance may be caused by new infarction or an unmasking of an old infarction as a result of improved coronary perfusion in areas opposite old scar. The disappearance of Q waves is postulated to result from improved perfusion and electrical activity in the by-passed area.[87] Permanent Q waves may form when the infarction is limited to the subendocardial region; Q waves may, on occasion, be absent with a proven transmural infarction.[86,90,91] There is a good correlation between Q waves on the standard ECG and leads recording directly from the epicardial surface, although significant scarring may be present, particularly in the apical area, producing epicardial Q waves without corresponding Q waves on the external ECG. Other pathologic studies have also found more extensive infarction to be present than is revealed by the ECG.[89,92]

With many exceptions the ECG furnishes a fair, but not quantitative, anatomic localization of inferior and anterior infarctions. The comprehensive study by Horan and associates, correlating 1184 autopsies with the QRS, found that the presence or absence of an abnormal Q wave ≥ 0.03 s in the presence of normal conduction provides a sensitivity of 61 percent and a specificity of 89 percent of infarction. An abnormal Q wave limited to either the V_1-V_4 leads or leads II, III, and aV_F predicted the anatomic site in less than half the patients and allowed a false positive incidence of 46 percent.[93] Abnormal Q waves residing in more than one electrocardiographic zone or in the V_5, V_6 area were far more reliable for infarction, with a false positive incidence of only 4 percent. In contrast, an excellent correlation between the ECG predicted area and the pathologic findings was observed by Savage and associates in a postmortem study of 24 patients.[89] They were, however, unable to separate posterior from inferior infarctions on the basis of the anatomic-electrocardiographic correlations; poor correlation was also present in the extent of inferior-posterior infarctions.

The diagnostic value of inferior Q waves has been correlated with the angiogram by Shettigar et al.[94] In this group of 48 patients with inferior infarction by history, total or subtotal obstruction of the right coronary artery, and/or inferior wall contraction abnormalities, 15 percent had diagnostic Q waves in all three inferior leads and 29 percent did not have Q waves in any leads. Diagnostic Q waves were most frequent in lead III and least frequent in lead II. Because lead III displays an abnormal Q wave in 4 percent of a normal population and because a Q wave may be seen in this lead with COLD, cor pulmonale, right bundle branch block (RBBB), and LVH, these workers concluded that lead aV_F was more reliable in diagnosing myocardial infarction. Inferior wall asynergy was seen in 76 percent of patients with abnormal inferior Q waves, as well as in 74 percent of patients without diagnostic Q waves. The finding of a fairly broad Q wave isolated to lead III is a common dilemma. This is not resolved by the common practice of using deep inspiration to see if the Q wave persists. An extensive electrocardiographic and vectorcardiographic study in patients with inferior infarctions and in normal controls shows the inspiratory effects on the Q wave to be extremely unreliable in separating the two groups.[95]

The apical, posterior, and lateral areas of the left ventricular anatomy, both atria, and the right ventricle are poorly represented by the ECG, while the anterior, septal, and inferior surfaces are more adequately sampled. A posterior infarction, located beneath the posterior atrioventricular groove and often called a "true posterior" to distinguish it from an inferior infarction, is the most inaccessible area to the ECG.[93] The diagnosis is deduced by analyzing the anterior leads V_1, V_2 for reciprocal changes—an increase in the amplitude and width of the R wave, an RV_1 duration of ≥ 0.04 s, and an R/S ratio in $V_1 \geq 1$.[96,97] A slurred or notched RV_1 is suggestive. Inferior wall involvement often accompanies posterior infarction. Acutely, ST depression and an upright T wave may be noted in V_1. An R/S ratio ≥ 1 in V_2 is present in 12 percent of a normal population and is therefore not helpful. Other causes of an abnormal R wave in V_1, including RBBB, and type A W-P-W syndrome have to be excluded.[92]

Isolated apical infarctions usually produce inferior Q waves and are inseparable from inferior infarctions unless there is evidence of simultaneous anterior (V_3, V_4) and inferior involvement.

Abnormal Q waves in leads I, aV_l, V_5, and V_6 are fairly specific for lateral wall infarction if obstructive cardiomyopathy is excluded; however, the ECG is very insensitive to recognizing infarction in this area. The term "high lateral" infarction is no longer acceptable.[35]

Infarction of the atria and the right ventricle are also commonly missed by the ECG although present at postmortem. Atrial infarction does produce an abnormality of atrial repolarization, the PT_a segment. This is witnessed as a depressed PR segment in leads II, III, aV_F, V_1, and V_2, atrial arrhythmia, and pulmonary emboli.[98] Right ventricular infarction is usually a component of an extensive inferior infarction and is suspected by finding significant right ventricular dysfunction with a relatively low left ventricular filling pressure.

Angiographic correlations An entirely normal resting ECG is quite compatible with severe coronary artery disease.[99] Severe double- or triple-vessel obstruction can be present in 65 percent of patients with a normal resting ECG who have been found to have abnormal coronary arteriograms.[100] The incidence of this discrepancy in the general population is unknown. In the population referred for coronary angiography, the vast majority of these patients have angina pectoris and an extensive collateral circulation.[99]

On the other hand, the presence of a Q wave does not certify that coronary artery disease is the malefactor. Hilsenrath and associates found normal coronary arteries in 25 of 47 patients with isolated patterns of anterior wall infarction (false positive rate of 53 percent) and 11 of 41 patients with inferior infarction patterns (false positive rate of 27 percent).[101] Horan and associates discovered an 11 percent false positive rate in 768 patients with Q waves.[102] Both investigators found that the predictive value of Q waves is greatly enhanced when multiple areas are involved. So-called pseudoinfarction patterns are, of course, well known.[101] Recognized causes are listed in Table 2.[103]

Angiograms have also been correlated with the presence or absence of Q waves to see if the ECG is helpful in predicting the specific coronary artery involved and the presence, extent, and site of ventricular asynergy. The evidence in one study is that the left anterior descending coronary artery is significantly diseased in 96 percent of hearts with anterior infarction, while the right coronary artery, with or without the circumflex artery, is greatly obstructed in 87 percent with inferior infarction.[104] Multiple areas of infarction indicated multivessel disease in 93 percent.

Q waves were also highly associated with ventricular asynergy in the anticipated area in two studies (95 percent and 81 percent), but the correlation was only fair (64 percent) in another study.[105] Disappointingly, 49 percent had ventricular asynergy without an

TABLE 2

Conditions that may produce a pseudoinfarction pattern

Left ventricular hypertrophy
Right ventricular hypertrophy
Chronic lung disease
Pulmonary embolus
Pneumothorax
Congestive cardiomyopathy
Hypertrophic obstructive cardiomyopathy
Hypertrophic nonobstructive cardiomyopathy
Myocarditis
Friedreich's ataxia
Muscular dystrophy
Amyloidosis
Primary and metastatic tumors to the heart
Left bundle branch block
Left anterior hemiblock
Wolff-Parkinson-White syndrome
Intracranial hemorrhage
Traumatic heart disease
Hyperkalemia

abnormal Q wave, although the degree of asynergy was less severe and often reversible when Q waves were absent.[105]

Correlation with old and recurrent myocardial infarction The possibility that a normal ECG can be recorded during the initial and succeeding stages of an acute myocardial infarction is well known, although the knowledge is frequently disregarded. The long-term fate of the ECG that is originally diagnostic of an acute infarction is less appreciated.[106] Various studies have found that the ECG may return entirely to normal in 2 to 10 percent of patients with abnormal Q waves and in 34 percent of those with ST-T changes only.[107-110] The return to normal is completed by 1 year in the majority, but others may continue to resolve over several years.[108] In a much higher percentage, the ECG becomes nondiagnostic, though still abnormal. The incidence of reinfarction in the group returning to normal appears to be similar to those with a persistent abnormality. It is estimated that more than 70 percent of single old infarctions present at autopsy are missed by the ECG.[111,112] The vectorcardiogram has a superior performance to the ECG in diagnosing old infarctions but yields a higher incidence of false positive results. The reasons for the disappearance of the evidence of infarction include shrinkage of the infarcted area into a shell of normal tissue during healing; infarction occurring in opposing areas, cancelling the imbalance in forces produced by the original infarction; small size of the infarction; collateral circulation in the surrounding area;[87] and the development of a bundle branch block or conduction defect.

The presence of ventricular hypertrophy and both right and left bundle branch block drastically reduces the accuracy of the ECG in diagnosing infarction. In the extensive study by Horan and associates, an abnormal Q wave was found in 69 percent of patients with myocardial infarction plus RBBB, in 70 percent with LBBB plus infarction, and in 62 percent with incomplete LBBB plus infarction.[102] However, there was a false positive rate of 25 percent with RBBB, 39 percent with LBBB, and 40 percent with incomplete LBBB. In a small group of 8 patients with LBBB and inferior Q waves, there were no false positive results. This was not true for RBBB and inferior Q waves. In an evaluation of the ECG, Simonson and associates found an incidence of a false positive diagnosis of infarction of 13 percent with LVH, 13 percent with RBBB, and 9 percent with LBBB.[63]

A recurrence of myocardial infarction in the same area as a previous infarction may also be difficult to recognize. Merrill and Pearce, in a study of 21 patients who died from acute myocardial infarction superimposed on a prior infarction, were able to make the diagnosis in 81 percent by observing further increases of preexisting ST-segment elevation or depression, deeper inversion of already inverted T waves, and further deepening and widening of pathologic Q waves.[113] They admitted that a smaller second infarction might be more difficult to detect.

ST-T Wave Correlation Acute and evolving ST-T wave changes provide the major electrocardiographic evidence of fresh ischemia or infarction. The ST-segment deviation may be evanescent, however, and not present at the time the patient arrives for an ECG. Ambulatory monitoring has documented ST elevation or depression occurring without chest pain or other symptoms. With Prinzmetal's variant angina, ST elevation results from intense myocardial ischemia in the area predicted by the ST vector. Spasm of a "normal" coronary artery or spasm superimposed upon severe coronary artery obstruction has been documented in these patients. This form of ischemia differs from typical angina pectoris in which ST depression is often manifest. In a recent study, a 12-lead ECG was recorded during chest pain in 41 patients with unstable angina pectoris.[114] ST or T wave changes were observed in 83 percent of the 29 patients who were subsequently found to have significant coronary artery disease by angiography. ST-segment elevation and depression occurred with equal frequency and were associated with a similar degree of coronary artery disease and ventricular contraction abnormalities. In 5 patients with coronary artery disease, no electrocardiographic changes occurred, while ST depression was noted in 2 of 12 patients with normal coronary arteries. The authors concluded that an ECG taken during chest pain is of limited diagnostic potential because of the number of false positives (16.6 percent) and false negatives (17.2 percent) findings. They did not try to document coronary artery spasm but did note that the ST elevation with chest pain was more common in patients with old myocardial infarction. Our conclusion is that ST depression or elevation that comes with chest pain and is resolved when the patient is free of pain is highly suggestive of myocardial ischemia.

The natural history of ST elevation following myocardial infarction has been studied by Mills et al.[115] They concluded that the ST-segment elevation resolves in 95 percent of inferior and 40 percent of anterior infarctions within 2 weeks. ST-segment elevation that persists after 2 weeks usually does not resolve, is associated with more severe infarction, and indicates a ventricular aneurysm. Although highly specific for ventricular aneurysm, continuing ST elevation is not a very sensitive clue, since many hearts with an aneurysm do not have ST elevation.[105]

Prognostic correlations The ECG would indeed be valuable if it served as an oracle in predicting future cardiac events. Studies have shown that the ECG does have some prognostic capabilities. Recent studies comparing patients with ECG changes of nontransmural infarction to those with transmural infarction indicate that, although they differ in acute complications and ECG changes, they share a similar long-term prognosis. The Coronary Drug Project, a multicenter experience with 2,035 male survivors of myocardial infarction followed over 3 years, related the risk of death to the ECG at the time of entry into the study.[116] They found that patients with a normal ECG had one-third the mortality risk as those with residual abnormalities. Horizontal or downsloping ST depression of 1.0 mm or more was the most serious prognostic factor with a high risk of death—45 percent of patients with this finding died. Other findings associated with a high risk were presence, size, and site of Q waves; left ventricular conduction defects; atrial fibrillation; ventricular premature beats; high R wave amplitude in lead II; and T wave amplitude in lead V_5. They concluded that the ECG findings in infarct survivors effectively discriminate between men with vastly different degrees of risk and contribute to predicting the probability of dying in a given period. The Tecumseh, Michigan, study looked at 47 individuals over age 20 without evidence of heart disease who had nonspecific T wave inversion.[117] A follow-up 20 to 72 months later showed that this group had a high prevalence of hypertensive or coronary artery disease and an excess mortality over the expected age-related death rate.

Despite this good prognostic performance of the ECG, the report of a person dying suddenly from severe coronary disease shortly after a normal ECG has been recorded is a familiar one.

THE STRESS ELECTROCARDIOGRAM: ITS VALUE AND LIMITATIONS IN THE DIAGNOSIS OF ISCHEMIC HEART DISEASE

Introduction

The electrocardiographic response to exercise is a useful technique in the diagnosis and management of patients with coronary artery disease. Recently, however, the test has come under increased scrutiny because of the need for greater precision in the diagnosis of this disease.[118–119] A thorough understanding of the limitations of the stress test is essential to select the proper clinical setting for its use.

Methodology

The methods utilized in exercise testing have been well described in a number of recent reviews.[120–123] We feel the test should be multistaged with continuous progressive workload to a predicted maximal heart rate. We have utilized standard tables of predicted maximal heart rates by age for males and females.[124–125] Patients are exercised to fatigue, and the test is not considered adequate unless they reach 85 percent of their predicted maximal heart rate. The patient is tested after a 4-h fast, and careful attention is given to proper application of electrodes which are the silver-silver chloride type. A multiple lead ECG is used, and care is taken in positioning electrode leads to minimize deformity of the ECG signal.

The protocol should maximize test sensitivity. If patients are not maximally exercised, they may not achieve a heart-rate pressure product to produce ischemia. Improper electrodes enhance artifacts, and multiple leads increase diagnostic sensitivity by 10 to 15 percent.[126] Because drug and recent food ingestion alter the ST segment, they should be excluded prior to testing.[126a] Patients should always have base-line measurements made standing and following hyperventilation, since these activities may cause significant ST-segment depression and T wave inversion. The final interpretation of ST-segment depression should subtract any control abnormality.

The response of the ST segment to exercise is the

most sensitive aspect of the ECG in determining the presence of coronary artery disease. The ST-segment response to exercise-induced ischemia is a graduated phenomenon dependent upon left ventricular function and the extent and location of myocardial ischemia.[127,128] An ischemic response may be indicated by an ST segment which demonstrates only J-point depression, a depressed J point with a slow rising ST segment, depression of the J point with a horizontal or downsloping ST segment, or an ST segment which has a sagging or rounded contour.[129] The magnitude of the J-point depression and the direction of the ST segment correlate best with the severity of myocardial ischemia.[130]

J-point depression alone is considered a normal response to exercise. However, when the depression is ≥ 1.5 mm, there may be a significant association with coronary artery disease.[131] When coupled with a slow-rising ST segment, sensitivity for identifying coronary disease may exceed 90 percent.[132] There is, however, an incidence of false positivity as high as 33 percent.

Horizontal ST depression is a more specific, but less sensitive, indicator of coronary artery disease. Specificity will exceed 97 percent when a criteria of ≥ 2 mm of ST depression is utilized; however, sensitivity is low, approaching only 50 percent.[130] There is a progressive decrease in sensitivity with an increase in the magnitude of ST depression required. Most studies find that a 1 mm ST depression provides the best specificity with the least loss of sensitivity.

ST-segment elevation with exercise is a very specific sign of coronary artery disease. It reflects either previous myocardial infarction with ventricular wall dyskinesia or a severely stenosed coronary vessel in the distribution of the ECG area indicated by the ST-segment elevation.[133,134] This change appears to correlate better with ventricular wall motion abnormalities than with the development of myocardial ischemia.

Other electrocardiographic responses, such as T wave changes and conduction disturbances, have a low sensitivity and specificity for coronary artery disease. U wave inversion may be significant; while this is an insensitive indicator of coronary disease, inversion with exercise has been reported to be a fairly specific marker for ischemia.[135] R wave changes can be helpful, and Bonoris et al. have described an increase in sensitivity and specificity utilizing an index of the R wave and ST-segment response.[136] The R wave normally decreases with exercise but may remain unchanged or increased in amplitude with ischemia.

Computer techniques may permit a more precise quantification of the integrated area of the ST segment below the isoelectric line and identify criteria which provide better sensitivity without loss of specificity.[137]

Pretest Factors Utilized in Determining Sensitivity and Specificity

Patients with known atherosclerotic heart disease, as demonstrated by typical angina pectoris, previous myocardial infarction, or a positive coronary arteriogram, have a high sensitivity and specificity with treadmill exercise testing.[120] The stress test in these patients is utilized in assessing the extent of physical impairment and providing objective assessment of mechanisms which may produce symptoms.[138,139] The stress test is also utilized early in the postmyocardial infarction period to provide information concerning proper exercise prescription and prognosis.[143] Several studies have indicated that new ST-segment depression with exercise in the postmyocardial infarction period is associated with a higher incidence of future coronary events.[140–142]

When the stress test is utilized for screening individuals for latent coronary artery disease, there may be a high incidence of false positive responders. Borer and Froelicher found that false postive responders accounted for greater than two-thirds of positive tests in a population of asymptomatic individuals.[144,145] Erikssen, however, in a large screening study, found only one-third of the positive responders to be without significant coronary disease.[146]

The ST-segment response in women during exercise testing has been described as a less specific indicator of coronary artery disease.[147] Ksumi found that women have a greater rise in pulmonary and systemic pressures with exercise and suggested that this may account for the abnormal ST-segment response.[148] Linhart, in a study of 98 consecutive female patients, found no differences in sensitivity or specificity as compared to male responders.[149] The higher frequency of positive ST-segment responses in women may result because they are frequently being evaluated for chest pain associated with anxiety and are taking drugs which effect the central nervous system.[120] An abnormal resting ST-T wave does not exclude the use of the stress ECG in the evaluation for the presence of coronary artery disease. Linhart and Turnoff found the validity of stress exercise testing only slightly reduced when care was taken to exclude patients with nonischemic origin of the ST-segment changes.[150] Similar observations were noted by Kancell and are consistent with the higher incidence of coronary artery disease in a population with an abnormal resting ECG.[151]

The validity of the exercise response in diagnosing coronary artery disease and determining its severity is enhanced by utilizing additional parameters in describing a positive or negative response (Table 3). An early onset of an ischemic ST-segment response dur-

TABLE 3

Additional evidence supporting coronary artery disease as the cause of a positive exercise test

Onset of ST depression at low level exertion
Persistence of ST depression
Inability to reach maximal predicted heart rate
Fall in systolic blood pressure during exertion
ST depression of 2 mm or more
Exercise induced chest pain
Downsloping ST segment
Decreased exercise tolerance

ing the Bruce stage 1 carries a specificity of 97 percent and is associated with triple-vessel disease in 73 percent of the patients. Patients who exercise to Bruce stage 3 without ST-segment changes are unlikely to have triple-vessel disease (< 10 percent). However, a negative response to Bruce stage 4 has a low sensitivity in excluding single-vessel disease.[126,152]

ST depression persisting beyond 8 min into recovery, as well as exercise-induced hypotension, suggests severe multivessel disease.[153,154] It is unusual for patients with triple-vessel disease to have a heart-rate pressure product greater than 25,000.[126] An ST-segment depression of ≥ 4 mm is also associated with main left or multivessel disease, especially if the change occurs in Bruce stage 1 or 2.[155]

Sensitivity and specificity for detection of coronary artery disease by stress electrocardiography has been determined by correlation with coronary angiography. It must be appreciated that there are several limitations that are inherent in this method of analysis: (1) there is no general agreement about the amount of luminal narrowing on the arteriogram or the effect of multiple obstructions, long segments of narrowing, or distal vessel disease on coronary blood flow; (2) the significance of collaterals and the functional distribution of blood in the myocardium cannot be appreciated on the angiogram; (3) other disease states besides cor-

onary obstruction will produce myocardial ischemia; and (4) normal coronaries do not exclude the presence of anatomic coronary obstruction by spasm.

Table 4 describes the diagnostic value of exercise testing in patients who have been studied with coronary angiography, utilizing 1-mm horizontal ST depression as a criteria of a positive response. Sensitivity increases significantly with increasing severity of the disease. These studies, however, were done in selected patients; as noted earlier, there may be a significantly higher false positivity when a population with a low prevalence of coronary disease is tested.

A false positive finding may result from a number of conditions (Table 5). Care must be taken to question the patient carefully concerning drug usage, to exclude valvular and myopathic heart diseases, and to make sure that the click-murmur syndrome is excluded during auscultation. The patient should be evaluated with ECG recordings in the supine and standing positions and hyperventilated before exercise to evaluate ST-segment response.

A false negative finding may be related to poor patient effort, inadequate monitoring, or the presence of ventricular dyskinesia (Table 6).

Arrhythmias

Many normal individuals will develop ventricular ectopic activity at or near maximal exercise.[156] The suppression of ventricular ectopic activity with exercise or the development of ventricular ectopy in the postexercise period are insensitive indicators of coronary artery disease. The pattern most suggestive of this diagnosis is the development of ventricular ectopy at heart rates of less than 130 per minute, particularly if associated with complex ventricular arrhythmias such as multiform ventricular premature beats or ventricular tachycardia.[157]

TABLE 4

Studies evaluating the diagnostic value of exercise testing in patients who have been studied with coronary angiography*

Study	N	Specificity	Single vessel	Double vessel	Triple vessel	Total
Kassebaum et al.	68	97%	25%	38%	85%	53%
Martin and McConahay	100	89%	35%	67%	86%	62%
McHenry et al.	166	95%	61%	91%	100%	81%
Helfant et al.	63	83%	60%	83%	91%	79%
Bartel et al.	609	94%	39%	62%	73%	63%
Goldschlager et al.	110	93%	40%	63%	79%	64%
Mason et al.	84	89%	—	—	—	78%
Roitman et al.	100	82%	—	—	—	73%
Average		90%	43%	67%	86%	69%

* Used by permission of the authors and Year Book Medical Publishers.

REPOLARIZATION ABNORMALITIES

ST-Segment Elevation

Although the ST segment is usually close to the iso-electric line, a normal ST-segment elevation of less than 2.5 mm may occur in leads V_1 to V_3.[158] The repolarization abnormality of LVH, often referred to as a "strain pattern," produces ST elevation in the right precordial leads. A similar ST vector is seen in LBBB. Upward deviation of the ST segment as a result of infarction, pericarditis, coronary artery spasm, ventricular aneurysm, and early repolarization pattern (ERP) is covered elsewhere. The morphology of the ST-segment deviation is not very specific, although a concave contour is more likely to be caused by pericarditis or ERP, while a convex ST segment suggests infarction. An analysis of the ST segment height, vector, serial changes, and the associated QRS alterations will often reveal the reason.

ST-Segment Depression

ST segment depression[158] is a very nonspecific finding. Myocardial ischemia or injury, LVH, digitalis,[159] hyperkalemia and hypokalemia, and hypomagnesemia can produce a similar ST depression in the left precordial and sometimes inferior leads. ST-segment

TABLE 5

Conditions that may produce a false positive exercise test

Wolff-Parkinson-White syndrome
Lown-Ganong-Levine syndrome
Mitral valve prolapse
Left or right ventricular hypertrophy
Digitalis
Left bundle branch block
Diuretics
Cardiomyopathy
Hypertrophic obstructive cardiomyopathy
Valvular heart disease
Anemia
Hyperventilation
Vasoregulatory asthenia
Hypertension
Female sex
Hypokalemia
Sedatives
Anti-depressant drugs
Recent glucose or food ingestion
Pericardial disease
Excessive double product (heart rate × blood pressure)
Improper interpretation
Inadequate recording equipment

TABLE 6

Conditions that may produce a false negative exercise test

Submaximal test
Patient is on propranolol or nitrates
Post myocardial infarction
Right bundle branch block
Single lead monitored
Cancellation of forces
Single vessel disease
Slow upsloping ST (2 mm at 0.08 s)

depression in the right precordial leads may be more specific and is seen with posterior wall infarction and acute right-sided heart strain.

T Wave Abnormalities

The normal T vector is directed anteriorly, inferiorly, and to the left in the adult. Criteria for normal amplitude have never been established.

Numerous cardiac and systemic disorders, as well as physiologic influences such as hyperventilation, standing, smoking, recent food ingestion, emotion, and exercise, may lower the T wave amplitude or cause a nonspecific T wave inversion. This has recently been discussed by Surawicz and will not be detailed here.[160] Although the T wave inversion seen in ischemic heart disease is often in the nonspecific category, the presence of a deep, symmetrical T wave inversion can suggest the diagnosis, particularly if serial changes occur.

A tall precordial T wave that exceeds 10 mm in height is a more specific finding.[161] This occasionally occurs in a normal individual, often in association with ST elevation resulting from ERP, and is also a finding with acute myocardial ischemia or infarction, hyperkalemia, left ventricular hypertrophy, and anemia. Tall, broad (0.24–0.26 s) T waves may be the earliest ECG finding of infarction. Tall, thin, peaked (0.16 s) T waves warn of hyperkalemia. With LVH resulting from aortic stenosis or hypertension, the T waves are tall in leads V_1 to V_4, while leads V_4 to V_6 are the preference for the tall T waves associated with aortic regurgitation, patent ductus arteriosus, and ventricular septal defect.

Q-T Interval

A short Q-T interval corrected for heart rate can be a manifestation of digitalis, hypercalcemia, and hyperkalemia.

A prolongation of the Q-T interval may be related to the hereditary prolonged Q-T interval syndrome, subarachnoid hemorrhage or stroke, hypokalemia, mitral valve prolapse, myocardial infarction, and drugs, including quinidine, procainamide (Pronestyl), and phenothiazines.[162] Giant U waves may also be present. This is important to recognize, since patients with these problems are susceptible to ventricular arrhythmias and sudden death.

The U wave

A prominent U wave is often seen with slow heart rates as well as with disorders that cause Q-T prolongation and papillary muscle dysfunction. An inverted U wave is considered a sign of myocardial ischemia.

The Pre-excitation Syndrome

Pre-excitation is present when the normal AV nodal pathway is bypassed and early excitation of the ventricle occurs. Three anatomic variants are described.[163–166] They include the Wolff-Parkinson-White syndrome (W-P-W), in which AV conduction occurs over an accessory pathway located away from the AV node, the Lown-Ganong-Levine syndrome (L-G-L), in which a specific intraatrial tract enters the lower aspect of the AV node (permitting premature activation of the His bundle) and the Mahaim fibers, a discrete muscle bundle which connects the lower AV node, His bundle, or bundle branches directly to ventricular myocardium. These three forms of pre-excitation deform the electrocardiogram in characteristic ways. In the W-P-W syndrome a short P-R interval, a prolonged QRS, and an initial slow slurring of the first component of the QRS, referred to as a delta wave, are the diagnostic features. The QRS in the W-P-W syndrome is a fusion beat reflecting the combined conduction through the accessory pathway and the AV node. The L-G-L syndrome is characterized by a short P-R interval, less than 0.11 s in adults and 0.08 to 0.09 s in children, and a normal QRS complex. Pre-excitation via the Mahaim fibers results in a normal P-R interval with a prolonged QRS preceded by a delta wave.

In the W-P-W syndrome, a shortened P-R interval is a necessary element of the diagnostic criteria. In children, however, the normal P-R interval is shorter than in adults.[163] The P-R interval also changes with heart rate, lengthening with slower sinus rates. In patients with relatively long refractory periods in the accessory pathway, the P-R interval may be greater than 0.12 s.

Accessory pathways may be present at any point in the AV ring. When the pathways are distant from the sinus node or enter the ventricular septum near the His bundle, there may be only a slight deformity of the QRS complex.[167] The vectorial direction of the delta wave also depends upon the location of the bypass tract. It can be confused with a notch on the initial portion of the QRS complex. The concertina effect represents variation in the fusion complex with a shortening or lengthening of the delta wave. The duration of the P wave to the end of the QRS remains the same, while the P-R interval and QRS complex change in their duration. This may result in variation of the P-R interval, the QRS complex, and the ST and T segments.[166,167]

These electrocardiographic variants are not rare and are seen frequently in any busy ECG reading station.[165] The significance of these conduction defects lies in the manner in which they deform the ECG, causing confusion with bundle branch block and ischemic heart disease, and their association with tachyarrhythmias.[163,164]

The following difficulties occur in diagnosis as a result of pre-excitation syndrome:

1 Bundle branch block: Pre-excitation may simulate bundle branch block with prolongation of the QRS complex and abnormalities in repolarization. Similarly, the presence of bundle branch block may be difficult to determine in the presence of pre-excitation.

2 Ischemic heart disease: As a general rule, the electrocardiogram is not helpful in the diagnosis of ischemic heart disease or myocardial disease when pre-excitation exists. Q waves may be related to the accessory pathway and may mimic myocardial infarction.[163,164] Pathways have been described which cause Q waves in the inferior, anterolateral, or anteroseptal leads and tall R waves simultating posterior infarction in lead V_1.

3 Repolarization abnormalities: ST-T waves may be altered from the anomalous depolarization. Changes in these segments should not be confused with ischemic or metabolic abnormalities. Variations in the ST and T wave segments, including ST elevation, may be related to the concertina effect and not to myocardial ischemia.

4 Arrhythmias: Intermittent conduction along the accessory pathway may be misinterpreted as ventricular ectopic beats. This often occurs with atrial fibrillation and is misinterpreted as ventricular tachycardia unless the grossly irregular rhythm, periods of extremely rapid ventricular rate, and normally conducted impulses are recognized.[163–170]

5 Latent pre-excitation: Evidence for pre-excitation may never be seen on the ECG even when anomalous pathways can be demonstrated at autopsy. Some patients manifest pre-excitation only on an infrequent or isolated ECG with normal conduction the rest of the time. Pre-excitation may not be appreciated in patients with long refractory periods of the accessory pathway unless the patient develops AV block. In these patients the pre-excitation may occur when there is prolonged conduction over normal AV pathways.[171] Patients may conduct over the anomalous pathway in a retrograde, but not antegrade, direction. They remain subject to tachyarrhythmias. In these patients, pre-excitation can only be appreciated by electrophysiologic evaluation showing retrograde conduction over an accessory pathway.[172]

Pericarditis

The ECG changes in pericarditis vary depending on the presence of acute or chronic inflammation, the presence and size of pericardial effusion and the degree and location of constriction.

A Acute pericarditis
  1 The ST vector is directed anteriorly, inferiorly, and to the left—toward the apex.[173–176] This results in widespread ST elevation, usually of less than 5 mm, in leads I, II, aV_L, aV_F, V_2 to V_6.
  2 Evolutionary ST changes last from a few days to a few weeks until the ST segment returns to the isoelectric line.[173]
  3 PR segment deviation, oriented superiorly and to the right, produces an elevated PR segment in aV_R and a depressed PR segment in the midprecordial leads.[177]
  4 The T vector points superiorly and rightward, producing widespread T inversion, particularly in the left precordial leads.[173–176] A notched or diphasic T wave is often present.[174]
  5 Atrial arrhythmias.
B Pericardial effusion[173,176]
  1 Decreased QRS and T voltage.
  2 Electrical alternans of the QRS or QRS-T amplitudes.[173,176,178]
C Pericardial constriction[173,176]
  1 Decreased QRS and T voltage
  2 Wide, notched P waves
  3 Widespread low voltage, flat or inverted T waves
  4 Atrial arrhythmias, usually atrial fibrillation
  5 Right axis deviation, a LAA and posterolateral T inversion with scarring predominately of the left ventricle and left AV groove[179]

CORRELATIONS

Acute pericarditis, documented by friction rubs, produces ECG alterations in 80 to 96 percent of patients.[173,175] The incidence of ECG findings in asymptomatic patients or patients without friction rubs is unknown. The ECG may show characteristic evolutionary ST-T changes or nonspecific T wave changes only. PR-segment deviation is a relatively subtle finding and was present 82 percent of the time in 50 patients with pericarditis studied by Spodick.[177] This may be the only ECG evidence of pericarditis and should be carefully searched for. PR-segment deviation was also found in 9 of 48 patients with an early repolarization pattern. In 8 of 9 patients, this was limited to the limb leads, in contrast to pericarditis, where it was always present in both the limb and precordial leads.[180]

The ST-segment elevation of an early repolarization pattern is frequently included in the differential diagnosis of pericarditis. In a study of 1,188 normal USAF flying personnel with ST-segment elevation thought to be caused by ERP, the ST vector was directed anteriorly, inferiorly, and to the left.[181] ST elevation was usually less than 2 mm, never more than 4 mm, and was confined to the precordial leads (usually V_4 to V_6) in 37.3 percent, only to the limb leads (usually lead II or aV_F) in 42 percent, and was present in both limb and precordial leads in 58.1 percent. The pattern included tall, peaked precordial T waves in the majority and remained fairly constant, with some exceptions, over 8 years. Spodick carefully compared records of 48 patients with pericarditis to those of 48 patients with ERP and concluded that the morphology of the ST-segment elevation was not often helpful; however, pericarditis was favored by PR-segment deviation or ST-segment elevation or both occurring simultaneously in precordial and limb leads and an ST vector oriented leftward of the QRS vector.[180] When ST elevation was limited to either the limb or precordial leads and the ST vector was to the right of both the QRS and T vector, then ERP was suspected.

Low voltage is so insensitive a finding that it is not very helpful in diagnosing pericardial effusion or constriction. However, electrical alternans of the QRS or QRS-T complex is almost diagnostic of a very large pericardial effusion with an unrestrained heart swinging in a pendular fashion. Malignancy involving the pericardium or, far less likely, tuberculosis and rheumatic pericarditis, is the cause.[178]

Virtually all patients with chronic constrictive pericarditis have an abnormal ECG. This is usually nonspecific except with constriction primarily involving the left ventricle and left AV groove when a characteristic pattern of RAD, a LAA, and posterolateral T inversion occurs.[179]

MITRAL AND AORTIC VALVE DISEASE

The P Wave

The P wave provides a helpful electrocardiographic marker for assessing the hemodynamic significance of valvular heart disease. As described previously, the LAA correlates best with interatrial conduction defects, and conduction is influenced by increased atrial volume and increased atrial pressure. In rheumatic valvular disease the LAA may be more a result of the fibrosis and scarring of the atrial wall than of significant hemodynamic abnormalities. In patients with mitral stenosis, the LAA correlates with atrial size, atrial pressure, diastolic mitral valve gradient, and mitral valve area.[182-185] A sensitivity and specificity exceeding 90 percent for identifying increased LA volume is described in one study.[183] The LAA in mitral regurgitation does not correlate with mean left atrial pressure or the height of the regurgitant V wave; however, it is associated with the severity and chronicity of the regurgitation.[183-186] This is most often dependent on left atrial size, with a 77 percent sensitivity and only 11 percent false negativity.[183]

Atrial fibrillation is common in mitral valve disease. The reversibility of this rhythm may be correlated with the degree of structural wall damage demonstrated by pathology. In mitral stenosis, atrial fibrillation increases progressively with age, approximately 50 percent of patients developing this rhythm by the age of 45 years.[188] When fibrillatory waves exceed 1 mm in amplitude, they are suggestive of rheumatic valvular disease.[189] After surgery for mitral stenosis, the LAA returns to normal.[190] The mechanism is unclear but may be related to improved conduction at lower pressures.

A LAA occurs frequently in patients with aortic valve disease, occurring in 84 percent of patients with severe aortic stenosis in one study.[191] This change appears unrelated to left atrial size, pressure, or hypertrophy but does correlate with hypertrophy of the left ventricle and aortic valve gradient.[182,192] One study noted a LAA in 11 of 12 patients with a valvular gradient equal to or greater than 50 mm Hg. However, a 31 percent false positive rate was described when correlated with left atrial size.[182] The type of LAA correlates with the anatomic and hemodynamic defect present. A PTF-V$_1$ appears most sensitive to increased left atrial pressure, while P wave duration and the P/PR ratio correlate best with left atrial size.[185] Atrial fibrillation is rare in aortic stenosis and may suggest coexisting mitral valve disease.[184]

The QRS-T Complex[193-207]

The ventricular contribution to the ECG is of limited value in the diagnosis and assessment of mitral stenosis. Cancellation of right ventricular forces by opposing left ventricular forces does not allow for the expression of RVH until it is quite advanced. Only 20 percent of patients with mild pulmonary hypertension have ECG evidence of RVH.[205] However, when right ventricular systolic pressure is equal to or greater than 70 mm Hg, 54 percent of patients exhibit RVH, and all patients demonstrate ECG evidence for RVH when this pressure is greater than 110 mm Hg or exceeds systemic pressure.[205] A less specific, but more sensitive, sign may be a shift in QRS axis, which, with increasing pulmonary artery pressure, moves right-

ward in the frontal plane. One study noted that 88 percent of patients with a mitral valve area equal to or less than 1.3 cm^2 had an axis greater than +60°.[206] Several studies suggest that vectocardiographic analysis is more sensitive than the ECG. One study found that the evidence for RVH in patients with mitral stenosis is 63 percent with the vectorcardiograph but only 43 percent with the ECG. When patients with significant pulmonary hypertension only are included, the sensitivity of the vectorcardiograph is 86 percent as compared to 67 percent for the ECG.[207] Multivariate analysis with computer techniques increases sensitivity even further, and one study noted a 74 percent recognition rate with only 6 percent false positive results.[207]

The ECG in aortic stenosis is normal in all patients with trivial obstruction and in most patients with moderate obstruction.[193] In congenital aortic stenosis, even a very severe valvular gradient may not alter the ECG. The recent natural history study of 422 patients under age 22 found that the severity of aortic stenosis was unrelated to the R wave amplitude in lead V$_6$ or to the S wave depth in lead V$_1$. The only discriminating parameter was the T wave in lead V$_6$, which is always upright if the gradient is equal to or less than 50 mm Hg, but is flat, biphasic, or inverted in 50 percent of patients with a gradient equal to or greater than 80 mm Hg.[194] Although the pattern of LVH is present in 90 percent of patients with severe disease, false negative results occur.[184] Correlative autopsy studies of left ventricular weight and size, reviewed in the previous section, describe the reasons for the imperfect correlation. The specificity of voltage criteria for LVH increases with age and is quite high over 60 years of age.[195] The ST-T pattern of pressure overload is also quite specific but may be mimicked by ischemia, particularly in the elderly. Sudden death may occur in patients with a normal ECG and aortic stenosis but is more common when LVH and ST changes are present.[196] The ECG of severe aortic regurgitation typically shows a pattern of LVH with related ST-T changes. The R wave amplitude in leads V$_4$ to V$_6$ may be huge.

ECG abnormalities are reported in 60 percent of patients with mitral leaflet prolapse.[197,198] The most common finding is a superior orientation of the T wave in the frontal axis with an abnormally wide QRS-T angle. This results in a T wave inversion in leads II, III, and AV$_F$.[199] Less commonly, there is a posterior direction of the T wave in the horizontal axis with T wave inversion in leads V$_4$ and V$_6$. The ST segment is usually normal but may be depressed in the inferior leads. Q-T prolongation may occur and is described in 26 percent of patients in one study.[198] There is a high association of ventricular tachyarrhythmia with Q-T prolongation. Many arrhythmias are ascribed to this disorder, and sudden death as a result of ventricular arrhythmias is a recognized complication.[197,200] The most common arrhythmias are sinus arrest, atrial fibrillation, ventricular premature beats, and ventricular tachycardia.

The QRS-T in mitral regurgitation is of limited value in assessing the anatomic or physiologic abnormalities present. The presence of ECG abnormalities increases with duration of disease and severity of the regurgitation. In spite of the chronic left ventricular volume overload, LVH is reported in only 30 to 70 percent of patients.[186] Unlike other causes of LVH, the frontal axis is more to the right, averaging 52°, and maximum QRS voltage is less than in aortic valve disease.[184] Patients with severe acute mitral regurgitation from a ruptured chordae tendinea do not exhibit ECG changes; the diagnosis may be suggested by the incongruity of a severe hemodynamic abnormality and a near normal ECG.

The ECG findings in papillary muscle dysfunction are variable and nonspecific. Infarction limited to the papillary muscle or subendocardial region may not be reflected on the ECG or cause only nonspecific ST-T wave changes.[201] A specific ST and T wave pattern is described which includes (1) moderate depression of the J-junction with concave upward deformity of the ST segment, (2) slight to moderate depression of the J-junction with convex upward deformity of the ST segment and terminal inversion of the T wave, and (3) marked J-junction depression with either convex or concave upward deformity of the ST segment.[202] These patterns are nonspecific, however, and occur in many forms of subendocardial ischemia including LVH, intraventricular conduction defects, and digitalis effect. However, one study found evidence of infarction in 75 percent of 20 patients,[203] and in another study of 187 patients with acute myocardial infarction, papillary muscle dysfunction was noted in 63 percent.[204] Inferior or posterior infarction occurs most commonly and accounts for approximately 75 percent of patients.

CARDIOMYOPATHY[209–228]

Congestive Cardiomyopathy

The ECG is usually abnormal, although nonspecific, in patients with congestive cardiomyopathy (CCM). An atrial abnormality, usually LAA, occurs in 33 to 52 percent of patients.[212] A LAA pattern provides an insight into both left ventricular end-diastolic pressure (LVEDP) and left atrial size, with an LVEDP greater than or equal to 26 mm Hg in 89 percent and an increased radiographic size of the left atrium in 70 percent of patients.[209] P-R prolongation may occur with an incidence of 6 to 30 percent.[210–212] Complete heart block is rare, however, except in Chagas' disease, where it is present in 25 percent of patients.[213] The

block in Chagas' disease results from fibrosis of the right and left bundles and not involvement of the AV node.[214] Left axis deviation is reported in 18 to 58 percent of CCM patients as a result of fibrosis of the left anterior fascicle.[215] Complete LBBB is reported in 10 to 40 percent of these patients;[208] one study noted that 92 percent of patients with this finding had a left ventricular ejection fraction less than or equal to 30 percent.[209] Right bundle branch block is uncommon in CCM except in Chagas' disease. When it does occur, it is frequently associated with left axis deviation. Low voltage is reported in 25 percent of patients[212] and is suggestive of amyloidosis when present in all leads.[216] Conversely, LVH is also frequent, occurring in one-third of CCM patients.[209]

Pathologic Q waves are reported in 8 to 13 percent of patients involving leads I and AV_L in 75 percent and leads II, III and AV_F in 25 percent.[209] The absence of a septal Q wave in leads I, AV_L, and V_5, and V_6 occurs in 35 to 70 percent of CCM patients and may represent confluent fibrosis in the septum or an incomplete block of the left bundle branch.[217]

ST-T abnormalities are present in almost every patient. However, these are nonspecific and frequently related to conduction defects or secondary changes of LVH. Arrhythmias are common—premature ventricular contractions are described in 20 to 80 percent and atrial fibrillation in 3 to 50 percent of patients.[208,209,218,219] No correlation exists for the presence of mitral regurgitation, increased LVEDP, or decreased left ventricular function with these arrhythmias.[209]

The ECG is frequently abnormal in acute and chronic alcoholism.[211,220] One study demonstrated ECG abnormalities in 54 percent of patients admitted to a psychiatric facility with alcoholism.[221] Findings are similar to those in patients with CCM. A characteristic cloven, dimpled, or inverted T wave abnormality described by Evans in alcoholic patients is not supported by other studies, in which the T wave changes are nonspecific and frequently associated with digitalis effects or LVH.[220,222] LVH occurs more frequently in alcoholics than in patients with CCM and is reported in 66 percent of patients in one study. Pathologic Q waves are uncommon and more suggestive of hypertrophic cardiomyopathy. Conduction defects, including LAD, first-degree AV block, LBBB, and RBBB are frequent.

Hypertrophic Obstructive Cardiomyopathy

An abnormal ECG occurs in 70 percent of asymptomatic and 90 percent of symptomatic patients with hypertrophic obstructive cardiomyopathy (HOCM).[223] An atrial abnormality, usually LAA, is present in 30 to 50 percent of these patients.[209,224] However, a biatrial or a right atrial abnormality is frequent, and one study noted a 46 percent incidence of RAA in HOCM.[210] The presence of a RAA with LVH is considered highly suspicious of HOCM and occurs rarely in valvular aortic stenosis.[226] LVH is present in approximately 70 percent of these patients with HOCM and is associated with secondary ST-T wave changes more than 90 percent of the time.[208,224,225] Abnormal Q waves occur in 25 to 35 percent of patients and may be caused by myocardial fibrosis creating electrical dead zones or septal hypertrophy leading to an increased amplitude of the septal vector with reciprocal Q waves in the inferior and lateral leads. When present, they are always in leads II, III and AV$_F$, with 25 percent of patients demonstrating Q waves in both inferior and anterior leads.[209] No relationship of Q waves to echocardiographic septal thickness or outflow tract obstruction is described.[223] There is an association between increased septal thickness and left atrial dimension on the echocardiogram with LVH, LAA by ECG, and repolarization abnormalities. A significantly higher LVEDP was present with LAA or LVH, and LAA correlated with an elevated mean left atrial pressure.[223]

No significant ECG differences are noted between obstructive and nonobstructive hypertrophic cardiomyopathy.[223] Age may alter the prevalence of ECG findings. One study noted that only 30 percent of asymptomatic children with HOCM had an abnormal ECG, and pathologic Q waves tend to occur less frequently in affected patients over 60 years of age.[227,228] The W-P-W syndrome may be present in some patients with HOCM. Arrhythmias are a late finding and are poorly tolerated.

THE ECG IN DIAGNOSIS OF CARDIAC INVOLVEMENT IN NEUROMYOPATHIC DISEASE

Duchenne's muscular dystrophy is a sex-linked recessive disorder which affects males in the first decade of life. The onset is characterized by weakness of the pelvic girdle, and the course is constant and often rapid. The disorder is associated with typical ECG changes that indicate cardiac involvement. There are tall right precordial R waves with an increased R/S ratio in lead V and deep Q waves in the limb and lateral precordial leads.[228a] Affected siblings have identical tracing, and female carriers may demonstrate similar features.

Erb's limb-girdle dystrophy is an autosomal recessive disorder with onset in the second decade. Cardiac involvement is uncommon, but there may be disturbances in rhythm or conduction and abnormal Q waves or minor T wave abnormalities.[228b] Friedreich's ataxia is a familial disorder with ataxia from degen-

eration of the spinocerebellar tracts. The ECG may demonstrate T wave inversion, especially in the left precordial leads and in leads I, II, and aV$_F$.[228a] There may be right and left ventricular hypertrophy, and acute changes resembling myocardial ischemia can occur.

Myotonic dystrophy is a slow progressive degenerative autosomal dominant disorder. ECG abnormalities occur in two-thirds of patients usually late in the course of the disease.[228b] P-R prolongation and conduction defects occur. P waves are low in voltage, and ST-segment changes and flattening or inversion of the T wave are seen.[228b] Infarct patterns, RBBB, LBBB, complete heart block, and ventricular tachycardia or fibrillation may occur in the course of the disease. Sinus bradycardia is more common in myotonic dystrophy, while sinus tachycardia is more frequent in Duchenne's dystrophy and in Friedreich's ataxia.

MYOCARDITIS

Myocardial inflammation has been described with almost every known bacterial, viral, rickettsial, mycotic, and parasitic disease. ECG abnormalities are frequent but nonspecific. Acute viral myopericarditis represents one of the most common infectious illnesses affecting the heart. Changes in the ECG in the absence of other clinical evidence of myocarditis occurs in 10 to 33 percent of patients with common infectious diseases.[229,230] The following outline describes the ECG abnormalities reported in viral infections:[229]

A ST-T wave changes
   1 Coxsackie
   2 Poliomyelitis
   3 Mumps
   4 Rubella
   5 Rubeola
   6 Rabies
   7 Lymphocytic choriomeningitis
   8 Herpes simplex

B Conduction disturbances including P-R prolongation, AV block, and bundle branch block
   1 Poliomyelitis
   2 Mumps
   3 Influenza
   4 Infectious mononucleosis
   5 Rubella
   6 Rubeola
   7 Varicella

C Arrhythmias
   1 Poliomyelitis
   2 Coxsackie
   3 Infectious Hepatitis
   4 Rubeola
   5 Herpes zoster

The electrocardiographic changes in acute myocarditis are usually T wave changes, either reduced amplitude or inversion, often occurring in the left precordial leads. The ECG usually reverts to normal as the illness subsides; however, T wave inversion may remain for weeks to months after the acute illness.[231] Sinus tachycardia may be the only arrhythmia present and is usually suggestive of myocarditis when there is persistence of the tachycardia during the convalescent phase.[231] Premature ventricular contractions are the most common arrhythmia and may occur in the absence of any other ECG abnormalities. Conduction defects are unusual in mild forms of myocarditis and usually occur in more widespread severe disease.[231] Conduction defects are associated with a less favorable prognosis and may persist after the acute illness has subsided. Occasional patients develop ECG changes simulating myocardial infarction. ST and T segments are abnormal, and there may be deep symmetrical inversion of the T wave. Changes consistent with pericarditis may occur and are more common with the enteroviruses.[231]

Myocarditis may also result from bacterial, spirochetal, rickettsial, protozoal, and helminthic infections. The ECG abnormalities characteristic of these infections are noted in the following list:[229]

Bacterial Myocarditis

1 ST-T wave changes
   Diptheria
   Typhoid fever
   Scarlet fever
   Meningococcemia
   Staphylococcus
   Pneumococcus
   Gonococcus
   Brucellosis
   Tetanus

2 AV conduction disturbances or bundle branch block
   Diptheria
   Tuberculosis
   Typhoid fever
   Acute rheumatic fever
   Scarlet fever

3 New Q waves or changes that mimic myocardial infarction
   Tuberculosis
   Bacterial endocarditis
   Melioidosis

Tertiary syphilis is associated with AV block, bundle branch block, and changes mimicking myocardial infarction. These result from diffuse gummatous lesions involving the myocardium. Leptospirosis is frequently associated with myocarditis. T wave changes are common, as is bradycardia, and complete heart block can occur. There is usually prolongation of the P-R and Q-T interval. Rickettsial myocarditis results from typhus, Rocky Mountain spotted fever, or Q fever and is associated with nonspecific ST and T wave changes. Both leptospirosis and rickettsia infections may result in congestive heart failure, hypotension, and circulatory collapse. Mycotic infections of the myocardium usually result in necrotizing lesions with focal myocardial granulomas or abscesses. ECG abnormalities may be limited to T wave changes. Pericarditis is common, as are arrhythmias. Chagas' disease is the most common protozoal infection involving the heart. ECG features are very characteristic and include right bundle branch block, left anterior hemiblock, asymmetrically inverted T waves, and frequent and multiform ventricular premature beats.

Helminthic infections may involve the myocardium. They are associated with focal muscle necrosis, myocardial abscess formation, and cyst formation which may develop from larvae in the myocardium.

ST-T wave changes are associated with (1) trichinosis, (2) echinococcosis, (3) strongyloidiasis, and (4) cysticercosis.[229] Schistosomiasis may produce cor pulmonale with associated ECG changes.

Myopericarditis can often be a difficult disease to diagnose. Besides the classic features of myocarditis or pericarditis, it may present as a coronary mimic with chest pain typical of myocardial ischemia, progressive heart failure that follows a relentless course with a fatal termination, or an influenza-like illness with fever of uncertain origin. While the ECG changes are nonspecific, it is helpful to remember that new Q waves are rare. ST elevation over 5 mm is unusual. There are usually no reciprocal ST changes when ST elevation is present, and T wave inversion over 7 mm is uncommon.[232] Myocarditis can be suspected when T wave changes are transient or variable and are associated with prolonged severe pain that bearing no relationship to the rather mild ECG changes and absence or small enzyme rise.

CONGENITAL HEART DISEASE[233–250]

The ECG can be a useful tool in the evaluation of congenital heart disease. However, there are many limitations and few specific patterns. In the newborn, the ECG is especially difficult to interpret and may not reflect any anomalies, if present. A few specific ECG findings do suggest developmental abnormalities, such as left axis deviation in endocardial cushion defects, W-P-W syndrome in Ebstein's anomaly, or the abnormal orientation of the QRS axis with single ventricle.

The following discussion highlights ECG findings occurring after the newborn period that occur in association with various congenital defects.

Congenital Defects Associated with Abnormalities of the P Wave

Right atrial abnormality occurs with:

1 Atrial septal defect

2 Pulmonic stenosis

3 Ebstein's anomaly

4 Tricuspid atresia

5 Tetralogy of Fallot

6 Eisenmenger's complex

7 Primary pulmonary hypertension

8 Total anomolous pulmonary venous connection

9 Transposition of the great vessels

10 Pulmonary atresia

11 Hypoplastic left heart syndrome

Left atrial abnormality occurs with:

1 Ventricular septal defect

2 Patent ductus arteriosus

3 Mitral stenosis

4 Aortic stenosis

5 Endocardial fibroelastosis

The P wave is helpful in identifying the position of the heart within the chest as well as significant right ventricular or left ventricular pressure overload. When the atria are in their normal positions, the P wave is directed inferiorly and to the left in the frontal plane. When the atria are reversed, as in situs inversus or levoversion, the P wave becomes negative in lead I; the direction of depolarization in the frontal plane is directed downward and to the right.[233–235] The direction of the P wave is also altered in a sinus venosus atrial septal defect. In this anomaly the P wave is leftward in the frontal axis, usually less than +15°, and is associated with inversion of the P wave in lead III.[236] A similar orientation of the P wave may occur with a common atrium where the leftward shift tends to be quite marked, -50° in some cases.[237]

The presence of a RAA in other congenital defects is usually associated with a pressure overload of the right atrium. Therefore, patients with cor triatriatum, congenital mitral stenosis, pulmonic stenosis, and tricuspid atresia have P wave abnormalities which may reflect the degree of right atrial hypertension.[235] RAA also occurs in double outlet right ventricle with pulmonic stenosis and may be useful in separating this condition from cyanotic tetralogy of Fallot where a RAA is less common.[235] A RAA is not common in corrected transposition but does occur with complete transposition and truncus arteriosus with large pulmonary arteries.[235,238] The P wave is usually normal in atrial septal defect. However, in patients with an ostium primum, an atrial abnormality may be evidence of pulmonary hypertension with associated mitral regurgitation.[239]

A LAA in patients with congenital heart disease is associated with either a pressure overload of the left ventricle, as in aortic outflow obstruction of the supravalvular, valvular, or subvalvular type, or with volume overload of the left ventricle as seen in patients with ventricular septal defect, patent ductus arteriosus, transposition of the great vessels, and truncus arteriosus.[235] The LAA in ventricular septal defects is suggestive of a relatively large left-to-right shunt.[239]

Congenital Defects Associated with QRS Axis Deviation

Left axis deviation (LAD) occurs with:

1 Endocardial cushion defect

2 Tricuspid atresia

LAD is present in most patients with an endocardial cushion defect.[235] LAD is distinctive for this lesion and is felt to be related to a congenital alteration of the excitation pathway.[240] The LAD persists even in the presence of a right ventricular pressure overload due to mitral regurgitation from an ostium primum defect. In tricuspid atresia, LAD is present in up to 85 percent of patients and is part of the ECG triad which includes RAA and LVH.[241] A leftward deviation in the QRS axis may also occur in congenital conditions that result in volume or pressure overload to the left ventricle, such as aortic stenosis, patent ductus arteriosus, and coarctation of the aorta.[242] LAD may also exist in corrected transposition of the great vessels when the arterial ventricle is the dominant ventricle.[235] In older patients and in adults with anomalous origin of the left coronary artery from the pulmonary artery, the QRS axis may shift to the left.[243]

Right axis deviation occurs with:

1 Pulmonic stenosis

2 Atrial septal defect, secundum type

3 Tetralogy of Fallot

4 Ebstein's anomaly

5 Eisenmenger's complex

6 Pulmonary atresia

7 Mitral stenosis

8 Cor triatriatum

Patients with situs inversus may have a mirror-image ECG, so that right precordial leads will resemble corresponding sites in the left precordium. True RAD is usually associated with a pressure and volume overload of the right ventricle. In pulmonic stenosis the axis shift is a clinically useful sign, and the degree reflects the severity of the right ventricular hypertension. An axis from $+120°$ to $+269°$ is progressively more common with increasing severity of the stenosis.[244]

Congenital Defects Associated with Ventricular Hypertrophy

Right ventricular hypertrophy occurs with:

1 Pulmonic stenosis

2 Tetralogy of Fallot

3 Eisenmenger's complex

4 Transposition of the great vessels

5 Truncus arteriosus

6 Atrial septal defect

7 Hypoplastic left-sided heart syndrome

8 Primary pulmonary hypertension

9 Cor triatriatum

10 Congenital mitral stenosis

RVH reflects significant pressure or volume overload of the right ventricle. It is most severe in patients with an intact ventricular septum and pulmonary hypertension or pulmonary valvular stenosis. In patients with pulmonic stenosis, the severity of the RVH, as measured by the ECG, corresponds to the degree of obstruction. An RV_1 of ≥ 20 mm and an SI of ≥ 10 mm correlated with a pressure gradient across the pulmonary valve greater than 50 mm Hg.[244] SI and SV_6 showed a progressive increase in voltage with increasing gradient. An SI greater than 15 mm deep was present only when the pressure gradient was ≥ 80 mm Hg.[244] A Q wave in lead V_1 was present with a gradient ≥ 80 mm Hg. When the R wave in V_1 was less than 10 mm, an upright T wave was associated with more severe disease than an inverted T wave; when the R wave exceeded 10 mm, an inverted T wave reflected a larger pressure gradient.[244] In atrial septal defect, a dominant R wave in lead V_1 is associated with a large shunt and an initial R wave of large amplitude or Rs configuration is found with increased pulmonary vascular resistance and RVH.[239] In ventricular septal defect, an R wave of great amplitude in lead V_1 is usually associated with increased pulmonary vascular resistance and possibly a reverse shunt (Eisenmenger's syndrome).[245] In patients with RVH and an associated ventricular septal defect, as seen in te-

tralogy of Fallot, double outlet right ventricle, or truncus arteriosus, deeply inverted right precordial T waves are unusual. This is more suggestive of severe right ventricular pressure overload, as occurs in pulmonic stenosis with intact ventricular septum, where the right ventricular pressure can exceed systemic pressure.[235]

Left ventricular hypertrophy occurs with:

1 Aortic stenosis

2 Tricuspid atresia

3 Coarctation of the aorta

4 Endocardial fibroelastosis

5 Ventricular septal defect

Lesions resulting in volume or pressure overload of the ventricle produce a pattern of LVH. This pattern is characteristic of patients with left ventricular outflow obstruction or primary myocardial disease. When coarctation of the aorta in infancy is associated with a hypoplastic left-sided heart syndrome, a prominent right ventricular pattern, rather than LVH, may be seen.[235] Patients with a volume overload of the left ventricle, as in ventricular septal defect or patent ductus arteriosus, will demonstrate prominent Q waves in the lateral precordial leads and tall R waves in leads V_5 and V_6.[239,245] An RV_6 greater than two standard deviations from normal occurred most frequently in patients with larger shunts and was present in 27 percent in spite of normal pulmonary artery pressures.[245] A QV_6 that was ≥ 4 mm was more common in patients with increased pulmonary blood flow. ST depression and T wave inversion in these leads is usually consistent with a marked pressure overload of the left ventricle. A pattern simulating LVH may occur in anomalous origin of the left coronary artery from the pulmonary artery. In these patients, the posterior basilar portion of the left ventricle is supplied by the normal right coronary artery, and this zone tends to hypertrophy.[243] Tall R waves may occur in AV_L and the left precordial leads with T wave inversion in I, AV_L, V_5, and V_6.

Combined ventricular hypertrophy occurs with:

1 Ventricular septal defect

2 Patent ductus arteriosus

3 Transposition of the great vessels

4 Truncus arteriosus

Combined ventricular hypertrophy may occur with a significant right-to-left shunt and volume overload of both the right and left ventricles. This is characterized by tall R waves in the right precordial leads and a prominent Rs pattern with increased voltage in the left precordial leads. An equiphasic RS complex of great amplitude (Katz-Wachtel phenomenon) is seen in leads V_3 through V_5 in children who have moderate to severe left-to-right shunts.[239]

Conduction Defects and Arrhythmias Associated with Congenital Heart Disease

Bundle branch blocks are uncommon in congenital heart disease. However, the pattern of right bundle branch block in atrial septal defect occurs in more than 90 percent of patients with this anomaly.[235] This distinctive feature is not thought to be related to a conduction abnormality but rather to localized hypertrophy of the crista supraventricularis.[246] Therefore, the presence of the defect has a significant association with the magnitude of the left-to-right shunt—a tall R' in V_1 is associated with a large shunt, and the absence of an R' usually indicates insignificant shunting. A complete block of the right or left fascicle may be produced during surgical correction of congenital lesions, particularly with total correction of tetralogy of Fallot.[250] Patients with postoperative total correction for tetralogy of Fallot who have LAD, RBBB, and complete AV block at the time of surgery may have a significant late incidence of sudden death. P-R prolongation is described in atrial septal defect, patent ductus arteriosus, and corrected transposition of the great vessels. Varying degrees of second- and third-degree block may occur in Ebstein's anomaly.[247] A pre-excitation syndrome of the W-P-W syndrome type B occurs in 10 percent of these patients.[235]

Arrhythmias are uncommon in congenital heart disease except in Ebstein's anomaly, where repetitive supraventricular tachycardias may occur.[247] These arrhythmias are not necessarily associated with the pre-excitation syndrome. Atrial fibrillation often occurs late in congenital heart disease. In atrial septal defect, atrial fibrillation occurs in 13 percent of patients between 40 and 65 years of age and in 50 percent of patients over the age of 65.[248] After surgery for transposition of the great vessels (Mustard procedure), only 57 percent of patients remain in sinus rhythm.[249] A sick sinus syndrome may be a consequence of this surgery.

In summary, the ECG is a highly complex measurement resulting from an interaction of biologic and technical factors as influenced by various disease processes. Truly normal values for each age group, sex, body weight, and numerous other variables that can affect the ECG have never been derived, and therefore differentiation between the normal and abnormal is fraught with difficulty. Interpretation of the ECG must be based on an understanding of these limitations and an appreciation of the statistical meaning of sensitivity, specificity, and disease prevalence. The ECG is a very helpful diagnostic test, but the information must be used with caution and incorporated into other available clinical measurements in the total assessment of the patient.

REFERENCES

1 Simonson, E.: "Differentiation between Normal and Abnormal in Electrocardiography," The C. V. Mosby Company, St. Louis, 1961.

2 Simonson, E.: The Effect of Age on the Electrocardiogram, *Am. J. Cardiol.*, 29:64, 1972.

3 Mihalick, M. J., and Fisch, C.: Electrocardiographic Findings in the Aged, *Am. Heart J.*, 87:117, 1974.

4 Nemati, M., McCaughan, D., Doyle, J., et al.: The Influence of Constitutional Variables on Orthogonal Electrocardiograms of Normal Women, *Circulation*, 56:989, 1977.

5 Simonson, E., Blackburn, H., Puchner, T. C., et al.: Sex Differences in the Electrocardiogram, *Circulation*, 22:598, 1960.

6 Nemati, M., Doyle, J., McCaughan, D., et al.: The Orthogonal Electrocardiogram in Normal Women. Implications of Sex Differences in Diagnostic Electrocardiography, *Am. Heart J.*, 95:12, 1978.

7 Ishekawa, K.: Correlation Coefficients for Electrocardiographic and Constitutional Variables, *Am. Heart J.*, 92:152, 1976.

8 Dougherty, J. D.: The Relation of the Frontal QRS Axis to the Anatomic Position of the Heart, *J. Electrocardiol.*, 3:267, 1970.

9 Goldberg, E.: Mechanical Factors and the Electrocardiogram, *Am. Heart J.*, 93:629, 1977.

10 Pipberger, H. V., Arzbaecher, R. C., Berson, A. S., et al.: Recommendations for Standardization of Leads and of Specifications for Instruments in Electrocardiography and Vectorcardiography, *Circulation*, 52:11, 1975.

11 Caceres, C. A.: Limitations of the Computer in Electrocardiographic Interpretation, *Am. J. Cardiol.*, 38:362, 1976.

12 Burchell, H. B., and Reed, J.: A Test Experience with a Machine-processed Electrocardiography Diagnosis: The Recognition of "Normal" and Some Specific Patterns, *Am. Heart J.*, 92:773, 1976.

13 Caceres, C. A.: Present Status of Computer Interpretation of the Electrocardiogram: A 20-Year Overview, *Am. J. Cardiol.,* 41:121, 1978.

14 Willems, J. L., Poblete, P. F., and Pipberger, H. V.: Day-to-Day Variation of the Normal Orthogonal Electrocardiogram and Vectorcardiogram, *Circulation,* 45:1057, 1972.

15 Sokolow, M., and Lyon, T. P.: The Ventricular Complex in Left Ventricular Hypertrophy as Obtained by Unipolar Precordial and Limb Leads, *Am. Heart J.,* 37:161, 1949.

16 Johnson, J. C., Horan, L. G., and Flowers, N. C.: "Diagnostic Accuracy of the Electrocardiogram," in A. N. Brest (ed.), "Clinical Electrocardiographic Correlations, Cardiovascular Clinics," Vol. 8, F. A. Davis Company, Philadelphia, 1977, p. 25.

17 Rautaharju, P. M., Blackburn H. W., and Warren, J. W.: The Concepts of Sensitivity, Specificity and Accuracy in Evaluation of Electrocardiographic, Vectorcardiographic and Polarcardiographic Criteria, *J. Electrocardiol.,* 9:275, 1976.

18 Refkin, R. D., and Hood, W. B., Jr.: Bayesian Analysis of Electrocardiographic Exercise Stress Testing, *N. Engl. J. Med.,* 297:681, 1977.

18a Grant, R. P.: "Clinical Electrocardiography: The Spatial Vector Approach," McGraw-Hill Book Company, New York, 1957.

18b Chow, T., Helm, R. A., and Kaplan, S.: "Clinical Vectorcardiography," 2d ed., Grune & Stratton, Inc., New York, 1974.

19 Redwood, D. R., Borer, J. S., and Epstein, S. E.: Whither the ST Segment during Exercise?, *Circulation,* 54:703, 1976.

20 Simonson, E.: Principles and Pitfalls in Establishing Normal Electrocardiographic Limits, *Am. J. Cardiol.,* 33:271, 1974.

21 Massie, E., and Walsh, T. J.: "Clinical Vectorcardiography and Electrocardiography," Year Book Medical Publishers, Inc., Chicago, 1960.

22 Hurst, J. W., and Myerburg, R. J.: "Introduction to Electrocardiography," McGraw-Hill Book Company, New York, 1973.

23 Puech, P.: The P Wave: Correlation of Surface and Intraatrial Electrograms, *Cardiovasc. Clin.,* 6:44, 1974.

24 Kasser, I., and Kennedy, J. W.: The Relationship of Increased Left Atrial Volume and Pressure to Abnormal P Waves on the Electrocardiogram, *Circulation,* 39:339, 1969.

25 Morris, J. J., Estes, H. E., and Whalen, R. E.: P-Wave Analysis in Valvular Heart Disease, *Circulation,* 29:242, 1964.

26 Macruz, R., Perloff, J. K., and Case, R. B.: A Method for the Electrocardiographic Recognition of Atrial Enlargement, *Circulation,* 17:882, 1958.

27 Saunders, J. L., Calatayud, J. B., Schulz, K. J., et al.: Evaluation of ECG Criteria for P-Wave Abnormalities, *Am. Heart J.,* 74:757, 1967.

28 Termini, B. A., and Lee, Y.: Echocardiographic and Electrocardiographic Criteria for Diagnosing Left Atrial Enlargement, *South. Med. J.,* 68:161, 1975.

29 Brown, O. R., Harrison, D. C., and Popp, R. L.: An Improved Method of Echographic Detection of Left Atrial Enlargement, *Circulation,* 50:58, 1974.

30 Waggoner, A. D., Adyanthaya, A. V., Quinones, M. A., et al.: Left Atrial Enlargement, *Circulation,* 54:553, 1976.

31 Romhilt, D. W., Bove, K. E., Conradi, S., et al.: Morphologic Significance of Left Atrial Involvement, *Am. Heart J.,* 83:322, 1972.

32 James, T. N.: P Waves, Atrial Depolarization, and Pacemaking Site, in R. C. Schlant and J. W. Hurst (eds.), "Advances in Electrocardiography," Vol. 1, Grune & Stratton, Inc. New York, 1972. Chap. 5.

33 Josephson, M. E., Kastor, J. A., and Morganroth, J.: Electrocardiographic Left Atrial Enlargement, *Am. J. Cardiol.,* 39:967, 1977.

34 Chou, T., and Helm, R. A.: The Pseudo P Pulmonale, *Circulation,* 32:96, 1965.

35 Surawicz, B., Uhley, H., Borun, R., et al.: Task Force 1: Standardization of Terminology and Interpretation, *Am. J. Cardiol.,* 41:130, 1978.

36 Rios, J. C., Schatz, J., and Meshel, J. C.: P Wave Analysis in Coronary Artery Disease: An Electrocardiographic-Angiographic and Hemodynamic Correlation, *Chest,* 66:146, 1974.

37 Tarazi, R. C., Miller, A., Frohlich, E. D., et al.: Electrocardiographic Changes Reflecting Left Atrial Abnormality in Hypertension, *Circulation,* 34:818, 1966.

38 Brohet, C. R., Liedtke, C. E., and Tuna, N.: P Wave Abnormalities in the Orthogonal Electrocardiogram, Correlation with Ventricular Overload in Pulmonic and Aortic Valvular Heart Disease, *J. Electrocardiol.,* 8:103, 1975.

39 Abraham, A. S.: P-Wave Analysis in Myocardial Infarction, Pulmonary Edema, and Embolism, *Am. Heart J.,* 89:30, 1975.

40 Romhilt, D. W., and Scott, R. C.: Left Atrial Involvement in Acute Pulmonary Edema, *Am. Heart J.,* 83:328, 1972.

41 Heikkila, J., Hugenholtz, P. G., and Tabakin, B. S.: Prediction of Left Heart Filling Pressure and Its Sequential Change in Acute Myocardial Infarction from the Terminal Force of the P Wave, *Br. Heart J.,* 35:142, 1973.

42 Romhilt, D. W., Bove, K. E., and Norris, R. J.: A Critical Appraisal of the Electrocardiographic Criteria for the Diagnosis of Left Ventricular Hypertrophy, *Circulation,* 40:185, 1969.

43 Romhilt, D. W., and Estes, H. E.: A Point-Score System for the ECG Diagnosis of Left Ventricular Hypertrophy, *Am. Heart J.*, 75:752, 1968.

44 Scott, R. C., Seiwert, V. J., Simon, D. L., et al.: Left Ventricular Hypertrophy, *Circulation*, 11:89, 1955.

45 Chou, T., Scott, R. C., Booth, R. W., et al.: Specificity of the Current Electrocardiographic Criteria in the Diagnosis of Left Ventricular Hypertrophy, *Am. Heart J.*, 60:371, 1960.

46 Carter, W. A., and Estes, E. H.: Electrocardiographic Manifestations of Ventricular Hypertrophy; a Computer Study of ECG-Anatomic Correlations in 319 cases, *Am. Heart J.*, 68:173, 1964.

47 Dower, G. E., Horn, H. E., and Ziegler, W. G.: On Electrocardiographic-Autopsy Correlations in Left Ventricular Hypertrophy. A Simple Postmortem Index of Hypertrophy Proposed, *Am. Heart J.*, 74:351, 1967.

48 Abbasi, A. S., MacAlpin, R. N., Eber, L. M., et al.: Left Ventricular Hypertrophy Diagnosed by Echocardiography, *N. Engl. J. Med.*, 289:118, 1973.

49 Bennett, H., and Evans, D. W.: Correlation of Left Ventricular Mass Determined by Echocardiography with Vectorcardiographic and Electrocardiographic Voltage Measurements, *Br. Heart J.*, 36:981, 1974.

50 Morganroth, J., Maron, B. J., Krovetz, L. J., et al.: Electrocardiographic Evidence of Left Ventricular Hypertrophy in Otherwise Normal Children, *Am. J. Cardiol.*, 35:278, 1975.

51 Bahler, A. S., Teichholz, L. E., Gorlin, R., et al.: Correlations of Electrocardiography and Echocardiography in Determination of Left Ventricular Wall Thickness: Study of Apparently Normal Subjects, *Am. J. Cardiol.*, 39:189, 1977.

52 Browne, P. J., Dresser, K. B., Benchimol, A., et al.: The Echocardiographic Correlates of Left Ventricular Hypertrophy Diagnosed by Electrocardiography, *J. Electrocardiol.*, 10:105, 1977.

53 Dunn, F. G., Chandraratna, P., deCarvalho, J. G., Basta, L. L., et al.: Pathophysiologic Assessment of Hypertensive Heart Disease with Echocardiography, *Am. J. Cardiol.*, 39:789, 1977.

54 Dolgin, M., Fisher, V. J., Shah, A., et al.: The Electrocardiographic Diagnosis of Left Ventricular Hypertrophy: Correlation with Quantitative Angiography, *Am. J. Med. Sci.*, 237:301, 1977.

55 McFarland, T. M., Alam, M., Goldstein, S., et al.: Echocardiographic Diagnosis of Left Ventricular Hypertrophy, *Circulation*, 57:1140, 1978.

56 Scott, R. C.: Ventricular Hypertrophy, *Cardiovasc. Clin.*, 5:220, 1973.

57 Mazzoleni, A., Wolff, R., Wolff, L., et al.: Correlation between Component Cardiac Weights and Electrocardiographic Patterns in 185 Cases, *Circulation*, 30:808, 1964.

58 Kilty, S. E., and Lepeschkin, E.: Effect of Body Build on the QRS Voltage of the Electrocardiogram in Normal Men, *Circulation*, 31:77, 1965.

59 Walker, C. H., and Rose, R. L.: Importance of Age, Sex and Body Habitus in the Diagnosis of Left Ventricular Hypertrophy from the Precordial Electrocardiogram in Childhood and Adolescence, *Pediatrics*, 28:705, 1961.

60 Ishikawa, K., Berson, A. S., and Pipberger, H. V.: Electrocardiographic Changes Due to Cardiac Enlargement, *Am. Heart J.*, 81:635, 1971.

61 Dunn, R. A., Zenner, R. J., and Pipberger, H. V.: Serial Electrocardiograms in Hypertensive Cardiovascular Disease, *Circulation*, 56:416, 1977.

62 Holt, J. H., Barnard, A. C., and Kramer, J. O.: A Study of the Human Heart as a Multiple Dipole Source, *Circulation*, 56:392, 1977.

63 Simonson, E., Tuna, N., Okamoto, N., et al.: Diagnostic Accuracy of the Vectorcardiogram and Electrocardiogram, *Am. J. Cardiol.*, 17:829, 1966.

64 Selzer, A.: Limitations of the Electrocardiographic Diagnosis of Ventricular Hypertrophy, *J.A.M.A.*, 195:175, 1966.

65 Walker, I. C., Helm, R. A., and Scott, R. C.: Right Ventricular Hypertrophy, *Circulation*, 11:215, 1955.

66 Walker, I. C., Scott, R. C., and Helm, R. A.: Right Ventricular Hypertrophy, *Circulation*, 11:223, 1955.

67 Scott, R. C.: The Electrocardiographic Diagnosis of Right Ventricular Hypertrophy: Correlation with the Anatomic Findings, *Am. Heart J.*, 60:659, 1960.

68 Scott, R. C.: The Correlation between the Electrocardiographic Patterns of Ventricular Hypertrophy and the Anatomic Findings, *Circulation*, 21:256, 1960.

69 Roman, G. T., Walsh, T. J., and Massie, E.: Right Ventricular Hypertrophy, *Am. J. Cardiol.*, 7:481, 1961.

70 Ray, C. T., Horan, L. G., and Flowers, N. C.: An Early Sign of Right Ventricular Enlargement, *J. Electrocardiol.*, 3:57, 1970.

71 Goodwin, J. F., and Abdin, Z. H.: The Cardiogram of Congenital and Acquired Right Ventricular Hypertrophy, *Br. Heart J.*, 21:523, 1959.

72 Booth, R. W., Chou, T., and Scott, R. C.: Electrocardiographic Diagnosis of Ventricular Hypertrophy in the Presence of Right Bundle-Branch Block, *Circulation*, 18:169, 1958.

73 Littmann, D.: The Electrocardiographic Findings in Pulmonary Emphysema, *Am. J. Cardiol.*, 5:339, 1960.

74 Scott, C. R.: The Electrocardiogram in Pulmonary Emphysema and Chronic Cor Pulmonale, *Am. Heart J.*, 61:843, 1961.

75 Phillips, J. H., and Burch, G. E.: Problems in the Diagnosis of Cor Pulmonale, *Am. Heart J.*, 66:818, 1963.

76 Fowler, N. O., Daniels, C., Scott, R. C., et al.: The Electrocardiogram in Cor Pulmonale with and without Emphysema, *Am. J. Cardiol.,* 16:500, 1965.

77 Oram, S., and Davies, P.: The Electrocardiogram in Cor Pulmonale, *Prog. Cardiovasc. Dis.,* 9:341, 1967.

78 Kamper, D., Chou, T., Fowler, N. O., et al.: The Reliability of Electrocardiographic Criteria of Chronic Obstructive Lung Disease, *Am. Heart J.,* 80:445, 1970.

79 Ferrer, M. I.: Clinical and Electrocardiographic Correlations in Pulmonary Heart Disease (Cor Pulmonale), in J. C. Rios (ed.): "Clinical-Electrocardiographic Correlations, Cardiovascular Clinics," F. A. Davis Company, Philadelphia, 1977, p. 215.

80 Scott, R. C., Kaplan, S., Fowler, N. O., et al.: The Electrocardiographic Pattern of Right Ventricular Hypertrophy in Chronic Cor Pulmonale, *Circulation,* 11:927, 1955.

81 Spodick, D. H.: Electrocardiographic Responses to Pulmonary Embolism, *Am. J. Cardiol.,* 30:659, 1972.

82 McIntyre, K. M., Sasahara, A. A., and Littmann, D.: Relation of the Electrocardiogram to Hemodynamic Alterations in Pulmonary Embolism, *Am. J. Cardiol.,* 30:205, 1972.

83 Stein, P. D., Dalen, J. E., McIntyre, K. M., et al.: The Electrocardiogram in Acute Pulmonary Embolism, *Prog. Cardiovasc. Dis.,* 17:247, 1975.

84 The Urokinase-Pulmonary Embolism Trial, *Circulation,* 47 (suppl.): 2, 1973.

85 Smith, M., and Ray, C. T.: Electrocardiographic Signs of Early Right Ventricular Enlargement in Acute Pulmonary Embolism, *Chest,* 58:205, 1970.

86 Helfant, R. H.: Q Waves in Coronary Heart Disease: Newer Understanding of Their Clinical Implications, *Am. J. Cardiol.,* 38:662, 1976.

87 Conde, C. A., Meller, J., Espinoza, J., et al.: Disappearance of Abnormal Q Waves after Aortocoronary Bypass Surgery, *Am. J. Cardiol.,* 36:889, 1975.

88 Sternberg, L., Wisneski, J. A., Ullyot, D. J., et al.: Significance of New Q Waves after Aortocoronary Bypass Surgery, *Circulation,* 52:1037, 1975.

89 Savage, R. M., Wagner, G. S., Ideker, R. E., et al.: Correlation of Postmortem Anatomic Findings with Electrocardiographic Changes in Patients with Myocardial Infarction, *Circulation,* 55:279, 1977.

90 Boineau, J. P., Blumenschein, S. D., Spach, M. S., et al.: Relationship between Ventricular Depolarization and Electrocardiogram in Myocardial Infarction, *J. Electrocardiol.,* 1:233, 1968.

91 Durrer, D., Van Lier, A. W., and Buller, J.: Epicardial and Intramural Excitation in Chronic Myocardial Infarction, *Am. Heart J.,* 68:765, 1964.

92 Bodenheimer, M. M., Banka, V. S., Trout, R. G., et al.: Correlation of Pathologic Q Waves on the Standard Electrocardiogram and the Epicardial Electrogram of the Human Heart, *Circulation,* 54:213, 1976.

93 Hilsenrath, J., Hamby, R. I., and Hoffman, I.: Pitfalls in the Prediction of Coronary Artery Disease from the Electrocardiogram or Vectorcardiogram, *J. Electrocardiol.,* 6:291, 1973.

94 Shettigar, U. R., Hultgren, H. N., Pfeifer, J. F., et al.: Diagnostic Value of Q-Waves in Inferior Myocardial Infarction, *Am. Heart J.,* 88:170, 1974.

95 Mimbs, J. W., deMello, V., and Roberts, R.: The Effect of Respiration on Normal and Abnormal Q Waves, *Am. Heart J.,* 94:579, 1977.

96 Benchimol, A., and Desser, K. B.: The Electrovectorcardiographic Diagnosis of Posterior Wall Myocardial Infarction, *Cardiovasc. Clin.,* 5:184.

97 Perloff, J. K.: The Recognition of Strictly Posterior Myocardial Infarction by Conventional Scalar Electrocardiography, *Circulation,* 30:706, 1964.

98 Levine, H. D., Young, E., and Williams, R. A.: Electrocardiogram and Vectorcardiogram in Myocardial Infarction, *Circulation,* 45:457, 1972.

99 Martinez-Rios, M. A., Bruto Da Costa, B. C., Cencena-Seldner, F. A., et al.: Normal Electrocardiogram in the Presence of Severe Coronary Artery Disease, *Am. J. Cardiol.,* 25:320, 1970.

100 Redy, K., Hamby, R. I., Hilsenrath, J., et al.: Severity and Distribution of Coronary Artery Disease in Patients with Normal Resting Electrocardiograms, *J. Electrocardiol.,* 7:115, 1974.

101 Hilsenrath, J., Hamby, R. I., Glassman, E., et al.: Pitfalls in Prediction of Coronary Arterial Obstruction from Patterns of Anterior Infarction on Electrocardiogram and Vectorcardiogram, *Am. J. Cardiol.,* 29:164, 1972.

102 Horan, L. G., Flowers, N. C., and Johnson, J. C.: Significance of the Diagnostic Q Wave of Myocardial Infarction, *Circulation,* 43:428, 1971.

103 Chou, T.: Pseudo-infarction (Noninfarction Q Waves), *Cardiovasc. Clin.,* 5:200, 1973.

104 Williams, R. A., Cohn, P. F., Vokonas, P. S., et al.: Electrocardiographic, Arteriographic and Ventriculographic Correlations in Transmural Myocardial Infarction, *Am. J. Cardiol.,* 31:595, 1973.

105 Bodenheimer, M. M., Banka, V. S., and Helfant, R. H.: Q Waves and Ventricular Asynergy: Predictive Value and Hemodynamic Significance of Anatomic Localization, *Am. J. Cardiol.,* 35:615, 1975.

106 Madias, J. E., and Gorlin, R.: The Myth of Acute "Mild" Myocardial Infarction, *Ann. Intern. Med.,* 86:347, 1977.

107 Toutouzas, P., Avgoustakis, D., Koroxenides, G., et al.: The Electrocardiogram and Vectorcardiogram in the Diagnosis of the Old Inferior Myocardial Infarction, *J. Electrocardiol.,* 6:319, 1973.

108 Burns-Cox, C. J.: The Occurrence of a Normal Electrocardiogram after Myocardial Infarction, *Am. Heart J.,* 75:572, 1968.

109 Willems, J., Draulans, J., and DeGeest, H.: An Appraisal of the Minnesota Code in "Inferior" Myocardial Infarction, *J. Electrocardiol.,* 3:147, 1970.

110 Skjaeggestad, O., and Molne, K.: Electrocardiogram on Patients with Healed Myocardial Infarction Disclosed at Autopsy, *Acta. Med. Scand.,* 179:23, 1966.

111 Woods, J. D., Lawne, W., and Smith, W. G.: The Reliability of the Electrocardiogram in Myocardial Infarction, *Lancet,* 2:205, 1963.

112 Canner, P. L., Berge, K. G., and Klimt, C. R.: The Coronary Drug Project, *Circulation,* 67:1, 1973.

113 Merrill, S. L., and Pearce, M. L.: An Autopsy Study of the Accuracy of the Electrocardiogram in the Diagnosis of Recurrent Myocardial Infarction, *Am. Heart J.,* 81:48, 1971.

114 Rahim, A., Parameswaran, R., and Goldberg, H.: Electrocardiographic Changes During Chest Pain in Unstable Angina, *Br. Heart J.,* 39:1340, 1977.

115 Mills, R. M., Young, E., Gorlin, R., et al.: Natural History of S-T Segment Elevation after Acute Myocardial Infarction, *Am. J. Cardiol.,* 35:609, 1975.

116 Blackburn, H.: The Prognostic Importance of the Electrocardiogram after Myocardial Infarction, *Ann. Intern. Med.,* 77:677, 1972.

117 Ostrander, L. D.: The Relation of "Silent" T Wave Inversion to Cardiovascular Disease in an Epidemiologic Study, *Am. J. Cardiol.,* 25:325, 1970.

118 Exercise Tests before Exercise, *Med. Lett.,* 20:12, 1978.

119 Sheffield, C. T., Reeves, T. J., Blackburn, H., et al.: The Exercise Test in Perspective, *Circulation,* 55:681, 1977.

120 Koppes, G., McKiernan, T., Bassan, M., et al.: Treadmill Exercise Testing, Part II, in W. P. Harvey et al. (eds.), *Curr. Probl. Cardiol.,* 7(8): 1977.

121 Fortuin, N. J., and Weiss, J. L.: Exercise Stress Testing, *Circulation,* 56:699, 1977.

122 Ellestad, M. H.: "Stress Testing: Principles and Practice," F. A. Davis Company, Philadelphia, 1975.

123 Amsterdam, E. A., Wilmore, J. H., and DeMaria, A. N. (eds.): "Symposium on Exercise in Cardiovascular Health and Disease," Yorke Medical Books, 1977.

124 Sheffield, L. T., Maloof, J. A., Sawyer, J. A., et al.: Maximal Heart Rate and Treadmill Performance of Healthy Women in Relation to Age, *Circulation,* 57:79, 1978.

125 AHA Committee on Exercise: "Exercise Testing and Training of Apparently Healthy Individuals," American Heart Association, New York, 1972.

126 Chaitman, B. R., Bourassa, M. G., Wagniart, P., et al.: Improved Efficiency of Treadmill Exercise Testing Using a Multiple Lead ECG System and Basic Hemodynamic Exercise Response, *Circulation,* 57:71, 1978.

126a Simonson, E., and Keys, H.: The Effect of an Ordinary Meal or the Electrocardiogram, *Circulation,* 1:1000, 1950.

127 Tonkon, M. J., Miller, R. R., DeMaria, A. N., et al.: Multifactor Evaluation of the Determinants of Ischemic Electrocardiographic Response to Maximal Treadmill Testing in Coronary Disease, *Am. J. Med.,* 62:339, 1977.

128 Simoons, M. L., VanDenBrand, M., and Hugenholtz, P. G.: Quantitative Analysis of Exercise Electrocardiograms and Left Ventricular Angiocardiograms in Patients with Abnormal QRS Complexes at Rest, *Circulation,* 55:55, 1977.

129 Stuart, R. J.: Significance of ST Depression Patterns in Treadmill Stress Testing, *J. Cardiovasc. Pulmonary Technol.,* 2:14, 1978.

130 Martin, C. M., and McConahay, D. R.: Maximal Treadmill Exercise Electrocardiography, *Circulation,* 46:956, 1972.

131 Kurita, A., Chaitman, R. B., and Bourassa, M. G.: Significance of Exercise-induced Junctional ST Depression in Evaluation of Coronary Artery Disease, *Am. J. Cardiol.,* 40:492, 1977.

132 Stuart, R. J., and Ellestad, M. H.: Upsloping ST Segments in Exercise Stress Testing: Six-Year Follow-up Study of 438 Patients and Correlation with 248 Angiograms, *Am. J. Cardiol.,* 37:19, 1976.

133 Fortuin, N. J., and Friesinger, G. C.: Exercise-Induced ST Segment Elevation, *Am. J. Med.,* 49:459, 1970.

134 Chahine, R. A., Raizner, A. E., and Ishimori, T.: The Clinical Significance of Exercise-induced ST-Segment Elevation, *Circulation,* 54:209, 1976.

135 Master, A. M., and Rosenfeld, I. L.: Two-Step Exercise Test, *Mod. Concepts Cardiovasc. Dis.,* 36(4):19, 1967.

136 Bonoris, P., Greenberg, P. S., Christison, G. W., et al.: Evaluation of R Wave Amplitude Changes versus ST-Segment Depression in Stress Testing, *Circulation,* 57:904, 1978.

137 McHenry, P. L., Phillips, J. F., and Knoebel, S. B.: Correlation of Computer-quantitated Treadmill Exercise Electrocardiogram with Arteriographic Location of Coronary Artery Disease, *Am. J. Cardiol.,* 30:747, 1972.

138 Patterson, J. A., Naughton, J., Pietras, R. J., et al.: Treadmill Exercise in Assessment of the Functional Capacity of Patients with Cardiac Disease, *Am. J. Cardiol.,* 30:757, 1972.

139 Bruce, R. A.: Exercise Testing of Patients with Coronary Heart Disease, *Ann. Clin. Res.,* 3:323, 1971.

140 Shaeffer, C. W., Jr., Daly, R. G., and Smith, S. C.: Maximal Treadmill Exercise Testing in the Management of the Postmyocardial Infarction Patient, *Chest,* 68:20, 1975.

141 Markiewicz, W., Houston, N., and DeBusk, R. F.: Exercise Testing Soon after Myocardial Infarction, *Circulation,* 56:26, 1977.

142 Granath, A., Sodermark, T., Winge, T., et al.: Early Workload Tests for Evaluation of Long-term Prognosis of Acute Myocardial Infarction, *Br. Heart J.,* 39:758, 1977.

143 Haskell, W. L.: Physical Activity after Myocardial Infarction, *Am. J. Cardiol.,* 33:776, 1974.

144 Borner, J. S., Rrensike, J. F., Redwood, D. R., et al.: Limitations of the Electrocardiographic Response to Exercise in Predicting Coronary Artery-Disease, *N. Engl. J. Med.,* 293:367, 1975.

145 Froelicher, V. F., Thompson, A. J., Longo, M. R., Jr., et al.: Value of Exercise Testing for Screening Asymptomatic Men for Latent Coronary Artery Disease, *Prog. Cardiovasc. Dis.,* 18:265, 1976.

146 Erikssen, J., Enge, I., Forfang, K., et al.: False Positive Diagnostic Tests and Coronary Angiographic Findings in 105 Presumably Healthy Males, *Circulation,* 54:371, 1976.

147 Cumming, G. R., Dufresne, C., and Kich, L., et al.: Exercise Electrocardiogram Patterns in Normal Women, *Br. Heart J.,* 35:1055, 1973.

148 Kusumi, F., Bruce, R. A., Ross, M. A., et al.: Elevated Arterial Pressure and Post-exertional ST-Segment Depression in Middle-aged Women, *Am. Heart J.,* 92:576, 1976.

149 Linhart, J. W., Laws, J. G., and Satinsky, J. D.: Maximum Treadmill Exercise Electrocardiography in Female Patients, *Circulation,* 50:1173, 1974.

150 Linhart, J. W., and Turnoff, H. B.: Maximum Treadmill Exercise Test in Patients with Abnormal Control Electrocardiograms, *Circulation,* 49:667, 1974.

151 Kansal, S., Roitman, D., and Sheffield, L. T.: Stress Testing with ST-Segment Depression at Rest: An Angiographic Correlation, *Circulation,* 54:636, 1976.

152 McNeer, J. F., Margolis, J. R., Lee, K. L., et al.: The Role of the Exercise Test in the Evaluation of Patients for Ischemic Heart Disease, *Circulation,* 57:64, 1978.

153 Goldschlager, N., Selzer, A., and Cohn, K.: Treadmill Stress Tests as Indicators of Presence and Severity of Coronary Artery Disease, *Ann. Intern. Med.,* 85:277, 1976.

154 Thomson, P. D., and Kelemen, M. H.: Hypotension Accompanying the Onset of Exertional Angina, *Circulation,* 52:28, 1975.

155 Goldman, S., Tselos, S., and Cohn, K.: Marked Depth of ST-Segment Depression during Treadmill Exercise Testing: Indicator of Severe Coronary Artery Disease, *Chest,* 69:729, 1976.

156 Kennedy, H. L., and Underhill, S. J.: Frequent to Complex Ventricular Ectopy in Apparently Healthy Subjects, *Am. J. Cardiol.,* 38:141, 1976.

157 McHenry, P. L., Morris, S. N., and Kavalier, M.: Clinical Significance of Treadmill Exercise-induced Ventricular Arrhythmias, *Am. J. Cardiol.,* 33:154, 1974. (Abstract.)

158 Caskey, T. D., and Estes, E. H.: Deviation of the S-T Segment, *Am. J. Med.,* 36:424, 1964.

159 Kini, P. M., Willems, J. L., Batchlor, D., et al.: ST-T Changes Induced by Digitalis and Ventricular Hypertrophy: Differentiation by Quantitative Analysis, *J. Electrocardiol.,* 5:101, 1972.

160 Surawicz, B.: The Pathogenesis and Clinical Significance of Primary T-Wave Abnormalities, in R. C. Schlant and J. W. Hurst (eds.), "Advances in Electrocardiography," Vol. 1, Grune & Stratton, Inc., New York, 1972.

161 Pinto, I. J., Nanda, N. C., Poiswas, A. K., et al.: Tall Upright T Waves in the Precordial Leads, *Circulation,* 36:708, 1967.

162 Reynolds, E. W., and Vander Ark, C. R.: Quinidine Syncope in the Delayed Repolarization Syndromes, *Mod. Concepts Cardiovasc. Dis.,* 45:117, 1976.

163 Ferrer, M. I.: "Pre-excitation," Futura Publishing Company, Mount Kisco, N.Y., 1976.

164 Chung, E. K.: Wolff-Parkinson-White Syndrome: Current Views, *Am. J. Med.,* 62:252, 1977.

165 Narula, O. S.: Wolff-Parkinson-White Syndrome: A Review, *Circulation,* 47:872, 1973.

166 Gallagher, J. J., Gilbert, M., Svenson, R. H., et al.: Wolff-Parkinson-White Syndrome: The Problem, Evaluation and Surgical Correlation, *Circulation,* 51:767, 1975.

167 Boineau, J. P., Moore, E. N., Spear, J. F., et al.: Basis of Static and Dynamic Electrocardiographic Variations in Wolff-Parkinson-White Syndrome, *Am. J. Cardiol.,* 32:32, 1973.

168 Wellens, H. J., and Durrer, D.: Patterns of Ventriculoatrial Conduction in the Wolff-Parkinson-White Syndrome, *Circulation,* 49:22, 1974.

169 Wellens, H. J., and Durrer, D.: Wolff-Parkinson-White Syndrome and Atrial Fibrillation, *Am. J. Cardiol.,* 34:777, 1974.

170 Becker, A. E., Wellens, H. J., and Durrer, D.: Pathologic Electrocardiographic Correlations in Wolff-Parkinson-White Syndrome, *Circulation,* 48(suppl. 4):142, 1973.

171 Goel, B. G., and Han, J.: Manifestation of the Wolff-Parkinson-White Syndrome after Myocardial Infarction, *Am. Heart J.,* 87:633, 1974.

172 Sung, R. J., Gelband, H., Castellanos, A., et al.: Clinical and Electrophysiologic Observations in Patients with Concealed Accessory Atrioventricular Bypass Tracts, *Am. J. Cardiol.,* 40:839, 1977.

173 Fowler, N. O.: The Electrocardiogram in Pericarditis, *Cardiovasc. Clin.,* 5:256, 1974.

174 Surawicz, B., and Lasseter, K. C.: Electrocardiogram in Pericarditis, *Am. J. Cardiol.,* 26:471, 1970.

175 Spodick, D. H.: Electrocardiogram in Acute Pericarditis, *Am. J. Cardiol.,* 33:470, 1974.

176 Spodick, D. H.: Pathogenesis and Clinical Correlations of the Electrocardiographic Abnormalities of Pericardial Disease, in J. C. Rios (ed.), "Clinical Electrocardiographic Correlations," F. A. Davis Company, Philadelphia, 1977.

177 Spodick, D. H.: Diagnostic Electrocardiographic Sequences in Acute Pericarditis, *Circulation,* 48:575, 1973.

178 McGregor, M., Ch, B., and Baskind, E.: Electric Alternans in Pericardial Effusion, *Circulation,* 11:837, 1955.

179 Kazemias, T. M., and Wasserburger, R. H.: Pericarditis Revisited, *J. Electrocardiol.,* 4:62, 1971.

180 Spodick, D. H.: Differential Characteristics of the Electrocardiogram in Early Repolarization and Acute Pericarditis, *N. Engl. J. Med.,* 295:523, 1976.

181 Parisi, A. F., Beckmann, C. H., and Lancaster, M. C.: The Spectrum of ST Segment Elevation in the Electrocardiograms of Healthy Adult Men, *J. Electrocardiol.,* 4:137, 1971.

182 Morris, J. J., Estes, E. H., Whalen, R. E., et al.: P Wave Analysis in Valvular Heart Disease, *Circulation,* 29:242, 1964.

183 Kasser, I., and Kennedy, J. W.: The Relationship of Increased Left Atrial Volume and Pressure to Abnormal P Waves on the Electrocardiogram, *Circulation,* 39:339, 1969.

184 Rios, J. C., and Goo, W.: Electrocardiographic Correlates of Rheumatic Valvular Disease, *Cardiovasc. Clin.,* 5(2):247, 1973.

185 Rios, J. C., and Leet, C.: Electrocardiographic Assessment of Valvular Heart Disease, *Cardiovasc. Clin.,* 8:161, 1977.

186 Bentrvogleo, L. G., Urricchio, J. F., Waldou, A., et al.: An Electrocardiographic Analysis of Sixty-five Cases of Mitral Regurgitation, *Circulation,* 38:572,

187 Bailey, G. W. H., Brau, A. B. A., Hancock, W. E., et al.: Relationship of Left Atrial Pathology to Atrial Fibrillation in Mitral Valvular Disease, *Ann. Intern. Med.,* 69:13, 1968.

188 Rolue, J. C., Bland, F. F., Sprague, H. B., et al.: The Course of Mitral Stenosis without Surgery: Ten and Twenty Years Perspective, *Ann. Intern. Med.,* 52:741, 1960.

189 Skoulos, A., and Horlick, L.: The Atrial F Wave in Various Types of Heart Disease and Its Response to Treatment, *Am. J. Cardiol.,* 14:174, 1964.

190 Calatagud, J. B., Saunders, J. L., Schultz, A. J., et al.: P Wave Changes after Open Heart Mitral Commissuratory for Isolated Mitral Stenosis, *Angiology,* 19:1238, 1968.

191 Gooch, A. S., Calatagud, J. B., Rogers, P. A., et al.: Analysis of the P Wave in Severe Aortic Stenosis, *Chest,* 49:459, 1966.

192 Morris, J. J., Dunlop, W. H., Thompson, H. K., et al.: P Wave Analysis in the Electrocardiographic Diagnosis of Left Ventricular Hypertrophy, *Circulation,* 32(suppl. 11):154, 1965.

193 Wood, P.: Aortic Stenosis, *Am. J. Cardiol.,* 1:553, 1958.

194 Wagner, H. R., Weidman, W. H., Ellison, R. C., et al.: Indirect Assessment of Severity in Aortic Stenosis, *Circulation,* 56(2)(suppl. 1):20, 1977.

195 Shah, P. M.: Clinical-Electrocardiographic Correlations: Aortic Valve Disease and Hypertrophic Subaortic Stenosis, *Cardiovasc. Clin.,* 8:151, 1977.

196 Schwartz, L. S., Goldfischer, J., Sprague, G. J., et al.: Syncope and Sudden Death in Aortic Stenosis, *Am. J. Cardiol.,* 23:647, 1969.

197 Jeresaty, R. M.: Mitral Valve Prolapse-Click Murmur Syndrome, *Prog. Cardiovasc. Dis.,* 15:623, 1973.

198 Malcolm, A. D., Boughner, D. R., Kostuk, W. J., et al.: Clinical Features and Investigative Findings in Presence of Mitral Leaflet Prolapse, *Br. Heart J.,* 38:244, 1976.

199 Pocock, W. A., and Barlow, J. B.: Postexercise Arrhythmias in the Billowing Posterior Mitral Leaflet Syndrome, *Am. Heart J.,* 80:740, 1970.

200 Wei, J. Y., Bulkley, B. H., Schaeffer, A. H., et al.: Mitral Valve Prolapse Syndrome and Recurrent Ventricular Tachyarrhythmias, *Ann. Intern. Med.,* 89:6, 1978.

201 Harrison, D. C., Isaeff, D. M., and DeBusk, R. F.: Papillary Muscle Syndrome, *D.M.* No. 1, 1972.

202 Burch, G. E., DePasquale, N. P., and Phillips, J. H.: The Syndrome of Papillary Muscle Dysfunction, *Am. Heart J.,* 75:399, 1968.

203 Bashaur, F. A.: Mitral Regurgitation Following Myocardial Infarction, *Chest,* 48:113, 1965.

204 Heikkila, J.: Mitral Incompetence as a Complication of Acute Myocardial Infarction, *Acta Med. Scand.,* (suppl. to V),182:475, 1967.

205 Cueto, J., Toshima, J., Armyo, G., et al.: Vectorcardiographic Studies in Acquired Valvular Disease with Reference to the Diagnosis of Right Ventricular Hypertrophy, *Circulation,* 33:588, 1967.

206 Hugenholtz, P. G., Ryan, T. J., Stein, S. W., et al.:

The Spectrum of Pure Mitral Stenosis-Hemodynamic Studies in Relation to Clinical Disability, *Am. J. Cardiol.*, 10:773, 1962.

207 Walston, A., Harley, A., and Pipberger, H.: Computer Analysis of the Ortho-Electrocardiogram and Vectorcardiogram in Mitral Stenosis, *Circulation*, 50:472, 1974.

208 Bahl, O. P., and Massie, E.: Electrocardiographic and Vectorcardiographic Patterns in Cardiomyopathy, *Cardiovasc. Clin.*, 4:95, 1972.

209 McMartin, D. E., and Flowers, N. C.: Clinical Electrocardiographic Correlations in Diseases of the Myocardium, *Cardiovasc. Clin.*, 8:191, 1977.

210 Hollister, R. M., and Goodiver, J. F.: The Electrocardiogram in Cardiomyopathy, *Br. Heart J.*, 25:357, 1963.

211 McDonald, C. D., Burch, G. E., and Walsh, J. J.: Alcoholic Cardiomyopathy Managed with Prolonged Bed Rest, *Ann. Intern. Med.*, 74:681, 1971.

212 Hamby, R. I., and Raia, F.: Electrocardiographic Aspects of Primary Myocardial Disease in 60 Patients, *Am. Heart J.*, 76:316, 1968.

213 Pinto Cima, F. X., Spiritus, O., and Tranchesi, J.: Arrhythmias and Vector Electrocardiographic Analysis of Complete Bundle Branch Block in Chagas' Disease, *Am. Heart J.*, 56:501, 1958.

214 Rosenbaum, M. R.: Myocardiopathy, *Prog. Cardiovasc. Dis.*, 7:142, 1964.

215 Corne, R. A., Parkin, T. W., Brandenburg, R. O., et al.: Significance of Marked Left Axis Deviation, *Am. J. Cardiol.*, 15:605, 1965.

216 Brigden, W.: Cardiac Amyloidosis, *Prog. Cardiovasc. Dis.*, 7:142, 1964.

217 Burch, G., and DePasquale, N.: A Study at Autopsy of the Relation of Absence of the Q Wave in Lead I, aV_L, V_5 and V_6 to Septal Fibrosis, *Am. Heart J.*, 60:336, 1960.

218 Massumi, R. A., Rios, J. G., Gooch, A. S., et al.: Primary Myocardial Disease, *Circulation*, 31:19, 1965.

219 Marriott, H. J. L.: Electrocardiographic Abnormalities, Conduction Defects and Arrhythmias in Primary Myocardial Disease, *Prog. Cardiovasc. Dis.*, 7:99, 1964.

220 Bashour, T. T., Fahdul, H., and Cheng, T. O.: Electrocardiographic Abnormalities in Alcoholic Cardiomyopathy, *Chest*, 68:24, 1975.

221 Priest, R., Binn, J., and Kitchin, A.: Electrocardiogram in Alcoholism and Accompanying Physical Disease, *Br. Med. J.*, 1:1453, 1966.

222 Evans, W.: The Electrocardiogram of Alcoholic Cardiomyopathy, *Br. Heart J.*, 21:445, 1959.

223 Savage, D. D., Seides, S. F., Clark, C. E., et al.: Electrocardiographic Findings in Patients with Obstructive and Nonobstructive Hypertrophic Cardiomyopathy, *Circulation*, 58:402, 1978.

224 Frank, S., and Braunwald, E.: Idiopathic Hypertrophic Subaortic Stenosis. Clinical Analysis of 126 Patients with Emphasis on the Natural History, *Circulation*, 37:759, 1968.

225 Estes, E. H., Wholer, R. E., Roberts, S. R. et al.: Electrocardiographic and Vectorcardiographic Findings in Idiopathic Hypertrophic Subaortic Stenosis, *Circulation*, 26:714, 1962.

226 Goodwin, J. F., Hollman, A., Cleland, W. P., et al.: Obstructive Cardiomyopathy Simulating Aortic Stenosis, *Br. Heart J.*, 22:403, 1960.

227 Maron, B. J., Henry, W. L., Clark, C. E., et al.: Asymmetric Septal Hypertrophy in Childhood, *Circulation*, 53:9, 1976.

228 Whiting, R. B., Powell, W. J., Dinsmore, R. E., et al.: Idiopathic Hypertrophic Subaortic Stenosis in the Elderly, *N. Engl. J. Med.*, 285:196, 1971.

228a Perloff, J. K.: Cardiomyopathy Associated with Heredofamilial Neuromyopathic Disease, *Mod. Concepts Cardiovasc. Dis.*, 40:5, 1971.

228b Perloff, J. K.: Cardiac Involvement in Heredofamilial Neuromyopathic Disease, *Cardiovasc. Clin.*, 4:334, 1974.

229 Wenger, N. K.: Infectious Myocarditis, *Cardiovasc. Clin.*, 4:107, 1972.

230 Weinstein, L.: Cardiovascular Manifestations in Some of the Common Infectious Diseases, *Mod. Concepts Cardiovasc. Dis.*, 23:229, 1954.

231 Stapleton, J. F., Segal, J. P., and Harvey, W. P.: The Electrocardiogram of Myocardiopathy, *Prog. Cardiovasc. Dis.*, 13:217, 1970.

232 Gardiner, A. J. S., and Short, D.: Four Faces of Acute Myopericarditis, *Br. Heart J.*, 35:433, 1973.

233 Campbell, M., and Reynolds, G.: Significance of the Direction of the P Wave in Dextrocardia and Isolated Levocardia, *Br. Heart J.*, 14:481, 1952.

234 Mirowski, M., Neill, C. A., and Taussig, H. B.: Left Atrial Ectopic Rhythm in Mirror Image Dextrocardia and in Normally Placed Malformed Hearts, *Circulation*, 27:864, 1963.

235 Perloff, J. K.: "The Clinical Recognition of Congenital Heart Disease," W. B. Saunders Company, Philadelphia, 1970.

236 Hancock, E. W.: Coronary Sinus Rhythm in Sinus Venous Defect and Persistent Left Superior Vena Cava, *Am. J. Cardiol.*, 14:608, 1964.

237 Munoz-Amos, S., Gorrin, J. R. D., Anselm, G., et al.: Single Atrium, *Am. J. Cardiol.*, 21:639, 1968.

238 Corvocho, A.: Transposition of the Great Vessels, *Am. J. Cardiol.*, 21:797, 1968.

239 Gooch, A. S., and Kini, P. M.: Electrocardiogram in Adults with Congenital Heart Disease, *Cardiovasc. Clin.*, 8:171, 1977.

240 Burchell, H. B., Dushane, J. W., and Brandenburg, R. O.: The Electrocardiogram of Patients with Atrioventricular Cushion Defects, *Am. J. Cardiol.*, 6:575, 1960.

241 Guller, B., Titus, J. L., and DuShane, J. W.: Electrocardiographic Diagnosis of Malformations Associated with Tricuspid Atresia: Correlation with Morphologic Features, *Am. Heart J.*, 78:180, 1969.

242 Moss, A. J., and Emmanouilides, G. C.: "Practical Pediatric Electrocardiography," J. B. Lippincott Company, Philadelphia, 1973.

243 Ulsar, I., Criley, J. M., and Lewis, K. B.: Anomalous Left Coronary Artery Arising from the Pulmonary Artery in an Adult, *Circulation,* 33:727, 1966.

244 Ellison, R. C., Freedom, R. M., Keane, J. F., et al.: Indirect Assessment of Severity of Pulmonary Stenosis, *Circulation,* 56(suppl. 1):14, 1977.

245 Weidman, W. H., Gersony, W. M., Nugent, E. W., et al.: Indirect Assessment of Severity in Ventricular Septal Defect, *Circulation,* 56(suppl. 1):24, 1977.

246 Burch, G. E., and DePasquale, N. P.: "Electrocardiography in the Diagnosis of Congenital Heart Disease," Lea & Febiger, Philadelphia, 1967.

247 MaChuy, R., Trouchesi, J., Ebard, M., et al.: Ebstein's Disease, *Am. J. Cardiol.,* 21:653, 1968.

248 Gault, J. H., Morrow, A. G., Gay, W. A., et al.: Atrial Septal Defect in Patients Over the Age of Forty Years, *Circulation,* 37:261, 1968.

249 Takahashi, M., Lindesmith, G. G., Lewis, A. B., et al.: Long-term Results of the Mustard Procedure, *Circulation,* 56(suppl. 55):85, 1977.

250 Gotsman, M. S., Beck, W., Bernard, C. N., et al.: Results of Repair of Tetralogy of Fallot, *Circulation,* 40:803, 1969.

Mark E. Silverman and Barry D. Silverman express their deep appreciation to Mrs. Patricia Kirby, Mrs. Sam Ray, and Mrs. Barbara Green for their expert secretarial assistance, and to Mrs. Cindy Timm and Ms. Janan Henry for their library skills in finding much of the reference material.

The Value and Limitations of Echocardiography[*]

JOEL M. FELNER, M.D.

Pulse-reflected ultrasound has found wide application in cardiology because it is safe and has considerable diagnostic value. Standard M-mode or single dimension echocardiography is now an established diagnostic tool in clinical cardiology. It is extremely useful in measuring distances and dimensions of cardiac chambers as well as patterns of motion of the walls and valves, but the tracing does not resemble the heart because there is no spatial orientation. With the development of two-dimensional real-time scanning systems, greater understanding of anatomic space relations and ease of diagnosis should be forthcoming.

Echocardiography is of great value in the evaluation of a wide variety of cardiac symptoms, signs, and laboratory abnormalities. Chest pain, a common cardiac symptom, frequently occurs secondary to coronary atherosclerosis. Although echocardiography is of limited value in establishing the diagnosis of angina pectoris resulting from coronary atherosclerotic heart disease in the absence of segmental abnormalities in wall motion, it is extremely important in identifying the noncoronary causes of chest pain, such as aortic stenosis, hypertrophic cardiomyopathy, mitral valve prolapse, and pericarditis in the presence of a pericardial effusion. The presence of a heart murmur may be suggestive of organic heart disease. Echocardiography is frequently valuable in the differential diagnosis of the systolic murmur resulting from atrial septal defect and hypertrophic cardiomyopathy and the diastolic murmurs of mitral stenosis, left atrial tumor, and Austin Flint; it is also useful in confirming the absence of organic heart disease in patients with functional murmurs.

Enlargement of the cardiac shadow on chest x-ray is a common cardiac abnormality. By virtue of its ability to distinguish pericardial effusion from intrinsic cardiac enlargement, to accurately identify the specific cardiac chamber enlarged, and to distinguish cavitary dilatation from wall hypertrophy, echocardiography can detect both the presence and the etiology of cardiac enlargement. Occasionally it can distinguish cardiac enlargement from an extracardiac mass.

The characteristics of the majority of cardiac conditions have been delineated by M-mode echocardiography. More information is needed, however, to establish sensitivity and specificity for even accepted diagnostic criteria. It is generally acknowledged that in some disease states echocardiography is very sensitive and specific. In adults who have mitral stenosis, left atrial myxoma, hypertrophic cardiomyopathy, or pericardial effusion, echocardiography can diagnose (rule in) or exclude (rule out) these conditions virtually every time. On the other hand, echocardiography is specific but not entirely sensitive for the diagnosis of mitral valve prolapse because if the pathognomonic abnormality is not visible, as it may not be in 10 to 20 percent of cases, prolapse cannot be excluded. In other applications, such as the diagnosis of valvular pulmonic stenosis, the detection of valvular vegetations, and the assessment of prosthetic valve function, the sensitivity of echocardiography is poor.

In this chapter, we will attempt to place in perspective the sensitivity and specificity of M-mode echocardiography, discuss the false positive and false negative results for the diagnosis of various cardiac abnormalities, and enumerate some of the limitations of this relatively new method for evaluation of the heart.

INSTRUMENTATION, TECHNIQUE, AND TRAINING

Echocardiography has its problems as well as its advantages. Ultrasound travels poorly through lung, ribs, sternum, and thick chest walls, and since the record reflects sound waves, the beam angle is extremely critical. Realizing these limitations, it is not surprising that the examination is difficult and that reliability and reproducibility cannot always be guaranteed.

The quality of the echocardiographic examination is more dependent on the expertise of the technician than on any other single factor. The echocardiographer must be thoroughly familiar with the ultrasonic cardiac anatomy and the various intracardiac landmarks because the recording methods require exceptional skill and the interpretation is deceptively complex. Most technical problems result from the examiner's lack of experience and inadequate under-

---

[*] From the Department of Medicine, Emory University School of Medicine, and Grady Memorial Hospital, Atlanta.

standing of the clinical considerations in the individual patients. Since certain clinical information is required in each case to provide a useful recording, professional interpretation of the echocardiogram should not be separated from the individual conducting the study. Interpretation should be based only on what can be definitely identified. Making judgments from incomplete echoes or in the absence of electrocardiographic reference should be avoided.

The most important consideration in performing an echocardiogram is in the choice of a transducer. It is very difficult to achieve recordings in the very obese or in individuals with large barrel-shaped chests. In these patients, where the heart is located at a greater distance from the chest wall, a lower frequency transducer with greater penetration but poorer resolution (e.g., a 1.6 MHz transducer) is better than the conventional 2.25 MHz transducer.

The standardization of transducer position is also a crucial consideration, especially when attempting to achieve comparability of echocardiograms. Because ultrasound travels poorly through bone and air, certain conditions, such as chronic obstructive lung disease, pectus excavatum, and recent chest surgery, can prohibit using the standard approach, which is through the third or fourth intercostal space adjacent to the sternum. Techniques for avoiding ribs and lung include placing the transducer in the subxyphoid area, in the suprasternal notch, or at the cardiac apex. Caution must be exercised in utilizing these different acoustic windows. For instance, in using the subxyphoid approach, it is imperative that the patient be supine rather than semirecumbent and that the transducer be placed a few centimeters below and to the right of the xyphoid process and pointed in the direction of the midclavicular line. In addition, the depth and controls must be readjusted to accommodate the increased distance between the transducer and the heart when this approach is used.

The use of echocardiographic controls must be understood in order to fully appreciate the diagnostic capabilities of the equipment. Appropriate use of the "near-gain" and "time-gain compensation" controls are necessary because sound waves lose their intensity (attenuate) as they travel deeper into the body tissue. If all echoes were dsplayed without selective modification of their intensity according to depth, those structures near the chest wall would be very intense relative to those from more distant structures of similar density. The greatest artifactual error introduced by incorrect use of these controls is the elimination of a portion of the echoes from the right side of the interventricular septum or even the entire septum itself.

A potential technical error is the poor lateral resolution (the ability to distinguish structures lying in close proximity to each other) that results from the finite beam width of current ultrasonic devices.[1] Ultrasonic energy cannot be accurately focused over the entire depth range of the beam and in fact spreads over a finite angle, causing some echoes to appear as if they

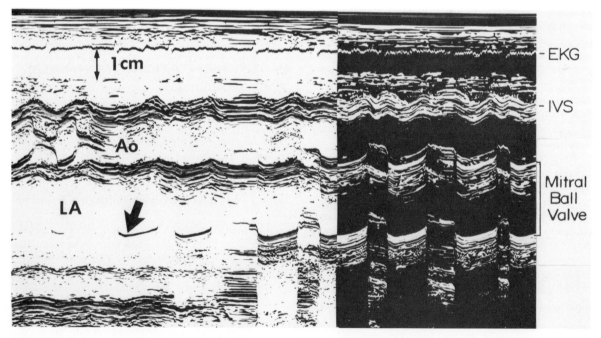

FIGURE 1 Echocardiographic sweep from the aorta to the Starr-Edwards mitral valve prosthesis. At left, the posterior ball echo is displayed in the left atrium (arrow), although the ball remains in its cage in the left ventricle. Ao, aorta; LA, left atrium; IVS, interventricular septum.

are from structures in the central beam, whereas in fact they are echoes from structures off the main or display axis. These ''spurious'' echoes are displayed at a sight where there is no directly corresponding anatomic structure and may result in misinterpretation of clinical tracings. For example, in Fig. 1, echoes of a Starr-Edwards prosthesis are shown at a sight where there is no corresponding structure. In addition, structures as much as 10 to 15 mm apart may be imaged on the axis of the beam and present confusion. Extraneous echoes from the papillary muscle or aorta may therefore be imaged simultaneously with the mitral valve and produce apparently abnormal systolic bulges in the motion pattern. Since this effect also depends on the sonic frequency and element size of the transducer, this problem can be reduced for structures at a given depth by the use of a focused transducer.

Potential problems in technique must be taken into account in every echocardiographic interpretation. Technical limitations of echocardiography include (1) drop-out phenomenon, i.e., the sudden loss of echoes from an anatomic structure in the ultrasound beam; (2) reverberations, i.e., false impressions of a second interface twice as far from the transducer as the first interface, since sound waves can be reflected more than once before returning to the transducer;[2] this delays the reflected wave and gives the appearance of a structure behind the heart; and (3) measuring distance—the greater the distance from the chest wall of a cardiac structure, the greater the error in measurement.[3]

The degree of interobserver variability, especially when making echocardiographic measurement in the 2- to 3-mm range, among experienced echocardiographers independently reading the same high-quality tracings is considerable.[4] If small changes in echocardiographic dimensions are assigned significance (e.g., left ventricular wall thickness), this potential error could be minimized and validity and objectivity ensured if each tracing is interpreted by at least two independent echocardiographers. In addition, if millimeter markers were placed on all recording paper and all measurements reported to the nearest whole number, this would reduce interpreter error. Computer analysis of echocardiographic data and the addition of cross-sectional echocardiographic studies should significantly improve the sensitivity of various echocardiographic techniques.

INTERPRETATION

Left Ventricle and Interventricular Septum

Much of the enthusiasm for echocardiography stems from the claim that it can be used to evaluate left ven-

tricular performance. Left ventricular size and function, however, are derived from measurement of only the minor axis of the chamber, since it is not possible to measure the long axis by M-mode echocardiography. One of the problems in using this single cavity dimension is that it has to be standardized so that it is comparable in all patients, since more than one dimension through the left ventricle can be obtained. For example, in a normal left ventricle which tapers toward the apex, a dimension taken near the left ventricular apex at the level of the papillary muscles would be smaller than one through the body of the left ventricle (Fig. 2). In order to make certain that the ultrasonic dimension was taken through the body of the left ventricle, it was determined that parts of both mitral valve leaflets or chordae tendineae should be present in the echocardiographic tracing.[5]

The left ventricular dimension by echo is influenced by the interspace in which the transducer is placed. A good quality M-mode scan is possible from various transducer positions on the chest wall. Therefore, if one desires reproducibility, the relationship of the transducer to the heart must be the same in each patient. This requires that the ultrasonic beam be essentially perpendicular to the mitral valve echogram and that the septum and the anterior wall of the aorta be equidistant from the transducer.[6] If the transducer is too high, then the aortic wall will be closer to the transducer than the septum, producing false overriding of the septum by the aorta. This could produce an echocardiogram that might be confused with the echocardiogram from patients with tetralogy of Fallot.

One of the more common errors is the assumption that echocardiography measures left ventricular volumes. The fact is that echocardiography does not measure left ventricular volumes but provides an internal left ventricular dimension. If one assumes that the ventricle is contracting symmetrically, there is a statistical relationship between the dimensions and the corresponding volumes. However, it is preferable to use the echocardiographic dimension itself as a correlate of volume rather than cube the left ventricular dimension and risk a threefold error when extrapolating to the left ventricular volume. Ejection fraction can be estimated by echocardiography. Since the estimation is created by extrapolation, it is best avoided. Determining the fractional shortening of the left ventricle or ΔD [$(LVID_d - LVID_s)/LVID_d$, where $LVID_d$ = the left ventricular internal dimension at end-diastole (d) and $LVID_s$ = the left ventricular internal dimension at end-systole (s)] provides the same information as the more familiar ejection fraction. The mean velocity of circumferential fiber shortening is a useful measure of myocardial contractility and is capable of accurately distinguishing normal from abnormal left ventricular function, whereas posterior wall velocities do not consistently make this distinction.

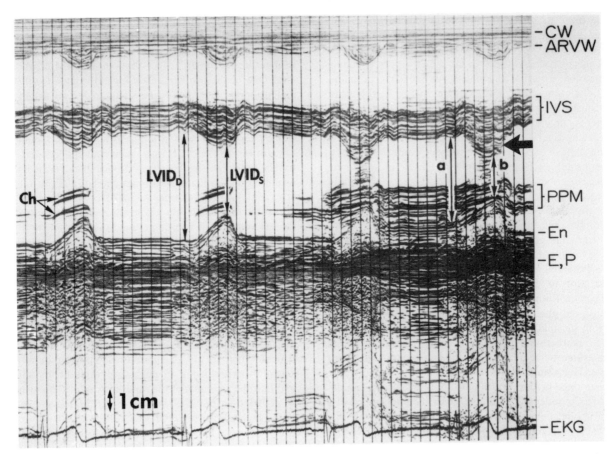

FIGURE 2 The echocardiogram shows the left ventricle as the ultrasound beam crosses the chordae on the left and the papillary muscle on the right. The left ventricular internal diameters would be significantly underestimated if measurements were made at the level of the papillary muscles (diameters a and b). The conventional measurement is made at the level of the chordae as shown. The endocardial echo of the left side of the interventricular septum (heavy arrow) spuriously extends into the left ventricular cavity. Therefore, echocardiographic measurements should always be made from the onset of the echoes. Ch, chordae tendineae; LVIDd, left ventricular internal diameter, end-diastole; LVIDs, left ventricular internal diameter, end-systole; CW, chest wall; PPM, posterior papillary muscle; ARVW, anterior right ventricular wall; IVS, interventricular septum; En, endocardium; E,P, epi-pericardium

When the ventricle is segmentally diseased, however, as occurs with coronary artery disease, the situation is quite different, and the area of the ventricle examined by the standard echocardiographic approach may no longer be representative of the entire ventricle.[7] In addition, since the plane of the echocardiographic beam traverses only the interventricular septum and posterior wall, apical and anterior motion disorders may be totally missed.

Of fundamental importance in determining left ventricular function is the ability to record clear endocardial echoes both from the left side of the interventricular septum and from the posterior free wall. Since the endocardium-blood interface is a poor reflector of ultrasound, higher gain settings are often required. When the gain is increased, however, the length of the echoes from the endocardial surface of the septum is increased and extend into the left ventricular cavity, thus introducing an error in measuring the left ventricular internal dimension (Fig. 2). This results in a threefold error when the cube law is used to calculate the estimated volumes. It is now clear that the location of the interface in the display is determined by the location of the first, rather than the last, deflection produced by the echo;[1] therefore, one should always measure dimensions from the onset of the echoe in M-mode recordings. Obtaining echoes from the interventricular septum requires considerable expertise. Optimally, both the right and left sides of the septum should be visualized in order to avoid the error of recording only one side, usually the right, since this will spuriously enlarge the minor axis. In analyzing the interventricular septum, remember that there is a hinge or pivot point between its upper one-third and lower two-thirds. Above the hinge, the septum moves anteriorly during systole, and below this point, it moves posteriorly in systole.[8]

Patients with diffuse left ventricular dysfunction can be readily identified echocardiographically.[9] For instance, depressed myocardial contractility may be evident even before clinical heart failure is detectable in patients receiving an increasing drug regimen with the cardiotoxic agent doxorubicin (Adriamycin).[10] In some patients with essential hypertension, echocardiography reveals changes in left ventricular structural function before definite clinical symptoms or signs of congestive heart failure develop, sometimes even before changes occur in the electrocardiogram or chest x-ray. Echocardiography may thus prove to be our most sensitive and most specific noninvasive technique for evaluating the hearts of patients with essential hypertension.[11] There are patients, however, with lesser degrees of ventricular malfunction who may not have abnormal echocardiograms. No one has adequately demonstrated just how sensitive the echocardiographic examination is in this situation.

Right Ventricle

The echocardiographic examination of the right ventricle has many limitations. The right ventricle lies directly behind the sternum; therefore, the echocardiogram measures only that portion of the right ventricle which lies anterior to the interventricular septum corresponding primarily to the right ventricular outflow tract. Furthermore, the internal dimension of the right ventricle varies considerably among normal persons and is affected by cardiac rotation, transducer angulation, and respiration. Unless the right ventricular cavity is moderately enlarged, estimation of the cavity size by echocardiography is unpredictable and unreliable.

The anterior wall of the right ventricle maybe impossible to measure either because its anterior border is inseparable from the chest wall echoes or because the endocardial surface is indistinct. Assessment of the right ventricular free wall remains outside the scope of echocardiographic study (except in infants and young patients who have a thin wall) unless a special high frequency transducer is used, because of interference by the gaseous tissues of the lung and because of problems caused by the physical properties of ultrasound.

Right Atrium

The ability of M-mode echo to provide data regarding the right atrium has been limited. Two-dimensional echocardiography may allow one to identify an increase in size of the right atrium and right ventricle.

Left Atrium

There is a good correlation between the left atrial dimension obtained by echocardiography and that obtained by angiography. Although the echocardiographic measurement is easily obtainable and useful, the wide range of normal values and the various methods used to determine left atrial size may lead to false positive and false negative results. The most useful method appears to be the ratio of left atrial dimension at end-systole to aortic root dimension at end-diastole.[2] In normal patients, this ratio is 0.87:1.11, whereas in patients with left atrial enlargement it is above 1.17. This ratio has proved particularly useful in following the magnitude of a left-to-right shunt through the patent ductus arteriosus of premature infants with respiratory distress syndrome. Ratios within the normal range, however, may be obtained in patients with large left atria and in the presence of aortic root dilatation. As with the right ventricular measurement, the left atrial dimension is not valid with the transducer in the subxyphoid position.

The combination of parasternal and suprasternal transducer positions has allowed a bidimensional (anteroposterior and superoinferior) evaluation of left atrial size which often detects enlargement of the left atrium that cannot be detected when only the single parasternal transducer position is used. Furthermore, a spuriously small left atrial dimension will be obtained in patients wth pectus excavatum if only the parasternal transducer position is used.

Linear and fuzzy echoes of unknown origin observed in the left atrium should not be mistaken for the posterior left atrial wall. It has been shown by green dye studies that only the dense echoes represent the true posterior left atrial wall. The etiology of these fuzzy echoes is not clear. They could originate from relatively stagnant blood which layers along the left atrial wall, or they may arise from the pulmonary veins as they enter the left atrium. Parallel or punctate echoes are frequently observed within the left atrial cavity and can be mistaken for left atrial clots or tumors. Clear-cut echocardiographic evidence of left atrial clots is seldom encountered, since most intra-atrial thrombi are in the left atrial appendage and not in the path of the transducer beam. Besides finding bands of echoes within the left atrium, one occasionally can see parts of the mitral annulus, the mitral prosthesis, the transverse sinus of the pericardium, and left atrial tumors.

DIAGNOSTIC APPLICATIONS

Mitral Stenosis

The initial diagnostic application of cardiac ultrasound was the recognition of mitral stenosis.[13] The echocar-

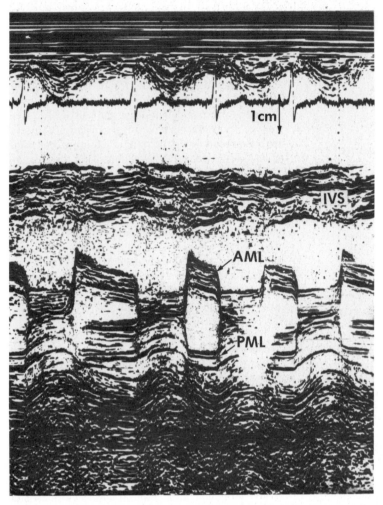

FIGURE 3 The mitral valve echogram is characteristic of mitral stenosis; however, the posterior leaflet uncharacteristically moves in a posterior direction. The thickened leaflets, diminished excursion of the valve, and reduced diastolic (EF) slope confirm the diagnosis. IVS, interventricular septum; AML, anterior mitral leaflets; PML, posterior mitral leaflet.

diogram is now considered to be diagnostic for mitral stenosis and no false negative results have been reported. The characteristic echocardiographic features include thickened leaflets and diminished excursion of the valve, a reduced diastolic (EF) slope and A wave amplitude of the anterior leaflet, and paradoxical motion of the posterior leaflet. The most specific echocardiographic finding was reported to be paradoxical or anterior motion of the posterior leaflet in diastole. Patients with mitral stenosis have been described who have normal or posterior motion in the leaflet in diastole. This occurred in 10 percent of patients in one study.[14] The diagnosis of mitral stenosis, however, does not present a problem in most of these cases, since the leaflets are markedly thickened and virtually always abnormal in motion (Fig. 3).

Standard M-mode echocardiographic techniques

are not reliable in assessing the severity of mitral stenosis.[14] The diastolic (EF) slope of the anterior leaflet, the excursion of the valve, and the calculated valve orifice have not proved useful in quantitating the severity of stenosis. Since the diastolic (EF) slope reflects the rate of left atrial emptying and left ventricular filling, many entities can result in slow filling of the left ventricle and therefore reduce the EF slope (Table 1). Reduced valve mobility is generally the result of fibrosis and shortening of fused chordae tendineae and papillary muscles and is not necessarily a reflection of the severity of the lesion. Other conditions such as low output states and severe aortic regurgitation may also result in decreased amplitude of valve movement. Furthermore, any conclusions based on the degree of EF slope or valve mobility presupposes optimal transducer angulation, since even small changes in beam

TABLE 1

Causes of decreased diastolic EF slope of the anterior mitral valve leaflet

1 Decreased mitral valve flow
   a Mitral stenosis
   b Mitral stenosis and regurgitation
   c Left atrial tumors

2 Decreased ventricular compliance
   a Systemic arterial hypertension
   b Idiopathic hypertrophic subaortic stenosis
   c Aortic stenosis
   d Restrictive cardiomyopathy

3 Pulmonary artery hypertension
   a Primary
   b Secondary

direction may produce an erroneous tracing. Therefore, when calculating the velocities and amplitude of the valve, multiple motion recordings must be examined and only the maximum slope and excursion used. Even alterations in cardiac rate and rhythm may have a significant effect on the diastolic EF slope of the anterior mitral leaflet.

Reliance on the valve thickness or the presence of calcification of the leaflets in the assessment of the severity of mitral stenosis is also unwise. The degree of thickening is a poor index of the severity of the stenosis because orifice size is affected by the amount of commissural fusion rather than by the degree of leaflet thickening. Furthermore, if aortic regurgitation is also present, some leaflet thickening may occur as a result of that alone. Since there are no objective criteria for quantitating the amount of calcium present, judgment of the degree of leaflet calcification may be inadvertently underestimated or overestimated. A major discrepancy encountered in attempting to assess the severity of mitral stenosis by echocardiography probably arises from the coexistence of left ventricular disease or the presence of concomitant mitral regurgitation.

Echocardiography is not only the most sensitive and specific noninvasive method for diagnosing mitral stenosis but is also useful in confirming mitral stenosis when associated abnormalities are present such as aortic or tricuspid valve disease. Echocardiography is extremely valuable in differentiating the diastolic apical rumble of rheumatic mitral stenosis from that of Austin Flint.

Mitral Regurgitation

Only limited success has been achieved in detecting mitral regurgitation by M-mode echocardiography because the structural changes that result in mitral regurgitation, such as failure of the leaflet edges to coapt

during ventricular systole, make it impossible to diagnose this condition with certainty. In general, the echocardiographic features of mitral regurgitation are nonspecific (hyperdynamic left ventricular wall motion, increased left ventricular and left atrial dimensions) unless there is evidence of mitral valve prolapse, a flail mitral leaflet, or mitral annular calcification. If there is coexistent aortic regurgitation or other evidence of a left ventricular volume overload lesion, echocardiography is not useful. The diagnosis of mitral regurgitation may be made convincingly when there is systolic expansion of the left atrial wall, a relatively rare occurrence.

Pathologic changes from a chronic rheumatic process results in a fixed fibrotic, often heavily calcified mitral valve. The echocardiogram clearly mirrors this abnormal structure, and it is often difficult to differentiate predominant valve stenosis from predominant regurgitation by observing the mitral valve echogram alone. Because of the similarity of the echocardiographic patterns of rheumatic mitral stenosis and mitral regurgitation, it has been our policy to interpret echocardiograms that exhibit these findings as demonstrating merely rheumatic mitral valve disease, since the mitral valve echogram may demonstrate the classical features of mitral stenosis even though the patient may show clinical and hemodynamic evidence of predominant mitral regurgitation (Fig. 4).

Mitral Valve Prolapse Syndrome

Echocardiography is one of the primary methods of diagnosing mitral valve prolapse, and yet the precise sensitivity and specificity of echocardiography remains unresolved. The major difficulty in defining the presence or absence of mitral valve prolapse appears to be a lack of a definitive "gold standard." The "gold standard" is difficult to determine because of the problems of defining valve prolapse by ventriculography and because there is rarely any pathologic confirmation in this usually benign condition.[16]

Mitral prolapse has been observed within a large group of asymptomatic patients.[17] This finding makes us concerned as to the true incidence of this abnormality and also whether the echocardiographic criteria are inaccurate and too sensitive (providing many false positive results). At the present time, it is uncertain whether the mitral valve prolapse syndrome is a common disorder, the prevalence of which has been recognized only by the advent of echocardiography, or whether the echocardiographic abnormalities observed represent a variant of the normal mitral valve motion. Even with relatively sensitive criteria, there are still patients with clinical evidence of mitral valve prolapse in whom echocardiographic examination discloses no abnormalities and others with echocardi-

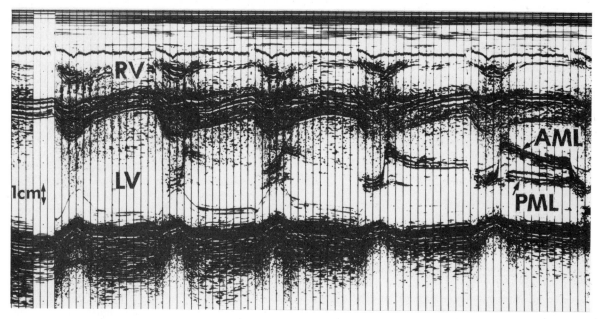

FIGURE 4 This echocardiogram is from a 33-year-old woman with rheumatic mitral regurgitation. The thickened mitral valve leaflets and abnormal motion of the posterior leaflet is consistent with the rheumatic etiology. Although the mitral valve appearance is identical to that of pure mitral stenosis, the slightly enlarged left ventricle and hyperkinetic wall motion is consistent with mitral regurgitation. RV, right ventricle; LV, left ventricle; AML, anterior mitral leaflet; PML, posterior mitral leaflet.

ographic evidence of prolapse who have no clinical evidence of the syndrome. Based on our experience of mitral valve prolapse, we can accurately confirm by echocardiography only 80 percent of clinically suspected cases.

In order to diagnose mitral valve prolapse by echocardiography, it is important to have a clear understanding of the echocardiographic pattern observed in normal individuals and to realize that mitral valve prolapse is represented by a variable spectrum of abnormalities on the echocardiogram. The echocardiographic pattern that is considered to be specific for mitral valve prolapse is midsystolic "buckling" (greater than 2 to 3 mm from the C point) of the posterior and/or anterior leaflet into the left atrium (Fig. 5). The mitral leaflets first come together at the onset of systole and pursue a horizontal or slightly anterior course until midsystole, when they manifest an abrupt posterior motion.[18] A second pattern, continuous pansystolic posterior bowing or hammocking of the mitral leaflets throughout systole, is a useful but not a specific sign of mitral valve prolapse provided that adequate care has been taken to avoid excessive inferior angulation of the transducer. Abnormally high transducer placement (e.g., in the second left intercostal space) may produce holosystolic posterior motion in normal subjects.[19] Caution should be used in diagnosing mitral valve prolapse from this echocardiographic pattern in the absence of ancillary findings, such as

increased amplitude of excursion of the mitral valve in diastole as well as multiple echoes in systole, since the same pattern may be seen in patients with congestive cardiomyopathy.

The echocardiographic diagnosis of mitral valve prolapse is difficult. This may in part reflect the geometric limitations of a one-dimensional view of the relatively copious mitral leaflet tissue. Certainly, prolapse of an isolated scallop of the posterior leaflet could be missed if the ultrasonic beam fails to pass through that particular portion of the valve. In addition, this failure might be caused by technically poor visualizations of the most severely prolapsed portion of the leaflet, which is virtually parallel to the sound beam and in apposition to the atrioventricular wall, making it more difficult to image. The posterior mitral leaflet is a tri-scalloped structure. Since the scallops may prolapse at different degrees, the echocardiogram may not always accurately assess the severity of prolapse. Furthermore, the ultrasound beam has a limited width and probably does not transect all the scallops. Therefore, the mitral echocardiogram may appear normal with one transducer angulation and reveal abnormalities only when the beam traverses a specific portion of the leaflets.

Certain provocative maneuvers, such as having the patient inhale amyl nitrite to reduce left ventricular end-diastolic volume, should be employed to "bring out" prolapse in all clinically suspected cases.

The diagnosis of mitral prolapse should be made with caution in patients with large pericardial effusions, since the presence of cardiac swinging may introduce motion artifacts that are indistinguishable from those seen with true prolapse (see ''Pericardial Diseases'' below).

Flail Mitral Valve Leaflet Syndrome

The echocardiogram may be useful in detecting torn chordae tendineae, which results in a flail mitral valve leaflet. Using the criteria considered to be characteristic of flail posterior leaflet, M-mode echocardiography is neither very sensitive nor specific for detecting the flail posterior leaflet. Every echocardiographic abnormality may be entirely absent, and the multiple diastolic echoes of the posterior leaflet created by the flail edge are frequently indistinguishable from those of atrial myxoma, mitral valve prolapse, or an infec-

tive vegetation. Two-dimensional echocardiography allows a clear identification of a vegetative mass that moves along with the flail posterior leaflet and thus provides advantages over M-mode echocardiography.[20]

The M-mode echocardiographic diagnosis of a flail anterior leaflet is even less satisfactory. This abnormality is suggested by the chaotic diastolic fluttering and exaggerated excursion of the anterior leaflet. Chaotic fluttering, however, may not be appreciated in the case of rheumatic heart disease with fibrotic or thickened leaflets, and coarse diastolic fluttering may be seen in aortic regurgitation, atrial flutter, and atrial fibrillation.

Infective Endocarditis

Echocardiography is not a sensitive method for detecting vegetations in patients with infective endocar-

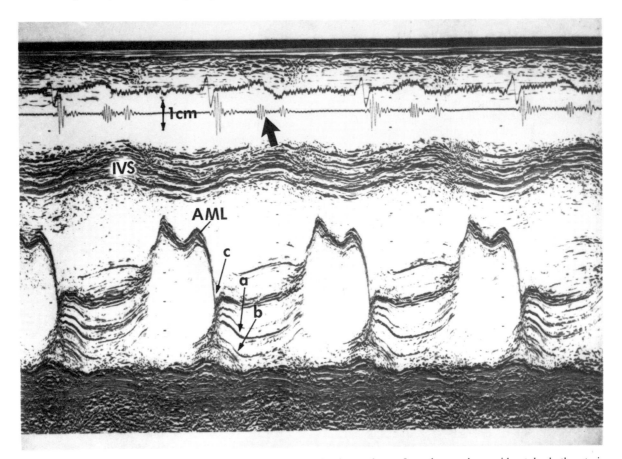

FIGURE 5 This echophonocardiogram is diagnostic of mitral valve prolapse. In early systole to midsystole, both anterior (arrow a) and posterior (arrow b) leaflets of the mitral valve move abruptly posterior [3 mm from the closure point (arrow c) of the mitral valve] toward the left atrial wall. Multiple echoes from both leaflets of the mitral valve are evident. The midsystolic click (arrowhead) occurs in midsystole and does not coincide with the initial posterior buckling of the leaflets. IVS, interventricular septum; AML, anterior mitral leaflet.

ditis, since only those lesions with vegetations greater than 2 to 3 mm are visible. In patients with clinically proven endocarditis, only about one-third show echocardiographic evidence of vegetations.[21] Although echocardiography may be helpful in the early detection of a changing pattern, it cannot distinguish between active and healed vegetations. We have followed patients who have had unchanging vegetations for 6 months despite bacteriologic cures.[22]

Visualization of vegetations is important from a prognostic viewpoint. It seems likely that the ability to record vegetations on the leaflets signifies an advanced degree of destruction of the valve structure and/or an extremely large vegetation.[23] There is evidence to suggest that the clinical course of patients with echocardiographic evidence of vegetations is much more ominous than that of those without vegetations. In one series, all but 2 of 22 patients with demonstrable vegetations either died or required heart surgery, whereas none of those without vegetations died from heart disease or required an emergency surgical procedure.[24]

Although vegetations have been recorded on all four cardiac valves, the dense, thickened, shaggy echoes originally thought to be specific for vegetations can also be seen with fibrosis and/or calcification of the valve leaflets. Mitral valve vegetations must be distinguished from mitral stenosis with a severely fibrosed or calcified valve, atrial myxoma, and myxomatous transformation of the mitral valve. Large aortic valve vegetations may be confused with the findings of a flail aortic valve. A particularly difficult problem occurs in trying to make the echocardiographic diagnosis of vegetations on a prosthetic valve. The prosthetic valve usually produces so many echoes by itself that it is difficult to identify any additional echoes from possible vegetations.

Echocardiography may be valuable in the patient wih suspected endocarditis who has negative blood cultures. Although a positive diagnosis cannot be made from the echocardiogram alone, the finding of a vegetation may be helpful in substantiating the diagnosis.

Mitral Annular Calcification

The sensitivity and specificity of ultrasound in identifying calcification in general and the mitral valve annulus in particular is excellent. The echocardiographic pattern of mitral annular calcification is virtually diagnostic. Echocardiography is even more sensitive than chest roentgenography or fluoroscopy in detecting mitral annular calcification.

The characteristic pattern of mitral valve calcification on echo consists of a broad band of dense echoes lying just posterior to the mitral leaflet and just anterior to the endocardium of the left ventricular posterior wall. The explanation for the presumably intracavitary appearance of this structure is not totally understood, but it is undoubtedly related to the beam width of the ultrasound signal. The separation of structures produced by this dense band of echoes must not be misdiagnosed as a pericardial effusion (Fig. 6).

Atrial Myxoma

The echocardiographic features of atrial myxoma are virtually diagnostic. The echocardiographic detection of cardiac tumors, especially a mobile left atrial myxoma, can be very reliable, since the actual tumor can be visualized. Echocardiography may therefore replace cardiac catheterization as the major tool in identifying this condition. Long-term postoperative results in these patients have been excellent.[25]

The echocardiographic diagnosis of left atrial myxoma is dramatic and frequently obvious, but it is not always simple. Atrial myxomata may have a variety of appearances depending upon their location and histologic character. Echocardiographic detection of a left atrial myxoma is principally contingent upon the tumor extending through the mitral orifice during mitral valve opening. Such protrusion probably occurs in the majority of cases (90 percent), but sessile tumors may not prolapse behind the mitral valve and for this reason may not be visualized.[26] If the technician is not informed of the possibility of a myxoma, is unfamiliar with its echocardiographic appearance and attempts to "clean up" the echoes of the tumor by reducing intensity, or does not realize that these echoes may only be seen in the left atrium, the diagnosis may be missed if the tumor is not traversing the valve orifice at the time of the examination. Therefore, in order to avoid missing a left atrial myxoma, a complete echocardiographic examination should encompass several gain settings with long, uninterrupted recordings of the mitral valve at the level of the left ventricle and left atrium and through the aorta and left atrium. Some authors have recommended using several views, including the suprasternal approach to visualize the left atrium, in order to increase the specificity and sensitivity of this technique.[27] These multiple views, however, cannot always be adequately performed owing to the variability of the shape of the thorax.

There are several conditions which may simulate myxoma, including a large left atrial thrombus, the redundant and voluminous leaflets in mitral valve prolapse, a vegetation on a flail posterior mitral leaflet, and severely calcified leaflets in mitral stenosis. To the experienced echocardiographer, these conditions do not pose a very difficult differential problem, however.

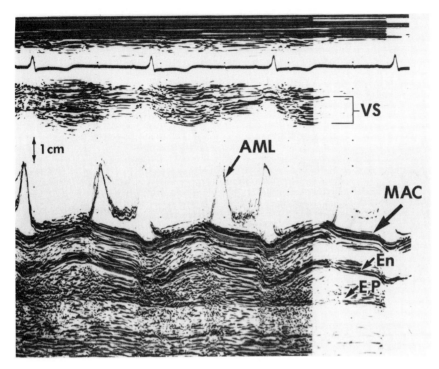

FIGURE 6 The echocardiogram is from a patient with a calcified mitral annulus. A posterior pericardial effusion may be misdiagnosed if the calcified annulus is inadvertently interpreted as the endocardium, if the endocardium is misinterpreted as the epicardium, and if the epi-pericardial echo is misinterpreted as the pericardium. AML, anterior mitral leaflet; VS, interventricular septum; MAC, mitral annular calcification; En, endocardium; E,P, epi-pericardium.

Valvular Prostheses

Assessing the functional status of the multitude of various prosthetic valves is a difficult clinical as well as echocardiographic problem. The optimal application of echocardiography in prosthetic valve assessment appears to be serial evaluation with control recordings made after the immediate postoperative period. Studies obtained during the recovery period, however, appear to be useful only in the detection of gross abnormalities of valve function and must be interpreted with exceptional caution. Paradoxical septal motion, for instance, is expected following cardiopulmonary bypass and is unrelated to the diagnosis or surgical procedure. In general, echocardiography is an insensitive method for detecting prosthetic valve malfunction.

The combination of phonocardiography and echocardiography and occasionally spectroanalysis provides much more information than any one study alone and has been successfully used to assess prosthetic valve function.[28] Long recording strips are needed because sticking of valves may be intermittent and short recording strips may miss intermediate abnormalities of valve motion.

The exact model and size of the prosthetic valve should be known to the technologist before any attempt is made to record the valve. The motion of the prosthetic valve is determined not only by the valve characteristics themselves but also by the motion of the entire cardiac structure and by the hemodynamics on either side of the valve. These variables should be taken into account when studying prosthetic valve echograms.

The best recording for analysis of prosthetic valve echograms is one that clearly defines the time of valve opening and closure and most closely approximates the normal excursion and amplitude of the heterograft, disk, or poppet. The transducer angle relative to the position of the valve is critical for measuring the amplitude of excursion. Unless the beam parallels the axis of the opening and closing movements, measurements of amplitude are not of value, except when the relative position of the beam to the valve remains absolutely fixed and the amplitude definitely changes from beat to beat. The mitral disk prosthesis is best recorded with the transducer at the cardiac apex and the beam angled toward the mitral annulus along the long axis of the valve. The aortic valve is more difficult to evaluate. The transducer is generally placed in the right supraclavicular fossa, especially with a ball-

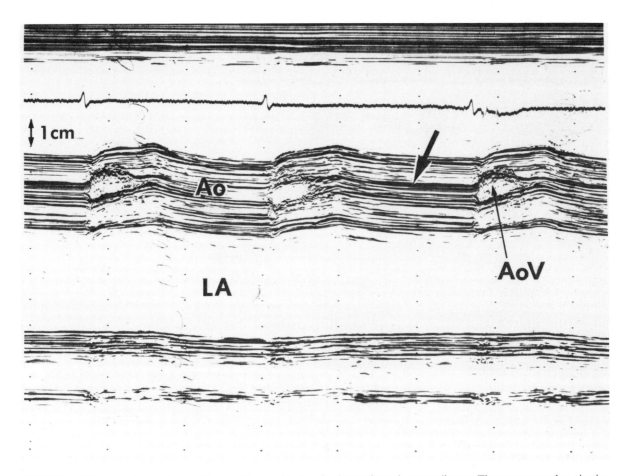

FIGURE 7 Echocardiogram from a 68-year-old man with chronic obstructive pulmonary disease. There was no catheterization evidence of aortic stenosis despite the presence of dense, centrilinear echoes suggestive of aortic valve calcification (arrow) and reduced opening of and thickened aortic leaflets. Ao, aorta; AoV, aortic valve; LA, left atrium.

valve prosthesis, directing the beam to travel along the longitudinal axis of the valve. With tilting disk valves, various echo patterns can be obtained depending upon the position of the transducer.

Measurements that are potentially useful in assessing prosthetic valve function are the interval from the beginning of systole to mitral valve opening (A_2 to MVO) and the duration of the opening of the aortic valve. These parameters can be measured easily and are not dependent on aligning the beam with the poppet axis but are more often altered by changes in left ventricular function than by changes in the prosthesis itself.

Tricuspid Valve

Criteria for optimal tricuspid valve recordings have not yet been developed to determine when technical errors such as transducer angulation are having a significant effect. The tricuspid valve echogram must not

be mistaken for the pulmonic valve echo or for the echo of a Swan-Ganz catheter. The images of the tricuspid and pulmonic valves bear a striking resemblance to each other and could easily be confused if associated echocardiographic anatomy and beam angulation are not taken into consideration.

Cardiac diseases that primarily affect the tricuspid valve are uncommon. Tricuspid stenosis may be suggested by echocardiography because of the slow diastolic (EF) slope of the anterior tricuspid leaflet. The reliability of this finding is uncertain, since a reduced slope may occur because of transducer angulation or other right ventricular problems such as reduced compliance. The diagnosis of tricuspid stenosis can be excluded in the presence of mitral stenosis, however, if a normal tricuspid echogram is present.

The tricuspid valve may exhibit high-frequency diastolic fluttering, similar to that of the mitral valve in aortic regurgitation, in the presence of pulmonic regurgitation. This finding is nonspecific, however, since

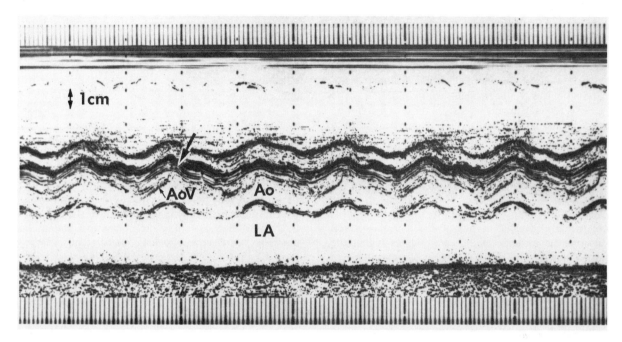

FIGURE 8 There is a dense multicentrilinear echo (arrow) which represents calcification in either the aortic valve, the aorta, or the coronary arteries, since it is stronger than either wall of the aorta. The aortic valve does not open fully. These findings may be seen in patients with aortic stenosis. This echocardiogram, however, is from a 54-year-old man with calcification in his right coronary artery but without catheterization evidence of aortic stenosis. Ao, aorta; AoV, aortic valve; LA, left atrium.

fluttering may also be seen in atrial septal defect, tricuspid regurgitation, and in some normal subjects, especially infants. The reliability of echocardiography in demonstrating tricuspid valve prolapse, which may be associated with concomitant mitral prolapse, is limited by the fact that the valve is technically more difficult to record and cannot be examined from various transducer positions as effectively as the mitral valve.

Aortic Stenosis

M-mode echocardiography has many deficiencies with respect to evaluating patients with valvular aortic stenosis. The echocardiographic finding of a dense band of echoes in the aortic root obscuring the valve cusps is suggestive evidence of calcific aortic stenosis. It may be difficult to determine whether these findings represent aortic stenosis (obstruction to outflow) or aortic sclerosis (cusp calcification without obstruction) (Fig. 7). The echocardiographic criteria proposed for the diagnosis of aortic stenosis have been disappointing, although echocardiography is a sensitive means of assessing the presence of valvular calcification. Mild aortic stenosis can probably be satisfactorily separated from severe aortic stenosis, but moderate degrees of aortic stenosis may be badly misinterpreted if one tries to quantitate them. If the aortic cusps open to the periphery of the aortic root, one can reliably

rule out significant rheumatic or calcific aortic stenosis. This, however, does not apply to patients with congenital aortic stenosis.

In an elderly patient, the absence of calcification on the echogram and/or fluttering of the aortic leaflets virtually excludes the presence of hemodynamically significant aortic stenosis. Extensive multilayering or a thick conglomerate of echoes signifying calcium in association with diminished aortic cusp excursion may indicate aortic stenosis. In mild and moderate forms of aortic stenosis, the diminished leaflet excursion may be equivocal and limited to only one leaflet. Since aortic valve orifice dimension is related to cardiac output, diminution in orifice alone is not a sufficient criteria for a diagnosis of aortic stenosis. In addition, calcification in contiguous structures such as the proximal coronary arteries may mimic calcific aortic valve disease, and heavily calcified cusps may be seen in severe aortic regurgitation with no gradient across the aortic valve (Fig. 8). Attempts at quantitating the degree of stenosis by the appearance of the aortic valve echoes can be frustrating and misleading. One must exert great caution not to diagnose aortic stenosis unless at least some leaflet motion is seen, since merely directing the transducer eccentrically through the aortic root or excess gain setting can produce spurious echoes within the aorta. In order to optimize the echocardiographic study of aortic stenosis the patient should be examined in the supine position, 30° to 60° left lateral, and sitting up leaning on the transducer.

M-mode echocardiography is relatively insensitive in detecting congenital aortic stenosis at a time when there is minimal fibrosis and no calcification. Echocardiograms in younger adults with congenital aortic stenosis are indistinguishable from those in individuals with normal aortic valves. This finding results from the passage of the ultrasonic beam through the base of a doming valve in which the valvular elements are in close proximity to the aortic walls, resulting in apparently brisk opening and closing movements of the cusp images.[29]

Echocardiography can confirm the presence of a congenitally bicuspid aortic valve if there is marked diastolic eccentricity of the cusp echoes within the aortic lumen. This echocardiographic appearance of the aortic valve is believed to be very specific, but it is not a highly sensitive sign of a bicuspid valve, since the aortic valve diastolic closure line may be central and not eccentric when a bicuspid valve is present. Nanda et al. developed an eccentricity index to aid in the diagnosis of a bicuspid valve and showed marked diastolic eccentricity of the aortic valve in all 21 patients with a bicuspid aortic valve proved by surgery and angiography.[30] Radford et al. found that 75 percent of patients with proved bicuspid aortic valve had characteristic eccentricity.[31] Despite its high degree of specificity, caution should be exercised in making the diagnosis of a bicuspid aortic valve, since abnormal eccentricity has also been seen in a high membranous ventricular septal defect and a sinus of Valsalva aneurysm. False negative results have been reported in patients with bicuspid aortic valves who had tetralogy of Fallot. Abnormal eccentricity of the aortic leaflets is of no value in estimating the severity of stenosis, since the M-mode echocardiographic appearance of functionally normal stenotic and incompetent bicuspid valves is similar unless calcification has developed.

There are several problems involved in determining the presence or absence of a bicuspid aortic valve by echocardiography. First, only when the diastolic closure of the aortic cusps and the presence of both the anterior and posterior aortic walls are clearly recorded should an eccentricity index be determined. In addition, the aortic leaflet measurement must be made at a precise and constant point at end-diastole, and the internal aortic root diameter should be measured (posterior surface of the anterior wall to the anterior surface of the posterior wall) rather than the more conventional aortic root measurement. Second, it is important to be aware of the many anatomic variations that may exist when studying the aortic valve; three cusps of unequal size may cause an eccentric diastolic position, whereas a bicuspid valve with two symmetrical cusps may not demonstrate eccentricity. Therefore, absence of eccentricity does not exclude the

presence of a bicuspid valve, and an eccentric valve does not invariably confirm the presence of a bicuspid valve. Third, the angle of the beam passing through the aorta and closed aortic leaflets may vary from patient to patient and from transducer position to transducer position, leading to an erroneous appearance of one small and one large cusp. It is, therefore, important to try to normalize the diastolic position of the aortic leaflets by using several transducer positions and angles before concluding that the aortic valve is indeed bicuspid. Fourth, successful aortic commissurotomy does not alter the eccentricity index, the presence of multilayered diastolic echoes, or the systolic motion of the aortic valve.[32] Fifth, the echocardiographic diagnosis of a bicuspid valve cannot be made in the presence of calcific aortic stenosis.[32a]

Aortic Regurgitation

Fine diastolic fluttering of the mitral valve is characteristic of chronic aortic regurgitation, and yet there are several problems in the echocardiographic diagnosis. First, systematic studies to determine the incidence of false positive and false negative diagnoses have not been done. Second, fine diastolic fluttering is not pathognomonic of aortic regurgitation, since patients with right-to-left shunts in the absence of semilunar valve incompetence may show similar fluttering. Third, diastolic fluttering is not a constant observation, since the direction rather than the severity of regurgitation dictates whether the flow strikes the mitral valve. Fourth, the presence or absence of diastolic fluttering of the mitral valve is of no predictive value in the quantification of the regurgitant flow in aortic regurgitation. Fifth, the failure to observe oscillations of the mitral valve in patients with documented aortic regurgitation may be due to coexistent mitral stenosis, since the high atrial pressure in mitral stenosis may distend the valve and probably dampen any tendency to flutter. Proper use of the gain control may avoid this problem (Fig. 9). It is also worthwhile to look for fluttering of the ventricular septum, since it is also characteristic of aortic regurgitation.

Chronic aortic regurgitation and acute aortic regurgitation have different echocardiographic findings. Severe aortic regurgitation of recent onset frequently causes premature closure of the mitral valve, which is a useful prognosticator of the need for valve replacement. It is neither specific, since it may be seen in bradycardia, nor highly sensitive for the diagnosis of acute aortic regurgitation.

Aortic Root Disease

The echocardiographic diagnosis of dissection of the aorta depends on a combination of several features and meticulous attention to technical details rather

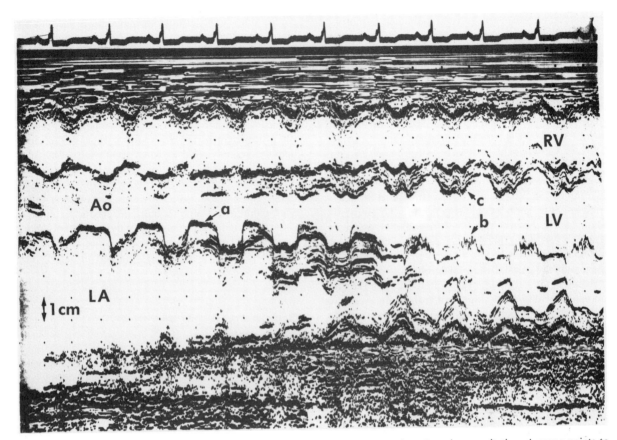

FIGURE 9 This echocardiogram is from a patient with combined mitral stenosis and aortic regurgitation. Arrow a points to the mitral valve characteristic of mitral stenosis. Without appropriate use of the gain control or angling the ultrasound beam toward the body of the left ventricle, the fine oscillations on the calcified mitral valve (arrow b) and on the interventricular septum (arrow c) would not be apparent. RV, right ventricle; LV, left ventricle; Ao, aorta; LA, left atrium.

than on a single specific observation. Nevertheless, there is high incidence of false positive and false negative results. When a clinical diagnosis of aortic dissection is suspected, abnormalities on echo may provide noninvasive confirmation. It is clearly apparent that the absence of the characteristic echocardiographic findings do not exclude aortic dissection, especially since a dissection that does not involve the aortic annulus cannot be detected by echo.

There are important limitations to the diagnosis. Brown et al. demonstrated the classic echocardiographic features of aortic root dissection in some patients without clinical findings of aortic root dissection or aortic valve disease.[33] False positive separation of aortic root walls was recorded in patients with increased thickness of the aortic walls as a result of severe generalized atherosclerosis from a large focal anterior wall plaque or syphilis.[34] False positive echocardiograms can be created by the manner in which the ultrasonic beam transects the aortic root. Aortic valve disease per se may cause false widening of one or both sides of the aorta.

Pulmonary Valve Disease

The pulmonary valve is technically the most difficult of the cardiac valves to record. It is also difficult to interpret the recording. Only portions of the posterior pulmonary leaflet are consistently recorded, and even these are recorded only in about 60 to 70 percent of patients. Therefore, caution must be used in examining the echoes of one leaflet and trying to apply the data to the entire valve itself. The patterns of motion of the pulmonary valve echogram are not specific for any particular clinical disorder but nevertheless may provide valuable indirect information concerning local pressure and flow characteristics in response to the structured disorder of the valve and, as such, may prove useful when applied to a specific clinical situation.

The echocardiographic findings in valvular pulmonic stenosis may be useful, but their reliability and sensitivity have not yet been tested. It was originally believed that an exaggerated *a* dip amplitude (presystolic opening of the pulmonary valve) was diagnostic of moderate to severe valvular pulmonic stenosis.[35] These echocardiographic abnormalities, however, reflect the relative pressure existing across the pulmonary valve after atrial contraction and are not specific for valvular pulmonic stenosis. Peak inspiration, for instance, can increase the depth of the *a* wave, and the *a* dip can vary in amplitude depending upon the position of the transducer, the heart rate, and the stroke volume (Fig. 10). Premature opening of the pulmonary valve has been observed occasionally in constrictive pericarditis and sinus of Valsalva aneurysm with rupture into the right atrium. The presystolic motion of the pulmonary valve is absent in atrial fibrillation. Furthermore, patients with an absent or diminished *a* dip may have severe valvular pulmonic stenosis related to thickened or deformed cusps which do not respond to the small positive-pressure gradient generated by atrial systole. Therefore, the ability to reliably demonstrate an exaggerated *a* dip on the pulmonary valve appears to depend both on the ability to record the pulmonary valve and on the pliability of the valve. The presence of an exaggerated *a* dip (greater than 10 mm) is characteristic of valvular pulmonic stenosis; however, the absence of an exaggerated *a* dip does not exclude this diagnosis.

No single echocardiographic finding is specific for pulmonary hypertension, because there is considerable overlap in all measurements of the pulmonary valve echogram between normal subjects and patients with pulmonary hypertension.[36] In contrast to pulmonic stenosis, however, pulmonary hypertension is extremely reliable in the presence of a constellation of echocardiographic abnormalities, including diminished or absent *a* dip, decreased E to F slope, rapid opening velocity, and elevated right ventricular systolic time intervals. In the presence of right heart failure, however, there may be a considerable increase in right ventricular diastolic pressure which may influence pulmonary valve motion and produce a large *a* wave in patients with pulmonary hypertension. Thus, one may get a false negative echogram even in the face of pulmonary hypertension when the right ventricle fails.

Coronary Atherosclerotic Heart Disease

The use of echocardiography to study patients with coronary atherosclerotic heart disease has significant

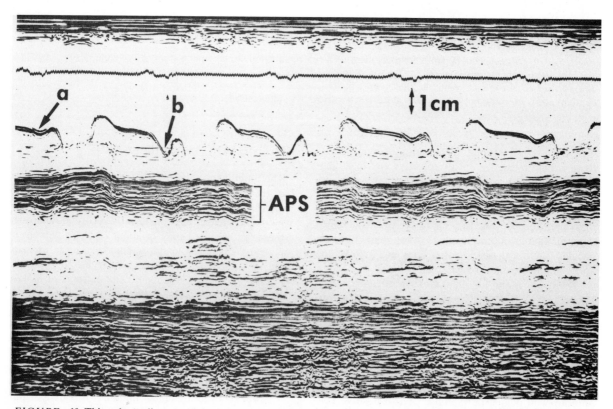

FIGURE 10 This echocardiogram of the pulmonary valve is from a normal teenager. The presystolic opening of the valve (*a* dip) is in the acceptable range for patients with valvular pulmonic stenosis. The *a* dip varies in amplitude during respiration from a normal 2 mm (arrow a) at end-expiration to a moderately increased 10 mm (arrow b) during peak inspiration. APS, atriopulmonary sulcus.

limitations. The extremely accurate echocardiographic studies of left ventricular function are based on the assumption that the view obtained is representative of the entire left ventricle. This is true in most of the conditions but is not true in coronary artery disease where the motion abnormalities are segmental and not uniform and the area of involvement is generally unknown in the absence of invasive study. The exact area of ventricular myocardium transversed by the ultrasound beam and, therefore, the beam's relationship to normal or ischemic myocardium are difficult to define. The examination is also extremely difficult and frequently suboptimal in quality because of the middle-aged, obese, emphysematous patient, who comprises a significant part of the population of patients with coronary disease.

The sensitivity of M-mode echocardiography in coronary atherosclerotic heart disease is diminished because not every area of the left ventricle can be examined adequately. It is not possible in most cases to examine the truly inferior surface of the left ventricle by M-mode echocardiography because the ultrasound beam cannot be directed so that it strikes the surface perpendicularly; therefore, it is difficult to diagnose right coronary artery disease abnormalities. Because coronary disease affects only segments of the myocardium, multiple areas of the septum and free wall must be recorded before the echocardiographic evaluation can be considered adequate. Since normally contracting muscle can influence the motion of adjacent ischemic tissue, even if the echo beam transects an area of infarction, it is conceivable that this segment may be pulled in a normal direction by adjacent viable myocardium. An abnormally moving ischemic muscle will affect an immediately adjacent normal myocardium by reducing the motion of the adjoining muscle even though that muscle may still be normal. In addition, abnormalities of wall motion are not even specific for coronary atherosclerotic heart disease. Patients with congestive cardiomyopathy invariably have abnormal wall motions that may resemble the abnormal wall motion resulting from coronary atherosclerotic heart disease. Furthermore, ventricular wall contractility may be influenced by movement of the entire heart within the chest, by motion of the adjacent left ventricular segments, by relative diastolic volumes, by postoperative open heart surgery, and by conduction abnormalities.

The echocardiographic findings in acute infarction appear to be principally dependent on the position of the infarcted area relative to the echo beam. If the acutely infarcted area of the ventricle is remote from the portion recorded, the findings are nonspecific and are related primarily to depressed myocardial contraction or to compensatory increases in wall motion. If the echo beam intersects a hypermobile noninfarcted segment or a hypomobile infarcted segment of myocardium, the end-systolic and end-diastolic dimensions will not reflect the changes in the volume of the ventricle as a whole.[37]

A further limitation of echocardiography is noted when it is compared to the results of ventriculography, since the areas examined by these two procedures are not identical. The conventional sonar window used in echocardiography does not allow for an adequate view of the heart analogous to the right anterior oblique ventriculogram. In most patients the apical left ventricular structures are not well visualized below the papillary muscles. Limitations may be overcome by routinely recording sector and linear scans from multiple chest locations. In addition to scanning the ultrasonic beam in an arc sector between the cardiac base and apex from the conventional parasternal area, one should also record scans with the transducer laterally over the left precordium, at the cardiac apex, and in the subxyphoid position. These different transducer locations will enable more complete visualization of the left ventricular walls. In general, better estimates of left ventricular wall motion are obtained by scanning the ventricle from multiple positions with a slow, steady motion using a condensed scan (paper speed of 10 mm/s).[38] Two-dimensional echocardiography (sector scanning and multicrystal sonar systems) will offer better estimates of left ventricular wall motion because one obtains adequate views of the heart analogous to the right anterior oblique ventriculogram.

The absence of systolic septal wall thickening may provide information about left ventricular contractility. The ischemic myocardium is frequently associated with a thin but dense septum which fails to thicken during systole. Decreased systolic thickening of the ventricular septum in patients with coronary disease is an indicator of high-grade stenosis or complete occlusion in the proximal left coronary artery system.[39] Septal motion and systolic thickening may also be entirely normal in patients with critical stenosis or occlusion of the proximal portion of the left anterior descending (LAD) coronary artery. It is conceivable that in this group of patients, provocative measures such as isometric handgrip exercise or stress testing may convert a normal resting septal echo to an abnormal one. In patients with large anteroseptal infarcts with scarring and fibrosis of the septum, the septal echo may appear thin and dense because of fibrosis, and its motion may be hypokinetic, akinetic, or even dyskinetic. Systolic septal thickening, however, is seen in acute and chronic coronary artery disease as well as in patients with congestive cardiomyopathy.

The attempt to use echocardiographic location of abnormal septal motion in predicting the location of lesions in patients with coronary artery disease is also not specific. First, the echo beam must transect the muscular (not membranous) portion of the septum, and the ultrasound beam must be close to the septum

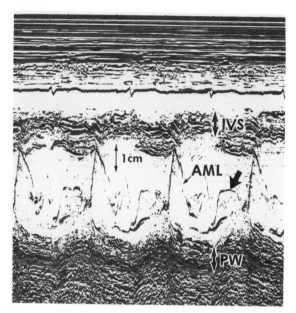

FIGURE 11 Echocardiogram from a presumably normal 14-year-old boy shows classic systolic anterior motion (arrow) of the mitral valve in the absence of asymmetric septal hypertrophy. IVS, interventricular septum; AML, anterior mitral leaflet; PML, posterior mitral leaflet; PW, posterior wall.

at 90°. Second, abnormal septal wall motion may imply disease of the LAD coronary artery but does not denote its location as being proximal or distal to the first septal perforating artery.

M-mode echocardiography cannot even consistently distinguish patients with coronary artery disease from normal subjects, since many patients with severe coronary artery obstruction have normal ventricular function at rest. With present techniques, it is also very difficult to obtain good echocardiograms from patients who are exercising. It appears that the primary indication for echocardiography in a patient with chest pain, whether it is typical of angina pectoris or not, is detection of a cause of ischemia other than coronary artery obstruction, such as mitral valve prolapse, asymmetric septal hypertrophy, aortic valve disease, or pericarditis (in the presence of an effusion).

The Cardiomyopathies

Echocardiography is extremely useful in the characterization of the various forms of cardiomyopathies, since it permits assessment of the dimensions of the left and right ventricles and the left atrium in addition to left ventricular wall thickness. The hypertrophic type of cardiomyopathy is diagnosed by an increase in muscle mass and asymmetric septal hypertrophy, with little or no increase in ventricular cavity size. The congestive type is associated with a moderate increase

in muscle mass without a change in wall thickness, hypokinetic wall motion, and an increase in ventricular cavity size. The restrictive type has a moderately increased cavity size and muscle mass but no distinguishing echocardiographic features, since the major defect is loss of compliance with restriction of diastolic filling of the ventricles.

IDIOPATHIC HYPERTROPHIC SUBAORTIC STENOSIS

Echocardiography is the "gold standard" for idiopathic hypertrophic subaortic stenosis (IHSS), also called hypertrophic cardiomyopathy. It is a sensitive and reliable technique for detecting asymmetric septal hypertrophy (ASH), which is considered the unifying link in the spectrum of hypertrophic cardiomyopathies. Asymmetric septal hypertrophy and systolic anterior motion (SAM) of the mitral valve are the two most important echocardiographic criteria for the diagnosis of IHSS. SAM without ASH has been reported in patients without detectable cardiovascular disease (Fig. 11),[40] and patients with familial hypertrophic cardiomyopathy can occasionally have concentric hypertrophy. These latter two findings are probably relatively uncommon and therefore modify but do not negate the commonly held concepts that patients with SAM usually have hypertrophic cardiomyopathy, and it is the rare patient with hypertrophic cardiomyopathy who does not have ASH on echocardiographic study.[41]

The thickness of the interventricular septum and posterior left ventricular wall must be measured accurately in order to make the diagnosis of IHSS. An accurate determination of the septal/posterior wall ratio requires that the endocardial surface of the right and left sides of the ventricular septum and the endocardial and the epicardial echoes of the posterior ventricular wall be well delineated (Fig. 12). The entire septum should be scanned and only the thinnest portion used for determining septal thickness.[42] Avoid identifying right ventricular trabeculations or portions of the tricuspid valve apparatus as the right side of the spectrum (Fig. 13). Improper beam angulation can result in a tracing suggestive of a thickened septum in normal subjects.

In the experience of Shah et al.,[43] asymmetric septal hypertrophy could be technically determined in no more than 75 percent of the patients with IHSS. Therefore, the diagnosis should only be made from echocardiograms of good diagnostic quality. ASH is not a specific echocardiographic sign for IHSS. An increase in the septal/posterior wall ratio has been described in normal newborns, in children with congenital heart disease, in adults with right ventricular pressure overload lesions, in professional athletes with

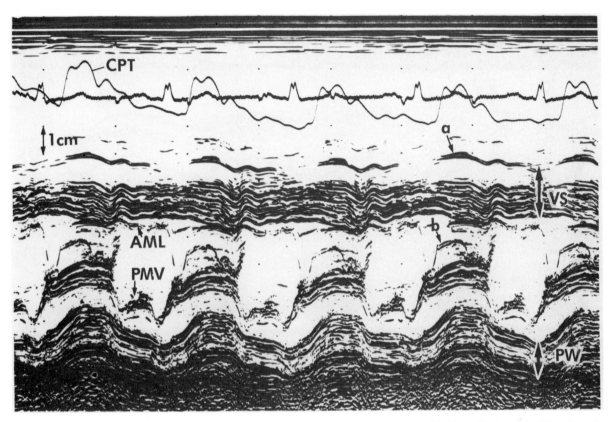

FIGURE 12 Echogram taken at the tips of the mitral valve leaflets from a patient with idiopathic hypertrophic subaortic stenosis. Asymmetric septal hypertrophy is confirmed by the almost 2:1 ratio of the ventricular septum to the posterior wall. The correct diagnosis of asymmetric septal hypertrophy must include accurate measurement of the true right side of the septum (arrow a). Systolic anterior motion of the mitral valve is demonstrated (arrow b). The carotid pulse shows the spike and dome pattern typical of IHSS. CPT, carotid pulse tracing; VS, ventricular septum; AML, anterior mitral leaflet; PW, posterior wall; PML; posterior mitral leaflet.

physiologic left ventricular hypertrophy, in patients with malignant hypertension, and in patients with inferior or true posterior myocardial infarction who have alterations in septal and left ventricular posterior wall thickness measurements.[44]

In order to detect SAM, the entire mitral valve must be recorded at its free edge where the ultrasound beam visualizes both the anterior and the posterior leaflets. The peak of the SAM should precede the peak of the posterior endocardium in actual cases. False negative diagnoses may occur if the anterior mitral valve leaflet is recorded too close to the annulus where only truncated motion may be seen and where the systolic anterior motion may be completely missed. False positive diagnoses of IHSS frequently result when the motion of the mitral annulus is mistaken for SAM, so-called pseudo-SAM. Pseudo-SAM is an exaggeration of the normal anterior motion of the mitral valve during systole that parallels the left ventricular posterior wall motion during systole and into diastole. It may be seen in pericardial effusion, atrial septal defect, mitral valve prolapse, and ventricular aneurysm.

If the following constellation of echo findings is obtained, erroneous echocardiography diagnoses of IHSS will be avoided:

1 Evidence of asymmetric septal hypertrophy with an interventricular septal/posterior left ventricular wall (IVS/PLVW) ratio in excess of 1.3.[42] Some echocardiographers prefer to diagnose ASH only when this ratio is greater than 1.5.[45] However, this definition would exclude patients with clear-cut IHSS hemodynamics and true anatomic septal hypertrophy.

2 Systolic anterior motion (SAM) of the anterior mitral valve leaflet.

3 Narrow left ventricular outflow tract.

4 Normal left ventricular hemodynamics.

5 Aortic valve preclosure.

Presence of any one echocardiographic sign should not, in itself, be considered diagnostic. For instance, early systolic closure of the aortic valve, which is a frequent finding in hypertrophic cardiomyopathy with

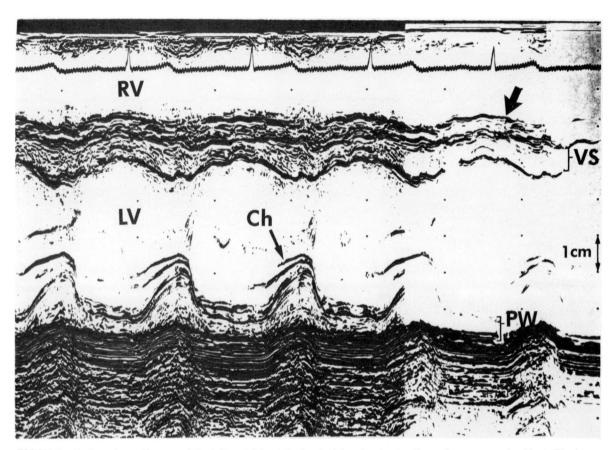

FIGURE 13 An echocardiogram of the left ventricle at the level of the chordae tendineae from a normal subject. The heavy arrow points to a structure anterior to the right side of the interventricular septum, which represents either a portion of the tricuspid valve apparatus or trabeculations within the right ventricle. If this structure is incorrectly included in the measurement of septal thickness, the ventricular septum will be spuriously thickened and asymmetric septal hypertrophy will be suspected. Correct use of the attenuation control, at the right portion of the tracing, reveals the true septal thickness. RV, right ventricle; LV, left ventricle; VS, ventricular septum; PW, posterior wall; Ch, chordae tendineae.

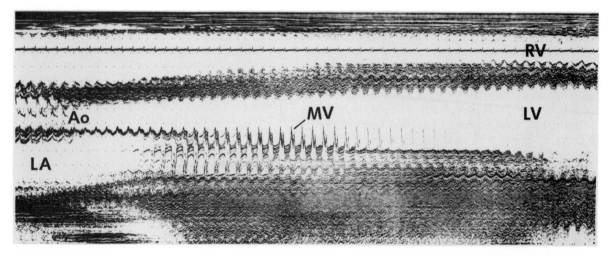

FIGURE 14 Condensed M-mode scan from a patient with congestive cardiomyopathy. The left ventricular cavity is markedly dilated and does not taper at the cardiac apex. Ventricular wall motion is decreased. Ao, aorta; LA, left atrium; MV, mitral valve; LV, left ventricle; RV, right ventricle.

a resting gradient, has occasionally been seen in discrete subaortic stenosis, in severe mitral regurgitation, and in congestive cardiomyopathy.

CONGESTIVE CARDIOMYOPATHY

The diagnosis of congestive cardiomyopathy is readily confirmed by echocardiography, obviating the need for cardiac catheterization in almost all cases. In patients presenting with congestive heart failure, the diagnosis can be made at the bedside and confirmed by echocardiography. The ability to assess left ventricular size and function, however, has permitted the echocardiographic diagnosis of cardiomyopathy to be made before congestive manifestations are apparent. The use of the condensed M-mode scan (Fig. 14) and analysis of all four heart valves (Fig. 15) with typical findings is virtually diagnostic. Confusion may occur in the patient who has ischemic heart disease with ventricular aneurysm. Furthermore, end-stage ischemic heart disease may be indistinguishable from end-stage congestive cardiomyopathy.

Pericardial Diseases

Echocardiography is currently the most sensitive and specific procedure for the diagnosis of pericardial ef-

fusion. The echocardiographic detection and serial follow-up of the presence and approximate size of pericardial fluid is more accurate than any other method and is associated with greater facility than radiographic and isotopic techniques.[46] Despite its usefulness, however, there are several pitfalls in the diagnosis of pericardial effusion:

1 Excess gain can mask the pericardial effusion by "filling in" the echo-free area.

2 One can mistake the mitral annulus for the posterior endocardial wall, especially with the transducer pointing medially, and mistake the relative echo-free endocardial-epicardial space (myocardium) for an effusion (Fig. 6). This can be avoided by first identifying the mitral valve and then sweeping toward the apex of the left ventricle to identify the chordae tendineae, endocardial, epicardial, and pericardial echoes. The pericardium is virtually a nonmoving flat line when there is significant pericardial effusion.

3 The presence of a left pleural effusion can complicate the demonstration of a pericardial effusion. The best means of distinguishing a pleural effusion from a pericardial effusion is a scan to the left atrium. The echo-free space representative of a pericardial effusion usually ends at the left ventricular-left atrial junction; at this level, the pericardium is tightly bound to the left atrial wall by its reflection on the pulmonary veins, preventing accumulation of fluid behind the left atrium. Occasionally, however, in the presence of large effusions, pericardial fluid may ex-

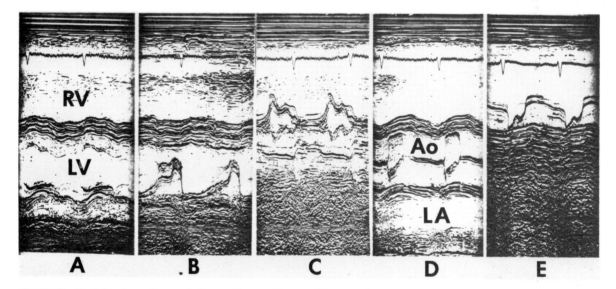

FIGURE 15 This echocardiogram is from a 34-year-old man with congestive cardiomyopathy. *A.* A dilated left ventricle and a markedly dilated right ventricle with dyskinetic motion of the septum and hypokinetic motion of the posterior wall. *B.* The mitral valve shows decreased excursion. The valve fails to open fully with the onset of diastole suggestive of elevated initial diastolic pressure; atrial systole causes the valve to open more completely. *C.* The tricuspid valve with diminished excursion. There is a prominent B point on the closing slope suggestive of elevated end-diastolic pressure. *D.* The reduced amplitude of the aorta and the aortic valve which gradually closes throughout systole are consistent with decreased forward cardiac output. The left atrium is enlarged. *E.* The pulmonic valve shows a diminished *a* dip, rapid systolic opening, and a significant notch in midsystole characteristic of pulmonary hypertension.

tend posteriorly to the left atrium and into the oblique pericardial sinus.

4 The presence of a large left atrium or left ventricular aneurysm extending inferiorly so that a portion of the atrium is posterior to the left ventricular wall may cause a false positive examination.

5 An anterior echo-free space of up to 50 mm in depth can be produced by having the patient in the left lateral position (and/or leaning forward); by an epicardial fat pad; by a homogeneous, localized thrombus; or by a pericardial cyst.[47] In general, it is unlikely that an anterior clear space results from a pericardial effusion in the absence of a posterior effusion.

6 The presence of a loculated effusion can cause a false negative diagnosis. This is most likely to occur in the presence of adhesions secondary to previous infection or cardiac surgery.

Pericardial fibrosis or a pericardial tumor may, by separating the posterior pericardium and epicardium, mimic a pericardial effusion. Several cases reaffirm that the diagnosis of a pericardial effusion should be made cautiously when the echogram shows separation of the epicardium and pericardium.

Although there have been some studies correlating the size of the effusion with the size of the sonolucent area behind the left ventricle, it is our experience that the quantity of pericardial fluid can be estimated in only a gross way (minimal, small, moderate, large).

A very large pericardial effusion may cause the heart to move freely within the pericardial sac. This type of excessive pendulous motion of the heart within a very large pericardial effusion causes the ventricles to move synchronously with high-amplitude oscillations and is referred to as the "swinging heart."[48] A considerable width of anterior and posterior echo-free space is visualized, between which the echoes arising from the heart itself exhibit oscillations or irregular sine-wave-like undulations of large amplitude (Fig. 16). When this occurs the anterior and posterior borders of the heart are sharply defined, but individual cardiac structures cannot be easily distinguished. This lack of proper definition of individual cardiac structures in a "swinging heart" has been attributed to (1) the large amplitude and high velocity of oscillations of the heart as a whole, which may obscure the details of individual valvular or endocardial echoes; and (2) the fact that most of the ultrasound energy is reflected back from the anterior pericardial effusion and the strong interface between it and the anterior right ven-

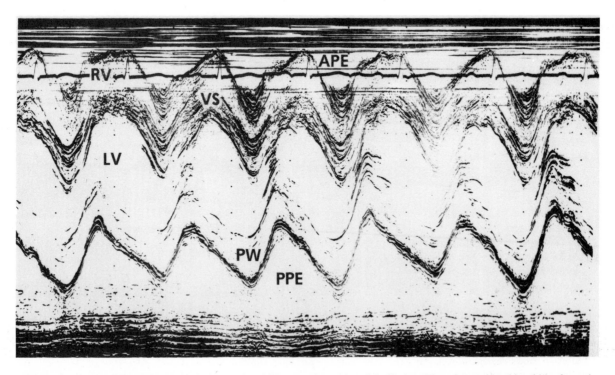

FIGURE 16 The echocardiogram is from a patient with a massive pericardial effusion. There is considerable width of anterior and posterior echo-free space visualized, between which echoes arising from the heart itself exhibit irregular sine-wave-like oscillations of large amplitude. The anterior and posterior borders of the heart are sharply defined. This abnormal oscillatory motion of the heart as a whole is referred to as a "swinging heart." APE, anterior pericardial effusion; RV, right ventricle; VS, ventricular septum; LV, left ventricle; PW, posterior wall; PPE, posterior pericardial effusion.

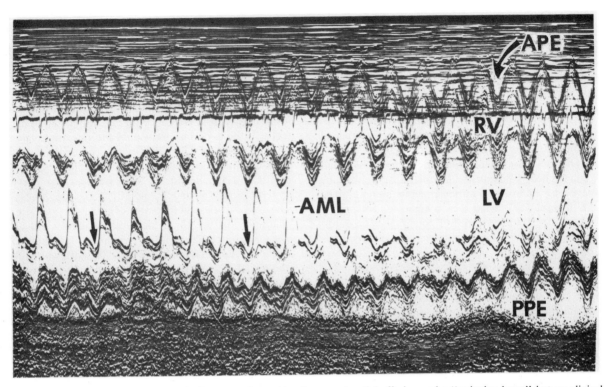

FIGURE 17 The echocardiogram is from a patient with a large pericardial effusion and a ''swinging heart'' but no clinical evidence of mitral valve prolapse. The heart may swing within the pericardial sac and distort the normal motion pattern of both walls of the heart and the mitral valve. The arrows point to holosystolic posterior motion of the mitral valve, so-called pseudo prolapse. APE, anterior pericardial effusion; PPE, posterior pericardial effusion; AML, anterior mitral leaflet; RV, right ventricle; LV, left ventricle.

tricular surface, so that relatively little ultrasound energy penetrates to the posterior cardiac structures.

It is not generally recognized that patients with large pericardial effusions may exhibit a classical ''swinging heart'' appearance in some scans, whereas in other scans at the same examination, an appearance suggestive of a moderate or even small effusion is obtained. When the transducer is directed caudally, the ''swinging heart'' appears as a narrow undulating band of indistinct echoes, with a large expanse of echo-free space anterior and posterior to it. On the other hand, with a cephalad transducer direction, the posterior echo-free space decreases markedly in width while the cardiac diameter (right ventricular anterior wall to left ventricular posterior wall) increases, the anterior echo-free space remaining the same. When a ''swinging heart'' appearance is detected by echocardiography, the transducer beam should be directed more cephalad toward the base of the heart, where it may result in diminution in the swinging motion and better visualization of individual cardiac structures. Conversely, in patients who apparently have only a moderate-sized pericardial effusion, aiming the transducer beam caudally (downward) and medially may reveal a ''swinging heart'' appearance, suggesting that the effusion is

probably larger than it was originally thought to be.

As a consequence of the free swinging of the heart, abnormal motion of various structures, including the ventricular walls, interventricular septum, and the heart valves, have been noted. Echoes of various cardiac structures, such as the ventricular septum and mitral valve, may show exaggerated motion, sometimes producing an apparent abnormality akin to that seen in various disease states. Thus, ''pseudo systolic anterior motion of the mitral valve,'' ''pseudo paradoxical'' septal motion and ''pseudo mitral prolapse'' have been described.[49] In addition, midsystolic notching or premature closure motion of the aortic or pulmonary valve has occasionally been noted.

The term ''pseudo prolapse'' refers to a posterior motion of the mitral valve in systole, associated with a corresponding posterior systolic motion of the whole heart (including the adjacent left ventricular posterior wall), in patients with large pericardial effusions (Fig. 17). After drainage of the effusion, such abnormal mitral and ventricular wall motion promptly disappears. Vignola et al. have noted that the contour of such ''pseudo mitral prolapse'' on the echogram depended on the heart rate.[50] The ''pseudo prolapse'' appeared in early or late systole if the heart rate exceeded 120 beats per minute, and a holosystolic "pseudo prolapse" appeared if the rate was below 120 beats per minute.

Echocardiography has not been especially helpful in determining the presence or absence of cardiac tamponade. Cardiac tamponade is a clinical syndrome, and the diagnosis should be made on the basis of clinical findings alone, since the hemodynamic significance of a pericardial effusion cannot be determined by the volume of pericardial fluid present.

The most consistent echocardiographic abnormality described in patients with constrictive pericarditis has been paradoxical ventricular septal motion. Since this abnormality may be seen in numerous conditions, echocardiographic evidence of constrictive pericarditis is tenuous.[22,24] Since restrictive cardiomyopathy is the major condition that must be differentiated from constrictive pericarditis, an estimate of pericardial thickness and/or calcification would be valuable; however, with present techniques, this has not been accomplished satisfactorily.

Congenital Heart Defects

Single-dimension M-mode echocardiography has proved to be a valuable noninvasive method in pediatric cardiology. It may provide valuable information so that cardiac catheterization and surgery can be planned with greater facility. Although M-mode scanning provides some spatial orientation, it is at best qualitative. When one is interested in the interrelationship of large structures, such as the ventricular chambers and great arteries, the accurate assessment of valve size and motion, and the demonstration of septal defects, it is possible that the newer two-dimensional imaging systems may prove to be superior.

ACYANOTIC LESIONS

A dilated right ventricle and abnormal interventricular septal motion are extremely sensitive echocardiographic findings for confirming the diagnosis of an atrial septal defect. Patients with small atrial septal defects, however, may not show these abnormalities. The combination of an enlarged right ventricle and paradoxic motion of the interventricular septum is evidence only for right ventricular volume overload and is a nonspecific finding. It must always be analyzed in light of the complete patient data base. A large right ventricular dimension and paradoxic motion of the interventricular septum may be seen in a variety of patients with right ventricular volume overload, including both secundum and primum atrial septal defects, anomalous pulmonary venous return, and tricuspid and pulmonic regurgitation. In addition, paradoxic

septal motion without right ventricular dilatation may be seen in patients with septal infarction, with left bundle branch block, and after open heart surgery.[51] The magnitude of the left-to-right shunt cannot be determined by echocardiography and the actual communication between the atria is rarely identified echocardiographically. Paradoxic motion of the septum is not invariable even in patients with large atrial septal defects. In fact, normal motion of the interventricular septum can be seen in patients with atrial septal defect in association with pulmonary/systemic flow ratios of less than 1.5, moderate to severe pulmonary artery hypertension, valvular pulmonic stenosis, or an associated left ventricular volume overload lesion. Demonstration of true paradoxic septal motion is not always accurate. False positive findings may occur if the upper septum is analyzed, since the aorta normally moves anteriorly with systole, dragging this superior portion of the septum along with it. The motion of the interventricular septum is therefore best evaluated just inferior to the edge of the mitral valve at the level of the chordae tendineae. The entire septum should be studied to ensure that the midportion of the septum at the level of the chordae is recorded. It appears that enlargement of the right ventricle and ventricular outflow tract is a more reliable sign of right ventricular volume overload, than is paradoxic movement of the septum.

The secundum and primum types of atrial septal defects are readily distinguishable by echocardiography.[22,32,51] The major distinguishing feature between a secundum type of atrial septal defect (ASD) and an ostium primum type of endocardial cushion defect is the mitral valve echogram. In secundum ASD, the mitral valve is normal. In the primum variety, the mitral valve is grossly abnormal. It is displaced anteriorly by abnormal attachment to the septum, causing the anterior leaflet to approximate the septum in diastole and the tricuspid valve in systole. Echocardiography is virtually diagnostic for the presence of an endocardial cushion defect, but it cannot reliably differentiate the partial type (ostium primum ASD) from the complete type. However, the integrity of the ventricular septum is well preserved in the primum defect, but septal dropout frequently occurs in the complete variety.[52]

M-mode echocardiography is insensitive in many common acyanotic lesions such as ventricular septal defect, coarctation of the aorta, and patent ductus arteriosus, since the primary abnormality cannot be visualized.

CYANOTIC LESIONS

M-mode echocardiography has been very helpful in the infant with cyanosis. It is very sensitive and specific for the diagnosis of the hypoplastic left-sided heart syndrome. It is also very reliable in differentiating the hypoplastic left-sided heart syndrome from noncardiac causes with similar shocklike features and from critical aortic stenosis in the first week of life.

Although sensitivity and specificity of M-mode echocardiography have not been determined for the majority of cyanotic lesions, a characteristic constellation of echocardiographic findings is virtually diagnostic. Failure to record the characteristic echocardiographic abnormalities, however, does not exclude the condition in question. For instance, the echocardiographic findings of a large right ventricle and a huge tricuspid valve with delayed closure after the mitral valve are virtually diagnostic of Ebstein's anomaly of the tricuspid valve. The absence of these findings, however, does not exclude the diagnosis. The absence of a recordable tricuspid valve in a newborn infant is virtually diagnostic of tricuspid atresia, but failure to record a structure is not always proof of its absence.

The most sensitive and most characteristic echocardiographic finding in tetralogy of Fallot is an abrupt ending of echoes from the interventricular septum together with significant overriding of the septal defect by the aorta.[53] Although this echocardiographic feature can separate patients with tetralogy of Fallot from normal subjects if the transducer is not placed in an unusually high position on the chest wall (e.g., in the second left intercostal space), a similar echocardiogram can be produced by truncus arteriosus or pulmonary atresia. These latter conditions, however, can be excluded if the pulmonary valve can be demonstrated by echo. It should not be assumed, however, that failure to identify the pulmonary valve excludes tetralogy of Fallot, since in tetralogy, the pulmonary valve may be small or immobile and difficult to record.

Although the M-mode ultrasound pattern can be used to demonstrate the altered spatial relationship of the great vessels in patients with *d*-transposition of the great arteries, it is a one-dimensional system which visualizes only a narrow portion of the heart. The anatomic relationship of adjacent structures is therefore not well defined, and the recording gives no information regarding simultaneous movement of contiguous structures which occasionally are quite different from the actual anatomy. Two-dimensional real-time echocardiographic systems, however, should greatly improve the accuracy of diagnosing anatomic abnormalities. Contrast echocardiography is a sensitive method for detection of intracardiac right-to-left shunt. When combined with M-mode and two-dimensional echocardiography, contrast echocardiography assumes an invaluable role in the recognition of cardiac anatomy and the hemodynamic status of patients with various congenital lesions.[54]

Although most of the echocardiography literature referable to cyanotic heart defects has emphasized the recognition of anatomic features, the most sensitive use of echocardiography appears to be in the preoperative and postoperative evaluation of ventricular performance. Because these anomalies are global in nature, regional wall function assessed by M-mode echocardiography will adequately reflect total left ventricular function.

CONCLUSION

Single-dimension M-mode echocardiography is definitely limited by beam width and lack of spatial orientation. Despite these limitations the technique has become a valuable diagnostic tool. The value and limitations of M-mode echocardiography have been highlighted in this chapter. With the addition of real-time two-dimensional systems (sector scanning and phased array equipment) and pulse Doppler systems to standard M-mode echocardiography, the scope of noninvasive methods in cardiology will be greatly increased.

REFERENCES

1 Roelandt, J., Van Dorp, W. C., and Bom, M.: Resolution Problems in Echocardiography: A Source of Interpretation Error, *Am. J. Cardiol.,* 37:256, 1976.

2 Kotler, M. N., Segal, B. L., Mintz, G. S., Parry, W. R. et al.: Pitfalls and Limitations of M-mode Echocardiography, *Am. Heart J.,* 94:227, 1977.

3 Linhart, J. W., Mintz, G. S., Segal, B. L., Dawai, N., and Kotler, M. N.: Left Ventricular Volume Measurement by Echocardiography: Fact or Fiction?, *Am. J. Cardiol.,* 36:114, 1975.

4 Felner, J. M., Blumenstein, B. A., and Schlant, R. C.: Variability in Echocardiographic Measurements, in press.

5 Feigenbaum, H.: "Echocardiography," 2d ed., Lea & Febiger, Philadelphia, 1976, p. 297.

6 Popp, R. L., Filly, K., Brown, O. R., and Harrison, D. C.: Effects of Transducer Placement on Echocardiographic Measurements of Left Ventricular Dimensions, *Am. J. Cardiol.,* 35:537, 1975.

7 Teichholz, E., Kreulen, T. H., Herman, M. V., and Gorlin, R.: Problems in Echocardiographic Volume Determinations: Echocardiographic-Angiographic Correlations in the Presence or Absence of Asynergy, *Am. J. Cardiol.,* 37:7, 1976.

8 Hagan, A. D., Francis, G. S., Sahn, D. J., Karliner,

J. S., Friedman, W. F., and O'Rourke, R. A.: Ultrasound Evaluation of Systolic Anterior Septal Motion in Patients with and without Right Ventricular Volume Overload, *Circulation,* 50:248, 1974.

9 Fortuin, N. J., and Pawsey, C. G.: The Evaluation of Left Ventricular Function by Echocardiography, *Am. J. Med.,* 63:1, 1977.

10 Ewy, G. A., Jones, S. E., and Friedman, M. J.: Echocardiographic Detection of Adriamycin Heart Disease, *Proc. Am. Soc. Clin. Oncol.* 16:228, 1975.

11 Schlant, R. C., Felner, J. M., Heymsfield, S. B., Gilbert, C. A., Shulman, N. B., Tuttle, E. P., and Blumenstein, B. A.: Echocardiographic Studies of Left Ventricular Anatomy and Function in Essential Hypertension, *Cardiovasc. Med.,* 2:477, 1977.

12 Brown, O. R., Harrison, D. C., and Popp, R. L.: An Improved Method for Echographic Detection of Left Atrium Enlargement, *Circulation,* 50:58, 1974.

13 Edler, I., and Gustafson, A.: Ultrasound Cardiogram in Mitral Stenosis, *Acta Med. Scand.,* 159:85, 1957.

14 Levisman, J. A., Abbasi, A. S., and Pearce, M. L.: Posterior Mitral Leaflet Motion in Mitral Stenosis, *Circulation,* 51:511, 1975.

15 Cope, G. D., Kisslo, J. A., Johnson, M. L., and Behar, V. S.: A Reassessment of the Echocardiogram in Mitral Stenosis, *Circulation,* 52:664, 1975.

16 Sahn, D. J., Wood, J., Allen, H. D., Peoples, W., and Goldberg, S. J.: Echocardiographic Spectrum of Mitral Valve Motion in Children with and without Mitral Valve Prolapse: The Nature of False Positive Diagnosis, *Am. J. Cardiol.,* 39:422, 1977.

17 Markiewicz, W., Stoner, J., London, E., Hunt, S. A., and Popp, R. L.: Mitral Valve Prolapse in One Hundred Presumably Healthy Young Female, *Circulation,* 53:464, 1976.

18 Popp, R. L., Brown, O. R., and Silverman, J. F.: Echocardiographic Abnormalities in the Mitral Valve Prolapse Syndrome, *Circulation,* 49:428, 1974.

19 Brown, O. R., and Kloster, F. E.: Echocardiographic Criteria for Mitral Valve Prolapse. Effect of Transducer Position, *Circulation,* 52 (suppl. 2): 165, 1975. (Abstract.)

20 Gilbert, B. W., Haney, R. S., Crawford, F., McClellan, J., Gallis, H. A., Johnson, M. L., and Kisslo, J. A.: Two-dimensional Echocardiographic Assessment of Vegetative Endocarditis, *Circulation,* 55:346, 1977.

21 Wann, L. S., Dillon, J. C., Weyman, A. E., and Feigenbaum, H.: Echocardiography in Bacterial Endocarditis, *N. Engl. J. Med.,* 295:135, 1976.

22 Felner, J. M., and Schlant, R. C.: "Echocardiography: A Teaching Atlas," Grune & Stratton, Inc., New York, 1976.

23 Pratt, C., Whitcomb, C., and Neumann, A.: Relationship of Vegetations on Echocardiogram to the Clinical Course in Systemic Emboli and Bacterial Vegetations, *Am. J. Cardiol.,* 41:384, 1978.

24 Roy, P., Tajik, A. J., Giuliani, E. R., Schattenberg, T. T., Gau, G. T., and Frye, R. L.: Spectrum of Echocardiographic Findings in Bacterial Endocarditis, *Circulation,* 53:474, 1976.

25 Mercier, L. A., Sutton, M. G., and Lie, J. T.: A Review of 40 patients with Atrial Myxoma Seen Over a 20-Year Period, *Am. J. Cardiol.,* 41:437, 1978.

26 Goodwin, J. F.: Symposium on Cardiac Tumors. Introduction: The Spectrum of Cardiac Tumors, *Am. J. Cardiol.,* 21:307, 1968.

27 Petsas, A. A., Gotlieb, S., Kingsley, B., Segal, B. L., and Myerburg, R. L.: Echocardiographic Diagnosis of Left Atrial Myxoma, *Br. Heart J.,* 38:627, 1976.

28 Kotler, M. N., Segal, B. L., and Parry, W. R.: Echocardiographic and Phonocardiographic Evaluation of Prosthetic Heart Valves, in M. N. Kotler, and B. L. Segal (eds.), "Clinical Echocardiography," F. A. Davis Company, Philadelphia, 1978, p. 187.

29 Johnson, M. L., Warren, S. G., Waugh, R. A., Kisslo, J. A., Sabistan, D. C., and Lester, R. G.: Echocardiography of the Aortic Valve in Nonrheumatic Left Ventricular Outflow Tract Lesions, *Radiology,* 112:677, 1974.

30 Nanda, N. C., Gramiak, R., Manning, J., Mahoney, F. B., Lipchik, E. O., and DeWeese, J. A.: Echocardiographic Recognition of the Congenital Bicuspid Aortic Valve, *Circulation,* 49:870, 1974.

31 Radford, D. J., Bloom, K. J., Kzukawa, T., Moes, C. A. F., and Rowe, R. D.: Echocardiographic Assessment of Bicuspid Aortic Valves. Angiographic and Pathological Correlates, *Circulation,* 33:80, 1976.

32 Felner, J. M.: Echocardiography: Acyanotic Congenital Heart Lesions, in M. N. Kotler and B. L. Segal (eds), "Clinical Echocardiography," F. A. Davis Company, Philadelphia, 1978, p. 251.

32a Shah, P. M.: Echocardiography of the Aortic and Pulmonary Valves, *Prog. Cardiovasc. Dis.,* 20:457, 1978.

33 Brown, C. R., Popp, R. L., and Kloster, F. E.: Echocardiographic Criteria for Aortic Root Dissection, *Am. J. Cardiol.,* 36:17, 1975.

34 Krueger, S., Starke, H., Forker, A. D., Eliot, R. S.: Echocardiographic Mimics of Aortic Root Dissection, *Chest,* 67:441, 1975.

35 Weyman, A. E., Dillon, J. C., Feigenbaum, H., and Chang, S.: Echocardiographic Patterns of Pulmonic Valve Motion in Valvular Pulmonic Stenosis, *Am. J. Cardiol.,* 34:644, 1974.

36 Kaku, R., Neumann, A., Bommer, W., Weinert, L., and Mason, D. T.: Sensitivity and Specificity of the Pulmonic Valve Echogram in the Detection of Pulmonary Hypertension, *Am. J. Cardiol.,* 41:436, 1978.

37 Rasmussen, S., Corya, B. C., Feigenbaum, H., and

Knoebel, S. B.: Detection of Myocardial Scar Tissue by M-mode Echocardiography, *Circulation,* 57:230, 1978.

38 Chang, S., Feigenbaum, H., and Dillon, J.: Condensed M-mode Echocardiographic Scan of the Symmetrical Left Ventricle, *Chest,* 68:93, 1975.

39 Corya, B. C., Rasmussen, S., and Feigenbaum, H.: Systolic Thickening and Thinning of the Septum and Posterior Wall in Patients with Coronary Artery Disease, Congestive Cardiomyopathy and Atrial Septal Defect, *Circulation,* 55:109, 1977.

40 Mintz, G. S., Kotler, M. N., Segal, B. L., and Parry, W. R.: Systolic Anterior Motion of the Mitral Valve in the Absence of Asymmetric Septal Hypertrophy, *Circulation,* 57:256,1978.

41 Maron, B. J., Gottdiener, J. S., Roberts, W. C., Henry, W. L., Savage, D. D., and Epstein, S. E.: Left Ventricular Outflow Tract Obstruction Due to Systolic Anterior Motion of the Anterior Mitral Leaflet in Patients with Concentric Left Ventricular Hypertrophy, *Circulation,* 57:527, 1978.

42 Henry, W. L., Clark, E. C., and Epstein, S. E.: Asymmetric Septal Hypertrophy. Echocardiographic Identification of Pathognomonic Anatomic Abnormality of IHSS, *Circulation,* 47:225, 1973.

43 Shah, P. M., and Sylvester, L. J.: Echocardiography in the Diagnosis of Hypertrophic Obstructive Cardiomyopathy, *Am. J. Cardiol.,* 62:830, 1977.

44 Henning, H., O'Rourke, R. A., Crawford, M. H., Righetti, A., and Karliner, J. S.: Inferior Myocardial Infarction as a Cause of Asymmetric Septal Hypertrophy, *Am. J. Cardiol.,* 41:817, 1978.

45 Abbasi, A. S., MacAlpin, R. N., Eber, L. M., and Pearce, M. L.: Left Ventricular Hypertrophy Diagnosed by Echocardiography, *N. Engl. J. Med.,* 289:118, 1973.

46 Felner, J. M.: Echocardiography: Pericardial Diseases, in J. W. Hurst (ed.), "The Heart," 4th ed., McGraw-Hill Book Company, New York, 1978, p. 473.

47 Felner, J. M., Franch, R. H., and Fleming, W.: Echocardiographic Identification of a Pericardial Cyst, *Chest,* 68:386, 1975.

48 Warren, B. H., Lynn, R. R., and Allen, F. H.: Echocardiographic Observation of Ventricular Volume Changes and Swinging Septal Position in Massive Pericardial Effusion, *J. Clin. Ultrasound,* 3:383, 1975.

49 Levisman, J. A., and Abbasi, A. S.: Abnormal Motion of the Mitral Valve with Pericardial Effusion: Pseudo-Prolapse of the Mitral Valve, *Am. Heart J.,* 91:18, 1976.

50 Vignola, P. A., Pohost, G. M., Curfman, G. E., and Meyers, G. S.: Correlation of Echocardiographic and Clinical Findings in Patients with Pericardial Effusion, *Am. J. Cardiol.,* 37:701, 1976.

51 Felner, J. M.: Echocardiography: Congenital Heart Disease, in J. W. Hurst (ed.), "The Heart," 4th ed., McGraw-Hill Book Company, New York, 1978, p. 456.

52 Williams, R. G., and LaCorte, M. A.: Echocardiographic Evaluation of Valvular and Shunt Lesions in Children, *Prog. Cardiovasc. Dis.,* 20:423, 1978.

53 Morris, D. C., Felner, J. M., Schlant, R. C., and Franch, R.: Echocardiographic Diagnosis of Tetralogy of Fallot, *Am. J. Cardiol.,* 36:908, 1975.

54 Seward, J. B., Tajik, A. J., Spangler, J. G., and Ritter, D. G.: Echocardiographic Contrast Studies. Initial Experience, *Mayo Clin. Proc.,* 50:163, 1975.

The Use and Misuse of Digoxin Blood Levels*

THOMAS W. SMITH, M.D., GREGORY D. CURFMAN, M.D., and
LAURENCE H. GREEN, M.D.

It is much easier to write upon a disease than upon a remedy. The former is in the hands of nature, and a faithful observer, with an eye of tolerable judgment, cannot fail to delineate a likeness. The latter will ever be subject to the whims, the inaccuracies, and the blunders of mankind.

WILLIAM WITHERING, 1785[1]

Cardiac glycosides have been used in the management of congestive heart failure and certain cardiac rhythm disturbances for 200 years. Nevertheless, the clinician, as well as the research investigator, continues to face important challenges regarding the optimal use of this class of drugs. The narrow margin between therapeutic and toxic doses of digitalis, resulting in a high incidence of digitalis toxicity in clinical practice, has stimulated the development of improved methods for measuring the circulating concentrations of these drugs. A competitive binding radioimmunoassay using specific antibody is now widely used in clinical laboratories for this purpose.[2] Although cardiac glycoside serum or plasma levels† measured in this way have important clinical applicability, misuse of the serum level and errors of judgment in its interpretation may limit its usefulness or even result in suboptimal patient management. In this chapter we review the available data on proper use and interpretation of serum cardiac glycoside concentrations in the clinical context.

CARDIAC GLYCOSIDE RADIOIMMUNOASSAY

It is evident that the clinical value of serum digitalis glycoside measurements will be limited by the accuracy of the assay technique itself. The radioimmunoassay for cardiac glycosides, like other radioimmunoassays, is subject to certain pitfalls that may yield erroneous results if careful attention is not paid

---

* From the Department of Medicine, Harvard Medical School, and Peter Bent Brigham Hospital, Boston (Dr. Smith).

† Serum and plasma concentrations of cardiac glycosides studied to date are equivalent, and the term "serum" will be used for convenience to denote either serum or plasma concentrations.

to selection of antisera, to the accuracy of standards and the purity of tracers, and to appropriate counting techniques.[3] A relatively frequent cause of confusion is the presence of preexisting radioactivity in the serum sample. This is generally the result of a scanning procedure using a γ-ray-emitting isotope and may be recognized if one channel of the scintillation spectrometer is set to detect radiation of differing energy. When identified, the problem may be dealt with by prior extraction of the cardiac glycoside or by the method outlined by Butler.[4] Failure to select antisera of sufficient specificity may result in interference by endogenously or exogenously administered steroids or steroid antagonists such as spironolactone.

Further details of available techniques for measurement of circulating cardiac glycoside concentrations are provided in reviews of this subject.[5,6] With the proliferation of commercial kits for the measurement of cardiac glycoside concentrations, it is particularly important for the clinician and clinical investigator to be certain that the values reported by the laboratory are accurate. Furthermore, uncertainty can be introduced if sufficient time has not elapsed since the last previous dose to allow full equilibration of the drug between intravascular and peripheral compartments. In practice, a safe time for sampling of serum or plasma is 6 h or more after the last oral cardiac glycoside dose and 4 h or more after an intravenous dose.

RATIONALE FOR THE USE OF SERUM DIGITALIS CONCENTRATION MEASUREMENTS

Previous data suggest that a potentially useful relationship can be defined between serum digitalis concentrations and the pharmacologic effects of these drugs. First, both inotropic and toxic effects of cardiac glycosides are known to be dose-related phenomena. A large number of studies' have shown increasing serum digitalis concentrations with increasing dosage,[6] so that at least a statistical correlation would be expected between plasma levels and clinical state. Second, at least in the case of digoxin, studies in experimental animals and in man have documented a relatively constant ratio of digoxin concentration in serum or plasma to that in the myocardium.[7–10] The argument can be raised, however, that since total myocardial concentration includes drugs bound both nonspecifically and specifically to myocardial receptors, the total myocardial digitalis content cannot be assumed to bear a direct relationship to effect. Third, evidence continues to accumulate indicating that the monovalent cation transport enzyme complex (Na^+ + K^+)-adenosine triphosphatase (ATPase) is involved in at least some of the actions of cardiac glycosides.[11] This plasma membrane transport system is influenced by cardiac glycosides only when these agents are present at the outer cell surface.[12,13] Thus, at least one putative cardiac glycoside receptor is in close proximity to the extracellular compartment, providing a basis for the translation of plasma concentration to myocardial effect. Finally, experimental studies have documented a highly significant relationship between serum digoxin concentration and electrophysiologic effects on the heart.[14]

CLINICAL STUDIES ON SERUM GLYCOSIDE LEVELS

Studies continue to appear aimed at defining the relationship between serum or plasma digitalis concentrations and clinical effect. Table 1 summarizes digoxin concentration data from a number of studies, which, taken together, involve well over 1,000 patients. Mean serum digoxin concentrations in groups of patients without evidence of toxicity average about 1.4 ng/ml. Table 1 also provides data concerning the relationship between serum digoxin concentration and cardiac toxicity. Mean serum digoxin concentrations tend to be two or three times higher in patients with clinical evidence of digoxin toxicity, and the difference in mean levels between patients with evidence for toxicity and those without was statistically significant in the vast majority of studies. Analogous data regarding serum digitoxin levels are summarized in Table 2. We would emphasize that overlap of serum digitalis levels between groups with and without evidence of toxicity has been observed in most series and tends to be more pronounced in prospective, blind studies than in retrospective studies.[2,15,41] Thus, no single serum glycoside level can be selected that clearly separates toxic and nontoxic states in the usual clinical setting. Indeed, this is just what one would predict based on the many known factors which may influence individual sensitivity to the toxic effects of cardiac glycosides. For example, toxicity may be present with an average or low serum level in the setting of severe hypokalemia or advanced intrinsic heart disease, while high serum levels may not be accompanied by clinical evidence of cardiac toxicity in subjects without heart disease or in patients receiving antiarrhythmic drugs. Yet another problem exists in establishing an accurate diagnosis of digitalis toxicity, since essentially all the disturbances of cardiac impulse formation and conduction caused by digitalis excess can occur as a result of underlying heart disease, even in patients who have never received digitalis. Therefore, digitalis serum levels must be interpreted in the clinical setting of the individual patient, keeping in mind a number of variables (discussed below) that may modify the individual's response to cardiac glycosides.

FACTORS INFLUENCING INDIVIDUAL SENSITIVITY TO CARDIAC GLYCOSIDES

In some instances, discrepancies between the serum concentration and the clinical state may be caused by analytic problems in the assay procedure, but variation in individual sensitivity to the effects of cardiac glycosides for any given dose has long been appreciated on clinical grounds. Even though serum concentration data take into account variations in absorption and excretion of digitalis glycosides by individual patients, factors including severity and type of underlying heart disease, metabolic derangements, interactions with other drugs, and certain concurrent disease states further modify individual response at any given serum concentration of the drug. Several factors deserving the attention of the clinician in every instance where the cardiac glycoside dosage regimen is in question are listed in Table 3.

Underlying Heart Disease

Listed first in Table 3 because of its overriding importance is the type and severity of underlying heart disease. This is graphically demonstrated by otherwise healthy subjects who ingest massive doses of cardiac glycosides with suicidal intent.[55] Cardiac toxicity in this clinical setting is usually manifested by disturbances of atrioventricular conduction or sinoatrial exit block rather than by increased automaticity of ectopic pacemakers, as is commonly seen in patients with established heart disease. Common causes of heart disease including ischemia, cardiomyopathy, and valvular lesions may result in electrophysiologic instability that will decrease tolerance to cardiac glycosides. The more severe and advanced the heart disease, the more likely is the existence of factors such as myocardial

TABLE 1
Serum or plasma digoxin concentrations: Patients with and without toxicity

Source	Methods	Mean concentration (ng/ml)		Statistical significance
		Patients without toxicity	Patients with toxicity	
Beller et al.[15]	Radioimmunoassay	1.0	2.3	Yes
Bertler, Redfors[16]	^{86}Rb uptake	0.9	2.4	Yes
Bertler et al.[17]	^{86}Rb uptake	1.4	3.1	Yes
Brooker, Jelliffe[18]	Enzymatic displacement	1.4	3.1	Yes
Burnett, Conklin[19]	ATPase inhibition	1.2	5.7	Yes
Carruthers et al.[20]	Radioimmunoassay	1.21	2.76	
Chamberlain et al.[21]	Radioimmunoassay	1.4	3.1	Yes
Doering et al.[22]	Radioimmunoassay	1.02	3.07	Yes
Evered, Chapman[23]	Radioimmunoassay	1.38	3.36	Yes
Fogelman et al.[24]	Radioimmunoassay	1.4	1.7	No
Grahame-Smith, Everest[25]	^{86}Rb uptake	2.4	5.7	Yes
*Hayes et al.[26]	Radioimmunoassay			
Infants		2.8	4.4	Yes
Children		1.3	3.4	Yes
Hoeschen, Proveda[27]	Radioimmunoassay	0.8–1.3	2.8	Yes
Howard et al.[28]	Radioimmunoassay	0.97	0.91	No
Huffman et al.[29]	Radioimmunoassay	1.49	3.32	Yes
Iisalo, Dahl, Sundquist[30]	Radioimmunoassay	1.2	3.1	Yes
Johnston, Pinkus, Down[31]	Radioimmunoassay	1.0	3.15	Yes
*Krasula et al.[32]	Radioimmunoassay			
Infants		1.7	3.6	Yes
Children		1.1	2.9	Yes
Lader, Bye, Marsdin[33]	Radioimmunoassay	1.1	2.2	Yes
*McCredie et al.[34]	Radioimmunoassay			
Infants		3.45		
Children		1.41	3.81	Yes
Morrison, Killip, Stason[35]	Radioimmunoassay	0.76	3.35	Not stated
Oliver, Parker, Parker[36]	Radioimmunoassay	1.6	3.0	Yes
Park et al.[37]	Radioimmunoassay	1.1	3.8	Yes
Ritzmann et al.[38]	^{86}Rb uptake	1.2 (median)	5.5 (median)	Yes
Scherrmann and Bourdon[39]	Radioimmunoassay	1.37	4.58	Yes
Singh et al.[40]	Radioimmunoassay	2.91	4.79	Yes
Smith, Butler, Haber[2]	Radioimmunoassay	1.3	3.3	Yes
Smith, Haber[41]	Radioimmunoassay	1.4	3.7	Yes
Waldorff, Buch[42]	Radioimmunoassay	1.0	2.3	Yes
Weissel et al.[43]	Radioimmunoassay	1.38	2.97	Yes
Whiting et al.[44]	Radioimmunoassay	1.4	3.5	Yes
Zeegers et al.[45]	Radioimmunoassay	1.6	4.4	Yes

* Pediatric patients.

fibrosis, focal ischemia, and ventricular dilatation with stretching of subendocardial Purkinje fibers that predispose to rhythm disturbances.

Electrolyte and Acid-Base Disturbances

Disturbances of potassium balance are known to influence the action of cardiac glycosides. Cardiac uptake of digoxin is modified by serum potassium concentrations, tending to increase with decreasing serum potassium. This appears to be related, at least in part, to an allosteric effect on cardiac glycoside binding to $(Na^+ + K^+)$-ATPase.[56,57] Atrioventricular conduction disturbances can be caused or exacerbated by greatly elevated serum potassium concentrations.[58] Diuretic therapy, insulin administration or carbohydrate loading, renal disease, and acid-base imbalance are all potential causes of significant alterations in potassium homeostasis and deserve particular attention in patients receiving digitalis.

Changes in serum concentrations of other electrolytes may also affect individual sensitivity to digitalis.

TABLE 2
Serum or plasma digitoxin concentrations: Patients with and without toxicity

Source	Methods	Mean concentration (ng/ml)		Statistical significance
		Patients without toxicity	Patients with toxicity	
Beller et al.[15]	Radioimmunoassay	20	34	Yes
Bentley et al.[46]	ATPase inhibition	23	39	Yes
Brooker, Jelliffe[18]	Enzymatic displacement	31.8	48.8	Not stated
Chiche et al.[47]	Radioimmunoassay	25.4	57	Yes
Dessaint[48]	Radioimmunoassay	26.8	96	Yes
Hillestad et al.[49]	[86]Rb uptake	16.8	28.3	Yes
Lukas, Peterson[50]	Double isotope dilution derivative	20	43-67 (range)	Not stated
Morrison, Killip[51]	Radioimmunoassay	25 (0.1 mg/day)	53	Yes
Peters et al.[52]	Radioimmunoassay	28.8	56.4	Yes
Rasmussen et al.[53]	[86]Rb uptake	16.6	48.7	Not stated
Ritzmann et al.[38]	[86]Rb uptake	20.5 (median)	37 (median)	Yes
Smith[54]	Radioimmunoassay	17	34	Yes

Administration of magnesium ion can suppress digitalis-induced arrhythmias,[59] and there is evidence that digitalis-induced K^+ efflux from the myocardium is reduced by magnesium ion.[60] Hypomagnesemia has been reported to predispose to digitalis toxicity.[61] Although the epidemiologic importance of magnesium depletion as a cause of enhanced digitalis sensitivity has not been completely defined, the frequent occurrence of Mg^{2+} depletion with diuretic therapy should keep the clinician alert to the possible interactions of magnesium ion and digitalis.

Increased serum calcium may enhance ventricular automaticity, and this effect may be additive to or even synergistic with the effect of digitalis.[62] Conversely, patients with digitalis intoxication have been reported to respond successfully to calcium-chelating agents.[63] Although animal experiments have yielded somewhat variable results,[64,65] caution is advisable in view of the possibility of reduced digitalis tolerance

TABLE 3
Factors influencing individual sensitivity to digitalis

Type and severity of underlying cardiac disease
Serum electrolyte derangements
  Hypokalemia or hyperkalemia
  Hypomagnesemia
  Hypercalcemia
  Hyponatremia
Acid-base imbalance
Concomitant drug administration
  Anesthetics
  Catecholamines and sympathomimetics
  Antiarrhythmic agents
Thyroid status
Renal function
Autonomic nervous system tone
Respiratory disease

when treating patients with hypercalcemia or when administering calcium intravenously to digitalized patients.

Reports in the literature suggest that acid-base disturbances may cause increased sensitivity to digitalis. Certainly, alterations in potassium homeostasis that follow shifts in hydrogen ion concentration will affect myocardial binding of digitalis glycosides. Although disturbances of acid-base balance per se have not been convincingly shown to precipitate digitalis toxicity in clinical studies, the experimental literature suggests caution in the use of digitalis in patients with marked acidosis or alkalosis.

Drug Interactions

Other drugs that are being taken concurrently by the patient can affect the response to digitalis glycosides through several mechanisms. Drugs including cholestyramine, neomycin, antacids, and kaolin-pectin can decrease gastrointestinal absorption of digoxin, thereby altering the serum and myocardial levels ultimately achieved.[66,67] Other drugs including phenobarbital, phenytoin, and phenylbutazone have been reported to diminish serum digitoxin concentrations in some patients, presumably through induction of hepatic drug-metabolizing enzyme systems.[67] The magnitude of this effect at usual therapeutic doses of these drugs is often insignificant, but in certain sensitive subjects it may lead to inadequate levels of digitalization. Measurement of serum digitalis levels will be helpful in detecting these types of drug interactions. Diuretic agents may predispose to the development of digitalis toxicity, both through diminution in glomerular filtration rate with consequent reduction in renal digoxin clearance and through the various electrolyte and acid-base disturbances that result from their use. Concomitant administration of antiarrhythmic agents may mask digitalis toxicity by suppressing digitalis-induced dysrhythmias. Recently, a potentially important intraction between digitalis and quinidine has been described.[68] Quinidine tends to increase serum glycoside levels by an undefined mechanism, and digitalis toxicity may result. Finally, the interrelationship of catecholamine and cardiac glycoside effects on the myocardium is intriguing but incompletely characterized. Several experimental studies have demonstrated that catecholamine-induced increases in ventricular automatically are additive to the arrhythmogenic effects of digitalis.[69] However, detailed clinical correlation has not been forthcoming. It is reasonable for the clinician to assume that sympathomimetic agents will increase the likelihood of enhanced automaticity of ectopic pacemakers in patients receiving digitalis.

Concurrent Disease States

Several concurrent disease states have been reported to be associated with an increased frequency of digitalis toxicity. Renal failure, particularly in patients requiring hemodialysis, can cause difficulties in the clinical use of digitalis, both because of the decreased elimination of digoxin with reduced renal function and because of the electrolyte shifts that are prone to occur in this patient group.

Thyroid disease has long been known to have an important effect on cardiac glycoside sensitivity. Hypothyroid patients tend to have a prolongation of serum digoxin half-life, while hyperthyroid patients tend to have relatively reduced serum digoxin levels.[70] Changes in elimination rate and volume of distribution may both contribute to these alterations.[70,71] In addition, there is a strong clinical impression that thyrotoxic patients tend to respond less well to any given serum concentration of digoxin, particularly with regard to the slowing of ventricular response in the presence of supraventricular tachyarrhythmias such as atrial fibrillation or atrial flutter. Conversely, there is an impression that hypothyroid patients have a higher incidence of overt toxicity at cardiac glycoside concentrations that are usually well tolerated.

The autonomic nervous system, both parasympathetic[72] and sympathetic systems, plays a potentially important role in mediating the effects of cardiac glycosides, and underlying autonomic tone may have an important influence on the clinical response to digitalis. Recent research suggests a permissive or even triggering role for the nervous system in digitalis-induced arrhythmias characterized by increased automaticity of ectopic pacemakers.[73] Thus, drugs or clinical states that influence sympathetic or para-

sympathetic tone can be expected to cause alterations in apparent digitalis sensitivity.

The relationship of cardiac glycoside sensitivity to pulmonary disease is a particularly complex area.[74] Recent epidemiologic studies indicate that the incidence of digitalis toxicity is increased in patients with pulmonary disease.[15,75] Clinical reports are often difficult to interpret, however, since respiratory failure and hypoxemia may provoke arrhythmias identical to those associated with digitalis toxicity.[76] Indeed, it is by no means certain that the apparently increased incidence of digitalis toxicity in the setting of pulmonary disease can be attributed to the disturbance in pulmonary function; instead, it may result from such associated factors as excessive cardiac glycoside dosage, hypokalemia, concomitant renal impairment, and sympathomimetic drugs concurrently administered. Experimental studies on the influence of arterial oxygen tension suggest that hypoxemia is more likely to predispose to toxicity when present acutely than when it is a chronic condition.[77] Further investigation is needed to define the epidemiology of digitalis intoxication in patients with pulmonary disease, paying particular attention to the type of lung disease present, the severity and chronicity of disease, and the independent influences of factors such as hypoxemia, hypokalemia, and sympathetic tone.

CONCLUSION

A review of our own experience and of the available literature indicates that knowledge of serum cardiac glycoside concentrations can be quite helpful to the clinician in defining the state of digitalization and in assigning certain broad probabilities to the likelihood of digitalis intoxication. *However, the myriad factors that bear on individual responses to digitalis require that serum concentration data be interpreted in the overall clinical context and that an isolated serum concentration not be used as a sole arbiter of the presence or absence of toxicity.* The overlap in serum digitalis concentrations between toxic and nontoxic patients underlines this conclusion. Certainly not every patient taking a digitalis preparation needs periodic "routine" serum level measurements to monitor drug dosage. The clinical situations in which knowledge of the serum level may be most useful include suspected manifestations of digitalis intoxication in the absence of an adequate history, suspected problems of patient compliance in taking prescribed digitalis doses, fluctuating renal function, the presence of overt or suspected malabsorption, the use of preparations of uncertain bioavailability, and the need to estimate the state of digitalization in patients in complex clinical circumstances, such as following cardiac surgery. More generally, it is our opinion that the measurement of serum cardiac glycoside concentrations is indicated whenever an unanticipated response to these drugs (either suspected toxicity or absence of an expected therapeutic effect) is encountered. Above all, however, we would emphasize that no laboratory test should diminish the essential role of close clinical follow-up by a vigilant physician with a sound working knowledge of the clinical pharmacology of digitalis.

REFERENCES

1 Withering, W.: An Account of the Foxglove, in F. A. Willius and T. E. Keys (eds.), "Cardiac Classics," The C. V. Mosby Company, St. Louis, 1941, p. 232.

2 Smith, T. W., Butler, V. P., Jr., and Haber, T.: Determination of Therapeutic and Toxic Serum Digoxin Concentrations by Radioimmunoassay, *N. Engl. J. Med.*, 281:1212, 1969.

3 Smith, T. W., and Haber, E.: Clinical Value of the Radioimmunoassay of the Digitalis Glycosides, *Pharmacol. Rev.*, 25:219, 1973.

4 Butler, V. P., Jr.: Digoxin Radioimmunoassay, *Lancet*, 1:186, 1971.

5 Smith, T. W., and Curfman, G. D.: Radioimmunoassay of Cardiac Glycosides, in W. Strauss, and B. Pitt (eds.), "Diagnostic Nuclear Cardiology," 2d ed., The C. V. Mosby Company, St. Louis, in press.

6 Smith, T. W., and Haber, E.: The Current Status of Cardiac Glycoside Assay Techniques, in P. N. Yu, and J. F. Goodwin, (eds.), "Progress in Cardiology," Vol. II, Lea & Febiger, Philadelphia, 1973.

7 Doherty, J. E., Perkins, W. H., and Flanigan, W. J.: The Distribution and Concentration of Tritiated Digoxin in Human Tissues, *Ann. Intern. Med.*, 66:116, 1967.

8 Gullner, H. G., Stinson, E. B., Harrison, D. C., and Kalman, S. M.: Correlation of Serum Concentrations with Heart Concentrations of Digoxin in Human Subjects, *Circulation*, 50:653, 1974.

9 Hartel, G., Kyllonen, K., Markkallio, E., Ojala, K., Manninen, V., and Reissell, P.: Human Serum and Myocardial Digoxin, *Clin. Pharmacol. Ther.*, 19:153, 1976.

10 Carroll, P. R., Gelbart, A., O'Rourke, M. F., and Shortus, J.: Digoxin Concentrations in the Serum and Myocardium of Digitalized Patients, *Aust. N. Z. J. Med.*, 3:400, 1973.

11 Schwartz, A.: Is the Cell Membrane NaK-ATPase Enzyme System the Pharmacologic Receptor for Digitalis? *Circ. Res.*, 39:2, 1976.

12 Caldwell, P. C., and Keynes, R. D.: The Effect of Ouabain on the Efflux of Sodium from a Squid Giant Axon, *J. Physiol.*, 148:8P, 1959.

13 Hoffman, J. F.: The Red Cell Membrane and the Transport of Sodium and Potassium, *Am. J. Med.*, 41:666, 1966.

14 Barr, I., Smith, T. W., Klein, M. D., Hagemeijer, F., and Lown, B.: Correlation of the Electrophysiologic Action of Digoxin with Serum Digoxin Concentration, *J. Pharmacol. Exp. Ther.*, 180:710, 1972.

15 Beller, B. A., Smith, T. W., Abelmann, W. H., Haber, E., and Hood, W. B., Jr.: Digitalis Intoxication: A Prospective Clinical Study with Serum Level Correlations, *N. Engl. J. Med.*, 284:989, 1971.

16 Bertler, A., and Redfors, A.: Plasma Levels of Digoxin in Relation to Toxicity, *Acta Pharmacol. Toxicol.*, 29 (suppl. 3): 281, 1971.

17 Bertler, A., Gustafson, A., Ohlin, P., Monti, M., and Redfors, A.: Digoxin Intoxication and Plasma Glycoside Levels, in O. Storstein (ed.), "Symposium on Digitalis," Gyldendal Norsk Forlag, Oslo, 1973, p. 300.

18 Brooker, G., and Jelliffe, R. W.: Serum Cardiac Glycoside Assay Based upon Displacement of ^{3}H-Ouabain from Na-K ATPase, *Circulation*, 45:20, 1971.

19 Burnett, G. H., and Conklin, R. L.: The Enzymatic Assay of Plasma Digoxin, *J. Lab. Clin. Med.*, 78:779, 1971.

20 Carruthers, S. G., Kelly, J. G., and McDevitt, D. G.: Plasma Digoxin Concentrations in Patients on Admission to Hospital, *Br. Heart J.*, 3:707, 1974.

21 Chamberlain, D. A., White, R. J., Howard, M. R., and Smith, T. W.: Plasma Digoxin Concentrations in Patients with Atrial Fibrillation, *Br. Med. J.*, 3:429, 1970.

22 Doering, W., Konig, E., and Sturm, W.: Digitalis Intoxication: Specificity and Significance of Cardiac and Extracardiac Symptoms. Part I: Patients with Digitalis-induced Arrhythmias, *Z. Kardiol.*, 66:121, 1977.

23 Evered, D. C., and Chapman, D.: Plasma Digoxin Concentrations and Digoxin Toxicity in Hospital Patients, *Br. Heart J.*, 33:540, 1971.

24 Fogelman, A. M., LaMont, J. T., Finkelstein, S., Rado, E., and Pearce, M. L.: Fallibility of Plasma-Digoxin in Differentiating Toxic from Non-toxic Patients, *Lancet*, 2:727, 1971.

25 Grahame-Smith, D. G., and Everest, M. S.: Measurement of Digoxin in Plasma and Its Use in Diagnosis of Digoxin Intoxication, *Br. Med. J.*, 1:286, 1969.

26 Hayes, C. J., Butler, V. P., and Gersony, W. M.: Serum Digoxin Studies in Infants and Children, *Pediatrics*, 52:561, 1973.

27 Hoeschen, R. J., and Proveda, V.: Serum Digoxin by Radioimmunoassay, *Can. Med. Assoc. J.*, 105:170, 1971.

28 Howard, D., Smith, C. I., Stewart, G., Vadas, M., Tiller, D. J., Hensley, W. J., and Richards, J. G.: A Prospective Survey of the Incidence of Cardiac Intoxication with Digitalis In Patients Being Admitted to Hospital and Correlation with Serum Digoxin Levels, *Aust. N. Z. J. Med.*, 3:279, 1973.

29 Huffman, D. H., Crow, J. W., Pentikainen, P., and Azarnoff, D. L.: Association between Clinical Cardiac Status, Laboratory Parameters, and Digoxin Usage, *Am. Heart J.*, 91:28, 1976.

30 Iisalo, E., Dahl, M., and Sundquist, H.: Serum Digoxin in Adults and Children, *Int. J. Clin. Pharmacol.*, 7:219, 1973.

31 Johnston, C. I., Pinkus, N. B., and Down, M.: Plasma Digoxin Levels in Digitalized and Toxic Patients, *Med. J. Aust.*, 1:863, 1972.

32 Krasula, R., Tanagi, R., Hastreider, A. R., Levitsky, S., and Soyka, L. F.: Digoxin Intoxication in Infants and Children, *J. Pediatr.*, 84:265, 1974.

33 Lader, S., Bye, A., and Marsdin, P.: The Measurement of Plasma Digoxin Concentration: A Comparison in Two Methods, *Eur. J. Clin. Pharmacol.*, 5:22, 1972.

34 McCredie, R. M., Chia, B. L., and Knight, P. W.: Infant versus Adult Plasma Digoxin Levels, *Aust. N. Z. J. Med.* 4:223, 1974.

35 Morrison, J., Killip, T., and Stason, W. B.: Serum Digoxin Levels in Patients Undergoing Cardiopulmonary Bypass, *Circulation*, 42;110, 1970.

36 Oliver, G. C., Parker, B. M., and Parker C. W.: Radioimmunoassay for Digoxin. Technic and Clinical Application, *Am. J. Med.*, 51:186, 1971.

37 Park, H. M., Chen, I. W., Manitassas, G. T., Lowey, A., and Saenger, E. L.: Clinical Evaluation of Radioimmunoassay of Digoxin, *J. Nucl. Med.*, 14:531, 1973.

38 Ritzmann, L. W., Bangs, C. C., Coiner, D., Custis, J. M., and Walsh, J. R.: Serum Glycoside Levels by Rubidium Assay, *Arch. Intern. Med.*, 132:823, 1973.

39 Scherrmann, J. M., and Bourdon, R.: Dosage de la Digoxine par Methode Radioimmunologique, *Eur. J. Toxicol.*, 9:133, 1976.

40 Singh, R. B., Rai, A. N., Srivastav, D. K., Somani, P. N., and Katiyar, B. C.: Radioimmunoassay of Serum Digoxin in Relation to Digoxin Intoxication, *Br. Heart J.*, 37:619, 1975.

41 Smith, T. W., and Haber, E.: Digoxin Intoxication: The Relationship of Clinical Presentation to Serum Digoxin Concentration, *J. Clin. Invest.*, 49:2377, 1970.

42 Waddorff, S., and Buch, J.: Serum Digoxin and Empiric Methods in Identification of Digitoxicity, *Clin. Pharmacol. Ther.*, 23:19, 1978.

43 Weissel, M., Fritzsche, H., and Fuchs, G.: Salivary Electrolytes and Serum Digoxin in the Assessment of Digitalis Intoxication, *Wien. Klin. Wochenschr.*, 88:455, 1976.

44 Whiting, B., Sumner, D. J., and Goldbert, A.: An Assessment of Digoxin Radioimmunoassay, *Scot. Med. J.*, 18:69, 1973.

45 Zeegers, J. J. W., Maas, A. H. J., Willebrands, A. F., Kruyswijik, H. H., and Jambroes, G.: The Radioimmunoassay of Plasma-Digoxin, *Clin. Chim. Acta*, 44:109, 1973.

46 Bentley, J. D., Burnett, G. H., Conklin, R. L., and Wasserburger, R. H.: Clinical Application of Serum Digitoxin Levels—a Simplified Plasma Determination, *Circulation*, 41:67, 1970.

47 Chiche, P., Baligadoo, S., Larvelle, P., and Borgard, J. P.: Intoxications Digitaliques et Deviations de l'Activite Therapeutique de la Digitaline, *Coeur Med. Intern.*, 15:249, 1976.

48 Dessaint, J. P.: Dosage Radio-immunologique des Digitalique (Digitoxine et Digoxine) dans le Sang, *Lille Med.*, 19:156, 1974.

49 Hillestad, L., Hansteen, V., Hatle, L., Storstein, L., and Storstein, O.: Digitalis Intoxication, in O. Storstein, (ed.), "Symposium on Digitalis," Gyldendal Norsk Forlag, Oslo, 1973, p. 281.

50 Lukas, D. S., and Peterson, R. W.: Double Isotope Dilution Derivative Assay of Digitoxin in Plasma, Urine and Stool of Patients Maintained on the Drug, *J. Clin. Invest.*, 45:782, 1966.

51 Morrison, J., and Killip, T.: Radioimmunoassay of Digitoxin, *Clin. Res.*, 14:668, 1970.

52 Peters, U., Hausamen, T.-U., and Grosse-Brockhoff, F.: Serial Tests of Serum Digitoxin Levels during Digitoxin Treatment, *Dtsch. Med. Wochenschr.*, 99:1701, 1974.

53 Rasmussen, K., Jervell, J., and Storstein, O.: Clinical Use of a Bio-assay of Serum Digitoxin Activity, *Eur. J. Clin. Pharmacol.*, 3:236, 1971.

54 Smith, T. W.: Radioimmunoassay for Serum Digitoxin Concentration: Methodology and Clinical Experience, *J. Pharmacol. Exp. Ther.*, 175:352, 1970.

55 Smith, T. W., and Willerson, J. T.: Suicidal and Accidental Digoxin Ingestion: Report of Five Cases with Serum Digoxin Level Correlations, *Circulation*, 44:29, 1971.

56 Enselbert, C. D., Simmons, H. C., and Mintz, A. A.: The Effects of Potassium upon the Heart, with Special Reference to the Possibility of Treatment of Toxic Arrhythmias Due to Digitalis, *Am. Heart J.*, 39:713, 1950.

57 Sampson, J. J., Albertson, E. C., and Kondo, B.: The Effect on Man of Potassium Administration in Relation to Digitalis Glycosides with Special Reference to Blood

Serum Potassium, the Electrocardiogram and Ectopic Beats, *Am. Heart J.*, 26:692, 1963.

58 Davidson, S., and Surawicz, B.: Ectopic Beats and Atrioventricular Conduction Distrubances, *Arch. Intern. Med.*, 120:280, 1967.

59 Ghani, M. F., and Smith J. R.: The Effectiveness of Magnesium Chloride in the Treatment of Ventricular Tachyarrhythmias Due to Digitalis Intoxication, *Am. Heart. J.*, 88:621, 1974.

60 Neff, M. S., Medelssohn, S., Kim, K. E., et al.: Magnesium Sulfate in Digitalis Toxicity, *Am. J. Cardiol.*, 29:377, 1972.

61 Seller, R. H., Ramirez, O., and Brest, A. N. Digitalis Toxicity and Hypomagnesemia, *Am. Heart. J.*, 79:57, 1970.

62 Nalbandian, R. M., Gordon, S., Campbell, R., et al.: A New Quantitative Digitalis Tolerance Test Based upon the Synergism of Calcium and Digitalis, *Am. J. Med. Sci.*, 233:503, 1957.

63 Surawicz, B.: Use of the Chelating Agent, EDTA, in Digitalis Intoxication and Cardiac Arrhythmias, *Prog. Cardiovasc. Dis.*, 2:432 1959–1960.

64 Lown, B., Black, H., and Moore, F. D.: Digitalis, Electrolytes and the Surgical Patient, *Am. J. Cardiol*, 6:309, 1960.

65 Smith, P. K., Wintler, A. W., and Hoff, H. E.: Calcium and Digitalis Synergism: The Toxicity of Calcium Salts Injected Intravenously into Digitalized Animals, *Arch. Intern. Med.*, 64:322, 1939.

66 Binnion, P. F.: Absorption of Different Commercial Preparations of Digoxin in the Normal Human Subject, and the Influence of Antacid, Anti-diarrheal, and Ion-Exchange Agents, in O. Storstein, (ed.), "Symposium on Digitalis," Gyldendal Norsk Forlag, Oslo, 1973, p. 216.

67 Koch-Weser, J.: Drug Interactions in Cardiovascular Therapy, *Am. Heart J.*, 90:93, 1975.

68 Leahy, E. B., Reiffel, J. A., Drusin, R. E., et al.: Interaction between Quinidine and Digoxin, *J.A.M.A.*, 240:533, 1978.

69 Becker, D. J., Nankin, P. M., and Bennett, L. D.,: Effect of Isoproterenol in Digitalis Cardiotoxicity, *Am. J. Cardiol.*, 10:242, 1962.

70 Doherty, J. E., and Perkins, W. H.: Digoxin Metabolism in Hypo- and Hyperthyroidism: Studies with Tritiated Digoxin in Thyroid Disease, *Ann. Intern. Med.*, 64:489, 1966.

71 Croxson, M. S., and Ibbertson, H. K.: Serum Digoxin in Patients with Thyroid Disease, *Br. Med. J.*, 3:566, 1975.

72 Moe, G. K., and Farah, A. E.: Digitalis and Allied Cardiac Glycosides, in L. S. Goodman and A. Gilman, (eds.), "The Pharmacological Basis of Therapeutics," The Macmillan Company, New York, 1970, p. 677.

73 Gillis, R. A., Pearle, D. L., and Levitt, B.: Digitalis: A Neuroexcitatory Drug, *Circulation*, 52:739, 1975.

74 Green, L. H., and Smith, T. W.: The Use of Digitalis in Patients with Pulmonary Disease, *Ann. Intern. Med.*, 87:459, 1977.

75 Chung, E. K.: Digitalis-induced Cardiac Arrhythmias: A report of 180 Cases, *Jpn. Heart J.*, 10:409, 1969.

76 Hudson, L. D., Kurt, T. L., Petty, T. L., et al.: Arrhythmias Associated with Acute Respiratory Failure in Patients with Chronic Airway Obstruction, *Chest*, 63:661, 1973.

77 Beller, G. A., Giamber, S. R., Saltz, S. B., et al.: Cardiac and Respiratory Effects of Digitalis during Chronic Hypoxia in Intact Conscious Dogs, *Am. J. Physiol.*, 229:270, 1975.

Advances in Cardiac Pathology*

BERNADINE H. BULKLEY, M.D.

Something may be learned from the most ordinary case if it is presented with the special object of illustrating the relation of disturbed function to altered structure.

SIR WILLIAM OSLER[1]

INTRODUCTION

New disease entities, both natural and iatrogenic, are appearing regularly, such as asymmetric hypertrophy of the heart, Prinzmetal's angina, prosthetic valve disease, and saphenous vein coronary bypasses, and morphologic evaluation is essental to their characterizations and to quality control of the interventions that may have led to them. New approaches to old diseases and new diagnostic tools also necessitate a critical review of accepted morphologic information in the light of new information. The impact of "modern" therapy on the presentation of disease is another area where morphologic information needs frequent update. In the 1920s Cabot reviewed the cardiac pathology at the Massachusetts General Hospital for the previous 25 years and determined, first, that most heart disease was imaginary; second, that the major cause of manifest heart disease was valvular abnormality resulting from rheumatic fever or syphilis; and third, that coronary artery disease was rare.[2] We now see cardiovascular disease as responsible for over half of the deaths in this country, and coronary artery disease is responsible for the majority of deaths within that group. Thus, there is little doubt that cardiac pathology has changed over the years. Our success in understanding and treating one disease has allowed others to emerge dominant. It is especially useful in an area such as the heart, in which animal models are limited, to continually avail ourselves of the wealth of information on the pathogenesis of disease that can be culled from human autopsy pathology, the latter being one of our most readily available sources of human scientific data. In this regard we might also heed the words of two students of pathology, Drs. Pickering and Heptinstall, who over 25 years ago cautioned:

> We would make a plea that so far as any conclusions are drawn as to the mechanisms of human disease, the evidence derived from man should at least be considered.[3]

* From the Departments of Pathology and Medicine, The Johns Hopkins Hospital Baltimore, Maryland. Supported in part by NIH SCOR Grant 5 P50 HL17655 and the Peter Belfer Laboratory for Myocardial Research.

PATHOGENESIS OF CORONARY ARTERY DISEASE

It is widely recognized that the major disease causing inadequate blood supply to myocardium is coronary atherosclerosis. Atherosclerotic lesions have a characteristic morphology and on this basis may be broadly classified into fatty streaks, fibrous plaques, and complicated plaques. Fatty streaks, which are focal accumulations of lipid-laden intimal cells of probably smooth muscle origin, occur in human arteries of virtually all ages, sex, and origin. Fibrous plaques represent a more advanced lesion composed of lipid-laden myointimal cells and fibrous tissue and can cause arterial narrowing. The most advanced atherosclerotic lesion is the complicated plaque in which necrosis, fibrin, pultaceous debris, and calcification are present, and it is the complicated plaque which is most often associated with plaque rupture, hemorrhage, and mural thrombosis (Fig. 1). Central to all theories of the pathogenesis of atherosclerosis is the need to account for the components of these lesions. Although the morphology of the atherosclerotic plaques is straightforward and widely agreed upon, the development of these lesions remains unclear.

Numerous pathogenetic theories put forth include mechanical injury, intimal hemorrhage, lipid infiltration, and thrombosis or encrustation.[4-9] The *lipogenic theories* and the *thrombogenic theories* of atherosclerosis are the ones most widely held today. Epidemiologic and biochemical studies have strongly implicated lipids in the pathogenesis of atherosclerosis, and morphologically, atherosclerotic plaques virtually always show abnormal lipid deposition. The mechanism by which lipids interact with the arterial wall to form a plaque is not known, however, and whether the fatty streak is a precursor of the occlusive complicated plaque has not been established. Although the role of thrombus in the inception of the atherosclerotic plaque is unsettled, there is little doubt that thrombus plays an important role in the progression of atherosclerotic plaques.[4,5] Both of these theories of atherosclerosis have been the source of considerable research and controversy for over a century, and conceptually they have largely dominated the thinking in regard to atherosclerosis without solution or resolution. It is therefore refreshing that a new theory of the pathogenesis of atherosclerosis has arisen. The clonal theory of atherosclerosis was first proposed approximately 6 years

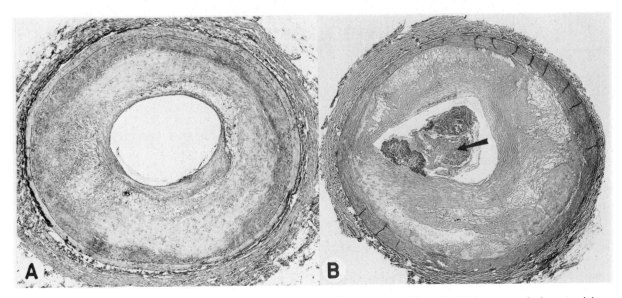

FIGURE 1 Atherosclerotic narrowing of coronary arteries by complicated plaque. Shown in (*B*) is a nonocclusive organizing fibrin platelet thrombus (arrow) being incorporated into the chronic plaque, suggesting the role of thrombus in plaque proliferation. (hematoxylin and eosin stain, *A*, × 25; *B*, × 20).

ago by Benditt and Benditt[10,11] and more recently has been advanced by other investigators.[12,13] The theory, in brief, states that atherosclerotic plaques develop from single precursor cells that proliferate much like benign tumors, and it is based on the observation that fibrous plaques from aortas of black women who are heterozygous for glucose 6-phosphate dehydrogenase (i.e., carry both A and B isoenzymes) are composed of cells that produce only one enzyme type. The finding of two isoenzymes in a given tissue would be compatible with derivation from multiple precursor cells, whereas the finding of only one isoenzyme, either A or B, in an atherosclerotic plaque would imply a single cell origin. Since the majority of atherosclerotic lesions studied in this fashion appear to have only one isoenzyme, it is suggested that plaques originate from single cells which have somehow been altered and stimulated to proliferate abnormally. Transforming or initiating agents might include viruses, drugs, and physical, chemical, or mechanical agents. Implied in this monoclonal concept of atherosclerosis is a genetic predisposition or susceptibility to these transforming agents.

Despite considerable controversy among proponents of one or the other school, the assorted theories, including the more recent monoclonal origin theory, are not necessarily mutually exclusive. Lipids may play a role in vascular injury resulting in intimal thromboses or possibly in direct stimulation of plaque proliferation. Proliferating thrombi have been shown to have monoclonal properties under certain conditions, and the host of risk factors including cigarette smoking, hypertension, and diabetes mellitus may be predisposing or accelerating conditions that affect intimal cells, lipid metabolism, or thrombogenicity.

PATHOGENESIS OF ISCHEMIC HEART DISEASE WITHOUT ATHEROSCLEROSIS

Large-Vessel Disease

Although in the Western world atherosclerosis is the cause of ischemic heart disease in the overwhelming majority of patients, there is increasing appreciation of nonatherosclerotic causes of myocardial ischemia and infarction. There are only a few reports of pathologically documented acute myocardial infarction with entirely normal coronary arteries at autopsy,[14,15] although clinical reports of this phenomenon are more common.[16–19]

The pathophysiology of myocardial infarction with normal coronary arteries is controversial. Some propose that infarction with angiographically normal coronary arteries reflects either coronary artery embolism with retraction, lysis, or recanalization, or an angiographically missed coronary lesion caused by an eccentric plaque.[20] More controversial is the role of coronary artery spasm in infarction. That spasm can be severe enough and sustained enough to lead to myocardial infarction has been questioned,[20,21] with arguments against spasm as a cause of infarction largely resting on the lack of an angiographically proven causal relationship between spasm and subsequent infarction, a proof which is difficult to obtain. There is little doubt, however, that coronary spasm does occur and may be a cause of myocardial insufficiency and, at least possibly, infarction in patients with and without atherosclerotic disease.[19,21–23] The occurrence of angina pectoris and myocardial necrosis and fibrosis in scleroderma patients suggests a coronary Raynaud's phenomenon in this disease (Fig. 2).[24,25] That coronary arterial embolism occurs mostly in patients with predisposing disease, including valvular abnormalities, cardiomyopathies, or arrhythmias,[26] and is infrequently associated with a clinical syndrome compatible with ischemic heart disease suggests that coronary thromboembolism de novo may not be the sole or primary explanation for nonatherosclerotic myocardial infarction.

It is likely that the infarction with normal coronary arteries will prove to be of heterogeneous origin, with etiologies including arrhythmias with hypoperfusion, coronary arterial spasm, and coronary emboli with lysis or retraction. Since there are few morphologic studies of patients coming to autopsy with this entity, further pathologic validation will be necessary to define and identify these assorted subgroups.

Small-Vessel Disease

Structural and possibly functional abnormalities of the small coronary arteries may also be important in the syndrome of angina pectoris with normal epicardial coronary arteries. The autonomic nervous system appears to play a role in vasomotion in the heart, as it does elsewhere in the body, with sympathetic stimulation of alpha receptors causing coronary vasocontriction, parasympathetic stimulation, and vasodilation.[28,29] There are few structural observations on the coronary microcirculation to correlate with the physiologic data. Structural abnormalities of small vessels have been studied in detail by James, who pointed out that patients with narrowed small coronary arteries and chest pain tend to have atypical chest pain which is less severe and less consistently related to exertion or stress than usual angina pectoris.[27] Detailed ultrastructural morphology of the human microcirculation has only recently been examined by Sherf et al., who described features of the terminal coronary arterioles and venules from biopsy specimens obtained from humans undergoing cardiac operation.[30] In addition to arterioles ranging from 100 μm down to 30 μm, precapillary "sphincters" measuring 30 to 15 μm were identified which were surrounded by numerous myoendothelial cells or bridges. It has been previously suggested that these myoendothelial bridges surrounding the precapillary vessels, which have been identified in many mammalian tissues, play a regulatory role by constricting and relaxing in response to a variety of stimuli. The pathophysiologic significance of these structures in the human coronary microcirculation is not known, but it is tempting to speculate that precapillary sphincters may be subject to both structural and functional abnormalities which could result in regional myocardial ischemia or necrosis in the setting of widely patent epicardial coronary arteries.[29]

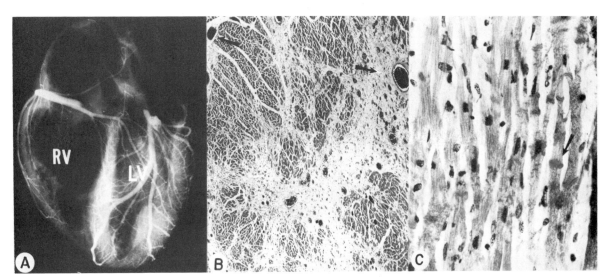

FIGURE 2 An example of myocardial necrosis and fibrosis that may occur in patients with scleroderma myocardial disease. *A.* Postmortem angiogram from a woman dying with biventricular heart failure as a result of scleroderma myocardial involvement. Although the epicardial coronary arteries are widely patent, extensive replacement fibroses (*B*) and foci of necrosis (*C*) were present throughout her heart. A Raynaud's phenomenon of the small vessels of her myocardium appears to best explain this process. [hematoxylin and eosin stain, *B,* × 45; *C,* × 60 (C)].

Another form of ischemia and at times infarction with normal epicardial coronary arteries is seen in conditions of severe left ventricular hypertrophy. Left ventricular hypertrophy, whether caused by long-standing hypertension, valvular obstructive disease, or an idiopathic process, when severe enough may be associated with symptoms of angina pectoris and with electrocardiographic changes compatible with diffuse subendocardial ischemia. At autopsy, subendocardial scars may be identified in the setting of widely patent coronary vessels, suggesting that infarction as well as ischemia may occur. The explanation for this is not entirely clear. As the heart hypertrophies (Fig. 3) the epicardial coronary arteries increase in caliber and length,[31] and there is no evidence that cardiac enlargement outstrips enlargement of the large coronary arteries. Under conditions of cardiac hypertrophy, the fate of the coronary microcirculation may be more important in determining regional tissue flow. Morpho-

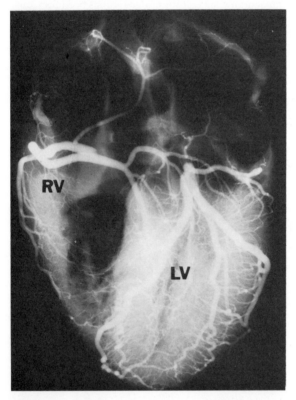

FIGURE 3 Postmortem coronary arteriogram of a heart from a patient with long-standing systemic hypertension. The heart was enlarged, weighing 550 g, and the left ventricle was hypertrophied, but no cavity dilation was present. The epicardial coronary arteries have also increased in size and caliber to "keep up" with the cardiac enlargement. Derangements in regional small-vessel coronary flow probably account for the angina and occasional infarction with normal coronary arteries that may occur under conditions of marked hypertrophy. LV, left ventricle. RV, right ventricle.

logic studies of the canine microvasculatures have demonstrated that under normal conditions the small vessels of the heart are arranged so as to maximize diffusion, with intercapillary distances close to myocardial fiber diameter.[32] The precise anatomic alterations that occur in the microvasculature of the endocardium and subendocardium consequent to hypertrophy have not been determined, although morphologic studies in human hearts with hypertensive left ventricular hypertrophy have shown increases in myocardial fiber diameter.[33] Physiologic studies on coronary blood flow in experimental hypertrophy have demonstrated that flow to the subendocardium may be inadequate and that during conditions of added myocardial stress necessitating maximal vasodilatation, the regional subendocardial underperfusion becomes even more accentuated.[34,35] Whether the abnormalities in regional perfusion reflect structural changes in the microcirculation or changes in the enlarging myocardial cell per se, the hypertrophied heart does appear to be a readily identifiable model of inadequate perfusion and ischemia with normal epicardial coronary arteries.

Much needs to be learned about the coronary circulation at all levels with regard to both structure and function and the interrelationship of the two. The difficulties inherent in sorting out these relationships have been well summarized by Dr. James:

> Nature is full of paradoxes and one of the most intriguing is the blood supply to the heart. While the heart cannot function normally without a good blood supply, it cannot receive an optimal blood supply unless it is functioning normally. Unlike any other organ in the body, the heart is absolutely dependent on its own normal function for its own normal blood supply. It is thus for purposes of blood supply both its sole provider and a major consumer, according to the laws of economics a sure example of conflict of interest.[36]

THE MYOCARDIUM IN ISCHEMIC DISEASE

Types of Acute Myocardial Infarction

The classic acute myocardial infarct as described by Mallory is a description of coagulation necrosis.[37] The coagulation infarct is a pale or white infarct and develops as a consequence of permanent interruption of coronary blood flow (Figs. 4 and 5). Although histologic evidence of coagulation necrosis is usually not evident before 6 h of coronary occlusion, Bouchardy and Majno have observed that thin, wavy fiber change may be one of the earliest signs of infarction, evident within 60 min after the acute ischemic event.[38] Ultra-

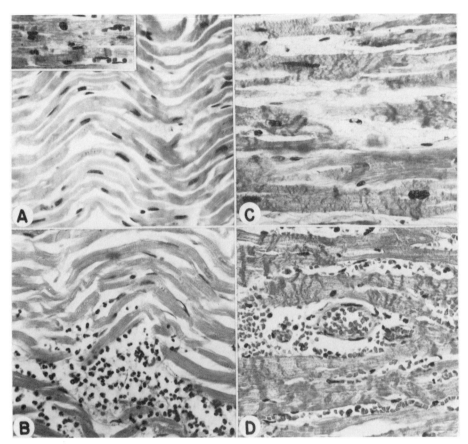

FIGURE 4 Shown are examples of coagulation (*A,B*) and contraction band (*C,D*) necrosis. *Coagulation necrosis* in its earliest stage within hours of coronary occlusion shows thin, wavy fiber formation and pyknosis of nuclei. *A*. After 48 h the nuclei are lost, and a heavy polymorphonuclear infiltrate is seen. *B*. The cell structure is otherwise minimally distorted. *Contraction band necrosis* shows considerable histologic distortion of cell structure within minutes of reperfusion. The muscle fibers show irregular transverse hypereosinophilic contraction bands with intervening cleared areas. The contraction bands represent accordion-like condensation of sarcomeres. *C*. By 48 h the contraction bands are still readily apparent, but the nuclei are gone (*D*) (hematoxylin and eosin stain, all × 220). (*From B. H. Bulkley and G. M. Hutchins, Myocardial Consequences of Coronary Artery Bypass Graft Surgery: The Paradox of Necrosis in Areas of Revascularization, Circulation, 56:906, 1977. Reproduced with permission of the American Heart Association.*)

structural changes in myocardium after coronary occlusion have suggested that signs of irreversible myocardial injury, including clumping of nuclear chromatin and mineralization of mitochondria, develop as early as 1 h after acute coronary occlusion.[39] It is generally believed that the appearance of electron-dense bodies within the swollen mitochondria correlate with irreversible cell death (Figs. 6 and 7). The precise nature of these granules is not fully established, but it appears that they are, at least in part, precipitates of calcium phosphate. It is likely that increased cell permeability to water and ions such as those of calcium plays an important role in the pathogenesis of irreversible cell death.[39,40] Studies with ionic lanthanum, the trivalent

ion which has properties similar to calcium, have shown abnormal intracellular deposits of this ion in myocardial cells subjected to hypoxia[41] and support the notion that membrane permeability changes are antecedent to structural changes of irreversible injury and therefore play an important pathogenetic role in the evolution of myocardial cell necrosis.

Another more recently recognized form of myocardial necrosis that can be distinguished from coagulation necrosis by light microscopy is contraction band or reperfusion necrosis. This latter form of necrosis is recognized histologically by dense transverse eosinophilic bands which ultrastructurally are observed to represent accordian-like condensations of

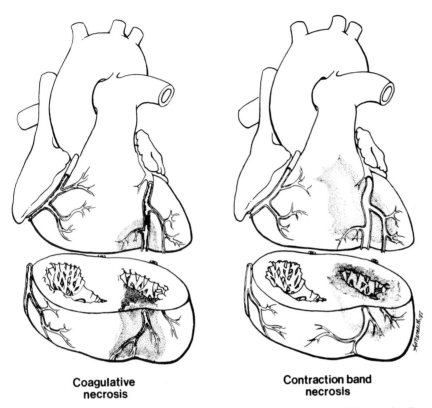

Coagulative necrosis

Contraction band necrosis

FIGURE 5 Schematic diagram illustrating the two forms of myocardial necrosis. Coagulative necrosis is most apt to occur in the setting of permanent coronary occlusion in previously narrowed atherosclerotic infarcts. The infarct is regional in the distribution of that vessel. Contraction band injury may be noted on the border of such infarcts and probably reflects collateral flow. Contraction band necrosis occurs in the setting of transient interruption in blood flow or hypoperfusion, as might occur as a result of transient hypotension or severe arrhythmias. In this setting, injury would be circumferential and mostly subendocardial.

sarcomeres (Figs. 4 and 8). At one time, contraction bands were thought to be artifacts. Their significance was first recognized in the majority of humans dying after cardiac surgery with cardiopulmonary bypass, a condition of necessary transient coronary nonperfusion. Subsequently, it was shown experimentally that contraction band necrosis occurred in myocardium reperfused after a 45-min occlusion, whereas coagulation necrosis resulted from permanent occlusion.[42] This distinction between patterns of myocardial necrosis is not merely an academic one, since the histologic type of injury is a dynamic pathologic marker of coronary perfusion. For example, the finding of subendocardial contraction band necrosis in a patient with a history of recurrent ventricular arrhythmias but normal coronary arteries is a reflection of transient coronary flow interruption, and the identification of contraction band necrosis in a large number of patients with scleroderma myocardial disease suggests that coronary spasm or myocardial Raynaud's phenome-

non may be a factor in the pathogenesis of this cardiomyopathy.[24,25] It should be noted that, experimentally, contraction band necrosis can also be induced by certain chemical agents such as high doses of catecholamines, potassium, and calcium.[43–45] Unrestrained calcium entry into cells injured by a variety of mechanisms has been suggested as a final common pathway in the pathogenesis of contraction band necrosis and may explain some of the success of calcium-blocking agents such as verapamil in the protection of myocardium from ischemic injury.[46]

Pathogenesis of Acute Myocardial Infarction

Clinical and pathologic studies are in general agreement that the coronary arteries in patients with angina pectoris and myocardial infarction, with rare exception, are narrowed by atherosclerosis.[47–51] What has come into question over the past several years, however, is the role of acute thrombotic occlusion of an atherosclerotic coronary artery in the pathogenesis of the acute myocardial infarction.[50,52-54] Evidence against the role of acute coronary thrombosis as a cause of myocardial infarction has included (1) the lower incidence of thrombosis observed in patients dying suddenly and in those with subendocardial infarction; (2) the greater incidence of coronary thrombi observed in patients with transmural myocardial infarction and especially cardiogenic shock; and (3) ^{125}I-labelled fibrinogen administered intravenously after clinical evidence of an acute myocardial infarct labels coronary thrombi.[52] These observations have led to the hypothesis that coronary artery thrombosis in acute infarction is a consequence and not a cause of the myocardial injury.[50-52]

These observations remain at variance with the bulk of morphologic studies, which identify an 80 to 90 percent incidence of recent coronary occlusion in the setting of histologically documented acute myo-

cardial infarction.[47,49,51,55-58] Autopsy studies utilizing postmortem angiography, which should increase sensitivity, generally reveal a greater incidence of cornary thrombi in relationship to myocardial infarction [47,51,59] (Fig. 9). Furthermore, many autopsy studies in which serial histologic examination of coronary lesions in the distribution of a myocardial infarct have identified an 80 to 90 percent incidence of plaque ulceration or intimal erosion underlying the acute coronary thrombus.[59,60] The difference among investigators, particularly with regard to identification of coronary thrombus in association with acute transmural infarction which ranges from 50 to 90 percent, may be in part methodologic.

There is little disagreement, however, that coronary thrombi are found more often in patients with transmural infarcts than in those with subendocardial infarcts or in those dying suddenly. With regard to subendocardial infarction, it is likely that many subendocardial infarcts occur in patients with only transient coronary occlusion, as might occur with hypo-

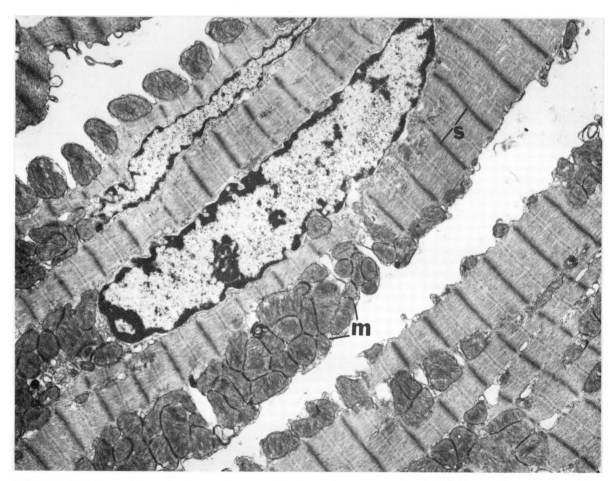

FIGURE 6 Electron micrograph of a normal myocardial cells showing orderly in-register arrangement of sarcomeres (s), and dense clusters of mitochondria (m) packed between them (× 17,640).

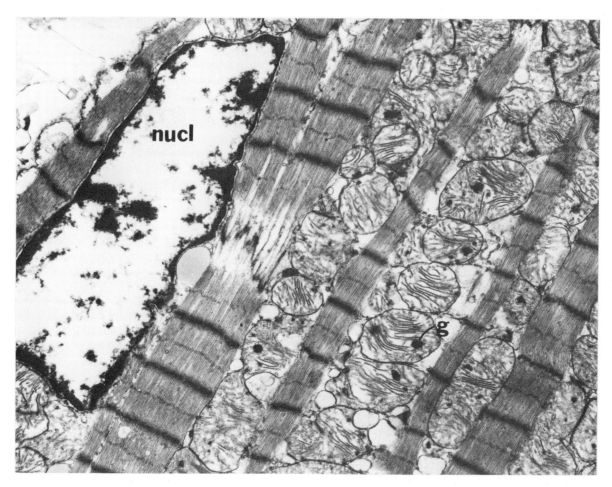

FIGURE 7 This cell has been injured by ischemia. There is margination clumping of nuclear (nucl) chromatin, the sarcomeres are separated, and the mitochondria are swollen with fragmented cristae and numerous large dense granules (g). These changes are compatible with irreversible cell death (× 25,000).

perfusion related to an arrhythmia, or as a result of rapid lysis or retraction of an occlusive thrombus. Accordingly, fewer identifications of occlusive thrombi at autopsy would be made. There is experimental evidence from the animal laboratory suggesting such an explanation. Reimer et al. have described a "wave front" phenomenon of ischemic cell death in dogs in which the extent to which myocardial infarction extended transmurally was a function of the duration of coronary occlusion; after a 40-min occlusion, necrosis was subendocardial, but after a 24-h occlusion, most infarcts were transmural.[61]

The general observation of a relatively low incidence of coronary thrombosis in patients dying suddenly with ischemic heart disease is no longer sufficient evidence against the causal role of coronary thrombus in acute infarction. Epidemiologic studies of sudden death both in this country and abroad have demonstrated that all survivors of "sudden death" do not go on to develop signs of acute myocardial infarction.[62-64] Rather, two populations appear to emerge:

those in which an acute infarct evolves and is the cause of the lethal arrhythmia and those in which severe stenotic coronary artery disease is present, but no new coronary arterial event or myocardial injury occurs. As Crawford has pointed out:

This failure to recognize that at least two mechanisms of sudden death may occur and a tendency to label all heart attacks as "myocardial infarction" has led to much of the prevailing confusion and difference of opinion regarding the role of coronary thrombosis. The facts to bear clearly in mind are that not every sudden ischemic heart disease death would have developed infarction if the patient had lived long enough; and that cases in which myocardial infarction develops almost always reveal a recent thrombosis in the coronary arteries if assiduously looked for.[51]

One of the strongest pieces of evidence against the causal role of thrombosis in the genesis of acute myocardial infarction was the identification of ^{125}I-labelled fibrinogen in thrombi associated with fatal acute infarcts when the ^{125}I fibronigen had been administered after the infarct had occurred.[52] This study demonstrated that at least some thrombotic deposition in the coronary artery in the distribution of an infarct occurred as a consequence of the infarct. A more recent study by Fulton and Summer[58] has reconciled these observations with the earlier studies. In this prospective clinicopathologic study, patients with acute infarcts also received ^{125}I-labelled fibrinogen. Autopsy studies on fatal acute infarcts studied with postmortem angiographic and serial histologic sectioning and autoradiography of the serial coronary sections demonstrated occlusive thrombus in all 32 cases in the artery of distribution to the infarct. In this study, however, all thrombi showed some ^{125}I activity, but the central core of the thrombus overlying ulcerated plaque was radionegative, except for 2 patients in whom the isotope had been administered during a period of unstable angina prior to the development of the infarct clinically. This elegant morphologic study not only provides strong evidence for the causal role of thrombotic occlusion in fatal acute infarcts but also demonstrates that propagation of the thrombus may continue after

the acute event whether or not cardiogenic shock is present.

In summary, the bulk of evidence to date suggests that an acute event—thrombosis usually overlying an eroded atherosclerotic coronary arterial plaque—is antecedent, and therefore likely causal, in the genesis of the majority of acute myocardial infarcts. What now remains unsettled and of great importance is not that thrombosis and plaque erosion occur but *why* they occur. Also, when thrombi occur, what factors determine the degree and duration of their acute occlusion? To date we remain woefully ignorant of the hemodynamic, mechanical, and metabolic events that predispose to, and precipitate, the acute coronary event.

Pathophysiologic Consequences of Acute Myocardial Infarction

The importance of the size of a myocardial infarct to the clinical outcome has been shown by the pathologic studies of Page et al.[65] and Alonso et al.[66] Their studies

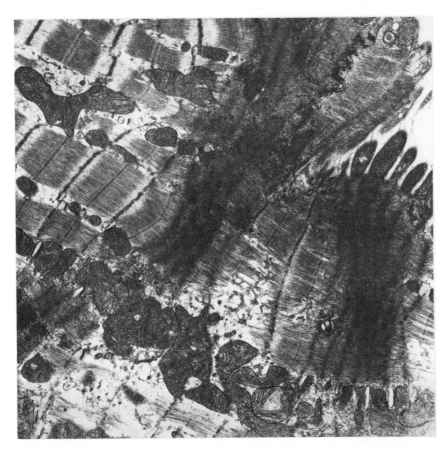

FIGURE 8 Electron micrograph showing contraction bands in a myocardial cell subjected to transient ischemia with reperfusion. Contraction bands represent accordion-like condensation of multiple sarcomeres (× 6300).

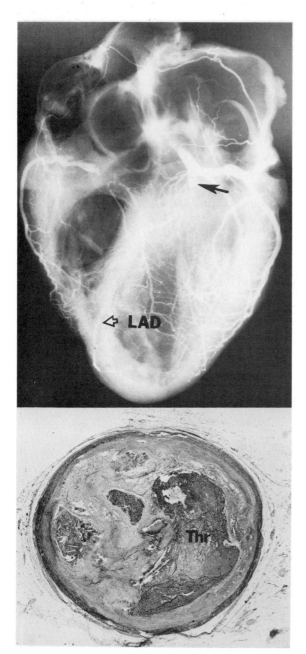

FIGURE 9 Postmortem arteriogram from a patient who died 4 days after a massive anteroseptal myocardial infarct. The left anterior descending (LAD) coronary artery is totally occluded proximally (closed arrow), and there is some distal retrograde filling of the LAD from collaterals (open arrow). The coronary artery was totally occluded by an acute thrombus (thr) superimposed on an ulcerated atherosclerotic plaque (below) (hematoxylin and eosin stain, × 14).

demonstrated that when hospitalized patients with fatal acute myocardial infarction died in cardiogenic shock, the shock almost always occurred in association with loss of a critical mass of myocardium. The

critical amount of infarct, including both old and new injury, was roughly 40 percent or more of left ventricular mass. Furthermore, these studies demonstrated that patients dying in cardiogenic shock consistently demonstrated evidence of extension of necrosis on the margins of the infarct and focally throughout both ventricles, probably reflecting hypoperfusion injury as a consequence of the shock state per se. Although the majority of patients in cardiogenic shock have lost a critical mass of myocardium, there are two important exceptions to this general rule. Acute papillary muscle rupture and rupture of the interventricular septum, both of which carry an 80 to 90 percent hospital mortality, generally lead to cardiogenic shock but are not necessarily associated with large infarcts. Fatal papillary muscle rupture, for example, which usually occurs in association with transmural posterior wall infarcts,[67,68] have been found to occur with infarcts involving approximately 20 percent or less of left ventricular myocardium. Since these infarcts generally occur away from the mitral annular area, mitral valve replacement is feasible even in the early period after infarction. The technical surgical problems associated with repair of a ventricular septal defect soon after infarction are, however, greater. Operative intervention is further complicated by the general association of severe triple-vessel disease with cardiac rupture.[69] Nevertheless, in an era of vasodilator therapy and mechanical cardiac assist devices, papillary muscle and septal rupture represent at least two potentially salvageable forms of cardiogenic shock after acute myocardial infarction.

Preservation of Ischemic Myocardium

Partly as an outgrowth of the recognition that survival after an acute infarct is, to a large degree, a function of the size of the infarction, considerable effort has been devoted to exploring interventions that might limit infarct size. Any intervention that could decrease the amount of myocardium lost after acute coronary occlusion would serve not only to improve early survival but also, hopefully, to preserve myocardial function, improving both early and late postinfarction morbidity and mortality.

A host of interventions have been shown to be effective in limiting the extent of myocardial necrosis resulting from acute coronary occlusion, including propranolol, verapamil, nephedipine, methylprednisolone, and hyaluronidase.[70–73] It is presumed that these agents work by favorably affecting the myocardial oxygen supply demand ratio through their effect on either myocardial metabolism, contractility, or collateral blood flow. Certain agents such as propranolol may exert a protective effect on the microvasculature during ischemia as well.[70] Not all of these protective agents have proved beneficial in the long run. Although methylprednisolone has been shown to diminish extent of myocardial injury in some studies, there is evidence from animal experiments[73] and from the human[74] that corticosteroid administration after acute infarction may inhibit infarct healing and increase the risks of infarct expansion, rupture, or aneurysm formation. Although anti-inflammatory agents such as cobra venom factor have been shown to decrease infarct size, other anti-inflammatory drugs such as indomethacin have been shown to result in increased myocardial necrosis in a canine infarct model.[75]

There is now a rapidly accumulating mass of data on agents that increase or decrease infarct size after coronary occlusion, most of which is still derived from the animal laboratory. Experimental data, to date, suggest that virtually all interventions—metabolic, pharmacologic, or mechanical—will likely prove effective in preserving ischemic myocardium only if the intervention is instituted within 6 to 9 h of the acute coronary event.[76] The actual amount of myocardium to be preserved in the human after an acute coronary event remains unclear and is likely a function of many factors not necessarily similarly operative in the experimental infarct, including collaterals, coronary spasm, extent and duration of coronary thrombosis, and myocardial hypertrophy.

Topographic Changes after Myocardial Infarction

Most efforts at myocardial preservation are directed at the first few hours following coronary occlusion. Autopsy studies have suggested that acute topographic changes may occur in the heart as a result of expansion of the myocardial infarct which might lead to a functional increase in infarct size.[77] The zone of acute infarction becomes akinetic almost immediately after interruption of blood flow and, in the days following the event, may undergo a progressive thinning and regional dilatation of the injured zone leading to "infarct expansion." Expansion may be a form of intramyocardial rupture in which stretching and disruption of myocardial cells leads to thinning of the infarct. This phenomena may be observed within a week of the acute infarct and at a time too early to be accounted for by macrophagic removal of dead tissue (Fig. 10). Infarct expansion occurs predominantly in large, transmural infarcts and in myocardium that has not been subjected to previous infarction. Patients with small subendocardial infarcts do not appear at risk for expansion. Thus, expansion shares many features with myocardial rupture, occurring primarily

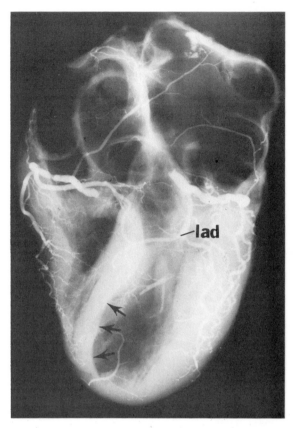

FIGURE 10 Expansion of an acute anteroseptal myocardial infarct of 7 days is seen in this postmortem radiograph. The left anterior descending (LAD) coronary artery is totally occluded in the distribution of the infarct. The infarcted segment (arrows) shows disproportionate thinning and dilatation, a regional alteration that led to net cavity dilatation within days of the acute event.

with transmural first infarcts and at an average of 5 to 7 days after the acute coronary event.

At autopsy, moderate to marked infarct expansion was observed in approximately one-quarter of transmural infarcts.[77] Serial two-dimensional echocardiographic study of selected acute infarcts has now demonstrated this phenomenon in several living patients with anterior transmural myocardial infarcts.[78] In the patients studied by echocardiography, infarct expansion resulted in a disproportionate dilatation of the region of infarction of close to 50 percent and in a net increase in left ventricular dimension of over 25 percent. It seems apparent that insofar as infarct expansion can lead to net left ventricular cavity dilatation, it will be deleterious to the acutely injured and ischemic heart. What remains to be determined is the extent to which infarct expansion may be a cause of clinical infarct extension with new necrosis, as a consequence of hemodynamic disadvantage associated with cavity dilatation, and the extent to which interventions in the acute setting may inhibit or aggravate the development of expansion.

Ischemic Cardiomyopathy

Viewed broadly, cardiomyopathy refers to disease of heart muscle, and its primary manifestation is an enlarged dilated heart most commonly associated with symptoms of pulmonary congestion. Dr. George Burch has pointed out that in the Western world in particular, and in the present era in which mortality from acute myocardial infarction appears to be falling, it is likely that ischemic rather than idiopathic cardiomyopathy will predominate in clinical practice.[79–81] The cardiac pathology of ischemic cardiomyopathy is severe three-vessel disease and extensive myocardial fibrosis in multiple vascular distributions leading to cardiac dilatation and secondary hypertrophy (Fig. 11). In some

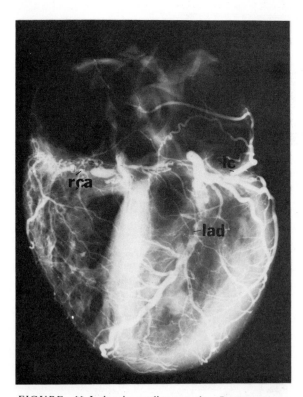

FIGURE 11 Ischemic cardiomyopathy. Postmortem radiograph of the intact heart shows significant biventricular dilation of this heart associated with severe triple-vessel disease with multiple near total occlusions of the left anterior descending (LAD) and left circumflex (LC) coronary arteries and a total occlusion of the right coronary (RCA) artery. This heart contained at least four separate infarcts in the distribution of the narrowed vessels. The heart dilated and hypertrophied in response to this injury, but no discrete left ventricular aneurysm had formed.

patients with ischemic cardiomyopathy, heart failure may predominate and chest pain may be minimal or absent, confusing the clinical picture with idiopathic congestive cardiomyopathy. Coronary angiography readily distinguishes the two entities, but more recently, myocardial perfusion scans with thallium 201 have proved useful in providing structural information on myocardium, often sufficient to distinguish ischemic from idiopathic congestive cardiomyopathy. Myocardial fibrosis or necrosis is rarely present in patients with idiopathic cardiomyopathy and the ^{201}Tl scan generally shows homogeneous tracer uptake (Figs. 12 and 13). This is in contrast to ischemic cardiomyopathy in which marked inhomogeneity in tracer uptake reflects regional myocardial injury characteristic of this condition.[82] The challenge of ischemic cardiomyopathy is whether or not surgical intervention is feasible to remodel and reperfuse the heart by infarct resection and coronary bypass. Since the scarring tends to be in multiple vascular distributions, however, and since a discrete left ventricular aneurysm is not present, the outlook for the surgical approach is not promising.

THE PATHOLOGY OF CORONARY ARTERY BYPASS GRAFT SURGERY

In the past decade a new form of coronary artery disease has appeared. Since the advent of coronary artery bypass graft surgery, we have been faced with an ever-increasing population that has undergone this procedure and in whom coronary anatomy has been drastically altered. Clinically, we know that this operation is almost always successful for relief of angina pectoris. Although individual patients or subsets may have achieved these benefits, abolition of myocardial ischemia, prevention of myocardial infarction, or prolongation of life have not been proved benefits of this procedure.[83] Important determinants of the outcome and success or failure of this procedure will be the early and the long-term changes in the implanted bypass graft, changes in the native coronary circulation, and the responses of myocardium to operation and to the implanted graft. Most of these answers will await detailed follow-up evaluation of patients clinically through postoperative angiographic studies. An important aspect of understanding the pathophysiology of coronary bypass grafting also will be the accumulation of morphologic information on early and late consequences of this procedure.[83,84] These late changes will of necessity be derived from studies of human morphology.

Although there is still limited information on the pathology of coronary artery bypass surgery, a number of studies have been performed that have provided

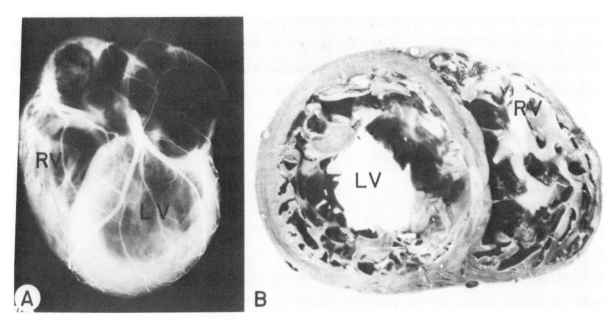

FIGURE 12 Here is an example of idiopathic dilated cardiomyopathy. Marked biventricular dilation is present, but the coronary arteries are widely patent. LV, left ventricle. RV, right ventricle. (*From B. H. Bulkley et al. Thallium 201 Imaging and Gated Blood Pool Scans in Patients with Ischemic and Idiopathic Congestive Cardiomyopathy: A Clinical and Pathologic Study, Circulation, 55:753, 1977. Reproduced with permission of the American Heart Association.*)

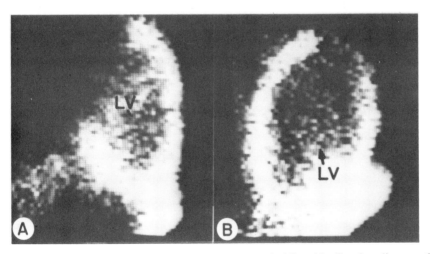

FIGURE 13 Thallium 201 myocardial perfusion scan in idiopathic dilated cardiomyopathy in the anterior (*A*) and left anterior oblique (*B*) position showing homogeneous tracer uptake and marked cavity dilatation. In diffuse cavity dilatation ischemic cardiomyopathy is evident, but perfusion defects are usually prominent. (*From B. H. Bulkley et al., Thallium 201 Imaging and Gated Blood Pool Scans in Patients with Ischemic and Idiopathic Congestive Cardiomyopathy: A Clinical and Pathologic Study, Circulation, 55:753, 1977. Reproduced with permission of the American Heart Association.*)

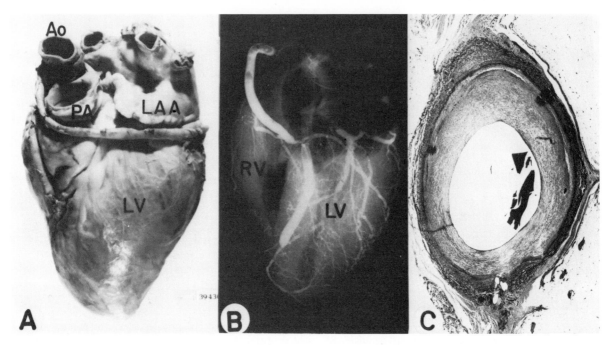

FIGURE 14 Pathology of coronary artery bypass graft surgery. *A*. A heart with saphenous vein bypass grafts from the aorta (Ao) to left anterior descending (LAD) and circumflex coronary arteries. *B*. A postmortem angiogram of a heart with patent bypass grafts to the LAD and right coronary arteries. *C*. A cross section of a saphenous vein implanted for 5 months. Although the lumen is widely patent, a thick layer of circumferential plaque is present (VvG, ×9). (*From B. H. Bulkley and G. M. Hutchins, Accelerated "Atherosclerosis": A Morphologic Study of 97 Saphenous Vein-Coronary Artery Bypass Grafts, Circulation, 55:163, 1977. Reproduced with permission of the American Heart Association.*)

information, particularly about the early effects of this procedure on the heart. To simplify the approach to the pathology of coronary bypass surgery, one should focus on at least three aspects of this procedure: the coronary artery graft anastomosis site, bypass graft iself, and the myocardium in the distribution of the grated vessel (Fig. 14).

Coronary Artery Bypass Graft Anastomosis

After a decade of coronary artery bypass surgery, the technical aspects of the anastomosis of the bypass graft to the coronary artery have been sufficiently developed so that most grafts are patent early after operation. Angiographic studies have suggested that well over 90 percent of grafts are patent within 6 months of this procedure. When grafts fail early, however, most of the time the failure is associated with a problem at the anastomosis site, most often at the coronary graft anastomosis site. A serial histologic study of the graft to coronary anastomoses by Griffith et al. (84) has demonstrated at least three mechanisms for occlusion in the anastomosis site: (1) compression or loss of arterial lumen by utilization of the bulk of arterial wall within the anastomosis; (2) thrombosis at the anas-

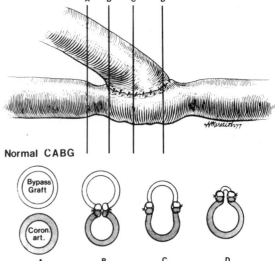

FIGURE 15 A schematic diagram of the vein-to-coronary artery bypass anastomosis. Serial histologic sectioning of the anastomotic site demonstrates three major mechanisms of narrowing. (See Fig. 16.) (*From B. H. Bulkley and G. M. Hutchins, Pathology of Coronary Artery Bypass Graft Surgery, Arch. Pathol., 102:273, 1978. Reproduced with permission of the American Medical Association.*)

tomosis site; (3) dissection of the native coronary artery at the site of anastomosis (Figs. 15 and 16). Compression and thrombosis are the most common causes of narrowing or occlusion at the anastomosis site. Compression or loss of circumference occurs most commonly as a result of anastomosis into a vessel with an internal diameter of less than 2 mm; as a result, with the necessary utilization of coronary wall for the anastomosis, the lumen become obliterated. The vessels may be intrinsically small, or they may have an eccentric atherosclerotic plaque at the site of the anastomosis that makes them functionally small. In the above autopsy study,[84] close to 50 percent of coronary arteries with internal diameters of less than 2 mm were occluded at autopsy, suggesting that coronary artery bypass graft into small vessels brings with it the inherent risk of graft failure.

Why grafts fail as a result of thrombosis is not entirely clear. Intimal injury has been shown to occur in almost all grafts that are removed from the leg and implanted in the heart. Ultrastructural studies have shown the endothelium to be denuded in the majority of these grafts. A normal response to vascular injury is intimal thrombosis. Why some patients should develop an occlusive thrombus as opposed to a thin layer of platelet fibrin deposition over the site is not clear, however. The role of anticoagulation in graft thrombosis and the potential for inhibition of graft thrombosis with anticoagulation remain to be determined.

Incontinuity Grafts

In the early years of coronary bypass surgery most patients received one or two bypass grafts. It is now the usual practice to attempt to bypass all critical stenoses, and as a consequence the need for as many as six or seven bypass grafts in a single patient has arisen. Since the aortic root is usually not large enough to accommodate more than two or three proximal vein-to-aorta anastomoses, incontinuity or jump grafts have been developed for multiple anastomoses (Fig. 17). Jump grafts utilize an end-to-end anastomosis at the aorta and distally in a coronary artery; in the midportion of the graft; and at sites of coronary artery narrowing; side-to-side anastomosis is performed between the graft and the coronary artery distal to a given occlusion. These "jumps" allow multiple grafts but also carry a risk of multiple anastomoses failure if one site becomes occluded. Furthermore, because these grafts are long and course for distances across the heart, they may be more prone to kinking and twisting. Although kinking and twisting may have no immediate consequence on graft patency, it remains to be seen whether or not, in the long run, the resulting hemodynamics stress may lead or predispose to atherosclerotic lesions.[85]

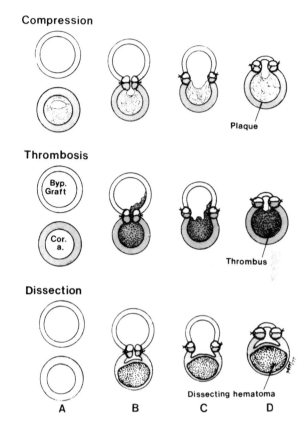

FIGURE 16 Diagram illustrating the three types of obstructive lesions that may occur at the graft-to-artery anastomosis site. Levels A, B, C, and D are the same as those shown in Figure 15. (*From B. H. Bulkley and G. M. Hutchins, Pathology of Coronary Artery Bypass Graft Surgery, Arch. Pathol., 102:273, 1978. Reproduced with permission of the American Medical Association.*)

Morphologic Changes of the Implanted Saphenous Vein Bypass Graft

It is now widely recognized that implanted saphenous vein bypass grafts undergo characteristic morphologic changes, which for the most part reflect the duration of their implantation.[86–93] In part as a consequence of the endothelial damage which probably always occurs with manipulation of the vein, virtually all grafts within 24 h of implantation show fibrin and platelet deposition on their surface. Laminar deposits of fibrin and platelet thrombi on the surface of the graft organize and within a 1- to 2-week period of time, grafts show intimal thickening or hyperplasia. The loose intimal fibrous plaques which develop circumferentially in the vascular lumen are characteristic of organizing thrombi and have been observed by most investigators in all grafts by 4 weeks and in most grafts by as early as 2 weeks after implantation.

Coronary Artery Bypass Grafts

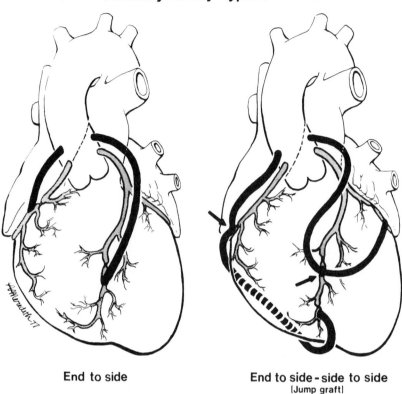

End to side   **End to side-side to side**
                                         [Jump graft]

FIGURE 17 Diagram illustrating coronary artery bypass grafts that have single and multiple anastomoses. (Left) Two single grafts with end-to-side anastomoses, (right) side-to-side (arrows) and end-to-side anastomoses in each of two separate grafts to left anterior descending and right coronary arteries, respectively. These are incontinuity or jump grafts. (*From B. H. Bulkley and G. M. Hutchins, Pathology of Coronary Artery Bypass Graft Surgery, Arch. Pathol., 102:273, 1978. Reproduced with permission of the American Medical Association.*)

Intimal and medial changes in late coronary artery bypass grafts, however, are considerably more variable and less predictable. Circumferential fibrous plaque of different grafts implanted for the same periods and often within the same heart varies in extent and in the degree to which it narrows the lumen (Fig. 18). Nevertheless, morphologic studies of grafts implanted for over 1 year have documented that greater than 75 percent lumenal narrowing of the coronary artery bypass graft by circumferential fibrous plaque may occur.[91] Angiographic studies in late survivors of coronary artery bypass graft surgery have also suggested the development of focal lumenal narrowings of the grafts both at and away from the anastomosis site. Although there is little histologic information in these very late grafts, it is suggested that a similar phenomenon of plaque proliferation within the graft leads to graft narrowing and, in some cases, failure.[94] This type of slow progressive development of graft lesions is to be distinguished from graft failure, which occurs early after

implantation and largely reflects sudden acute thrombosis of the graft.

The pathogenesis of the fibrous intimal plaque is not fully known. Some have suggested that the intimal proliferation is a normal response of a vein to arterial pressure, and to a certain extent, it reflects a reparative change as a consequence of hemodynamic alterations in pressure and flow. If the intimal proliferation were only an "arterialization" of the vein wall in response to the hypertensive stress, one might expect that the lesions would develop more or less to the same extent in all patients and that the lesions would not necessarily be focal. It is likely that fibrous plaque, which develops within weeks after implantation of the grafts, is a normal reparative phenomenon resulting from endothelial injury at the time of surgery, but that the continuation of the development of the fibrous plaque as time goes on represents continued traumatic injury related to increased pressure within the graft leading to endothelial damage, fibrin deposition, and subsequent plaque proliferation. Hemodynamic abnormalities within the graft per se, such as downstream graft narrowing creating a pressure gradient between the graft and the native vessels, may also accelerate endothelial injury and plaque proliferation. Histologically the fibrous intimal plaque that does develop in these grafts is virtually indistinguishable from atherosclerosis. Fibrous tissue infiltrated with lipid-laden macrophages and showing focal calcium deposition are all features of the intimal plaque that develops and, as such, may be viewed as an accelerated form of atherosclerosis in that it may develop as early as months after implantation. Whether or not risk fac-

tors important in the development and acceleration of atherosclerosis in the native coronary tree are the same for atherosclerosis within the graft is not known.

For the future it will be important to better characterize the morphology of late graft failures and to determine the effects of metabolic risk factors, including serum lipids and diabetes mellitus, and hemodynamic risk factors, including hypertension, disproportion between the graft and the coronary artery, and graft twisting, on the late outcome of this procedure. Whether or not anticoagulation has a role in the inhibition of plaque proliferation also remains to be determined. Only with angiographic and morphologic stud-

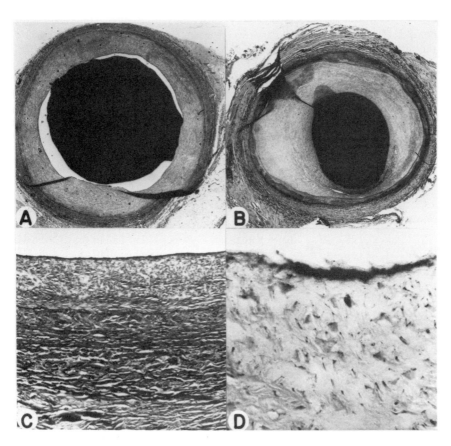

FIGURE 18 Saphenous vein bypass graft atherosclerosis. Two vein grafts are shown which have been in place for approximately 6 months and which contain different amounts of concentric fibrous plaque. *A*. Widely patent graft with circumferential plaque which is approximately four times as thick as the original vein wall (VvG, ×9). *B*. This graft has a focal narrowing by newly formed plaque which has comprised lumenal area by 75 percent (VvG, ×9). *C*. High-power magnification of vein wall shown in (*A*). Histologically the newly formed plaque has features of atherosclerosis with collagen fibers, mesenchymal cells and focal lipid laden macrophages, and calcium deposition. *D*. Focal fibrin deposits may also present on the intimal surface of the vein grafts. Black stained intimal fibrosis is shown here in this higher power magnification of a section of the graft shown in (*A*) and (*C*). Fibrin is still being deposited here after months of implantation (PTAH, × 300). (*From B . H . Bulkley and G . M . Hutchins, Accelerated ''Atherosclerosis'': A Morphologic Study of 97 Saphenous Vein-Coronary Artery Bypass Grafts, Circulation, 55:163, 1977. Reproduced with permission of the American Heart Association.*)

ies on the saphenous veins grafts implanted for periods of over 5 years will we be able to determine the extent to which this procedure is curative or merely palliative and the circumstances under which one or the other outcome prevails.

Myocardial Consequences of Coronary Artery Bypass Surgery

At the present time, myocardial infarction occurs in less than 5 percent of patients who undergo coronary artery bypass surgery when conventional techniques for detecting myocardial injury, i.e., the development of new Q waves, are utilized. Enzymatic analyses, myocardial imaging studies and autopsy studies have suggested the greater incidence of perioperative myocardial infarction. Regardless of the true incidence, which may range from 5 to 20 percent, the pathogenesis of myocardial infarction in the setting of coronary

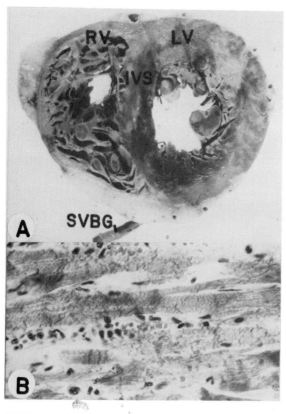

FIGURE 19 Myocardial necrosis after coronary bypass surgery. Despite a patent saphenous vein bypass graft (SVBG), hemorrhagic necroses (arrow) developed in the distribution of the bypass (A) and was of the contraction-band type (B) (hematoxylin and eosin stain, × 230). (Reproduced in part from B. H. Bulkley and G. M. Hutchins, Myocardial Consequences of Coronary Artery Bypass Graft Surgery, Circulation, 56:906, 1977, with permission of the American Heart Association.)

artery bypass surgery differs from that of the "usual" infarct.[94,96]

Coagulation necrosis is the predominant form of myocardial injury which occurs in patients with a natural history of coronary artery disease who develop myocardial infarction after coronary occlusion. As described above, this is to be distinguished from contraction band necrosis, which is the type of injury that develops in myocardium that has been reperfused after a period of lethal but transient nonperfusion. The myocardial necrosis that develops in the setting of bypass surgery is most apt to be contraction band in type (Fig. 19). By necessity the myocardium is subject to some degree of transient nonperfusion during operation. An autopsy study of 58 patients, accumulated over a 9-year period, who died within 1 month of coronary artery bypass surgery showed severe regional myocardial necrosis in 22 of them.[94] "Infarcts" in the 22 cases were predominantly contraction band necrosis or red infarcts, occurring most often in the distribution of a bypassed coronary artery that was widely patent and, to a certain extent, more often in patients with unstable angina and left main coronary artery disease. Only 4 patients showed the more classic coagulation infarct related to a new occlusion. Thus, in the majroity of patients with myocardial necrosis studied at autopsy, the injury developed in the setting of technically good myocardial revascularization. Furthermore, of the grafts that were totally occluded at autopsy, myocardial infarcts resulted in less than 20 percent. Thus, something of a paradoxical situation is present: most infarcts appear to occur in patients who have had technically good and patent grafts, and infarcts usually do not occur when grafts are occluded. The latter observation is not surprising, since collaterals are usually well developed in patients with chronic ischemic heart disease, and for the most part the bypassed narrowed vessel is still partially patent. That most injury occurs in relation to patent grafts is perhaps more surprising but has also been noted clinically. A postoperative angiographic study from the Cleveland Clinic demonstrated that when new wall motion abnormalities developed postoperatively, in 75 percent of the cases they developed in the distribution of patent grafts.[97]

The optimistic side of this observation is that the myocardial necrosis developing in the setting of patent grafts should be a treatable form of intraoperative myocardial injury. The ischemic myocardium in the distribution of a critically narrowed coronary artery is likely in particular jeopardy for necrosis during the stress of coronary artery bypass procedure, in which nonpulsatile mean perfusion pressures of 70 to 80 mm Hg are maintained. In the early days of coronary artery bypass graft surgery, normothermic anoxic arrest was used to induce a quiet operative field so that coronary anastomoses could be performed. More recently, hypothermia and the addition of a variety of cardioplegic solutions to induce a quiet field and a metabolically preserved myocardium have been introduced. It is likely that these improved techniques of intraoperative myocardial preservation will be successful in decreasing the intraoperative myocardial injury that occurs in some patients, particularly in those patients with the most severe coronary disease at the time of operation.[98-102] We might optimistically suggest that with improved methods of myocardial preservation, coronary artery bypass surgery may begin to show not only success in relief of angina but also improvement in myocardial contractility and possibly longevity.[83] Morphologic studies on the pathophysiology of the intraoperative injury will provide important feedback in understanding and preventing this type of myocardial loss.

IDIOPATHIC CARDIOMYOPATHIES

The cardiomyopathies can be broadly classified into two groups: primary idiopathic and secondary cardiomypathies. In the former group are the three categories of idiopathic dilated, hypertrophic and restrictive cardiomyopathy.[103,104] Secondary cardiomyopathies include the heterogeneous assembly of degenerative, metabolic, and infiltrative myocardial disease such as sarcoidosis, amyloidosis, and glycogen storage disease.[105-107] It is the primary cardiomyopathies that have been the focus of most clinical investigation.

Idiopathic Dilated
Congestive Cardiomyopathy

Although hypertrophic and congestive cardiomyopathies tend to be grouped under the broad heading of idiopathic cardiomyopathies, these two entities could not be further apart historically, functionally, or structurally. Idiopathic dilated congestive cardiomyopathy is an "old disease" which Sir William Osler described as "dilatation and hypertrophy of the heart due to over exertion and alcohol which occurs in able-bodied men at the middle period of life, [who] complain first of palpitations or irregularity of the action of the heart, shortness of breath, and subsequently the usual symptoms of cardiac insufficiency."[108] In contrast to hypertrophic cardiomyopathy, idiopathic dilated cardiomyopathy appears to be rarely heritable. Sporadic cases of dilated cardiomyopathy have been identified in families and, when studied, have suggested both dominant and recessive inheritance patterns.[109]

The characteristic morphologic finding in this disorder is a globe-shaped heart with dilatation generally out of proportion to hypertrophy (Fig. 12). Endocar-

dial thickening and mural thrombi in all four dilated chambers is common. Gross, microscopic, and ultrastructural findings in the myocardium in idiopathic congestive cardiomyopathy are usually disappointing. Grossly the myocardium appears normal, and histologically, nonspecific degeneration and hypertrophy of focal myocardial cells may be observed. Small foci of fibrosis may be present in subendocardium or at the tips of the papillary muscles, but necrosis or fibrosis of any significant amount does not occur. Acute or chronic inflammatory cells are also not a feature of this disorder. Ultrastructural changes in biopsies from patients with congestive cardiomyopathy have also identified no specific abnormalities of the myocardial cells.[104]

Although there is little new information on the pathogenesis of idiopathic dilated cardiomyopathy, there is continued evidence that a prior acute viral myocarditis may have somehow affected the heart and led to acute dilatation with subsequent chronic structural alteration.[110] Although this sequence of events has not been proved in the human, infection of mice hearts with Coxsackie B3 virus has suggested this sequence.[111] Other viral agents that have been implicated in human cardiomyopathy besides Coxsackie B are type A2 influenza virus and arboviruses. The role of the immune system as a cause or contributer to cardiomyopathy remains unclear. Recent immunofluorescent studies of human myocardial biopsies have detected deposits of complement and immunoglobulin on the surface of myocardial fibers,[112] alterations which may be primary or secondary to preexisting myocardial cell injury.

Other agents which have been implicated in the etiology of certain cardiomyopathies include heavy metals such as cobalt, alcohol, and a variety of drugs.[113,114] A relatively recent clinical and pathologic model of idiopathic cardiomyopathy in the human is the cardiomyopathy that may be produced by exposure to the antineoplastic drugs adriamycin and daunorubicin.[115,116] Usually observed in patients who have been exposed to over 550 mg/m² of these agents in a total dose, the antracyclene-induced cardiomyopathy occurs weeks to months after the drug administration. The hearts with this cardiotoxicity resemble the idiopathic dilated cardiomyopathies showing four-chamber cardiac dilatation and nonspecific focal myocardial degenerative lesions. Occasionally a hemorrhagic necrosis may be observed in this disease as well and is believed to reflect endothelial necrosis resulting from drug toxcity. The one distinctive morphologic abnormality that has been observed in this human "model" of cardiomyopathy is in the nucleus. Disorganization and decreased staining of chromatin have been attributed to binding of the antracyclene drug to nuclear DNA, which may subsequently lead to the cytoplasmic alterations and myocardial failure.[115]

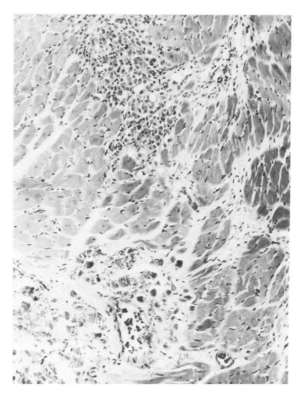

FIGURE 20 Photomicrograph of a section of myocardium from a strain of Syrian hamsters showing a heritable idiopathic dilated cardiomyopathy. Unlike human cardiomyopathy, this animal model shows marked focal necrosis, fibrosis, and calcification of myocardium (hematoxylin and eosin stain, × 160).

One form of cardiomyopathy of unknown etiology which is achieving increasing recognition is that observed in familial diabetes mellitus. Since much of the cardiac dysfunction observed in the adult diabetic is a consequence of atherosclerotic coronary disease, the suggestion that diabetes may also be associated with a nonatherosclerotic cardiomyopathy has been controversial. Regan et al. have recently provided further clinical and pathologic evidence, however, that a primary myocardial abnormality may develop in the diabetic.[117] They performed hemodynamic studies on 17 patients with familial diabetes mellitus and a history of dyspnea or chest pain, but with no prior history of myocardial infarction, systemic hypertension, or marked obesity, and observed normal coronary angiograms in 12 of them. Of this latter group, 8 showed left ventricular abnormalities suggestive of a preclinical cardiomyopathy with elevated end-diastolic pressures but normal ejection fractions. The 4 other patients who had a history of congestive heart failure showed more marked abnormalities, including diminished ejection fractions and diffuse hypokinesis. These investigators also did cardiac pathologic studies on 11

diabetics selected on the basis of adequate clinical evaluation. Nine of them had essentially normal epicardial coronary arteries, and none showed narrowings of the intramural coronary arteries, but the majority of them died of congestive heart failure.

The major postmortem abnormalities in the hearts of these latter patients were increased heart weights, deposition of periodic acid-Schiff-positive material in the interstitium, and increased concentrations of triglycerides and cholesterol in samples of myocardial tissue as compared to normal control hearts. Although other studies have pointed toward nonatherosclerotic coronary disease involving mainly small vessels as the cause of diabetic cardiomyopathy,[118,119] Regan et al. are suggesting that a diffuse extravascular abnormality of myocardial cell and interstitium may be responsible.[117] Clearly, more morphologic data needs to be acquired to better characterize this entity and to determine the relative contributions of vascular and extravascular abnormalities, when present, to the clinical syndrome of diabetic cardiomyopathy.

The major animal model for congestive cardiomyopathy is a genetic one which runs in a particular strain of Syrian hamsters.[120] The cardiomyopathy shows an autosomal recessive pattern of inheritance. In these hamsters a dilated and hypertrophied heart develops with age and results in death owing to congestive heart failure at approximately one-third the normal lifespan. These Syrian hamster strains have been exhaustively studied hemodynamically, biochemically, and structurally, and yet the precise mechanism for the cardiomyopathy has not yet been identified. Abnormalities of oxidative phosphorylation and calcium transport have been demonstrated, but these abnormalities tend to develop late in the course of the disease. Marked abnormalities of cell structure occur which are evident both histologically and ultrastructurally. Disruption of mitochondria and degeneration of sarcomeres may precede a local widespread necrosis, fibrosis, and calcification (Fig. 20). Although one of our best models, the hamster cardiomyopathy differs from most human congestive cardiomyopathies in which no consistent biochemical or structural abnormalities have been identified and in which genetic transmission is almost never present.

Hypertrophic Cardiomyopathy

In contrast to the idiopathic dilated form, hypertrophic cardiomyopathy is a relatively new disease which has been the subject of considerable focus, investigation, and controversy in recent years.[121] Hypertrophic cardiomyopathy was first described by the English pathologist Teare a little over 20 years ago as asymmetric hypertrophy of the heart associated with sudden death in young adults. Teare also observed the strikingly bizarre histologic features of the myocardium which led him to suspect a primary muscle tumor. The clinical significance of this morphologic observation became apparent with the observations of Lord Brock at almost the same time. Brock observed a patient with a clinical picture of valvular aortic stenosis who, at valve operation, was found to have a normal aortic valve but a greatly hypertrophied interventricular septum. Appropriately, he viewed this entity as an idiopathic cardiomyopathy with "functional obstruction." Subsequent studies of this disease from many centers characterized it as one that was most common in seemingly young healthy persons in their 20s and 30s; frequently familial; and associated with symptoms of syncope, heart failure, and left ventricular hypertrophy and with electrocardiograms often demonstrating a pseudoinfarct pattern. Sudden death was a recognized complication.[122] In symptomatic patients this disease appeared to carry an annual mortality as high as 4 percent, a figure quite as bad as that associated with symptomatic coronary disease but possibly worse in that a younger population was involved. Hemodynamic characterization of the disease demonstrated a variable subaortic pressure gradient as great as 75 to 100 mm Hg in some patients with this condition, which led to the early names for this disease: idiopathic hypertrophic subaortic stenosis (IHSS), hypertrophic

obstructive cardiomyopathy (HOCM), and muscular subaortic stenosis (MSS). In a short time, however, it became apparent that all patients with this disease did not have this gradient and that the presence or absence of the gradient did not appear to correlate with either symptoms or prognosis. The significance of the pressure gradient is also not fully understood. Since the gradient tends to be maximal in midsystole and late systole after much of the blood has been ejected, it is not clear whether the gradient reflects a true outflow tract obstruction or a pressure generated after outflow by virtue of cavity obliteration in late systole.

MORPHOLOGIC FEATURES OF HYPERTROPHIC CARDIOMYOPATHY

Detailed morphologic study of the heart in genetic hypertrophic cardiomyopathy[123–125] has demonstrated the occurrence of asymmetric hypertrophy in the majority of these hearts (Fig. 21). Not only are the hearts asymmetrically hypertrophied, particularly in the region of the septum, but there is also evidence that the septal curvature in the longitudinal plane is reversed, being convex to the left, resulting in an abnormally shaped left ventricular cavity. Since the transverse

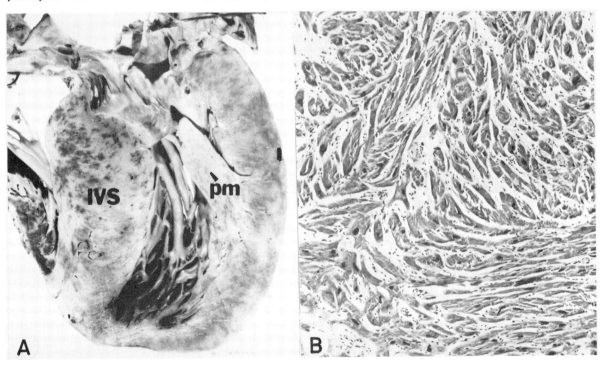

FIGURE 21 Genetic hypertrophic cardiomyopathy with asymmetric septal hypertrophy and marked reversal of septal curvature in the longitudinal plane, giving the septum a catenoid shape (*A*). Shown in (*B*) is the characteristic histologic finding of myocardium in the septum and sometimes in other portions of the left ventricle. The myocardial fibers have a disorganized pattern, giving a swirling and interlacing appearance. IVS, interventricular septum; pm, papillary muscle (hematoxylin and eosin stain, × 50).

plane is concave to the left as in the normal heart, the septum takes on a "catenoid" shape.[126] The occurrence of striking myocardial fiber disarray particularly in the septum, but also to a lesser extent in the left ventricular free wall, is also a feature of genetic hypertrophic cardiomyopathy.[123,127] Ultrastructural studies have shown that the disarray is also reflected at a subcellular level with abnormalities in orientation and branching of the sarcomeres. Striking abnormalities of the small vessels of the septum have been observed with overall enlargement of the vessels and with medial and intimal hypertrophy, but without compromise of the net lumen size.[124,128]

The gross morphologic findings in genetic hypertrophic cardiomyopathy have become especially useful in clinical diagnosis.[129,130] Asymmetric septal hypertrophy, which is one distinctive feature of this disease, can be detected noninvasively by the echocardiogram. The echocardiogram has been used to detect and identify asymptomatic disease in first-degree relatives and to identify an autosomal dominant pattern of inheritance.[131] What has become the subject of considerable study is the extent to which the rather striking morphologic findings in hypertrophic cardiomyopathy are specific and even pathognomonic for this entity. Initially, it was believed that both asymmetric septal hypertrophy (ASH) and myocardial fiber disarray were pathognomonic for hypertrophic cardiomyopathy and that virtually all patients with clinical

signs and symptoms of hypertrophic cardiomyopathy, and indeed, virtually all patients with idiopathic left ventricular hypertrophy, had these structural abnormalities of the heart.[121] ASH was viewed as the unifying link in the entire spectrum of hypertrophic cardiomyopathy.[132] However, this no longer appears to be the case. First, asymmetric septal hypertrophy and myocardial fiber disarray are not pathognomonic of hypertrophic cardiomyopathy, and second, all patients with hypertrophic cardiomyopathy do not appear to have the distinctive morphology initially described by Teare.

Evidence for the nonspecificity of asymmetry of septum and left ventricular free wall dimensions as a morphologic finding in the heart has come from many sources.[121,133–135] The human heart early in its embryonic and fetal development has a septum that is thicker than the free wall (Fig. 22). Many newborns also demonstrate asymmetry of septal thickness relative to the free wall. The septum may also be asymmetrically hypertrophied in conditions associated with severe right ventricular hypertrophy, including primary pulmonary hypertension and a host of congenital malformations associated with marked right ventricular hypertrophy. Similarly, the myocardial fiber disarray noted histologically is not pathognomonic of hypertrophic cardiomyopathy. Certain portions of the normal heart show branching muscle bundles similar in quality but not quantity to the disarray seen in the genetic form of

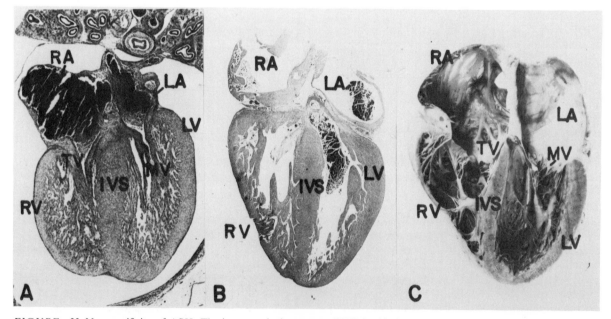

FIGURE 22 Nonspecificity of ASH: The interventricular septum (IVS) in this human embryo (*A*) and in this human fetus (*B*) is thicker than the left ventricular (LV) free wall. Shown in (*C*) is a normal adult heart showing the usual finding of an IVS equal to or slightly thinner than LV free wall. LA, left atrium; MV, mitral valve; RA, right atrium; RV, right ventricle; TV, tricuspid valve. (*From B. H. Bulkley et al., Asymmetric Hypertrophy and Myocardial Fiber Disarray, Circulation, 56:292, 1977. Reproduced with permission of the American Heart Association.*)

hypertrophic cardiomyopathy.[135] A variety of congenital heart diseases have also been observed to show marked myocardial fiber disarray in both septum and ventricular free wall and also to show striking small-vessel abnormalities.[134,136] Interestingly enough, salamander hearts grown in tissue culture also develop disorganized histology after several weeks, an observation which Ferrans et al.[123] suggested as pointing to the nonspecificity of this pattern.

These morphologic observations on ventricular configuration and myocardial histology do not mean that their occurrence in rather striking form in patients with clinical signs of hypertrophic cardiomyopathy is not an important and even characteristic and distinctive finding. It does mean, however, that their occurrence alone or in combination with conditions other than hypertrophic cardiomyopathy, such as congenital heart disease, acromegaly, valvular aortic stenosis, or the apparently healthy newborn, does not necessitate the diagnosis of a coexisting genetic cardiomyopathy.

HYPERTROPHIC CARDIOMYOPATHY: A SPECTRUM OF DISEASE

Some workers have suggested that all hypertrophic cardiomyopathy falls into a single disease category, virtually always showing the characteristic morphology outlined above.[132] Patients with idiopathic left ventricular hypertrophy and those with clinical signs and symptoms of hypertrophic cardiomyopathy have been lumped under this morphologic umbrella. There is increasing evidence, however, that the clinical spectrum of hypertrophic cardiomyopathy is more heterogeneous. All patients with this clinical presentation do not necessarily have asymmetric septal hypertrophy, myocardial fiber disarray, or abnormal systolic motion of the mitral valve; nor do they necessarily have a genetic disease carrying a rather imposing mortality. The hemodynamics and abnormal septal motion of mitral valve observed in hypertrophic disease can be created in an animal model by excess catecholamine administration[137] and have been observed in a variety of states, including volume depletion, during catecholamine infusion,[138] with long-standing hypertension, and valvular aortic stenosis.[139] Moreover, patients with hypercontractile states having clinical and echocardiographic features characteristic of a hypertrophic cardiomyopathy have been observed by noninvasive techniques to be free of asymmetric hypertrophy and have been noted at autopsy to show no asymmetric hypertrophy or abnormal myocardial histology.[140] Thus, although there is a distinctive form of hypertrophic disease described by Teare, not all hypertrophic disease appears to be Teare's disease. Since Teare's disease does show a characteristic asymmetric hypertrophy which allows ready noninvasive studies in those with or without prominent symptoms, we now know more about this disease than about other forms of hypertrophic disease, some of which may be true primary cardiomyopathies and some of which may represent "secondary" disease states.

PATHOGENESIS OF HYPERTROPHIC CARDIOMYOPATHY

Hypertrophic cardiomyopathy has only recently been defined, so it is not surprising that its pathogenesis is as yet unresolved. The form of hypertrophic cardiomyopathy associated with asymmetric hypertrophy and histologic abnormalities of myocardium may well reflect an underlying genetic defect which results in abnormal septal shape and myocardial fiber malalignment.[123] The septal configuration or the histologic disarray or both may be a primary manifestation of a genetic abnormality.[126,132] The histologic findings may also reflect abnormal wall stresses and wall tension created by a congenital abnormality of septal shape.[126,134] It is also possible that genetically determined functional abnormalities of contraction, as might be seen with abnormal beta receptors, could, if present early enough in embryonic life, result in the distinctive structural features of the heart as seen in genetic hypertrophic disease. Whether function dictates structure or structure dictates function is an issue that goes far beyond the discussion of hypertrophic cardiomyopathy and is not likely to be readily resolved. Nevertheless, it provides exciting avenues for speculation and thought.

SECONDARY CARDIOMYOPATHIES

Falling within the category of secondary cardiomyopathies are a host of disorders largely affecting myocardium, as opposed to coronary arteries, valves, or pericardium, that are secondary to a reasonably well identified pathogenetic process. Included therefore are a mixed assortment of disease such as sarcoidosis, amyloidosis, and glycogen storage disease. These three are identified in particular because they are examples of the "secondary cardiomyopathies" in that they may functionally behave, respectively, like dilated, restrictive, or hypertrophic cardiomyopathies.

A secondary cardiomyopathy which has been the subject of considerable recent study is that resulting from sarcoidosis (Fig. 23). Sarcoidosis is an infiltrative disease of myocardium which can mimic congestive

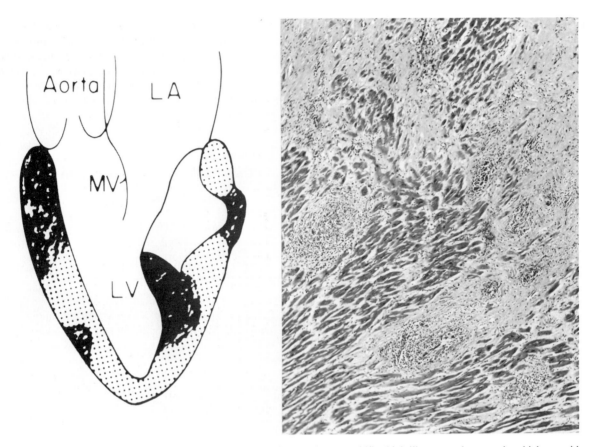

FIGURE 23 Shown in (*A*) is a schematic diagram adapted from Roberts et al.[141] which illustrates the ways in which sarcoid infiltration (black) of the myocardium can lead to cardiomyopathy. As seen in (*B*), sarcoid granulomas infiltrate and destroy myocardium (black areas). After the granulomatous process has healed, myocardial scars remain. LA, left atrium; LV, left ventricle; MV, mitral valve. (hematoxylin and eosin stain, × 60).

cardiomyopathy and lead to arrhythmias, including malignant ventricular arrhythmias, mitral incompetence, congestive heart failure, and sudden death.[105,141,142] Cardiac dysfunction is consequent to regional myocardial destruction by the granulomatous process with subsequent fibrosis. In addition to diffuse biventricular dilatation, regional aneurysm formation can result. The true incidence of cardiac sarcoidosis is not known, but a review of autopsy material from the Johns Hopkins Hospital suggests that well over 20 percent of patients with systemic sarcoidosis have some evidence of granulomatous infiltration of myocardium. In the majority of these patients, however, the infiltrative lesions are small and appear to have no clinical consequence. It is likely that only 5 percent or less of patients with systemic sarcoidosis have truly clinically significant disease.[105]

One of the obstacles to making this incidence assessment is that the diagnosis of myocardial sarcoidosis is difficult to make clinically, since the heart is not a readily biopsied organ; even if the latter were easier, there is no evidence that the yield would be great. Myocardial scans with isotopes such as ^{201}Tl allow noninvasive detection of myocardial infiltrative lesions and appear promising as a means of studying and possibly following this entity clinically. Thallium imaging in patients with cardiac sarcoidosis will be particularly useful in the younger patient in whom coronary disease as a cause of a given defect in myocardial tracer uptake is unlikely.[143]

VALVULAR HEART DISEASE

Rheumatic valvular disease and isolated aortic valvular stenosis are still the major causes of symptomatic valvular heart lesions. A recent study by Edwards et al. reexamined the pathogenesis of chronic rheumatic valvular disease, looking for evidence of ongoing smoldering active valvulitis.[144] They identified 10 cases of chronic rheumatic valvular disease in which active noninfective valvulitis coexisted, manifested by fibrinoid necrosis, edema, and inflammatory cellular infiltrates involving the aortic valve in all instances and the other three valves in 70 to 80 percent of the 10 patients. This study concluded that the active lesions represented an ongoing rheumatic endocarditis, consistent with the notion that recurrence is essential to the appearance of the chronic deforming rheumatic lesions. This study adds further support to the use of prophylactive penicillin in patients with a history of rheumatic heart disease.

Antibiotics are decreasing both the incidence and severity of rheumatic heart disease and the incidence and presentation of infective endocarditis, but the major change that is occurring in the area of valvular disease is iatrogenic. Considerable information has been gathered on the early and late changes in the prosthesis and the heart after valve replacement with the mechanical ball valve and tilting disk prostheses, which were the most popular type of artificial valve up until 3 to 4 years ago. Problems with ball variance, cloth wear, prosthetic-valve disproportion, thrombosis, endothelial proliferation, mechanical obstruction, dehiscence, and infection in these valves are by now well recognized.[145] Tissue valves have become increasingly popular as valve substitutes since they do not require anticoagulation. One reason for the current success of the present tissue valves is that they have undergone a special fixation process with stabilized glutaraldehyde, which essentially "tans" the valve and makes it antigenically inert and more durable. Earlier tissue valves fixed with formalin were prone to early degeneration, thickening, and infection.

The glutaraldehyde-fixed porcine heterograft is the tissue valve now most commonly used. The pig aortic valve sewn to cloth-covered stents demonstrates good hemodynamics after implantation with a minimal gradient and a central flow orifice. Widespread clinical use of these valves has given consistently good results at follow-up of over 5 years.[146] The major uncertainty of the porcine heterograft tissue valve is its long-term durability. Will the valve hold up indefinitely, and if not, what type of degenerative changes can we expect, and how soon? Answers to these and other questions about these valves will be dependent not only on meticulous clinical follow-up but also on careful morphologic analysis of structural changes in these valves after various periods of implantation and under various conditions.

To date, the latest and most in-depth analyses of the structural changes in the porcine valves have been performed by Spray and Roberts[147] and by Ferrans et al.[148] in which over 50 porcine heterografts were studied at autopsy after implantation periods of up to 75 months. The majority of these valves were normal by gross inspection; grossly evident abnormalities present in them included (1) cusp thrombus associated in some with commissural fusion and probable stenosis; (2) cusp degeneration with valvular incompetence,

presently found most often in those in place for close to 5 years or longer; and (3) prosthetic disproportion in which the stents appeared to compress and obstruct surrounding cardiac tissue. The most common and striking changes were observed histologically. The majority of valves demonstrated fibrin deposition and focal chronic inflammatory infiltrates. Giant cell formation was evident in close to half of the 18 late valves examined, suggesting a host reaction against the tissue valves. For the most part, these histologic abnormalities were focal and appeared not to impair valve function, but as the authors indicate, these observations clearly suggest that the porcine heterografts are not biologically inert. To what extent these structural changes will progress with time and be a source of valve dysfunction 5 to 10 years after implantation remains unknown, but this study strongly suggests that these valves may not be as durable as the currently available mechanical prostheses. Perhaps in no other area of cardiovascular disease is the need for human data to understand mechanisms and outcome of human disease so well exemplified.

Prosthetic Valve Endocarditis

One of the major and most life-threatening complications of prosthetic heart valves, regardless of type of prosthesis, is infective endocarditis. Infective endocarditis develops in as many as 4 percent of patients with prosthetic valves and may occur as a complication early in the postoperative period or late after valve replacement. It carries with it an unusually high mortality. Recent autopsy studies of the pathology of prosthetic valve endocarditis in patients who succumbed to prosthetic endocarditis have shown that annular infection, dehiscence, and prosthetic stenosis or incompetence frequently accompany prosthetic valve infection.[149–151] Incompetence of the valve usually results from dehiscence or from cusp destruction when tissue valves have been utilized and tends to occur most often with prostheses in the aortic position. Large vegetations leading to valvular stenosis were a relatively frequent finding in the mitral position, occurring in up to 70 percent of infected prosthetic mitral valves. Stenosis as a hemodynamic consequence of infective endocarditis is virtually unheard of when natural valves are infected. Another feature of prosthetic endocarditis which appears to differ from natural valve endocarditis is the relatively frequent occurrence of valve ring abscesses. Valve ring abscesses have been described in from 50 to 100 percent of patients dying with prosthetic endocarditis. It is a particularly forboding complication, since successful valve replacement becomes almost impossible if active infection involves the annulus, which is the sewing site. If the active infection can be eradicated with appropriate antibiotic treatment, replacement of the infected prosthesis, whether or not the infection involved the annulus, has a chance for success.

A major factor which appears to determine final outcome of prosthetic endocarditis is the severity of hemodynamic compromise. As with natural endocarditis, if severe heart failure has developed before surgical intervention, prognosis appears to be considerably poorer. Embolic phenomena are a frequent and often lethal complication of prosthetic endocarditis. Vegetations may be abundant, especially with staphylococcal and fungal infections, and necessitate surgical debridement. Conduction block is a relatively common accompaniment of aortic prosthetic endocarditis, and well over half the time it reflects deep infection that has involved the conduction tissue which is situated immediately beneath the aortic valve ring. Death usually results from intractable heart failure or embolism, and there is little doubt that, unlike its natural valve counterpart, surgical intervention is almost always necessary.

Natural Valve Infective Endocarditis

Recent autopsy studies on endocarditis have also focused on the valve ring abscess in natural valve infection. In a review of 95 autopsied patients with fatal active endocarditis, 27 patients were found to have ring abscesses,[152] a morphologic finding that implies deep-seated and refractory infections and that seriously complicates medical and surgical therapy. Major differences between the patients dying with valve ring abscess and those without annular involvement included a greater incidence of (1) aortic valve infection, (2) recent and severe valvular regurgitation, (3) atrioventricular block, (4) purulent pericarditis, and (5) short duration of symptoms prior to severe debility. Although these observations do not provide information as to how often they represent annular infection in the living and surviving patient with endocarditis, they do suggest clinical clues to deep-seated infection.

PERICARDIAL DISEASE

Infective Pericarditis

Infection of the pericardial sac is considerably less frequent but more lethal than valvular infection partly because recognition and therapy of purulent pericarditis is more difficult.[153] A recent review of the 200 consecutive cases of purulent pericarditis that have come to autopsy at the Johns Hopkins Hospital since 1889 has demonstrated the changing picture of this disease.[154] In the past, purulent pericarditis was more frequent than it is today and was almost universally

fatal; it tended to occur mainly in patients in their 20s as a complication of bacterial, predominantly pneumonococcal, pneumonia, who were otherwise healthy. Purulent pericarditis today is a new disease. It appears to occur most often in middle-aged debilitated patients as an infective complication of thoracic surgery, uremia, cancer, or other predisposing systemic disease.[154,155]

In close to 30 percent of patients with purulent pericarditis, other infections of the heart, either of the valve or of the myocardium, are also present. Infective pericarditis is associated with a thick fibrinopurulent epicardial exudate with adhesion formation. Pericardial effusions in excess of 100 ml are present about half the time, and very large pericardial effusions in excess of 300 ml and associated with cardiac tamponode may occur in up to 20 percent of patients with purulent pericarditis.

Although the epidemiology of purulent pericarditis has changed dramatically, largely as a result of antibiotics and the advent of cardiothoracic surgery, hemodialysis, and immunosuppressive therapy, what has not appeared to change is clinical success with diagnosis. Purulent pericarditis is still mainly an autopsy diagnosis, with as much as 80 percent of autopsy-recognized infection of the pericardium having been unrecognized during life. If unrecognized and therefore untreated, infective pericarditis is virtually always fatal.

The difficulty in recognizing purulent pericarditis is that the diagnosis can only be made with a pericardial aspiration, an invasive procedure which cannot be lightly undertaken in the debilitated or postoperative patient. With improved methods for detecting pericardial fluid, including echocardiography and nuclear scans, and with a high index of suspicion in the patient with a suggestive clinical picture combined with the presence of "risk factors" for infective pericarditis, we should be doing better. Once the diagnosis is made, therapy consists of appropriate antibiotic treatment combined with surgical drainage. Recent evidence suggests that treatment of purulent pericarditis can reduce its mortality to 40 percent. This striking improvement in mortality for this disease is to be strived for.

CONCLUSIONS

Cardiac pathology is one example of how the dead serve the living by continuing to teach us about pathogenesis of human disease. Much yet remains unsettled about fundamental pathophysiologic processes in the cardiovascular system that will sooner or later affect most of us, including atherosclerosis, mechanisms of acute vascular occlusions and irreversible ischemic injury, and the processes which determine success or failure of our medical and surgical interventions. The decline in rates of autopsies across the country[156] is a sad indication that the value of human pathology as a major source of data is not fully appreciated by both the physician and the lay population. We should not lose sight of the wise words of Dr. William Welch, the first pathologist-in-chief at the Johns Hopkins Hospital, who in an address to a local medical society, reminded: "Pathology must constitute the scientific basis of practical medicine."[157]

REFERENCES

1 Cushing, H.: "The Life of Sir William Osler," Oxford University Press, London, 1940, p. 249.

2 Cabot, R. C.: "Facts on the Heart," W. B. Saunders Company, Philadelphia, 1926.

3 Pickering, G. W., and Heptinstall, R. H.: Reversibility of Hypertension, *Lancet,* 2:1081, 1952.

4 Ross, R., and Glomset, J. A.: The Pathogenesis of Atherosclerosis, *N. Engl. J. Med.,* 295:369, 1976.

5 Ross, R., and Glomset, J. A.: The Pathogenesis of Atherosclerosis, *N. Engl. J. Med.,* 295:420, 1976.

6 Texon, M.: A Hemodynamic Concept of Atherosclerosis with Particular Reference to Coronary Occlusion, *Arch. Intern. Med.,* 99:418, 1957.

7 Smith, E. B.: The Relationship between Plasma and Tissue Lipids in Human Atherosclerosis, *Adv. Lipid Res.,* 12:1, 1974.

8 Mustard, J. F., Murphy, E. A., Rowsell, H. C., and Downie, H. G.: Platelets and Atherosclerosis, *J. Athero. Res.,* 4:1, 1964.

9 Roberts, W. C.: Does Thrombosis Play a Major Role in the Development of Symptom-producing Atherosclerotic Plaques?, *Circulation,* 43:1161, 1973.

10 Benditt, E. P., and Benditt, J. M.: Evidence for a Monoclonal Origin of Human Atherosclerotic Plaques, *Proc. Natl. Acad. Sci. USA.,* 70:1753, 1973.

11 Benditt, E. P.: Evidence for a Monoclonal Origin of Human Atherosclerotic Plaques and Some Implications, *Circulation,* 50:650, 1974.

12 Pearson, T. A., Wang, A., Solez, K., and Heptinstall, R. H.: Clonal Characteristics of Fibrous Plaques and Fatty Streaks from Human Aortas, *Am. J. Pathol.,* 81:379, 1975.

13 Pearson, T. A., Dillman, J. M., Solez, K., and Heptinstall, R. H.: Clonal Markers in the Study of the Origin and Growth of Human Atherosclerotic Lesions, *Circ. Res.,* 43:10, 1978.

14 Eliot, R. S., Baroldi, G., and Leone, A.: Necropsy Studies in Myocardial Infarction with Minimal or No Coronary Luminal Reduction Due to Atherosclerosis, *Circulation,* 50:1127, 1974.

15 Bulkley, B. H., Klacsmann, P. G., and Hutchins, G. M.: Angina pectoris, Myocardial Infarction and Sudden Cardiac Death with Normal Coronary Arteries: A Clinicopathologic Study of 9 Patients with Progressive Systemic Sclerosis, *Am. Heart J.,* 95:563, 1978.

16 Engel, H. J., Page, H. L., Jr., and Campbell, W. B.: Coronary Artery Spasm as the Cause of Myocardial Infarction During Coronary Arteriography, *Am. Heart, J.,* 91:501, 1976.

17 Khan, A. H., and Haywood, J. L.: Myocardial Infarction in Nine Patients with Radiologically Patent Coronary Arteries, *N. Engl. J. Med.,* 291:427, 1974.

18 Beary, J., Summer, W. L., and Bulkley, B. H.: Postpartum Acute Myocardium Infarction: A Rare Occurrence of Uncertain Etiology, *Am. J. Cardiol.,* 43:158, 1979.

19 Oliva, P. B., and Breckinridge, J. C.: Arteriographic Evidence of Coronary Arterial Spasm in Acute Myocardial Infarction, *Circulation,* 56:366, 1977.

20 Arnett, E. N., and Roberts, W. C.: Acute Myocardial Infarction and Angiographically Normal Coronary Arteries, *Circulation,* 53:395, 1976.

21 Maseri, A., Mimmo, R., Chierchio, S., Marches, C., Pesola, A., and L'Abbate, A.: Coronary Artery Spasm as a Cause of Acute Myocardial Ischemia in Man, *Chest,* 68:625, 1975.

22 Heupler, F. A., Jr., Proudfit, W. L., Bazavi, M., Shirey, E. K., Greenstreet, R., and Sheldon, N. C.: Ergonovine Maleate Provocative Test for Coronary Arterial Spasm, *Am. J. Cardiol.,* 41:631, 1978.

23 James, T. N.: Angina without Coronary Disease, *Circulation,* 42:189, 1970.

24 Bulkley, B. H., Ridolfi, R. L. Salyer, W. R., and Hutchins, G. M.: Myocardial Lesions of Progressive Systemic Sclerosis: A Cause of Cardiac Dysfunction, *Circulation,* 53:483, 1976.

25 Bulkley, B. H., Klacsmann, P. G., and Hutchins, G. M.: Angina Pectoris, Myocardial Infarction and Sudden Cardiac Death with Normal Coronary Arteries: A Clinicopathologic Study of 9 Patients with Progressive Systemic Sclerosis, *Am. Heart J.,* 95:563, 1978.

26 Prizel, K. R., Hutchins, G. M., and Bulkley, B. H.: Coronary Artery Embolism and Myocardial Infarction: A Clinicopathologic Study of 55 Patients, *Ann. Intern. Med.,* 88:155, 1978.

27 James, T. N.: Small Arteries of the Heart, *Circulation,* 56:2, 1977.

28 Feigl, E. O.: Control of Myocardial Tension by Sympathetic Coronary Vasocontriction in the Dog, *Circ. Res.,* 37:88, 1975.

29 Schaper, W., and Schaper, J.: The Coronary Microcirculation, *Am. J. Cardiol.,* 40:1008, 1977.

110

30 Sherf, L., Ben-Shaul, Y., Lieberman, Y., and Neufeld, H. N.: The Human Coronary Microcirculation: An Electron Microscopic Study, *Am. J. Cardiol.*, 39:599, 1977.

31 Hutchins, G. M., Bulkley, B. H., and Miner, M. M.: Correlation of Age and Heart Weight with Tortuosity and Caliber of Normal Human Coronary Arteries, *Am. Heart J.*, 94:196, 1977.

32 Bassingthwaighte, J. B., Yipintsoi, T., and Harvey, R. B.: Microvasculature of the Dog Left Ventricular Myocardium, *Microvasc. Res.*, 7:299, 1974.

33 Fuster, V., Danielson, M. A., Robb, R. A., Broadbent, J. C., Brown, A. L., and Elveback, L. R.: Quantitation of Left Ventricular Myocardial Fiber Hypertrophy and Interstitial Tissue in Human Hearts with Chronically Increased Volume and Pressure Overload, *Circulation*, 55:504, 1977.

34 O'Keefe, D. D., Hoffman, J. I. E., Cheitlin, R., O'Neill, M. J., Allard, J. R., and Shapkin, E.: Coronary Blood Flow in Experimental Canine Left Ventricular Hypertrophy, *Circ. Res.*, 43:43, 1978.

35 Rembert, J. C., Kleinman, L. H., Fedor, J. M., Wechsler, A. S., and Greenfield, J. C.: Myocardial Blood Flow Distribution in Concentric Left Ventricular Hypertrophy, *J. Clin. Invest.*, 62:379, 1978.

36 James, T. N.: The Delivery and Distribution of Coronary Collateral Circulation, *Chest*, 58:183, 1970.

37 Mallory, G. K., White, P. D., and Salcedo-Salgar, J.: The Speed of Healing of Myocardial Infarction. A Study of the Pathologic Anatomy in Seventy-two Cases, *Am. Heart J.*, 18:647, 1939.

38 Bouchardy, B., and Majno, G.: Histopathology of Early Myocardial Infarcts: A New Approach, *Am. J. Pathol.*, 74:301, 1974.

39 Jennings, R. B., Ganote, C. E., and Reimer, K. A.: Ischemic Tissue Injury, *Am. J. Pathol.*, 81:179, 1975.

40 Willerson, J. T., Scales, F., Mukerjee, A., Platt, M. R., Templeton, G. H., Fink, G. C., and Buja, L. M.: Abnormal Myocardial Fluid Retention as an Early Manifestation of Ischemic Injury, *Am. J. Pathol.*, 87:159, 1977.

41 Burton, K. P., Hagler, H. K., Templeton, G. H., Willerson, J. T., and Buja, L. M.: Lanthanum Probe Studies of Cellular Pathophysiology Induced by Hypoxia in Isolated Cardiac Muscle, *J. Clin. Invest.*, 60:1289, 1977.

42 Herdson, P. B., Sommers, H. M., and Jennings, R. B.: A Comparative Study of the Fine Structure of Normal and Ischemic Dog Myocardium with Special Reference to Early Changes following Temporary Occlusion of a Coronary Artery, *Am. J. Pathol.*, 46:367, 1965.

43 Reichenbach, D. D., and Benditt, E. P.: Myofibrillar Degeneration. A Response of the Myocardial Cell to Injury, *Arch. Pathol.*, 85:189, 1968.

44 Buja, L. M., Levitsky, S., Ferrans, V. J., Souther, S. G., Roberts W. C., and Morrow, A. B.: Acute and Chronic Effects of Normothermic Anoxia on Canine Hearts: Light and Electron Microscopic Evaluation, *Circulation*, 43(suppl. 1):44, 1971.

45 Bulkley, B. H., Nunnally, R. L., and Hollis, D. P.: Calcium Paradox and the Effect of Varied Temperature on Its Development. A Phosphorus Nuclear Magnetic Resonance and Morphologic Study, *Lab. Invest.*, 39:133, 1978.

46 Reimer, K. A., Lowe, J. E., and Jennings, R. B.: Effect of Calcium Antagonist Verapamil on Necrosis following Temporary Coronary Occlusion in Dogs, *Circulation*, 55:581, 1977.

47 Fulton, W. F. M.: "The Coronary Arteries," Charles C Thomas, Publisher, Springfield, Ill., 1965.

48 Rona, G.: The Pathogenesis of Human Myocardial Infarction, *Can. Med. Assoc.*, 95:1012, 1966.

49 Bouch, D. C., and Montgomery, G. L.: Cardiac Lesions in Fatal Cases of Recent Myocardial Ischaemia from a Coronary Care Unit, *Br. Heart J.*, 32:795, 1970.

50 Roberts, W. C., and Buja, L. C.: The Frequence and significance of Coronary Arterial Thrombi and Other Observations in Fatal Acute Myocardial Infarction, *Am. J. Med.*, 52:423, 1972.

51 Crawford, T.: "The Pathology of Ischaemic Heart Disease," Butterworth Co. (Publishers), Ltd., London, 1977.

52 Erhardt, L. R., Lundman, T., and Mellstedt, H.: Incorporation of ^{125}I-labelled Fibrinogen into Coronary Arterial Thrombi in Acute Myocardial Infarction in Man, *Lancet*, 1:387, 1973.

53 Erhlich, J. C., and Sinohara, Y.: Low Incidence of Coronary Thromboses in Myocardial Infarction. A Restudy by Serial Block Technique, *Arch. Pathol.*, 78:432, 1964.

54 Roberts, W. C.: Coronary Thrombosis and Fatal Myocardial Ischemia, *Circulation*, 49:1, 1974.

55 Chapman, I.: Morphogenesis of Occluding Coronary Artery Thrombosis, *Arch. Pathol.*, 80:256, 1965.

56 Chapman, I.: The Cause-Effect Relationship between Recent Coronary Artery Occlusion and Acute Myocardial Infarction, *Am. Heart J.*, 87:267, 1974.

57 Bulkley, B. H., and Hutchins, G. M.: Coronary Thrombosis: The Major Cause of Acute Myocardial Infarction in Athereosclerotic Coronary Artery Disease, *Circulation*, 55–56:64, 1977.

58 Fulton, W. F. M., and Summer, D. J.: Causal Role of Coronary Thrombotic Occlusion and Myocardial Infarction: Evidence of Stereo-arteriography, Serial Sections and [125]I Fibrinogen Autoradiography, *Am. J. Cardiol.*, 39:322, 1977.

59 Constantinides, P.: Plaque Fissures in Human Coronary Thrombosis, *J. Athero. Res.*, 6:1, 1966.

60 Friedman, M., and Vanden, B.: The Pathogenesis of a Coronary Thromboses, *Am. J. Pathol.*, 48:19, 1966.

61 Reimer, K. A., Lowe, J. E., Rasmussen, M. M., and

Jennings, R. B.: The Wavefront Phenomenon of Ischemic Cell Death: 1. Myocardial Infarct Size vs Duration of Coronary Occlusion in Dogs, *Circulation*, 56:786, 1977.

62 Pantridge, J. F., and Adgey, A. A.: Pre-hospital Coronary Care, *Am. J. Cardiol.*, 24:666, 1969.

63 Schaffer, W. A., and Cobb, L. A.: Recurrent Ventricular Fibrillation and Modes of Death in Survivors of Out-of-Hospital Ventricular Fibrillation, *N. Engl. J. Med.*, 293:259, 1975.

64 Weaver, W. D., Lorch, G. S., Alvarez, H. A., and Cobb, L. A.: Angiographic Findings and Prognostic Indicators in Patients Resuscitated from Sudden Cardiac Death, *Circulation*, 54:895, 1976.

65 Page, D. L., Caulfield, J. B., Kastor, J. A., DeSanctis, R. W., and Sanders, C. A.: Myocardial Changes Associated with Cardiogenic Shock, *N. Engl. J. Med.*, 285:133, 1971.

66 Alonso, D. R., Scheidt, S., Post, M., and Killip, T.: Pathophysiology of Cardiogenic Shock, Quantification of Myocardial Necrosis, Clinical Pathologic and Electrocardiographic Correlations, *Circulation*, 48:588, 1973.

67 Vlodaver, Z., and Edwards, J. E.: Rupture of Ventricular Septum or Papillary Muscle Complicating Myocardial Infarction, *Circulation*, 55:815, 1977.

68 Wei, J. Y., Hutchins, G. M., and Bulkley, B. H.: Papillary Muscle Rupture in Fatal Acute Myocardial Infarction: A Potentially Treatable Form of Cardiogenic Shock, *Ann. Intern. Med.*, 90:149, 1979.

69 James, T. N.: De Subitaneis Mortibus. XXIV. Ruptured Interventricular Septum and Heart Block, *Circulation*, 55:934, 1977.

70 Kloner, R. A., Fishbein, M. C., Cotran, R. S., Braunwald, E., and Maroko, P. R.: The Effect of Propranolol on Microvascular Injury in Acute Myocardial Ischemia, *Circulation*, 55:872, 1977.

71 Hillis, L. D., and Braunwald, E.: Myocardial Ischemia, *N. Engl. J. Med.*, 296:971, 1034, 1093, 1977.

72 Rasmussen, M. M., Reimer, K. A., Kloner, R. A., and Jennings, R. B.: Infarct Size Reduction by Propranolol before and after Coronary Ligation in dogs, *Circulation*, 56:794, 1977.

73 Maclean, D., Fishbein, M. C., Braunwald, E., and Maroko, P. R.: Long-term Preservation of Ischemic Myocardium after Experimental Coronary Artery Occlusion, *J. Clin. Invest.*, 61:541, 1978.

74 Bulkley, B. H., and Roberts, W. C.: Steroid Therapy during Acute Myocardial Infarction: A Cause of Delayed Healing and of Ventricular Aneurysm, *Am. J. Med.*, 56:244, 1974.

75 Jugdutt, B. I., Hutchins, G. M., Bulkley, B. H., Pitt, B., and Becker, L. C.: Effect of Indomethacin on Collateral Blood Flow and Infarct Size in the Conscious Dog, *Circulation*, in press.

76 Hillis, L. D., Fishbein, M. C., Braunwald, E., and Maroko, P. R.: The Influence of the Time Interval between Coronary Artery Occlusion and the Administration of Hyaluronidase on Salvage of Ischemic Myocardium in Dogs, *Circ. Res.*, 41:26, 1977.

77 Hutchins, G. M., and Bulkley, B. H.: Expansion versus Extension: Two Different Complications of Acute Myocardial Infarction, *Am. J. Cardiol.*, 41:1127, 1978.

78 Eaton, L. W., Weiss, J. L., Bulkley, B. H., Garrison, J. B., and Weisfeldt, M. L.: Regional Cardiac Dilitation After Acute Myocardial Infarction. Recognition by Two-Dimensional Echocardiography, *N. Engl. J. Med.*, 300:57, 1979.

79 Burch, G. E., Giles, T. D., and Cokolough, H. L.: Ischemic Cardiomyopathy, *Am. Heart J.*, 79:291, 1970.

80 Burch, G. E., Tsiu, C. Y., and Harb, J. M.: Ischemic Cardiomyopathy, *Am. Heart J.*, 83:340, 1972.

81 Schuster, E., and Bulkley, B. H.: Ischemic Cardiomyopathy: A Remodeling of the Heart Due to Severe Coronary Artery Disease, *Lab. Invest.*, in press.

82 Bulkley, B. H., Hutchins, G. M., Bailey, I., Strauss, H. W., and Pitt, B.: Thallium 201 Imaging and Gated Blood Pool Scans in Patients with Ischemic and Idiopathic Congestive Cardiomyopathy: A Clinical and Pathologic Study, *Circulation*, 55:753, 1977.

83 Bulkley, B. H., and Ross, R. S.: Coronary-Artery Bypass Surgery: It Works, but Why? *Ann. Intern. Med.*, 88:835, 1978.

84 Griffith, L. S. C., Bulkley, B. H., Hutchins, G. M., and Brawley, R. K.: Occlusive Changes at the Coronary Artery Bypass Graft Anastomosis: Morphologic Study of 95 Grafts, *J. Thorac. Cardiovasc. Surg.*, 73:668, 1977.

85 Hutchins, G. M., and Bulkley, B. H.: Mechanisms of Occlusion of Saphenous Vein-Coronary Artery "Jump" Grafts, *J. Thorac. Cardiovasc. Surg.*, 73:660, 1977.

86 Vlodaver, Z., and Edwards, J. E.: Pathologic Changes in Aortic-Coronary Artery Saphenous Vein Grafts, *Circulation*, 44:719, 1971.

87 Kern, W. H., Dermer, G. B., and Lindesmith, G. G.: The Intimal Proliferation in Aortic-Coronary Saphenous Vein Grafts: Light and Electron Microscopic Studies, *Am. Heart, J.*, 84:771, 1972.

88 Lawrie, G. M., Lie, J. T., and Morris, C. G.: Vein Graft Patency and Intimal Proliferation after Aortocoronary Bypass. Early and Long-term Angiographic Correlations, *Am. J. Cardiol.*, 38:856, 1976.

89 Bulkley, B. H., and Hutchins, G. M.: Pathology of Coronary Artery Bypass Graft Surgery, *Arch. Pathol.*, 102:273, 1978.

90 Unni, K. K., Kottke, B. A., Titus, J. L., Frye, R. L., Wallace, R. B., and Brown, A. L.: Pathologic Changes in Aortocoronary Saphenous Vein Grafts, *Am. J. Cardiol.*, 34:526, 1974.

91 Bulkley, B. H., and Hutchins, G. M.: Accelerated "Atherosclerosis": A Morphologic Study of 97 Saphenous Vein-Coronary Artery Bypass Grafts, *Circulation,* 55:163, 1977.

92 Lie, J., Lawrie, G. M., and Morris, G. C.: Aortocoronary Bypass Saphenous Vein Graft Atherosclerosis. Anatomic Study of 99 Vein Grafts from Normal and Hyperlipoproteinemic Patients Up to 75 Months Postoperatively, *Am. J. Cardiol.,* 40:906, 1977.

93 Bulkley, B. H., and Hutchins, G. M.: Acute Postoperative Graft Phlebitis: A Rare Cause of Saphenous Vein-Coronary Artery Bypass Failure, *Am. Heart J.,* 95:757, 1978.

94 Bulkley, B. H., and Hutchins, G. M.: Myocardial Consequences of Coronary Artery Bypass Graft Surgery: The Paradox of Necrosis in Areas of Revascularization, *Circulation,* 56:906, 1977.

95 Campeau, L., Lesperance, J., Corbara, F., Hermann, J., Grondin, C. M., and Bourassa, M. G.: Aortocoronary Saphenous Vein Bypass Graft Changes 5 to 7 Years after Surgery, *Cardiovasc. Surg.,* 58(suppl. 1):170, 1978.

96 Hutchins, G. M., and Bulkley, B. H.: Correlation of Myocardial Contraction Band Necrosis and Vascular Patency: A Study of Coronary Artery Bypass Graft Anastomoses at Branch-Points, *Lab. Invest.,* 36:642, 1977.

97 Phillips, D. F., Proudfit, W., Lim, J., and Sheldon, W. C.: Perioperative Myocardial Infarction: Angiographic Correlations, *Am. J. Cardiol.,* 39:269, 1977.

98 Hearse, D. J.: Reperfusion of the Ischemic Myocardium (editorial), *J. Mol. Cell Cardiol.,* 9:605, 1977.

99 Schaper, J., Hehrlein, F., Schlepper, M., and Thiedemann, K. U.: Ultrastructural Alterations during Ischemia and Reperfusion in Human Hearts during Cardiac Surgery, *J. Mol. Cell Cardiol.,* 9:175, 1977.

100 Schaff, H. V., Dombroff, R., Flaherty, J. T., Bulkley, B. H., Hutchins, G. M., Goldman, R., and Gott, V.: Effect of Potassium Cardioplegia on Myocardial Ischemia and Post Arrest Ventricular Function, *Circulation,* 58:240, 1978.

101 Bixler, T. J., Flaherty, J. T., Gardner, T. J., Bulkley, B. H., and Gott, V. L.: Effects of Calcium Administration during Post-ischemic Reperfusion on Myocardial Contractility, Stiffness, Edema, and Ultrastructure, *Circulation,* 58:240, 1978.

102 Englemen, R. M., Levitsky, S., O'Donoghue, and Auvil, J.: Cardioplegia and Myocardial Preservation during Cardiopulmonary Bypass, *Circulation,* 58(suppl. 1):107, 1978.

103 Burch, G. E., and DePasquale, N. P.: Recognition and Prevention of Cardiomyopathy, *Circulation,* 42:1, 1970.

104 Roberts, W. C., and Ferrans, V. J.: Pathologic Anatomy of the Cardiomyopathies. Idiopathic Dilated and Hypertrophic Types, Infiltrative Types, and Endocardial Disease with and without Eosinophilia, *Hum. Pathol.,* 6:287, 1975.

105 Silverman, K. L., Hutchins, G. M., and Bulkley, B. H.: Cardiac Sarcoid: A Clinicopathologic Study of 84 Unselected Patients with Systemic Sarcoidosis, *Circulation,* 58:1204, 1978.

106 Bulkley, B. H., and Hutchins, G. M.: Pompe's Disease Presenting as Hypertrophic Myocardiopathy with Wolff-Parkinson-White Syndrome, *Am. Heart J.,* 96:246, 1978.

107 Roberts, W. C., Dangel, J. C., and Bulkley, B. H.: Nonrheumatic Valvular Cardiac Disease: A Clinicopathologic Survey of 27 Different Conditions Causing Valvular Dysfunction, *Cardiovasc. Clin.,* 5:333, 1973.

108 Osler, W.: "The Principles and Practice of Medicine," D. Appleton and Co., Inc., New York, 1894, p. 639.

109 Ross, R. S., Bulkley, B. H., Hutchins, G. M., Harshey, J. S., Jones, R. A., Kraus, H., Liebman, J., Thorne, C. M., Weinberg, S., and Weech, A. A. Jr.: Idiopathic Familial Congestive Myocardiopathy: A Clinicopathologic Study in Three Generations, *Am. Heart J.,* 96:170, 1978.

110 Burch, G. E.: Ultrastructural Myocardial Changes Produced by Viruses, in "Recent Advances in Studies in Cardiac Structure and Metabolism," Vol. 6, University Park Press, Baltimore, 1975, p. 501.

111 Kawai, C., and Takatsu, T.: Clinical and Experimental Studies on Cardiomyopathy, *N. Engl. J. Med.,* 293:592, 1975.

112 Hatle, L., and Melbye, O. J.: Immunoglobulins and Complement in Chronic Myocardial Disease, *Acta Med. Scand.,* 200:385, 1976.

113 Kesteloot, H., Roelandt, J., Willems, H., Claes, J. H., and Joossens, J. V.: An Inquiry into the Role of Cobalt in the Heart Disease of Chronic Beer Drinkers, *Circulation,* 37:854, 1968.

114 Davies, M. J.: The Cardiomyopathies, in A. Pomerance and M. J. Davies (eds.), "The Pathology of the Heart," Blackwell Scientific Publications, Ltd., Oxford, 1975.

115 Buja, L. M., Ferrans, V. L., Mayer, R., Roberts, W. C., and Henderson, E. S.: Cardiac Ultrastructural Changes Induced by Daunorubicin Therapy, *Cancer,* 32:771, 1973.

116 Rinehart, J. J., Lewis, R. P., and Balcerzak, S. P.: Adriamycin Cardiotoxicity in Man, *Ann. Intern. Med.,* 81:475, 1974.

117 Regan, T. J., Lyons, M. M., Ahmed, S. S., Levinson, G. E., Oldewurtel, H. A., Ahmad, M. R., and Haider, B.: Evidence for Cardiomyopathy in Familial Diabetes Mellitus, *J. Clin. Invest.,* 60:885, 1977.

118 Rubler, S., Dlugash, J. Yareoglu, T. Z., Kumral, T., Branwood, A. W., and Grishman, A.: A New Type of Cardiomyopathy Associated with Diabetic Glomerusclerosis, *Am. J. Cardiol.,* 30:595, 1972.

119 Hamby, R. I., Zoneraich, S., and Sherman, L.: Diabetic Cardiomyopathy, *J.A.M.A.,* 229:1749, 1974.

120 Nadkarni, B. B., Hunt, B., and Heggtveit, H. A.: Early

Ultrastructural and Biochemical Changes in the Myopathic Hamster Heart, in "Recent Advances in Studies on Cardiac Structure and Metabolism," Vol. 1, University Park Press, Baltimore, 1972, p. 251.

121 Bulkley, B. H.: IHSS Afflicted: Idols of the Cave and the Marketplace, *Am. J. Cardiol.,* 40:476, 1977.

122 Braunwald, E., Lambrew, C. T., Rockoff, C. D., and Ross, J.: Idiopathic Hypertrophic Subaortic Stenosis. 1. A Description of the Disease Based on an Analysis of 64 Patients, *Circulation,* 30(suppl. 4):3, 1964.

123 Ferrans, V. J., Morrow, A. G., and Roberts, W. C.: Myocardial Ultrastructure in Idiopathic Hypertrophic Subaortic Stenosis: A Study of Operatively Excised Left Ventricular Outflow Tract Muscle in 14 Patients, *Circulation,* 45:769, 1972.

124 James, T. N., and Marshall, T. K.: De Subitaneis Mortibus: 12 Asymmetric Hypertrophy of the Heart, *Circulation,* 51:1149, 1975.

125 Davies, M. J., Pomerance, A., and Teare, R. D.: Pathological Features of Hypertrophic Obstructive Cardiomyopathy, *J. Clin. Pathol.,* 27:529, 1974.

126 Hutchins, G. M., and Bulkley, B. H.: Catenoid Shape of the Interventricular Septum: Possible Cause of Idiopathic Hypertorphic Subaortic Stenosis, *Circulation,* 58:392, 1978.

127 Wigle, E. D., and Silver, M. D.: Myocardial Fiber Disarray and Ventricular Septal Hypertrophy in Asymmetrical Hypertrophy of the Heart (editorial), *Circulation,* 58:398, 1978.

128 McReynolds, R. A., and Roberts, W. C.: The Intramural Coronary Arteries in Hypertrophic Cardiomyopathy, *Am. J. Cardiol.,* 35:154, 1975.

129 Henry, W. L., Clark, C. E., and Epstein, S. E.: Asymmetric Septal Hypertrophy. Echocardiographic Identification of the Pathognomonic Anatomic Abnormality of IHSS, *Circulation,* 47:225, 1973.

130 Bulkley, B. H., Rouleau, J., Strauss, H. W., and Pitt, B.: Idiopathic Hypertrophic Subaortic Stenosis: Detection by Thallium 201 Myocardial Perfusion Imaging, *N. Engl. J. Med.,* 293:1113, 1975.

131 Epstein, S. E., Henry, W. L., Clark, C. E., Roberts, W. C., Maron, B. L., Ferrans, V. J., Redwood, D. R., and Morrow, A. G.: Asymmetric Septal Hypertrophy, *Ann. Intern. Med.,* 81:650, 1974.

132 Henry, W. L., Clark, C. E., and Epstein, S. E.: Asymmetric Septal Hypertrophy (ASH): The Unifying Link in the IHSS Disease Spectrum: Observations Regarding its Pathogenesis, Pathophysiology and Course, *Circulation,* 47:827, 1973.

133 Larter, W. E., Allen, H. D., Sahn, D. J., and Goldberg, S. J.: The Asymmetrically Hypertrophied Septum. Further Differentiation of Its Causes, *Circulation,* 53:19, 1976.

134 Bulkley, B. H., Weisfeldt, M. L., and Hutchins, G. M.: Isometric Cardiac Contraction: A Possible Cause of the Disorganized Myocardial Pattern of IHSS, *N. Engl. J. Med.,* 296:135, 1977.

135 Bulkley, B. H., Weisfeldt, M. L., and Hutchins, G. M.: Asymmetric Septal Hypertrophy and Myocardial Fiber Disarray: Features of Normal, Developing and Malformed Hearts, *Circulation,* 56:292, 1977.

136 Jones, M., Ferrans, V. J., Morrow, A. G., and Roberts, W. C.: Ultrastructure of Crista Supraventricular Muscle in Patients with Congential Heart Diseases Associated with Right Ventricular Outflow Tract Obstruction, *Circulation,* 51:39, 1975.

137 Criley, J. M., Lennon, P. A., Abassi, A. S., and Blaufuss, A. H.: Hypertrophic Cardiomyopathy, in H. S. Levine (ed.), "Clinical Cardiovascular Physiology," Grune & Stratton, Inc., New York, 1976, p. 771.

138 Bulkley, B. H., and Fortuin, N.J.: Systolic Anterior Motion of the Mitral Valve without Asymmetric Septal Hypertrophy, *Chest,* 69:694, 1976.

139 Raizner, A. E., Chahine, R. A., Ishimori, T., and Awdeh, M.: The Clinical Correlates of Left Ventricular Cavity Obliteration, *Am. J. Cardiol.,* 40:303, 1977.

140 Come, P. C., Bulkley, B. H., Goodman, Z. P., Hutchins, G. M., Pitt, B., and Fortuin, N. J.: Hypercontractile Cardiac States Simulating Hypertrophic Cardiomyopathy, *Circulation,* 55:901, 1977.

141 Roberts, W. C., McAllister, H. A., Jr., and Ferrnas, V. J.: Sarcoidosis of the Heart. A Clinicopathologic Study of 35 Necropsy Patients (Group I) and a Review of 78 Previously Described Necropsy Patients (Group II), *Am. J. Med.,* 63:86, 1977.

142 James, T. N. De Subitaneis Mortibus XXV. Sarcoid Heart Disease, *Circulation,* 56:320, 1977.

143 Bulkley, B. H., Rouleau, J., Whitaker, J. Q., Strauss, H. W., and Pitt, B.: The Use of Thallium 201 Myocardial Perfusion Imaging in Sarcoid Heart Disease, *Chest,* 72:27, 1977.

144 Edwards, W. D., Peterson, K., and Edwards, J. E.: Active Valvulitis Associated with Chronic Rheumatic Valvular Disease and Active Myocarditis, *Circulation,* 57:181, 1978.

145 Roberts, W. C., Bulkley, B. H., and Morrow, A. G.: Pathologic Anatomy of Cardiac Valve Replacement: A Study of 224 Necropsy Patients, *Prog. Cardiovasc. Dis.,* 15:539, 1973.

146 Stinson, E. B., Griepp, R. B., Oyer, P. E., and Shumway, N. E.: Long-term Experience with Porcine Aortic Valve Xenografts, *J. Thorac. Cardiovasc. Surg.,* 73:54, 1977.

147 Spray, T. L., and Roberts, W. C.: Structural Changes in Porcine Xenografts Used as Substitute Cardiac Valves: Gross and Histologic Observations in 51 Glutaraldehyde-preserved Hancock Valves in 41 Patients, *Am. J. Cardiol.,* 40:319, 1977.

148 Ferrans, V. J., Spray, T. L., Billingham, M. E., and Roberts, W. C. Ultrastructure of Hancock Procine Val-

vular Heterografts, Pre-and Post-implantation Changes, *Circulation,* 58(suppl. I):10, 1978.

149 Madison, J., Wang, K., Gobel, F. L., and Edwards, J. E. Prosthetic Aortic Valvular Endocarditis, *Circulation,* 51:940, 1975.

150 Arnett, E. N., and Roberts, W. C.: Prosthetic Valve Endocarditis Clinicopathologic Analysis of 22 Necropsy Patients with Comparison of Observations in 74 Necropsy Patients with Active Infective Endocarditis Involving Natural Left-sided Cardiac Valves, *Am. J. Cardiol.,* 38:281, 1976.

151 Anderson, D. J., Bulkley, B. H., and Hutchins, G. M.: A Clinicopathologic Study of Prosthetic Valve Endocarditis in 22 Patients. Morphologic Basis for Diagnosis and Therapy, *Am. Heart J.,* 94:325, 1977.

152 Arnett, E. N., and Roberts, W. C.: Valve Ring Abscess in Active Infective Endocarditis. Frequency, Location and Clues to Clinical Diagnosis from the Study of 95 Necropsy Patients, *Circulation,* 54:140, 1976.

153 Rubin, R. H., and Moellering, R. C.: Clinical Microbiologic and Therapeutic Aspects of Purulent Pericarditis, *Am. J. Med.,* 59:68, 1975.

154 Klacsmann, P. G., Bulkley, B. H., and Hutchins, G. M.: The Changed Spectrum of Purulent Pericarditis: An 86-Year Autopsy Experience in 200 Patients, *Am. J. Med.,* 63:666, 1977.

155 Bulkley, B. H., Klacsmann, P. G., and Hutchins, G. M.: A Clinicopathologic Study of Postthoracotomy Purulent Pericarditis: A Continuing Problem of Diagnosis and Therapy, *J. Thorac. Cardiovasc. Surg.,* 73:408, 1977.

156 Roberts, W. C.: The Autopsy: Its Decline and a Suggestion for its Revival, *N. Engl. Med. J.,* 299:332, 1978.

157 Cushing, H.: "The Life of Sir William Osler," Oxford University Press, London, 1940, p. 324.

From Harvey to Coronary Bypass Surgery: An Exercise in Logic and Scientific Analysis*

J. WILLIS HURST, M.D. and SPENCER B. KING III, M.D.

If I have seen farther (than other men), it is because I have stood upon the shoulders of giants.

SIR ISAAC NEWTON, 1642–1727,[1]

The current views about coronary atherosclerotic heart disease have evolved over a time span of several centuries. In the past, new ideas were proclaimed only to be ignored by those who heard them. The purpose of this discussion is to highlight some of the time-tested concepts about this disease. We begin with the views of Harvey and end with a discussion of current ideas in an effort to visualize the step-by-step trend in thinking that has occurred during the last 400 years. In this way, we believe, we can be more assured that we are currently extending the same path that was so carefully laid by our predecessors. The views of today, as emphasized in the timeless quotation attributed to Sir Isaac Newton (see above), are merely extensions of the views of yesterday.[1] The question we must raise now is whether or not our current thoughts are *logical* extensions of previous thoughts and concepts. We believe they are. The discussion is divided into two parts: Part I deals with the evolution of our knowledge regarding the pathophysiology, recognition, and management of coronary atherosclerotic heart disease; and Part II discusses the modern recognition and treatment of coronary atherosclerotic heart disease.

PART I: THE EVOLUTION OF OUR KNOWLEDGE REGARDING THE PATHOPHYSIOLOGY, RECOGNITION, AND MANAGEMENT OF CORONARY ATHEROSCLEROTIC HEART DISEASE

Many people have contributed to our knowledge regarding the pathophysiology, recognition, and management of coronary atherosclerotic heart disease. We

will mention only a few of them here (see Table 1). The objective of the exercise is to show the growth of concepts and ideas that have been developed during the last four centuries. We must either extend them—believing that these ideas are, for the most part, correct—or dispense with them entirely—believing that they are not correct. We choose to believe that many of the ideas and concepts that have evolved are correct, and therefore we view current ideas in their light. The problem in coronary atherosclerotic heart disease is blockage of the coronary arteries with its associated decrease in coronary blood flow. The solution to the problem will be to prevent the blockage; decrease the myocardial need for oxygen; increase the blood flow; or use a combination of the three methods. The following discussion reveals how one is led to this point of view.

Sir William Harvey (1578–1657)

Harvey made many comments about the heart and circulation.[2] The one quoted here shows that he broke with tradition to suggest that arteries carried "nourishment" to the tissues. Others of his day thought that the venous blood carried nourishment and that the arteries supplied the tissues with vitality and heat. His view, that the coronary arteries supplied nourishment to the heart, was to be ignored for a hundred years or more. Allan Burns was destined to write the best account of the purpose of the coronary arteries (see later discussion). Harvey expressed his belief as follows:

> Besides, if the blood could permeate the substance of the septum, or could be imbided from the ventricles, what use were there for the coronary artery and vein, branches of which proceed to the septum itself, to supply it with nourishment?[2]

William Heberden, M.D.* (1710–1801)

Heberden wrote the following description of angina pectoris:

---

* From the Departments of Medicine and Radiology, Emory University School of Medicine, and Emory University Hospital, Atlanta.

* The original mention of angina pectoris was made by Heberden in a lecture before the Royal College of Physicians of London in July 1768 and published in their *Medical Transactions* in 1786 (Vol. 2, p. 59) under the title "Some Account of a Disorder of the Breast."

115

TABLE 1
From Harvey to coronary bypass surgery

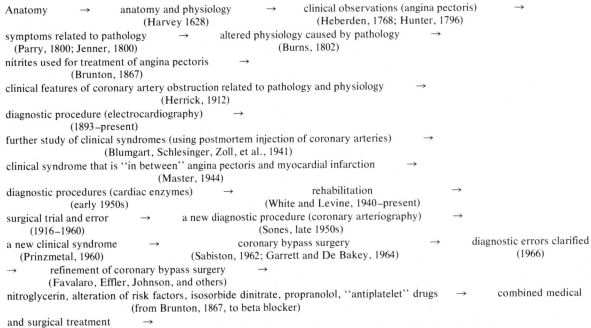

Anatomy → anatomy and physiology → clinical observations (angina pectoris) →
(Harvey 1628) (Heberden, 1768; Hunter, 1796)

symptoms related to pathology → altered physiology caused by pathology →
(Parry, 1800; Jenner, 1800) (Burns, 1802)

nitrites used for treatment of angina pectoris →
(Brunton, 1867)

clinical features of coronary artery obstruction related to pathology and physiology →
(Herrick, 1912)

diagnostic procedure (electrocardiography) →
(1893–present)

further study of clinical syndromes (using postmortem injection of coronary arteries) →
(Blumgart, Schlesinger, Zoll, et al., 1941)

clinical syndrome that is "in between" angina pectoris and myocardial infarction →
(Master, 1944)

diagnostic procedures (cardiac enzymes) → rehabilitation →
(early 1950s) (White and Levine, 1940–present)

surgical trial and error → a new diagnostic procedure (coronary arteriography) →
(1916–1960) (Sones, late 1950s)

a new clinical syndrome → coronary bypass surgery → diagnostic errors clarified
(Prinzmetal, 1960) (Sabiston, 1962; Garrett and De Bakey, 1964) (1966)

→ refinement of coronary bypass surgery →
(Favaloro, Effler, Johnson, and others)

nitroglycerin, alteration of risk factors, isosorbide dinitrate, propranolol, "antiplatelet" drugs → combined medical
(from Brunton, 1867, to beta blocker)

and surgical treatment →

Note: The dates shown in this illustration are, at best, mere approximations. It is not possible to identify the exact date a new concept occurred to the observer and its relationship to when the idea was published in a major journal or book or when it was communicated to some other person.

But there is a disorder of the breast marked with strong and peculiar symptoms, considerable for the kind of danger belonging to it, and not extremely rare, which deserves to be mentioned more at length. The seat of it, and sense of strangling, and anxiety with which it is attended, may make it not improperly be called angina pectoris.

They who are afflicted with it, are seized while they are walking, (more especially if it be up hill, and soon after eating) with a painful and most disagreeable sensation in the breast, which seems as if it would extinguish life, if it were to increase or to continue; but the moment they stand still, all this uneasiness vanishes.

In all other respects, the patients are, at the beginning of this disorder, perfectly well, and in particular have no shortness of breath, from which it is totally different. The pain is sometimes situated in the upper part, sometimes in the middle, sometimes at the bottom of the os sterni, and often more inclined to the left than to the right side. It likewise very frequently extends from the breast to the middle of the left arm. The pulse is, at least sometimes, not disturbed by this pain, as I have had opportunities of observing by feeling the pulse during the paroxysm. Males are most liable to this disease, especially such as have past their fiftieth year.

After it has continued a year or more, it will not cease so instantaneously upon standing still; and it will come on not only when the persons are walking, but when they are lying down, especially if they lie on the left side, and

oblige them to rise up out of their beds. In some inveterate cases it has been brought on by the motion of a horse, or a carriage, and even by swallowing, coughing, going to school, or speaking, or any disturbance of mind.

Such is the most usual appearance of this disease; but some varieties may be met with. Some have been seized while they are standing still, or sitting, also upon first waking out of sleep: and the pain sometimes reaches to the right arm, as well as to the left, and even down to the hands, but this is uncommon: in a very few instances the arm has at the same time been numbed and swelled. In one or two persons, the pain has lasted some hours, or even days; but this has happened when the complaint has been of long standing, and thoroughly rooted in the constitution: once only the very first attack continued the whole night.

I have seen nearly a hundred people under this disorder, of which number there have been three women, and one body twelve years old. All the rest were men near, or past the fiftieth year of their age.[3]

Heberden, a great clinical observer, did not seem to appreciate that the condition of angina pectoris was caused by a decrease in blood flow through obstructed coronary arteries. His contribution to medicine is timeless, and our respect for him is unbounded. We do humbly point out that all of his patients might not have had coronary atherosclerosis or myocardial ischemia, since he had no method of proving that they did. Heberden recognized this and wrote the following about it:

> An useful addition might have been made to these papers by comparing them with the current doctrine of diseases and remedies, as also with what is laid down in practical writers, and with the accounts of those who treat of the dissections of morbid bodies; but at my advanced age it would be to no purpose to think of such an undertaking.[3]

Heberden did mention the autopsy findings of one patient:

> On opening the body of one, who died suddenly of this disease, a very skillful anatomist could discover no fault in the heart, in the valves, in the arteries, or neighbouring veins, excepting small rudiments of ossification of the aorta.[3]

This message implies that he did not appreciate the role of obstructed coronary disease in the production of angina pectoris.

John Hunter, M.D. (1728–1793)

Hunter had said "that his life was in the hands of any rascal who chose to annoy and tease him." The following passage is reproduced in an effort to emphasize the role of emotional factors in the production of angina pectoris.[4] It was written in 1796, by Everard Home, who was the brother-in-law of John Hunter.

> Although evidently relieved from the violent attacks of spasm by the gout in his feet, yet he was far from being free from the disease, for he was still subject to the spasms, upon exercise or agitation of mind; the exercise that generally brought it on, was walking, especially on an ascent, either of stairs or rising ground, but never on going down either the one or the other; the affections of the mind that brought it on were principally anxiety or anger: it was not the cause of the anxiety, but the quantity that most affected him; the anxiety about the hiving of a swarm of bees brought it on; the anxiety lest an animal should make its escape before he could get a gun to shoot it, brought it on; even the hearing of a story in which the mind became so much engaged as to be interested in the event, although the particulars were of no consequence to him, would bring it on; anger brought on the same complaint and he could conceive it possible for that passion to be carried so far as totally to deprive him of life; but what was very extraordinary, the more tender passions of the mind did not produce it; he could relate a story which called up all the finer feelings, as compassion, admiration for the actions of gratitude in others, so as to make him shed tears, yet the spasm was not excited; it is extraordinary that he ate and slept as well as ever, and

his mind was in no degree depressed; the want of exercise made him grow unusually fat.

> In the autumn 1790, and in the spring and autumn 1791, he had more severe attacks than during the other periods of the year, but of not more than a few hours duration: in the beginning of October, 1792, one, at which I was present, was so violent that I thought he would have died. On October the 16th, 1793, when in his mind, and not being perfectly master of the circumstances, he withheld his sentiments, in which state of restraint he went into the next room, and turning round to Dr. Robertson, one of the physicians of the hospital, he gave a deep groan, and dropt down dead.[4]

Caleb Hillier Parry (1755–1822) and Edward Jenner (1749–1823)

Parry and Jenner were the first to understand that angina pectoris was related to disease of the coronary arteries. Home, the prosecutor of Hunter's body, hinted at this relationship, but Parry and Jenner firmed up the view. It is interesting to note that these great observers were friends. Parry went to grammar school with Jenner. Jenner was a friend of Heberden and a student of Hunter's. Allan Burns (see next discussion) gives Parry the credit for first understanding the cause of the condition.[5] Burns wrote the following statements regarding his views in this matter.

> To Drs. Heberden, Jenner, and Parry, we owe most of our information respecting this most fatal complaint. After the very able treatise which Dr. Parry has published on this subject, very little can now be added to the information he has communicated regarding the pathology of Syncope Anginosa. By a series of well related cases, he establishes the regular history of the disease, and by fair induction from a series of accurately performed dissections, he confirms his opinions respecting the cause of this affection; which I think, he has incontrovertibly proved to originate from some organic laesion of the nutrient vessels of the heart. In all patients who have died of Syncope Anginosa, where the body has been carefully examined, the coronary arteries have either been found ossified or cartilaginous.[5]

Allan Burns (1781–1813)

Allan Burns was not a physician, but during his short 31 years of life he learned medicine (see first article of this book). He was an original thinker. He understood the altered physiology that was produced by obstruction of a coronary artery. He was credited by Osler as the first to consider that coronary arteries might undergo spasm.[6] Burns discussed his views as follows:

> It has been long known, that although the heart is always full of blood, yet it cannot appropriate to its own wants

a single particle of fluid contained in its cavities. On the contrary, like every other part, it has peculiar vessels set apart for its nourishment. In health, when we excite the muscular system to more energetic action than usual, we increase the circulation in every part, so that to support this increased action, the heart and every other part has its power augmented. If, however, we call into vigorous action, a limb, round which, we have with a moderate degree of tightness applied a ligature, we find that then the member can only support its action for a very short time; for now its supply of energy and its expenditure, do not balance each other; consequently, it soon, from a deficiency of nervous influence and arterial blood, fails and sinks into a state of quiescence. A heart, the coronary vessels of which are cartilaginous or ossified, is in nearly a similar condition; it can, like the limb, be girt with a moderately tight ligature, discharge its functions so long as its action is moderate and equal. Increase however the action of the whole body, and along with the rest, that of the heart, and you will soon see exemplified, the truth of what has been said; with this difference, that as there is no interruption to the action of the cardiac nerves, the heart will be able to hold out a little longer than the limb.

If a person walks fast, ascends a steep, or mounts a pair of stairs, the circulation in a state of health is hurried, and the heart is felt beating more frequently against the ribs than usual. If, however, a person, with the nutrient arteries of the heart diseased in such a way as to impede the progress of the blood along them, attempts to do the same, he finds, that the heart is sooner fatigued than the other parts are, which remain healthy. When, therefore, the coronary arteries are ossified, every agent capable of increasing the action of the heart, such as exercise, passion, and ardent spirits, must be a source of danger.[5]

Brunton (1844–1916)

The use of amyl nitrite for the treatment of angina pectoris was first reported by Brunton.[7] He wrote the following in 1867:

On pouring from five to ten drops of the nitrite on a cloth and giving it to the patient to inhale, the physiological action took place in from thirty to sixty seconds; and simultaneously with the flushing of the face the pain completely disappeared, and generally did not return till its wonted time next night. Occasionally it began to return about five minutes after its first disappearance; but on giving a few drops more it again disappeared, and did not return. On a few occasions I have found that while the pain disappeared from every other part of the chest, it remained persistent at a spot about two inches to the inside of the right nipple, and the action of the remedy had to be kept up for several minutes before this completely subsided. In almost all other cases in which I have given it, as well as in those in which it has been tried by my friends, the pain has at once completely disappeared.[7]

The use of sublingual nitroglycerin came later. Nitroglycerin ointment was not used until about 20 years ago. Even then it was used for a while and discarded. Now the ointment is enjoying much success for the second time. The use of intravenous nitroglycerin has only recently been investigated and has now gained a firm place in the treatment of myocardial ischemia. Long-acting preparations have come and gone. Dinitro isosorbide is effective and will, we believe, be with us for a while.

Brunton did not do a scientific study on the effect of amyl nitrite. The patient's complaints were such that it was easy to determine that the effect of amyl nitrite was superior to other methods of treatment. His article on the subject would not be accepted for publication today.

James Herrick (1861–1954)

Herrick's observations are historic milestones. He broke with tradition which held that death occurred when a coronary artery was occluded and pointed out that a patient could live with an obstructed coronary artery. He described the clinical features of myocardial infarction, but few physicians listened to his brilliant admonition. Years passed before his views were known and accepted by members of the profession. In the meantime, patients were said to die of "acute indigestion" which, of course, was really a myocardial infarction. Even today, patients are seen with anterior chest discomfort and are said to have indigestion because the initial electrocardiogram shows no abnormality. It has been difficult for some to accept that the initial electrocardiogram may be normal in the patient with myocardial infarction. Herrick expressed his views as follows:

Obstruction of a coronary artery or of any of its large branches has long been regarded as a serious accident. Several events contributed toward the prevalence of the view that this condition was almost always suddenly fatal. . . . But there are reasons for believing that even large branches of the coronary arteries may be occluded—at times acutely occluded—without resulting death, at least without death in the immediate future. Even the main trunk may at times be obstructed and the patient live. It is the object of this paper to present a few facts along this line, and particularly to describe some of the clinical manifestations of sudden yet not immediately fatal cases of coronary obstruction.[8]

Herrick also called for the creation of a classification that defined the subsets that made up the clinical spectrum of coronary atherosclerotic heart disease. He wrote as follows:

The clinical manifestations of coronary obstruction will evidently vary, depending on the size, location and number of vessels occluded. The symptoms and end-results must also be influenced by blood-pressure, by the condition of the myocardium not immediately affected by the obstruction, and by the ability of the remaining vessels properly to carry on their work, as determined by their health or disease. *All attempts at dividing these clinical manifestations into groups must be artificial and more or less imperfect. Yet such an attempt is not without value, as it enables one the better to understand the gravity of an obstructive accident, to differentiate it from other conditions presenting* somewhat similar symptoms, and to employ a more rational therapy that may, to a slight extent at least, be more efficient.[8]

(See later discussion regarding the classification of the clinical spectrum of coronary atherosclerotic heart disease.)

Electrocardiography (1893 – present)

The electrocardiographic baton was passed from Lippman[9] to Marey[10] to Ader[11] to Waller[12] to Einthoven[13] to Lewis[14] to Wilson[15,16] to a group of modern thinkers including Grant.[17] The electrocardiogram can be used to assist in identifying coronary atherosclerotic heart disease. The problem, however, has been to learn the limitation of the method of examination. The tracing may reveal abnormal Q waves and abnormal ST and T wave changes of myocardial infarction. Infarction can, however, occur with only ST-T wave change, only T wave change, or no change. We now know that there are many causes of abnormal Q waves. These include cardiomyopathy, W-P-W syndrome, left ventricular hypertrophy, pulmonary embolism, emphysema, etc. We now know that most patients with angina pectoris have normal electrocardiograms and that the initial electrocardiogram is nondiagnostic in many patients with infarction. The exercise electrocardiogram has been refined since Master's early work.[17a] Even now the submaximal exercise electrocardiogram may give both false positive results (especially in women) and false negative results. Wilson showed his concern when he wrote the following passage in the preface of Lepeschkin's book:

In the last two decades there has been a tremendous growth of interest in electrocardiographic diagnosis and in the number and variety of electrocardiographs in use. In 1914, there was only one instrument of this kind in the state of Michigan and this was not in operation; there were probably no more than a dozen electrocardiographs in the whole of the United States. Now there is one or more in almost every village of any size, and there are comparatively few people who are not in greater danger of having their peace and happiness destroyed by an erroneous diagnosis of cardiac abnormality based on a

faulty interpretation of an electrocardiogram, than of being injured or killed by an atomic bomb.[18]

No cardiac examination is complete without an electrocardiogram, but the limitations of the method of examination are enormous. The other side of Wilson's coin is to remember that serious disease, especially coronary atherosclerotic heart disease, can be present even though the resting electrocardiogram may be normal. Coronary arteriography has brought this fact into clear focus.

Postmortem Injections of Coronary Arteries (Late 1930s and Early 1940s)

Many investigators had injected the coronary arteries of patients after death in an effort to gain more insight into the problem. None achieved the elegance of Blumgart and his group.[19] Much of our current understanding of the pathophysiology of obstructive coronary disease was initially pointed out by his dedicated group of investigators. Only one of their numerous scientific papers is highlighted here. It has been chosen because it deals with the collateral circulation and describes "coronary failure." The clinical syndrome popularized by Master as "coronary insufficiency" has its scientific basis in this work (see later discussion). Blumgart, Schlesinger, and Zoll wrote the following statements in 1941:

1 A detailed clinical and pathologic study of 355 consecutive cases examined post mortem has been made with particular reference to the role of coronary occlusions and the collateral circulation in angina pectoris, coronary failure and acute myocardial infarction.

2 In normal hearts intercoronary anastomoses larger than 40 microns are generally absent. Fine communications measuring less than 40 microns in diameter can be demonstrated by the injection of watery solutions but are probably of little functional significance in obviating the untoward effects of sudden coronary narrowing or occlusion.

3 Complete occlusion or considerable narrowing of one or more coronary arteries may exist without giving rise to any clinical signs or symptoms and without having produced myocardial damage.

4 The apparent inconsistency between the presence of long standing obstructive arterial lesions and the absence of significant pathologic or clinical evidence of myocardial damage was dispelled by the demonstration of a collateral circulation which served as a bypass in relation to the obstruction in each of these hearts.

5 Every patient suffering primarily from angina pectoris without evidence of valvular disease or arterial hypertension has shown old complete occlusion of at least one major coronary artery at postmortem examination; in the majority of instances at least two of the three main coronary arteries had been occluded before the terminal illness.

6 Attacks of cardiac pain more prolonged than those of angina pectoris but unattended by evidence of myocardial infarction are more accurately described as attacks of coronary failure.

7 A comparative study of the clinical characteristics of the coronary thrombosis and those of myocardial infarction forces the conclusion that coronary thrombosis and occlusion, per se, do not necessarily produce any characteristic clinical manifestations. The syndrome usually called "coronary occlusion", which consists of prolonged substernal oppression or pain, a fall in blood pressure, pallor and the other manifestations of shock, and is accompanied by electrocardiographic changes, fever, leukocytosis and an increased sedimentation rate, in reality signifies myocardial infarction and should be so termed.

8 In all three of the discussed syndromes, i.e. angina pectoris, coronary failure and acute myocardial infarction, the underlying mechanism seems to be a relative disproportion between the requirements of the heart for blood and the supply through the coronary arteries. The changes in the myocardium resulting from this disproportion depend solely on the extent and duration of the relative ischemia, not on the manner in which they are produced.

9 The absolute necessity for immediate and complete bed rest, sedation, reduction of excessively high cardiac rates and other measures designed to reduce the work of the heart in the presence of prolonged cardiac pain is emphasized as a means of limiting the extent of myocardial necrosis or even preventing its development. Such a regimen also affords an opportunity for the development of a more adequate collateral circulation.[19]

Arthur M. Master (1895–1973)

Heberden described angina pectoris. Herrick described acute coronary obstruction (myocardial infarction). Master, in 1944, emphasized that there was a spectrum of conditions that ranged from angina pectoris to myocardial infarction. He described the "in-between" group and applied the term "acute coronary insufficiency" to patients who had more than angina pectoris but did not have all the signs of infarction. Graybiel called the group "the intermediate coronary syndrome"[19a] and "coronary failure."[19] Blumgart et al. had used the latter term in 1941 (see earlier discussion).[19] Unfortunately, many physicians did not appreciate that many patients with "coronary insuf-

ficiency" were at great risk for subsequent infarction and sudden death. They continued to have great respect for the seriousness of infarction but viewed the patient with "coronary insufficiency" as having simply a "little warning." The patients that Master described are now said to have preinfarction angina or simply "unstable angina pectoris" or prolonged chest discomfort resulting from myocardial ischemia. Patients with such symptoms are no longer treated casually but are treated vigorously with drugs and bypass surgery when the conditions are right.

Herrick called for the creation of subsets of clinical syndromes in 1912. Master deserves the credit for emphasizing another group of patients—he added a subset. This definition of acute coronary insufficiency is reproduced below.

Master described coronary insufficiency as follows:

"Acute coronary insufficiency" is a syndrome of a more severe myocardial ischemia and is associated with myocardial damage. It is associated with a precipitating factor which decreases coronary flow or which increases the work of the heart and oxygen requirement of the heart muscle. . . .[20]

One of us (J.W.H.) has been interested in this important problem for 25 years and has been joined by the other (S.B.K.) to create the classification which is discussed in Chapter 62A of *The Heart* and in the latter part of this book.

Cardiac Enzymes (Early 1950s to Present)

Many investigators have reasoned that when a myocardial cell is injured, it leaks an intracellular enzyme. They further reasoned that if they could detect the enzyme in the peripheral venous blood, it would be possible to identify myocardial cellular damage by a blood test. The work in the field has been important, not only because the work has enormous practical application but also because it represented the entrance of chemistry into a field that had been previously studied by standard anatomic and physiologic techniques.

There are two major problems in utilizing the cardiac enzymes.

1 The enzyme (serum glutamic oxaloacetic transaminase) that was used early in the development of the field was not specific for myocardial damage.[21] Today, some of the enzymes (serum lactic dehydrogenase and creatine phosphokinase) that are now being measured are more specific for myocardial cellular damage than were those that were measured earlier.[22] (The MB fraction of creatine phosphokinase (CPK) is the most specific enzyme test for myocardial cellular damage).[23]

2 The serum level of cardiac enzymes may not be elevated when a patient with an acute cardiac event is first seen by the physician. Even when the serum level is elevated, the report of the test is not available for early decision making. Just as it has been difficult to teach the limitation of measuring the serum cardiac enzymes, many cardiac events that are potentially serious may have normal serum levels of cardiac enzymes. While the measurement may have prognostic value[24]—the higher the enzyme levels the poorer the prognosis—even this is limited, since one should be doing all that is possible for the patient despite the height of the enzyme level. Patients who have had previous infarcts may have only a small rise in the serum level of cardiac enzymes when a small new infarct occurs. A small new infarct—added to the old infarcts—compels one to view the new infarct as a very serious evident despite little rise in cardiac enzymes. In other words, a small infarct (with a small rise in cardiac enzymes) added to old infarcts may be more serious than a moderate-sized initial infarct (with a higher rise of cardiac enzymes). It has also become apparent that a small rise in serum enzymes in a patient with severe proximal coronary occlusion may herald a larger infarction with a worse prognosis than does a more marked enzyme rise in a patient with a completed infarction.

Rehabilitation (1940–Present)

Paul D. White and Samuel Levine deserve much credit in rehabilitating patients with myocardial infarction. Dr. White was a strong believer in having patients return to work after myocardial infarction. He had the thirty-fourth President of the United States return to work, and by his teaching, he encouraged one of us (J.W.H.) to do the same for the man who became our thirty-sixth President.

Dr. Levine pointed out that many patients with myocardial infarction rested their hearts more if they were allowed to sit in a chair rather than lie in bed. He and Bernard Lown wrote the following in 1951:

> The majority of patients were gotten out of bed during the first 2 days. They were helped out of bed and placed into a comfortable mobile chair with attention that no pressure was exerted on the popliteal spaces. They remained in a chair until they experienced fatigue. Our goal was to have these patients out of bed as much of the day as was comfortable. This was achieved in some who were up in the chair most of the day from the very beginning of their illness. In the majority, however, this usually meant that they were out of bed about one to two hours during the first day and increasing time intervals thereafter, so that by the end of the first week, they spent the larger portion of the day in a chair. The contraindications to the chair treatment were limited to patients with a continuing state of shock, those with marked debility and those with a concomitant cerebrovascular accident. High fever, severe pain, a friction rub, a diastolic gallop, heart block, cardiac arrhythmias, or the need for oxygen were not regarded as interdictions to the "chair" treatment. Nearly all patients fed themselves and were either permitted the use of the bedside commode or were granted toilet privileges.[26]

Now many more patients are advised to return to work after myocardial infarction than was true 30 and 40 years ago. The profession gradually explored the extent to which the patient with coronary atherosclerotic heart disease can enlarge in physical activity, and now many patients participate in carefully supervised "physical activity" programs.

Surgical Trial and Error (1916–1962)

Prior to coronary bypass surgery, many surgical procedures were devised to revascularize the heart.[27,28] Such procedures as cervical sympathectomy, abrasion to the epicardium, suturing adjacent tissue to the epicardium, internal mammary ligation, coronary sinus ligation, implantation of the internal mammary artery into the myocardium, coronary endarterectomy, and gas endarterectomy were tried and abandoned. Unfortunately, the claims made for the procedures were not substantiated, and this blunted the acceptance of coronary bypass surgery (see later discussion).

Coronary Arteriography (Late 1950s)

Coronary arteriography is synonymous with Mason Sones,[28a] who was the innovator. He persevered when many would not listen. He deserves the credit for the development of modern diagnosis and treatment. Sones first used coronary arteriography in the late 1950s, and the technique has now become an essential part of diagnostic work. As will be shown later, the technique has enabled us to correct our clinical opinion in many instances. It has also led to the development of coronary bypass surgery. Whereas Blumgart and his associates taught us a great deal by injecting the coronary arteries after death, Sones has made it possible to obtain the same information (and more) while the patient is still alive. Coronary arteriography will go down in history as one of the great medical advances of the twentieth century.

Myron Prinzmetal (1908–   )

Prinzmetal was an original thinker. He did not force all of his patients into the diagnostic pigeonholes created by his predecessors; instead, he identified a new syndrome. We now know that his syndrome of "variant angina pectoris" may result solely from coronary artery spasm or that a patient with obstructive coronary disease may have additional coronary artery spasm. The treatment for the two conditions is different. Prinzmetal and his coworkers wrote the following:

> The clinical, experimental, and therapeutic features of the variant form of angina pectoris described, to our knowledge, have not been previously delineated. Pain occurs at rest or during ordinary activity and is not precipitated by increased cardiac work. Emotional upset does not bring on the pain. The severity of the pain varies greatly, often being more severe than the pain of classic angina pectoris. Severe pain frequently is accompanied by arrhythmias, usually ventricular. The arrhythmias tend to occur at the peak of the pain and may be associated with faintness or syncope. The pain often is cyclic, with peaks of remarkable constancy every few minutes. If not cyclic, the increasing and decreasing periods of the pain frequently are of equal duration. The pain frequently occurs about the same time each 24 hours. After myocardial infarction there has been immediate and complete relief of the anginal pain.
>
> During severe pain, the electrocardiogram shows striking S-T segment elevation and reciprocal S-T segment depression in standard leads. The R wave may become significantly taller during the course of a severe attack. After the attack is over, the electrocardiogram immediately returns to its appearance prior to the pain. Failure to take a second electrocardiogram after the attack may lead to an erroneous diagnosis of myocardial infarction. There may be no change in the electrocardiogram at the onset or termination of a severe attack or at any time during a mild attack. The electrocardiogram may show spurious "improvement" during the course of the pain, if it has been abnormal prior to the onset of pain. This may lead to unwarranted optimism on the part of the physician, to the detriment of the patient. Exercise tests in these patients have not produced pain. In some instances exercise has led to S-T segment depression, but this has not been associated with pain.
>
> Myocardial infarction has occurred at the same site as that given rise to S-T elevation during the preceding anginal attacks. This sequence of events has made it possible to predict the site of future myocardial infarction. This is the only situation in which the site of a future myocardial infarction can be predicted.
>
> Basic intracellular and extracellular chemical changes in the variant form of angina have been identified and shown to be diametrically opposite to those occurring in classic angina pectoris. Basic pathophysiological differences between these two forms of angina also have been demonstrated. It has been shown that this syndrome has occurred only when a large coronary artery has been involved, such as that supplying the diaphragmatic area of the heart, or the anterior or the high lateral area.
>
> Nitroglycerin therapy has provided relief from pain in the variant form of angina as in classic angina. Anticoagulants have appeared to be indicated in the treatment of the variant form of angina to prevent the occurrence of myocardial infarction.
>
> These features of the variant form of angina pectoris have revealed it to be a distinct clinical entity. In typical cases, diagnosis without an electrocardiogram is possible. In atypical cases, the electrocardiographic changes during an attack are diagnostic.[29]

Coronary Bypass Surgery (1962 to Present)

Sabiston anastomosed the distal end of a saphenous vein graft to the end of the right coronary artery and anastomosed the proximal end of the vein to the aorta. This occurred in 1962. Sabiston wrote the following description of this historic event:

> I especially remember a 41-year-old gentleman with severe angina in whom a complete occlusion of the right coronary artery was demonstrated by arteriography. A right coronary endarterectomy was performed and the patient was relieved of the angina for a period of a year but then typical symptoms suddenly recurred. Repeat coronary arteriography demonstrated occlusion of the previously endarterectomized segment, a complication which was soon recognized as one of the limitations of this technique. On April 4, 1962, this patient was reoperated and a saphenous vein graft was obtained from the leg and anastomosed from the ascending aorta with the use of a partial occlusion clamp. This was illustrated at the time by Leon Schlossberg whose impact upon surgical teaching has been immense. The procedure was performed with the use of a partially occluding clamp on the aorta for the proximal anastomosis, thus allowing the heart to maintain the cardiac output. The distal end of the graft was anastomosed to the right coronary artery, and we were quite pleased with the immediate results and were hopeful that this technique might open a new approach in the management of patients with coronary atherosclerosis and myocardial ischemia. We were disappointed, however, that in the postoperative period the patient developed a cerebrovascular accident and died three days later. At autopsy, thrombus was present at the aortic end of the coronary anastomosis and we presumed that an embolus from this site had been swept into the cerebral circulation. Although in retrospect it is obvious that we should not have been discouraged by this initial experience, nevertheless we did not repeat it until the notable contributions of Favaloro and Johnson some six years later. Their successful use of vein grafts in the coronary circulation has greatly expanded the direct approach to the management of myocardial ischemia and they are deserving of much credit for this condition. This procedure currently constitutes the greatest single indication for cardiac surgery, and of the some 50,000 open heart cardiac operations performed in 1972 in a survey by the Joint Commission on the Accreditation of Hospitals, 25,000 were for coronary bypass surgery.[29a]

Garrett, Dennis, and DeBakey reported the successful use of end-to-side saphenous vein graft from the aorta to the coronary artery. This occurred in 1964. They wrote the following account of this event:

A 42 year old man had extensive occlusive disease of the coronary artery and angina pectoris. An autogenous saphenous vein bypass from the ascending aorta to the anterior descending coronary artery was performed on November 23, 1964. The patient suffered an asymptomatic anterior myocardial infarction during operation but made an uncomplicated recovery. Seven years after the operation, the graft functions with normal left ventricular hemodynamics, while the occlusive process has produced obstruction of the left main coronary artery and almost complete occlusion of the right coronary artery. To our knowledge, this is the first successful case of a saphenous vein-coronary artery bypass with the longest follow-up of a functioning coronary vein bypass graft.[30]

Favaloro, Effler, Johnson, Cooley, Spencer, Kirklin, Austen, and many others were instrumental in refining and developing coronary bypass surgery to its current state. They deserve our gratitude.

Coronary bypass surgery has stood the test of time. This procedure is extremely useful when patients are selected properly and when the experience of the surgical team reveals an operative risk of about 1 percent. The selection of patients is discussed in Part II of this discussion. This surgical procedure has been shown to increase coronary blood flow, improve myocardial performance, decrease the frequency of sudden death, relieve angina pectoris, and prolong life in properly selected patients. Our own interest in bypass surgery was greatly intensified when it became evident that the procedure increased coronary blood flow beyond an obstruction in a coronary artery.[31] We had been led by our predecessors to believe that the problem was related to a decreased blood flow in the coronary arteries. Therefore, we could not ignore any procedure that might correct such a serious fault.

Diagnostic Errors Clarified

The development of coronary arteriography made it possible to determine the accuracy of diagnoses made by clinicians. We have all diagnosed angina pectoris resulting from coronary atherosclerosis but were forced to change our mind when the coronary arteriogram showed no disease. We have also been surprised to find evidence of advanced coronary atherosclerotic heart disease demonstrated by coronary arteriography when we had doubted its existence. Proudfit, Shirey, and Sones studied the diagnostic error rate and wrote:

The clinical records of 1,000 patients who had adequate selective cine coronary arteriography were reviewed. The clinical diagnoses were made by a physician who had no knowledge of the arteriographic findings. Correlation of the clinical diagnoses with the arteriographic findings were made subsequently.

Symptomatic coronary disease was accompanied by arteriographic evidence of significant obstruction of major coronary arteries in most instances. A close correlation existed between the clinical diagnosis of angina pectoris without rest pain and significant arterial obstruction (95%). A similar correlation was found between QRS evidence of myocardial infarction and severe arterial obstruction (99%). The demonstrated arterial obstruction in patients who had angina pectoris almost always was severe and usually almost total or total in one or more major vessels. In myocardial infarction the demonstrated obstruction was always severe and generally almost total or total.

The correlation between clinical and arteriographic findings was moderately close in patients who had angina with symptoms at rest. The correlation between the arteriographic findings and less characteristic clinical syndrome (rest pain only, 79%, coronary failure, 78%, and especially atypical angina pectoris, 65%) was not so close. In congestive failure secondary to coronary disease, arterial obstruction was extensive unless ventricular aneurysm, mitral insufficiency, arrhythmia, arterial hypotension, or some other complication was present. Most patients thought to have noncoronary symptoms had no significant obstructive lesions.

In 37% of the entire group of patients, almost all of whom had been suspected of having coronary disease by some physicians, no significant arteriographic obstruction was demonstrated; in 27% the arteriograms were normal.

Diagnoses, based on appraisal of the clinical records without knowledge of the arteriographic findings, yielded 83% correlation with abnormal arteriographic findings in 700 patients thought to have coronary disease.[32]

Our own work on this subject is discussed in detail in the section of this book entitled "Limitations of symptoms in the Recognition of Coronary Atherosclerotic Heart Disease."

Nitroglycerin, Alteration of Risk Factors, Dinitro Isosorbide, Propranolol, and "Antiplatelet Drugs" (1867 to Present)

Nitroglycerin remains the best drug available for the immediate relief of angina pectoris.[32a] Nitroglycerin ointment applied to the skin is very useful in preventing attacks.[33] Intravenous nitroglycerin is useful in recurrent angina.[34] It is often used during and just after coronary bypass surgery to control hypertension, which is common with this procedure. Dinitro isosorbide is favored as the best long-acting preparation in decreasing the attacks of angina pectoris.[35] The harmful effects of smoking tobacco, eating a high fat, high cholesterol, high calorie diet, hypertension, inactivity, and emotional stress were highlighted in the 1940s. The benefit of the elimination of these "risk factors" are recommended but are still being studied.

Raymond Ahlquist conceived the idea of alpha and beta receptors in the early forties, and this led the development of beta blockers such as propranolol.[36] Propranolol reduces the myocardial requirements for oxygen, and many patients receive enormous benefit from its use.[37] Data are now appearing suggesting that patients who receive beta blockers may live longer than patients who do not.[38]

The use of Coumadin remains unsettled.[39] Recent data regarding the use of drugs which alter platelet function appear promising in the prevention of coronary events including arrhythmia and sudden death.[40,41] (See section in this book entitled "Antiplatelet Medication and Cardiovascular Disease.")

Combined Medical and Surgical Treatment

We have now arrived at the point where medical management is used in all patients, and medical treatment *plus* surgical treatment is offered to some patients. Part II of this article focuses on the current use of these methods.

We have not discussed the evolution of our knowledge of the etiology of coronary atherosclerosis in Part I. Rather, we chose to discuss the evolution of our knowledge of the ischemic process, the recognition of the disorder, and its management. The material that is discussed in Part II should encompass the time-tested principles laid down in Part I, and the new views that are suggested should be seen as logical extensions of the thoughts and actions of our predecessors.

PART II: THE MODERN RECOGNITION AND TREATMENT OF CORONARY ATHEROSCLEROTIC HEART DISEASE

Current Considerations

The interpretation of the results of scientific research that has been done since the development of coronary arteriography by Sones,[28a] combined with logic, has made it possible to extend the views and actions of the past. The following points seem pertinent now.

• The prevention of coronary atherosclerotic heart disease still alludes us.[42] Despite the lack of absolute proof of benefit, we recommend abstinence from smoking tobacco; the maintenance of normal body weight by controlling the intake of saturated fat, cholesterol, and refined sugar; the maintenance of normal blood pressure; the control of abnormal blood lipid (recognizing that the average serum cholesterol level for an adult male in this country is 225 mg/dl); a physical fitness program; and coping with emotional stress.

Although the death rate from coronary atherosclerotic heart disease is declining,[43] we must recognize that this disease still remains the primary killer in this country and is likely to remain so for many years.

We also recommend this approach to the problem after symptoms and signs of the disease have appeared. One must, of course, be reasonable. It is ridiculous to forbid the ingestion of eggs by a 75-year-old man with a destroyed ventricle. It is reasonable to hope that a 40-year-old man with angina pectoris who has broken all the rules of prevention might profit by changing his habits. While there is meager evidence to show that the atherosclerotic process may be reversed, it seems reasonable to hope that the process can be decelerated. We believe the patient who has undergone bypass surgery for coronary atherosclerotic heart disease should be urged to follow the rules of prevention and deceleration.

The role of platelet aggregation in the production of atheroma is now being investigated. Platelet aggregation may also play a role in the production of certain coronary events such as arrhythmias, sudden death, and infarction. The prevention of platelet aggregation by various drugs is now under careful study. In the meantime, some physicians are using the drugs without making definite claims as to their benefit.

The use of nitroglycerin, dinitro isosorbide, and propranolol are very useful and effective drugs. Their usage will be discussed later.

• There was a time when every physician believed he or she could identify angina pectoris resulting fron coronary atherosclerotic heart disease with considerable accuracy. Now, since we have coronary arteriography as the court of last appeal, it is clear that the diagnostic error rate is about 5 to 10 percent when classic Heberden angina is present.[32] (See section in this book entitled "Limitations of Symptoms in the Recognition of Coronary Atherosclerotic Heart Disease.") The diagnostic error rate is at least 30 percent when the patient gives a history of "angina pectoris" not directly related to effort. The diagnostic error rate is even greater when it is difficult to obtain a clear-cut history from the patient. Because of Bayes' rule the error rate is higher in women than it is in men. (See section entitled "Limitations of Symptoms in the Recognition of Coronary Atherosclerotic Heart Disease.")

• Coronary arteriography has become the court of last appeal in determining the presence or absence of coronary atherosclerotic heart disease. Like any court, it too may occasionally fail to clarify a problem. Coronary arteriography does not identify an ischemic myocardium per se but gives information that allows one to infer that ishcemia is present or could occur. For example, the chest discomfort experienced by a patient may not really be caused by the lesions found in the coronary arteries by coronary arteriography. Fortunately, this has not been a large problem. However, we need a method of identifying myocardial ischemia other than the indirect method of identifying symptoms and stress electrocardiography (with its false positive and false negative results) and coronary arteriography (which identifies abnormal anatomy). Radionuclide imaging may be further developed to the point where the technique will make it possible to identify ischemic myocardium in a reliable manner. (See article by Strauss in this book.) At the present time, radionuclide imaging is only in its infancy, and the equipment necessary for the test is not readily available. It should be made clear that radionuclide imaging will not replace coronary arteriography and left ventriculography which identifies anatomic abnormalities in the coronary arteries or ventricular muscle.

• Prior to the development of coronary arteriography, physicians believed that the prognosis of patients with severe angina pectoris was worse than it was for patients with mild angina pectoris. We now know that there is a rough relationship between the severity of symptoms and prognosis, but there are numerous exceptions. Certainly the prognosis of unstable angina is worse than it is for patients with stable angina pectoris.[44-46] (See discussion that follows.) Errors are made when one assumes that initial mild angina is always caused by mild disease; that a patient is better when he or she has less angina pectoris after the physician advises the patient to do less; that the patient will always tell the physician when angina is increasing; that patients seek medical advice whenever angina develops, and therefore one is able to prevent the more serious complications of obstructive coronary disease—myocardial infarction or sudden death.

The prognosis of a patient is determined more accurately by coronary arteriography and left ventriculography.[47] Patients who have evidence of considerable myocardial damage or obstruction of several coronary arteries have a poorer prognosis than do patients with good ventricular contractility and single vessel obstruction.

• Half of the patients who die of coronary atherosclerotic heart disease die suddenly.[48] Although patients may have chest discomfort as a result of myocardial ischemia prior to sudden death, they may not seek medical advice, and even when they do, it may not stimulate action on the part of the physician. This is a difficult group of patients to deal with, since the electrocardiogram is commonly normal and there are many noncoronary causes of chest discomfort.

Any form of treatment of coronary atherosclerotic heart disease must take into account the large group of patients that have sudden death. Obviously, an ideal form of treatment should prevent or decrease the incidence of sudden death.

• Blumgart, Schlesinger, and Zoll clarified the problem of intercoronary anastomoses.[19] Their postmortem injection of coronary arteries and their experimental work should be read by all students of coronary disease. Today, using coronary arteriography, intercoronary anastomoses (or collateral vessels) may be studied in the living patient. This information assists one in determining the need for coronary bypass surgery. For example, if there is subtotal obstruction of the left anterior descending artery and if collateral vessels from the right coronary artery are nourishing the myocardium ordinarily served by the left anterior descending artery, then one should be more concerned if there is 90 percent obstruction of the right coronary artery than if the right coronary artery is normal. The point is, it is useful to protect the source of collateral vessels. This protection is often accomplished by coronary bypass surgery (see later discussion).

Although collateral vessels may preserve the myocardium that is jeopardized by obstructive coronary disease, we know too little about the control of such collateral vessels. Will nature always produce a perfect balance between the decrease in coronary blood flow resulting from obstructive disease and the increase in blood flow through collateral vessels? Unfortunately, the answer to this question is no. If we were in perfect command of the collateral vessels, we could avoid infarction and sudden death, and bypass surgery would be needed less often.

• Some years ago the indication for coronary bypass surgery was disabling angina pectoris despite optimum medical management.[49] At that point in time the terms "disabling" and "despite optimum medical management" were poorly defined. The abuse of the concept became apparent when it became evident that some physicians used the term "disabled" to mean bedridden and others used the axiom "despite optimum medical management" to allow procrastination in order to try every combination of all the drugs that could be found. Accordingly, we now talk in terms of unacceptable angina pectoris despite medical management. The term "unacceptable" implies that the angina interferes with the desired life-style of the patient. We further define medical management as appropriate rest, nitroglycerin, isosorbide dinitrate in a dosage that is slightly less than the amount found by the patient

TABLE 2

Clinical syndromes not associated with "chest discomfort"

1 Sudden death and syncope
2 Pulmonary edema
3 Chronic heart failure
4 Abnormal electrocardiogram
5 Certain cardiac arrhythmias
6 Profound fatigue
7 An abnormal coronary arteriogram
8 Abnormal x-ray of the heart
9 Abnormal physical findings

SOURCE: Hurst and King.[53]

to cause headache and flushing, and propranolol in a dosage that is adjusted to give a heart rate of about 50 to 55 beats per minute.

• Myocardial ischemia can be managed in two ways. Certain drugs, such as propranolol,[37] decrease the myocardial need for oxygen, and coronary bypass surgery increases coronary blood flow and myocardial perfusion.[31] The two approaches are not in conflict; rather, they complement each other.

• Some of the current arguments assist in the manufacture of a controversy that does not exist.

Some observers would imply that obstruction of the left main coronary artery is not serious because they have found a few patients who did not have surgery who survived for several years.[51] Little mention is made of the risk the patients were taking, since the majority of patients will not be so lucky. The observers were identifying the survivors of a large group of desperately ill patients, the majority of whom died.

Some observers believe that triple-vessel disease is less serious than obstruction of the left main coronary artery. While this is occasionally true, it is not invariably true. For example, when there is 90 percent obstruction of the right coronary artery, 100 percent obstruction of the proximal circumflex coronary artery, and 90 percent obstruction of the proximal left anterior descending artery, common sense dictates that the condition is not vastly different from obstruction of the left main coronary artery.

Some observers have even said that "it is surprising how well patients with coronary disease do." When questioned, they have no idea of how many dropped out of their mentally compiled group of patients. In many instances the patients they are referring to have not been characterized by coronary arteriography and left ventriculography.

We believe that some patients with obstruction coronary disease have a poor prognosis (patients with left main coronary artery obstruction and patients with severe triple-vessel disease), that some patients have a good prognosis (patients with isolated obstruction of the right coronary artery and patients with isolated obstruction of the circumflex coronary artery), and that the prognosis for patients with less severe triple-vessel disease or double-vessel disease when one of the vessels is the left anterior descending artery or severe obstruction of the proximal left anterior descending artery is in between the prognoses for the two groups just mentioned.[52]

We believe that the prognosis for patients with poor left ventricular contraction and poor ejection fraction is worse than that for patients with normal left ventricular contraction and normal ejection fraction.[47,52] One objective in treatment is to prevent the development of poor left ventricular function (by large or small infarcts) as well as sudden death.[52]

Since patients with poor ejection fractions have poorer survival curves than do patients with normal ejection fractions, it is possible to identify the effect of treatment on the survival of this group in 3 to 4 years.[52] The effect of treatment on survival of patients with normal ejection fractions may not be detected for 4 or 5 years.[52]

• It seems proper to think in terms of a 10-year plan for a patient with coronary atherosclerotic heart disease. This need is highlighted by the fact that data are now available indicating that patients who qualify for and who have bypass surgery may have a 5-year survival rate that is within a few percentage points of the survival rate of a group of patients from the general population that has been matched for age and sex.[52] In the past, physicians made every effort to relieve

TABLE 3

Phases of decision making in pain syndromes due to coronary atherosclerotic heart disease

Phase I	Phase II	Phase III	Phase IV
Decisions based on physician's first encounter. Classification based on symptoms, complications, and abnormalities (if any) found in the initial electrocardiogram (if available). (See Table 4.)	Decisions based on subsequent encounters. Classification based on symptoms, complications, electrocardiographic findings, and level of cardiac enzymes.	Decisions based on results of submaximal exercise electrocardiogram test when test is indicated.	Decisions based on coronary arteriography and left ventriculography when study is indicated.

SOURCE: Hurst and King.[53]

TABLE 4
Clinical subsets identified in phase I (first encounter decision making)

Symptoms: Characterization based on analysis of patient's chest discomfort

1 Stable mild angina pectoris
2 Stable disabling angina pectoris
3 Recent onset angina pectoris without rest pain
4 Recent onset angina pectoris plus rest pain
5 Progressive angina pectoris without rest pain
6 Progressive angina pectoris with rest pain: not disabling
7 Progressive angina pectoris with rest pain: disabling
8 Any of the above in a patient with previous episodes of chest discomfort due to myocardial ischemia or with objective signs of previous coronary atherosclerotic heart disease
9 Prolonged chest discomfort attributed to myocardial ischemia in a patient without previous episodes of chest discomfort due to myocardial ischemia or objective signs of previous coronary atherosclerotic heart disease
10 Prolonged chest discomfort attributed to myocardial ischemia in a patient with previous episodes of chest discomfort due to myocardial ischemia or with objective signs of previous coronary atherosclerotic heart disease
11 Any of the above in a patient with previous coronary bypass surgery

Complications

1 No complications
2 Abnormal heart rhythm (state exact rhythm)
3 Heart failure (indicate degree)
4 Hypotension (indicate severity)

Initial electrocardiogram

1 Electrocardiogram not available
2 Normal
3 ST-segment displacement greater than 1 mm in leads I, II, III, aV_L, aV_F, and V_4–V_6 (subendocardial injury)
4 ST-segment elevation in leads II, III, and a V_F or leads I, aV_L, and V_1–V_6 (epicardial injury)
5 Tall, peaked T waves in leads I, aV_L, and V_4–V_6 (subendocardial ischemia)
6 T wave inversion in leads II, III, and aV_F or leads I, aV_L, and V_1–V_6 (epicardial ischemia)
7 Abnormal Q waves with ST- and T wave abnormality. State leads where abnormalities are found. (Dead zone effect, injury and ischemia.)

Definitions: Stable angina pectoris (categories 1 and 2 in table) implies that there has been no change in the frequency, duration, or precipitating factors of angina pectoris for 6 months.

Unstable angina pectoris refers to all other types of angina pectoris (Categories 3–7).

Prolonged chest discomfort attributed to myocardial ischemia. Angina pectoris usually lasts 1 to 5 min. Occasionally it lasts 10 to 15 min. Chest discomfort lasting longer than this may not be simply angina pectoris but may represent a more serious event.

SOURCE: Hurst and King.[53]

angina pectoris and to treat myocardial infarction and heart failure, but they did not think in terms of altering the future of the patient because there was little known

to be done. Now the hope of relieving angina pectoris plus preventing infarction, sudden death, and the progress of the disease during the next 5- to 10-year period must be considered.[52] We must plan ahead for the patient, not merely deal with the present.

Classification of Coronary Atherosclerotic Heart Disease[53]

Heberden recognized angina pectoris.[3] Herrick recognized myocardial infarction.[8] Master identified an "in-between" group that he called coronary insufficiency.[20] Now in 1979 we can extend the list of subsets. We are mindful that the list should be extended, but we are also mindful that any classification that is created must be teachable. We recommend a classification that is based on symptoms, abnormalities in the electrocardiogram and serum level of cardiac enzymes, coronary arteriography, and left ventriculography.[53]

Patients with coronary atherosclerotic heart disease may have chest, arm, and neck discomfort owing to myocardial ischemia, or they may present themselves with some other condition. Syndromes that may not be associated with chest, arm, and neck discomfort are shown in Table 2. Decisions must be made about patients with chest discomfort resulting from coronary atherosclerotic heart disease at four points in time (see Table 3). Syndromes that are associated with chest, arm, and neck discomfort are shown in Tables 4 through 6.

The subsets that can be identified based on the data that are available during the physician's first encounter with the patient are shown in Table 4. The subsets that can be identified based on the data that are available during the physician's subsequent encounter are shown in Table 5. The subsets that can be created based on the data collected after a stress electrocardiogram are shown in Table 6. The subsets that can be created based on data collected after performing a coronary arteriogram and left ventriculogram are shown in Table 7.

Table 3 emphasizes that the decision-making process is dynamic. It changes with the passage of time and the collection of new data. The selection of certain subsets is determined by information that the physician has at a given point in time. Furthermore, the selection of a certain subset should assist the physician in determining what he or she does for the patient at that point in time and what, if any, additional diagnostic procedures should be done. In other words, the subset by which the patient is identified should be linked to specific treatment. Whereas we have not yet achieved the goal, a great deal of progress toward it has been accomplished.

TABLE 5
Clinical studies identified in phase II (subsequent encounter decision making)

Symptoms: Characterization based on analysis of patient's chest discomfort

1 Chest discomfort no longer present
2 Chest discomfort improved (less severe or occurs less often)
3 Chest discomfort unchanged
4 Progressive chest discomfort (the chest discomfort has increased in frequency, becomes prolonged, or occurs at rest)

Complications: The development of complications must be identified and categorized

1 No complications
2 Normal rhythm
3 Abnormal heart rhythm (state exact rhythm)
4 Heart failure (indicate degree)
5 Hypotension (indicate severity)

Electrocardiogram

1 Electrocardiogram normal
2 No change since previous tracing
3 Further T-wave change of epicardial ischemia
4 Further ST-T change of subendocardial injury
5 Further ST-T change of epicardial injury
6 Development of abnormal Q waves (state where)
7 ST-segment abnormality of subendocardial injury occurring during chest discomfort
8 ST-segment abnormality of epicardial injury occurring during chest discomfort (Prinzmetal phenomenon)

Cardiac enzymes level

1 Enzyme blood levels not measured
2 No rise in blood level of cardiac enzymes
3 Slight rise in blood level of cardiac enzymes
4 Great rise in blood level of cardiac enzymes (CPK becoming four times normal value)

SOURCE: Hurst and King.[53]

Methods of Studying Subsets[52]

It is necessary to identify subsets when it becomes apparent that several different clinical syndromes make up the clinical spectrum caused by a disease process. Each subset should be defined in such a way that it is potentially linked to specific management and prognosis. This approach is of great value to practicing physicians, since we are interested in relieving the symptoms and prolonging the life of our patients.

The creation of such subsets makes it possible to study patients more scientifically. Since large numbers of patients are needed in order to study the value of a new drug or surgical procedure and since different subsets have different natural clinical courses, it is essential that similar subsets of patients be entered into any study group. One of the problems that has plagued the pursuit of knowledge about coronary atherosclerotic heart disease has been the failure of the clinical investigators to define the subsets of patients they have studied and reported.

At this point the clinical markers shown in Tables 2 through 7 are used to identify the subsets to be studied. Later, of course, other markers may be used if new markers are discovered, and this might lead to the creation of different subsets.

Different methods are needed to study the effect of a new treatment on the prolongation of life. The relief of angina pectoris can be studied by determining and comparing the amount (severity and frequency) of angina pectoris a patient has with one type of treatment with the amount of angina pectoris the same patient has with another type of treatment. The study can be designed so that a patient can serve as his or her own control. The reason for the superiority of one form of treatment over another may require further investigation. The comparison of one form of treatment over another in prolonging life cannot be studied by trying one method for a specified time and then trying another method for a specified period of time in a single patient. This type of study cannot be designed so that a patient can serve as his or her own control. The prolongation of life must be studied by comparing a specific treatment used for one group of patients with the results of a different treatment used for an identical group of patients.

We are not aware of a perfectly designed scientific study of nitroglycerin used for the relief of angina pec-

TABLE 6
Clinical subsets identified in phase III (decision making based on exercise electrocardiogram)

1 Exercise electrocardiogram not done (state reason)
2 Exercise electrocardiogram done but inadequate
3 Exercise electrocardiogram done and normal (record maximum heart rate and blood pressure achieved)
4 Exercise electrocardiogram done with equivocal results (record maximum heart rate and blood pressure achieved)
5 Exercise electrocardiogram done showing ST-segment depression of 1–1.9 mm occurring at stage 3 or 4 (record maximum heart rate and blood pressure achieved)
6 Exercise electrocardiogram done showing ST-segment depression greater than 2 mm at stage 3 or 4 (record maximum heart rate and blood pressure achieved)
7 Exercise electrocardiogram done showing ST segment greater than 2 mm at stage 1 or 2 (record maximum heart rate and blood pressure achieved)
8 Angina pectoris developed at stage _____ (record stage and also record maximum heart rate and blood pressure achieved)
9 Test stopped (state stage in which it was stopped and why; record maximum heart rate and blood pressure achieved)
10 Arrhythmia (state type)

SOURCE: Hurst and King.[53]

TABLE 7

Clinical subsets identified in phase IV (decision making based on coronary arteriography and left ventriculography)

Coronary arteriography

1 Not done
2 Normal
3 Less than 75% proximal cross-sectional obstruction* of a major vessel (state name of vessel)
4 Greater than 75% cross-sectional obstruction of a single vessel (state name of vessel)
5 Greater than 75% cross-sectional obstruction of two vessels (state names of vessels)
6 Greater than 75% cross-sectional obstruction of three vessels (state name of vessels)
7 Greater than 75% cross-sectional obstruction of left main coronary artery
8 All vessels bypassable
9 Some obstructed vessels not bypassable (state which vessels are not bypassable)

Left ventriculography

1 Normal left ventricle
2 Single area of hypokinesia with ejection fraction greater than 40% (the area involved should be specified)
3 Two areas of hypokinesia with ejection fraction greater than 40% (the areas should be specified)
4 Two areas of hypokinesia with ejection fraction less than 40% (the areas should be specified)
5 Generalized hypokinesia with ejection fraction greater than 20%
6 Ejection fraction less than 20%
7 Large ventricular aneurysm

* 75% cross-sectional obstruction is equivalent to 50% narrowing of the diameter of a vessel.

SOURCE: Hurst and King.[53]

toris, and yet every clinician can attest to the fact that patients believe the medication relieves them of the agonizing feeling they know so well. We hear no pleas now to discontinue the use of the drug even though there has been no carefully planned investigation of the matter.

Scientific studies have been done on the use of long-acting nitrites, and isosorbide dinitrate has been shown to prevent angina pectoris.[35] Propranolol has been studied extensively and has been shown to prevent angina pectoris.[37] No one doubts, however, that there is a placebo effect in addition to their pharmacologic effect. The method used to study the pharmacologic action of drugs that produce a beneficial effect is, of course, another matter.

Several methods have been developed to compare the effect of one type of treatment (coronary bypass surgery) with another type of treatment (drug therapy) on the prolongation of life. *None of the methods is perfect.*[52] The experimental design of the studies can usually be faulted, and the implementation of the stud-

ies is very difficult. Each study is filled with enormous problems that in the end leave the skeptical critics even more skeptical. We have recognized the difficulties and have looked at the results of all the studies in order to determine if a trend is present. We have looked for a trend that could be supported by logic—logic that extends the views of our predecessors. A gestalt, if you will. In the following pages we will express our views and support them with logic and scientific data.

There are four methods of comparing the effect of medical management with the effect of bypass surgery on the prolongation of life.[52] All the methods require that a coronary arteriogram and left ventriculogram be done on every patient in order to be as certain as possible that all the patients have obstructive coronary disease and to be able to establish subsets of disease depending on the location of the obstructions and the degree of ventricular contractility.

RETROSPECTIVE MATCHED METHOD

Early on, it was quite appropriate to compare the results of the medically treated patients of the sixties with the surgically treated patients of the early seventies. It was appropriate because it was the best that could be done at that point in time. Sones pioneered coronary arteriography at the Cleveland Clinic, and because of this development the group of clinical investigators there were able to establish the survival curves of subsets of patients with left main, triple-vessel, double-vessel, and single-vessel obstruction during an era prior to the extensive use of propranolol or the full development of coronary bypass surgery. Coronary bypass surgery was then developed at the Cleveland Clinic. Some would argue that it is not possible to arrive at an opinion if one compares the surgery of the early seventies with the prepropranolol era of the sixties. We believe it is not useless (as some have said) to compare the survival of patients treated surgically with a group of matched patients treated at an earlier point in time. After all, many patients still receive medical treatment today that resembles the medical treatment of the sixties.

The objection stated above was eliminated by comparing the effect of surgical treatment with the effect of medical management where the study groups were followed during the same time period. These studies suffered, as do all studies where one compares one treatment with another, in that one cannot be assured that all aspects of the study groups are perfectly matched. The problem of selection is introduced in this medical group as compared to the medical groups treated in the sixties when bypass surgery was not a choice. Despite this drawback, the studies cannot be totally discounted.

PROSPECTIVE MATCHED METHOD

The prospective matched method was the next method of study to be used. In this method a protocol is developed and the patients are entered in the study after the study begins. This method assures that the time frame for comparing the two groups is the same, but it does not eliminate the problem of perfectly matching patients, nor does it eliminate observer bias.

PROSPECTIVE RANDOMIZED METHOD

The prospective randomized method of study should offer the most reliable results. Assuming the experimental design is properly conceived and the number of patients studied is adequate, randomization should minimize both observer bias and the problem of perfectly matching the patients. The prospective nature of such studies guarantees that the two groups of patients are compared during the same time period. Unfortunately, the studies that have been conceived and implemented thus far have highlighted the problems of such studies. For example, a number of patients assigned to the medical group "cross over" to the surgical group when they elect to have bypass surgery. This occurred in 33 percent of patients in the National Institutes of Health Cooperative Study. In addition, the problem of observer bias is not totally eliminated by such a technique in that all eligible patients were not entered into the studies. Perhaps the most serious problem associated with this method of study occurs when many institutes are involved in an effort to increase the size of the study group. It is impossible to guarantee that the medical or surgical treatment is the same in all the institutions. Is each physician equally capable of assessing the amount of angina pectoris the patient has, and does each physician use propranolol in the same manner? Are the surgeons and anesthesiologists equally skilled in all of the participating hospitals? If one institution has results in favor of one method and another institution has results in favor of another method, then the summation of the results could indicate that the two methods of treatment have equal value. This actually happened in the Veterans Administration Cooperative Study (see later discussion)!

COMPARISON OF A STUDY GROUP WITH THE SURVIVAL OF A GROUP MATCHED FOR AGE AND SEX FROM THE GENERAL POPULATION

The Department of Health, Education and Welfare generates life tables that display the annual attrition rate (according to age and sex) of individuals in a study group and compare the survival curves for that group with the survival curve of a group of persons from the general population who have been matched for age and sex. Of course, the general population is made up of well people, known sick people, and people who have disease but do not know it. The survival curve for such a population is made up of a hodgepodge of different survival curves. One could argue that it is not proper to compare the survival curves of the study group, which is made up of a relatively small number of patients, with the survival curves of a large sample of persons from the general population.

There is no perfect method of comparing the survival time of patients treated with bypass surgery with the survival time of patients treated medically.[52] It is unlikely that new randomized studies will be initiated. There are two reasons for this. First, current data support the idea that there are subsets of patients who live longer as a result of bypass surgery. Therefore, it will be difficult for patients, physicians, and surgeons to randomize patients. Second, the problems associated with randomized studies have blunted the enthusiasm of clinical investigators.

Any opinion regarding the value of bypass surgery in prolonging life must be developed using acceptable logic and the scientific data that are available. As we will discuss later, we believe that the gestalt is in favor of bypass surgery at this point in time.

Relief of Angina Pectoris

Coronary bypass surgery will relieve angina pectoris in the majority of cases.[52,54-56] The follow-up of patients who have had coronary bypass surgery at Emory University Hospital reveals that 92 percent of patients had relief of their angina. Sixty-three percent of the patients had total relief, and 29 percent had partial relief. There was no change in 5 percent of patients, and the angina was worse in 3 percent.

Who should have surgery if one assumes that the only benefit is the relief of angina pectoris? To answer this question, one must consider the operative risk, the probability that bypass surgery will relieve the discomfort, and the severity of the angina. In general, bypass surgery should be performed when the angina pectoris is unacceptable to the patient despite optimum medical therapy and when the operative risk of the surgical team is 1 to 2 percent.[52] The term "unacceptable" is defined as angina pectoris that interferes with the life-style (work and pleasure) of a patient. The term "optimum medical management" is defined as appropriate rest, use of nitroglycerin, proper dosage of isosorbide dinitrate, and proper dosage of propranolol (achievement of a heart rate of 55 ± 5 beats per minute).

How often does medical management fail? Medical management did not relieve the angina pectoris to a satisfactory degree in 36 percent of the patients in the National Institutes of Health Cooperative Study of unstable angina.[45] Accordingly, this large percentage of patients "crossed over" from the group to which they were assigned (the medical group) and had surgery for unacceptable angina pectoris. Seventeen percent of the patients in the Veterans Administration Cooperative Study of stable angina pectoris "crossed over" from the medical group to have bypass surgery.[57] Fifty percent of these did so because of unacceptable angina pectoris.[57] These two studies were done in the recent past, and we must assume that optimum medical management was utilized. Since every effort would be made to keep the study groups "pure," we must also assume that the figures given would be an underestimation of the problem.

Propranolol is the most useful drug available for the prevention of angina pectoris.[37] There is evidence that the drug may also prolong the life of certain patients with coronary atherosclerotic heart disease.[38] Unfortunately, all patients cannot tolerate propranolol, since they develop extreme weakness and mental dullness on the drug.

As will be pointed out later, we do not require as much angina pectoris to prompt us to recommend bypass surgery for young patients as we do to recommend surgery for older patients. First, the operative risk is less in young patients than it is in patients who are beyond 65 to 70 years of age. Second, as we consider the likelihood that bypass surgery prolongs life in certain subsets of patients, it seems more logical to be more aggressive in young patients than in patients who are beyond 65 to 70 years of age. This is logical since the older patients have a shorter life expectancy and are more likely to develop additional diseases, such as carotid artery occlusive disease and cerebral atrophy, than are the younger patients.

The Dangers of Procrastination[52]

Some physicians believe that there is no urgency in moving with deliberate speed to have bypass surgery performed for patients with unstable angina pectoris. Plotnick and Conti's study on unstable angina pectoris revealed that the first-year mortality was 9.5 percent for those patients who could have had (but did not have) coronary bypass surgery.[58] During the follow-up period, 14 percent of the patients had myocardial infarction, and 50 percent had class III angina pectoris. The death rate during the first year was unacceptable, and one can infer that the large numbers of infarcts that occurred in the survivors would lead to poor myocardial contractility and inoperability. Sev-enteen percent of the patients were offered surgery at the end of the study period because of unacceptable angina pectoris. One of us (J. W. H.) studied a group of patients with unstable angina similar to those of Plotnick and Conti.[52] All patients had coronary bypass surgery. There were no operative deaths in the group, and no deaths occurred during the first 18 months after surgery. Because of such reports and our own experience, we favor moving with deliberate speed to have bypass surgery rather than trying every possible combination of rest and drugs, hoping that with the passage of time the patient will "get by."

It is often said that patients who have bypass surgery may not return to work. Although more data are needed on this matter, it is becoming evident that procrastination may play a role in whether or not patients return to work. Patients who have already retired at the time bypass surgery is performed may not return to work. Patients who are already receiving disability insurance or pensions because of coronary atherosclerotic heart disease may not return to work following bypass surgery. We have found that the group of professional people who are self-employed are likely to return to work if coronary bypass surgery is performed without delay. This prevents a claim of disability, retirement for the wrong reason, and the rearrangement of personnel in the office where the patient worked, leading him or her to feel rejected.

The Prolongation of Life[52]

As discussed earlier, it is difficult to compare the effect of two different methods of treatment on the survival of patients with coronary atherosclerotic heart disease. This is not simply the fault of the experimental design of the implementation of a study but results from the complex nature of the disease, which makes it difficult to match patients with precision (this is true whether the study is randomized or nonrandomized); requires that the patients be followed for many years; makes it difficult to retain all the patients in the medical treatment group, since unacceptable angina despite medical management forces some patients to "cross over" and have bypass surgery; makes it difficult to be certain that identical medical management is given to all patients in the medical group or that all patients in the surgical group receive equally good operations; and makes it difficult to compare medical treatment with surgical treatment, since the surgical patients also receive medical treatment. The question is, will bypass surgery plus medical management improve the survival of certain subsets of patients as compared to medical treatment alone? We believe that scientific data, imperfect as they are, and logic indicate that the answer is yes if the track record of the surgical team is such that the operative mortality is 1 to 2 percent.

The following material was written by one of us (J. W. H.) and published* in part in *Primary Cardiology*.[59]

We recommend coronary bypass surgery for the following subsets of patients with coronary atherosclerotic heart disease.

• Now in 1978, most observers believe that the logic and scientific data are sufficiently good to state that coronary bypass surgery will prolong the life of a patient with *high grade obstruction of the left main coronary artery*.[52] Obviously, most patients who are discovered to have this serious lesion will be studied because of symptoms of myocardial ischemia (one of the subsets with chest discomfort) or signs of ischemia (such as markedly positive exercise test). There are no studies of a large group of asymptomatic patients, but logic dictates that symptoms are a poor sign of this disease, since sudden death is common.

Several methods of study show that patients with obstruction of the left main coronary artery who have bypass surgery have better survival than patients who are treated medically. A study completed by the Veterans Administration deserves special emphasis, since there has been considerable confusion about the results of the Veterans Administration studies. The 3-year cumulative survival rate of patients with angina pectoris due to left main coronary artery obstruction who were operated on in the participating Veterans Administration Hospitals was about 83 percent, whereas the 3-year cumulative survival rate of patients treated medically was about 61 percent.[60] *The Veterans study was a prospective randomized study and the results are so conclusive that further trials will not be done.* The patients in the study received modern medical therapy, whereas surgical techniques have continued to improve and the operative mortality has been steadily reduced.

The 3-year survival rate of patients at Emory University Hospital who have had bypass surgery for left main coronary artery obstruction is about 88 percent.[52] The 18-month cumulative survival rate for the patients operated on during the last 2 years at Emory is about 94 percent.[52] This improvement reflects the constant improvement in surgical technique that most medical centers have experienced.

Several medical centers have data to support the assertion that the 5-year cumulative survival rate of patients who have bypass surgery for left main coronary artery obstruction will be about 87 percent if one assumes that the current operative risk of about 1 percent or less remains constant.[61-64] The expected 5-year survival rate of members of the general population whose age and sex are similar to an operated group is above 94 percent.[64]

• Another Veterans Administration study on *stable angina pectoris may also be used to show that the cumulative survival rate of patients who have bypass surgery for coronary obstruction (excluding left main coronary artery obstruction)* is superior to the survival rate of similar patients who are treated medically. Twenty percent of the patients in the Veterans Administration's clinical trial were contributed by the Hines Veterans Administration Hospital in Chicago.[65] The result of the Hines Veterans Administration Hospital Study shows a 5-year cumulative survival rate of about 90 percent for those who had bypass surgery compared to a cumulative survival rate of about 70 percent for those who were treated medically.[65] This study was a prospective randomized study and modern medical management was used, whereas more recent surgical techniques have produced an even lower operative mortality than reported in this study. When the good results of the Hines Veterans Administration Hospital Study is added to the results of the other hospitals that participate in the study, there appears to be no difference in medical and surgical treatment in survival. This suggests that some of the hospitals had poor surgical results. We have collected information on this study, and we believe that the Hines Veterans Administration study is a more accurate representation of the state of the art. In the subsequent discussion we will define the subsets of the group, which excludes left main coronary artery obstruction, and indicate the effect of surgery in each of the subsets.

• Common sense and logic dictate that there is not a great deal of difference in a patient with left main coronary artery obstruction and a patient with *high grade obstruction of three vessels*.[52] For example, the patient with total obstruction of the circumflex coronary artery, 90 percent obstruction of the left anterior descending artery, and 90 percent obstruction of the right coronary artery is at about the same risk as a patient with obstruction of the left main coronary artery. Note in the example just cited that the left coronary system is in great danger of being unable to supply blood to the left ventricle. There are many combinations of obstructions of the proximal portion of the three coronary arteries (right, circumflex, and left anterior descending arteries) that place a large portion of the left ventricle in great jeopardy.

There are many studies that show that patients who undergo bypass surgery for triple-vessel obstruction have a better survival than patients who receive medical therapy.[52] Since there has been some confusion about the results of the Veterans Administration clinical trial of patients with stable angina pectoris (excluding those with left main coronary artery obstruction), it seems proper to emphasize the results of their study here.[66] The results of this prospective randomized study showed that patients with stable angina pectoris, triple-vessel disease, and poor left ventricular function who had bypass surgery had a cumulative survival rate of about 85 percent at 54 months compared to the medically treated group that had a cumulative survival rate of about 76 percent at 54 months. This occurred despite the initial high operative mortality, which is no longer the case in most medical centers. Despite this, the crossover of the survival curves took place at about 3 years. If modern operative mortality is assumed for the surgically treated cases, then the difference would be even greater. Hultgren et al., writing for the Veterans Administration, has recently reported that *in patients with three-vessel disease and poor left ventricular function, 4-year follow-up data suggest a possible favorable effect of surgery.*[67]

The 3-year cumulative survival rate of patients with triple-vessel obstruction who were operated on at Emory University Hospital was about 88 percent.[52] With the improved surgical techniques of the last 2 years, the cumulative survival rate at 18 months is 93 percent.[52] The majority of these patients had unstable angina pectoris and were therefore more seriously ill than were the patients with stable angina pectoris reported by the Veterans Administration.[66] Despite this, which should place our surgical group at a disadvantage, the survival curve was better for the surgical group than it was for the medically treated group reported by the Veterans Administration which showed a 3-year cumulative survival rate of about 80 percent.[66]

Several groups are now reporting that if modern operative mortality is assumed (about 1 percent), it is possible to predict a 5-year cumulative survival rate of about 89 percent for patients who are operated on for triple-vessel obstruction.[62,64] This compares favorably to the 5-year cumulative survival rate of about 95 percent for a group of individuals from the general population whose age and sex match the surgical group.[64]

• Many studies suggest that the cumulative survival rate of patients who have coronary bypass surgery for *double-vessel obstruction* is better than the survival curve for patients treated medically. This is especially true when one of the obstructed arteries is the left anterior descending artery. The scientific data for this assertion comes by comparing modern surgery performed at one institution with similar patients who received modern medical treatment at another institution. The 3-year cumulative survival rate for patients with double-vessel obstruction who were operated on at Emory University Hospital was about 94 percent.[52] With improved surgical techniques of the past 2 years, the cumulative survival rate at 24 months is about 97 percent for the Emory surgical group.[52] The cumulative survival rate at 3 years for patients treated medically in the Veterans Administration study was about 88 percent.[57] Many of the Emory patients had unstable angina and the Veterans patients had stable angina. This should have placed the surgical group at a disadvantage compared to the medical group. Despite this, the surgical group fared better. The difference is even greater if one compares the survival of patients who have modern surgery with the survival of patients treated medically a decade ago (prior to the common use of propranolol). The Veterans Administration data for medical treatment is used because the Veterans study was carried out since propranolol was available for use in such patients.

Several medical centers have reported that if modern operative mortality is assumed (about 1 percent), it is possible to predict a 5-year survival rate of about 93 percent for patients who are operated on for double-vessel obstruction.[62,64] This compares favorably to the 5-year cumulative survival rate of about 95 percent for a group of individuals from the general population whose age and sex match the surgical group.[64]

• There are no data to support the assertion that patients with single-vessel disease who have bypass surgery live longer than patients who are treated medically.[52] Patients with single-vessel obstruction should be operated on if their angina pectoris is sufficiently troublesome to justify the operation. (Other signs of ischemia, such as a markedly positive exercise test or ventricular arrhythmia, might also prompt surgical intervention.) Common sense dictates that high grade obstruction of the left anterior descending artery is more serious than high grade obstruction of the right coronary artery, because the left anterior descending artery serves a large mass of the myocardium. Accordingly, when the obstruction is in the left anterior descending artery, bypass surgery should be performed when there is less angina than when the obstruction is in the right or the circumflex coronary arteries. The admonition set down by Abedin and Dack seems wise. They wrote:

For a single left anterior descending artery bypass, a competent surgical team should be able to achieve an operative mortality rate of less than 1%, a perioperative myocardial infarction rate of less than 4% and a patency rate of the bypass graft of more than 90%. Provided that such low morbidity and mortality rates can be achieved, it is logical to anticipate that surgery therapy will benefit a subgroup of symptomatic patients with an isolated proximal lesion of the left anterior descending coronary artery, without collateral vessels and with normally contracting myocardium in its distribution.[68]

• Patients with Prinzmetal angina (variant angina) should have coronary bypass surgery if the coronary arteriogram discloses persistent obstructive lesions. When the syndrome is due solely to coronary spasm, bypass surgery is not indicated.[52]

• Patients with myocardial infarction who continue to have episodes of myocardial ischemia despite medical management. Some patients with evidence of infarction continue to have chest pain despite nitroglycerin, propranolol, and opiates. Should this continue, one can assume that even more myocardium will be destroyed. Dead tissue does not hurt. Therefore, ischemic pain originates from muscle that will either recover or die. If the anatomic picture is suitable, coronary bypass surgery may prevent the death of such tissue. The Emory University Hospital experience shows that surgery can be performed with a very low operative risk.[69] (*Note:* we do not recommend coronary bypass surgery for patients who have just had a myocardial infarction but do not have recurrent ischemic chest pain.) *

SUMMARY AND CONCLUSIONS

The evolution of our knowledge regarding the modern recognition and modern management of coronary atherosclerotic heart disease has been traced from

---

* From J. W. Hurst, Coronary Bypass Surgery: The Evolution of a Personal View, *Primary Cardiol.,* in press. Reproduced with permission of J. W. Hurst and P. W. Communications, Inc.

"ancient" times to the present. (This article does not deal with the etiology of atherosclerosis.) Progress has been slow, and many of the currently accepted ideas were not accepted when the ideas were first published. As one views the sweep of history, one can sense the trend that knowledge has taken and is taking (see Table 1). The investigators during each era built on the solid ground of the observers that preceded them. It is reasonable, we believe, to accept the idea that the problem in coronary atherosclerotic heart disease is a decrease in coronary blood flow secondary to obstructive coronary disease (atherosclerosis). This leads to a decrease in myocardial perfusion. The problem can be corrected by preventing the obstruction from occurring in the coronary arteries; decreasing the myocardial need for normal myocardial perfusion; improving myocardial perfusion by removing the obstruction or placing a bypass graft beyond the obstructed area; or using a combination of all or some of the methods, We recognize that, at times, a conceptual trend that has been generated by history may be wrong. For example, Columbus broke with the historical trend when he proclaimed that the world was round. Maybe some new concept is just around the corner. Maybe we will be able to discard the previous ideas on this subject, and perhaps new relevations will solve the problem in another way. Maybe the myocardial ischemia comes first, as some creative person might postulate. But we doubt it. Therefore, until some new concept is created, we are on safe and reasonable ground when our current thought seems to be an extension of the thought that has gone before us. The scientific data, though imperfect, have been reviewed. These data, combined with logic, have led to the following conclusion. What has not been said is that progress made by many "disciplines" had to come together at a point in time in order that bypass surgery could be developed. Not the least of which was the technology that had its basis in physics and chemistry. For example, this article could not have been written had the artificial heart-lung machine and angiocardiographic equipment not been developed.

It is too early to state that coronary atherosclerotic heart disease can be listed as a preventable disease. However, the elimination of certain associated factors may be helpful in our efforts to prevent or decelerate the process. The same factors should also be dealt with vigorously in patients who have had bypass surgery.

Nitroglycerin, isosorbide dinitrate, and propranolol have already earned a permanent place in the management of angina pectoris. Propranolol may also prolong the life of certain patients with coronary atherosclerotic heart disease.

We recommend coronary bypass surgery for the following patients:

Patients who have angina pectoris that interferes with their desired life-style

Young patients with stable or unstable angina pectoris who have left main coronary artery obstruction, triple-vessel obstruction, double-vessel obstruction, and some patients with obstruction of the proximal portion of the left anterior descending artery

Older patients (65 to 70 or older) only if they have unacceptable angina pectoris despite modern medical therapy

Patients with Prinzmetal's angina when the coronary arteriogram shows that the syndrome is caused by persistent obstruction in the coronary arteries

Patients with myocardial infarction who continue to have episodes of myocardial ischemia despite medical management

Young patients without symptoms who have a coronary arteriogram performed because of a very positive exercise electrocardiogram or ventricular arrhythmia when the coronary arteriogram shows high grade obstruction in the left main coronary artery, triple-vessel obstruction, double-vessel obstruction, or obstruction of the left anterior descending artery

Patients with compelling coronary anatomy who are to have aortic or mitral valve surgery

These recommendations are predicated on the basis that the operative mortality of the surgical team selected to do the bypass procedure is about 1 to 2 percent. Teams who have an operative mortality in this range usually have a graft patency rate of about 90 percent and a perioperative infarction rate of 4 to 6 percent.

Since coronary atherosclerosis is the primary killer in this country, we recommend a combination of methods, imperfect as they are, for the management of this problem. We recommend the current methods of prevention and deceleration of atherosclerosis; the use of modern drugs; the use of bypass surgery for certain subsets of illness; and the use of current methods of prevention and deceleration following bypass surgery.

Let us hope some new and different breakthrough will solve the problem more easily and more perfectly.

REFERENCES

1 Burtt, E. A.: "The Metaphysical Foundations of Modern Physical Science. A Historical and Critical Essay." Harcourt, Brace and Company, Inc., New York, 1932, p. 202.

2 Willis, R.: "The Works of William Harvey, M.D., Translated from the Latin, with a Life of the Author," The Sydenham Society, 1906, London, 1847, p. 624.

3 Heberden, W.: Commentaries on the History and Cure of Diseases, in "Angina Pectoris," printed for T. Tayne, Mews-Gate, London, 1802.

4 Home, E.: "A Treatise on the Blood, Inflammation, and Gun Shot Wounds by the Late John Hunter. To Which Is Prefixed an Account of the Author's Life by His Brother-in-Law, Everard Home," Thomas Bradford, South Front Street, Philadelphia, 1796. (An earlier edition was published in England in 1794.)

5 Burns, A.: "Observations on Some of the Most Frequent and Important Diseases of the Heart," Hafner Publishing Company, New York, 1964, p. 137.

6 Osler, W.: "The Principles and Practice of Medicine," 3d ed., D. Appleton and Company, New York, 1899, p. 763.

7 Brunton, T. L.: On the Use of Nitrite of Amyl in Angina Pectoris, *Lancet*, 2:97, 1867.

8 Herrick, J. B.: Clinical Features of Sudden Obstruction of the Coronary Arteries, *J.A.M.A.*, 59:2015, 1912.

9 Lippmann, G.: Rélations entre les Phénomènes Électriques et Capillaires, *Ann. Chim. (Phys.), Ser. 5*, 5:494, 1875.

10 Marey, E. J.: Des Variations Électriques des Muscles et du Coeur en Particulier, Étudiées au Moyen de l'Électrometre de M. Lippman, *C.R. Acad. Sci. (Paris)*, 82:975, 1876.

11 Ader, C.: Sur un Nouvel Appariel Enregistreur pour Câbles Sousmarins, *C.R. Acad. Sci. (Paris)*, 124:1440, 1897.

12 Waller, A. D.: "An Introduction to Human Physiology," 2d ed., Longmans, Green & Co., Ltd., London, 1893.

13 Einthoven, W.: The Galvanometric Registration of the Human Electrocardiogram, Likewise a Review of the Use of the Capillary-Electrometer in Physiology, in F. A. Willius and E. Keys (eds.), in "Cardiac Classics," trans. by F. W. Willius, The C.V. Mosby Company, St. Louis, 1941.

14 Lewis, T.: "The Mechanism and Graphic Registration of the Heart Beat," 3d ed., Shaw, London, 1925.

15 Wilson, F. N. MacLeod, A. G., and Barker, P. S.: The Distribution of the Currents of Action and of Injury Displayed by Heart Muscle and Other Excitable Tissues, University of Michigan Press, Ann Arbor, 1933.

16 Wilson, F. N.: The Distribution of the Potential Differences Produced by the Heart Beat within the Body and at Its Surface, *Am. Heart J.*, 5:599, 1930.

17 Grant, R. P.: "Clinical Electrocardiography: The Spatial Vector Approach," McGraw-Hill Book Company, New York, 1957, p. 255.

17a Master, A. M.: Reminiscences of Fifty Years in Cardiology at Mount Sinai with Special Reference to the Two Step Test, *M. Sinai J. Med. N. Y.*, 39:486, 1972.

18 Wilson, F.: Foreword, in E. Lepeschkin, "Modern Electrocardiography," Vol. I, The Williams & Wilkins Company, Baltimore, 1951, p. 5.

19 Blumgart, H. L., Schlesinger, M. J., and Zoll, P. M.: Angina Pectoris, Coronary Failure and Acute Myocardial Infarction, *J.A.M.A.*, 116(2):91, 1941.

19a Graybiel, A.: The Intermediate Coronary Syndrome, *U.S. Armed Forces Med. J.*, 6:1, 1955.

20 Master, A. M.: Coronary Heart Disease: Angina Pectoris, Acute Coronary Insufficiency and Coronary Occlusion, *Ann. Intern. Med.*, 20:661, 1944.

21 LaDue, J. S., Wróblewski, F., and Karmen, A.: Serum Glutamic Oxaloacetic Transaminase Activity in Human Transmural Myocardial Infarction, *Science*, 120:497, 1954.

22 Wróblewski, F., Ross, C., and Gregory, K.: Isoenzymes and Myocardial Infarction, *N. Engl. J. Med.*, 263:531, 1960.

23 Roberts, R., Gowda, K. S., Ludbrook, P. A. and Sobel, B. E.: Specificity of Elevated Serum MB Creatine Phosphokinase Activity in the Diagnosis of Acute Myocardial Infarction, *Am. J. Cardiol.*, 36:433, 1975.

24 Coodley, E. L.: Prognostic Value of Enzymes in Myocardial Infarction, *J.A.M.A.*, 225:597, 1973.

25 White, P. D.: Personal communication (1947–1973).

26 Levine, S. A., and Lown, B.: The "Chair" Treatment of Coronary Thrombosis, *Trans. Assoc. Am. Physicians*, 64:316, 1951.

27 Litwak, R.: The Growth of Cardiac Surgery: Historical Notes, *Cardiovasc. Clin.*, 1951, pp. 3, 5.

28 Vansant, J. H., and Muller, W. H.: Surgical Procedures to Revascularize the Heart: A Review of the Literature, *Am. J. Surg.*, 100:572, 1960.

28a Sones, F. M.: Cine Coronary Arteriography, in J. W. Hurst and R. B. Logue (eds.), in "The Heart," McGraw-Hill Book Company, New York, 1966, p. 701.

29 Prinzmetal, M., Ekmekci, A., Kennamer, R., et al.: Variant Form of Angina Pectoris, *J.A.M.A.*, 174(14):102, 1960.

29a Sabiston, D. C., Jr.: The Coronary Circulation, *Johns Hopkins Med. J.*, 134:320, 1974.

30 Garrett, H. E., Dennis, E. W., and DeBakey, M. E.:

Aortocoronary Bypass with Saphenous Vein Grafts. Seven-Year Follow-up, *J.A.M.A.*, 223:729, 1973.

31 Marco, J. D., Barner, H. B., Kaiser, G. C., et al.: Operative Flow Measurements and Coronary Bypass Graft Patency, *J. Thorac. Cardiovasc. Surg.*, 71:545, 1976.

32 Proudfit, W. L., Shirey, E. K., and Sones, F. M.: Selective Cine Coronary Arteriography. Correlation with Clinical Findings in 1,000 Patients, *Circulation*, 33:901, 1966.

32a Aronow, W. S.: The Medical Treatment of Angina Pectoris. IV. Nitroglycerin as an Antianginal Drug, *Am. Heart J.*, 84:415, 1972.

33 Davis, J. A., and Wiesel, B. H.: The Treatment of Angina Pectoris with a Nitroglycerin Ointment, *Am. J. Med. Sci.*, 230:259, 1955.

34 Hurst, J. W.: Personal observations at Emory University Hospital.

35 Kattus, A. A., Alvaro, A. B., and Coulson, A.: Effectiveness of Isosorbide Dinitrate and Nitroglycerin in Relieving Angina Pectoris during Uninterrupted Exercise, *Chest*, 67:640, 1975.

36 Ahlquist, R. T.: Personal Communication in the early 1940s to J. Willis Hurst, M.D.

37 Dollery, C. T., and George, C.: Propranolol—Ten Years from Introduction, *Cardiovasc. Clin.*, 6:266, 1974.

38 Green, K. G. et al.: Multicentre International Study: Improvement in Prognosis of Myocardial Infarction by Long-term ß-Adrenoceptor Blockade Using Practotol, *Br. Med. J.*, 3:735, 1975.

39 Soffer, A.: Editorial comments, *Arch. Intern. Med.*, 136:1229, 1976.

40 Magenis, P. W.: Why Aspirin?, *Circulation*, 54:357, 1976.

41 Sherry, S.: Anturane and Heart Attacks, Coronary Club Inc. 3(4):

42 Schlant, R. C., and DiGirolamo, M.: Modification of Risk Factors in the Prevention and Management of Coronary Atherosclerotic Heart Disease, in J. W. Hurst (ed.), "The Heart," 4th ed., McGraw-Hill Book Company, New York, 1978, p. 1311.

43 Fox, S. M., III, and Robins, M.: Incidence, Prevalence and Death Rates of Cardiovascular Disease: Some Practical Implications, in J. W. Hurst (ed.), "The Heart'" 4th ed., McGraw-Hill Book Company, New York, 1978, p. 750.

44 Gazes, P. C., Mobley, E. M., Jr., Fairs, H. M., Jr., et al.: Preinfarction (Unstable) Angina. A Prospective Study. Ten-Year Follow-up: Prognostic Significance of Electrocardiographic Changes, *Circulation*, 48:331, 1973.

45 Hutter, A. M., Jr., Russell, R. O., Jr., Resnekov, L., et al.: Unstable Angina Pectoris. National Randomized Study of Surgical vs. Medical Therapy: Results in 1, 2 and 3 Vessel Disease, *Circulation*, 55, 56 (suppl. 3):60, 1977. (Abstract.)

46 Richards, D. W., Bland, E. F., and White, P. D.: A Completed Twenty-five-Year Follow-up Study of 456 Patients with Angina Pectoris, *J. Chronic Dis.*, 4:423, 1956.

47 Friesinger, G. C.: Prognosis of Coronary Atherosclerotic Heart Disease, in J. W. Hurst (ed.), "The Heart," 4th ed., McGraw-Hill Book Company, New York, 1978, p. 1211.

48 Scott, R. J., and Briggs, T. S.: Acute Myocardial Infarction and Sudden Death Due to Coronary Atherosclerosis (44th Scientific Sessions), *Circulation*, 43, 44 (suppl. 2):1971. (Abstract.)

49 Hurst, J. W., and Logue, R. B.: The Clinical Recognition and Management of Coronary Atherosclerotic Heart Disease, in J. W. Hurst (ed.), "The Heart," 3d ed., McGraw-Hill Book Company, New York, 1974.

50 Hurst, J. W., Logue, R. B., and Walter, P. F.: The Clinical Recognition and Medical Management of Coronary Atherosclerotic Heart Disease, in J. W. Hurst (ed.), "The Heart," 4th ed., McGraw-Hill Book Company, New York, 1978, p. 1156.

51 Goldberg, S., Grossman, W., Markis, J. E., et al: Total Occlusion of the Left Main Coronary Artery: A Clinical, Hemodynamic and Angiographic Profile, *Am. J. Med.*, 64:3, 1978.

52 Hurst, J. W., King, S. B., III, Logue, R. B., et al: The Value of Coronary Bypass Surgery: Controversies in Cardiology, Part I, *Am. J. Cardiol.*, 42:308, 1978.

53 Hurst, J. W., King, S. B., III: Definitions and Classification of Coronary Atherosclerotic Heart Disease, in J. W. Hurst (ed.), "The Heart," 4th ed., McGraw-Hill Book Company, New York, 1978, p. 1094.

54 Mundth, E. D., and Austen, W. G.: Surgical Measures for Coronary Heart Disease, *N. Engl. J. Med.*, 293:75, 124, 1975.

55 Hultgren, H. N., Peduzzi, P., Pfeiffer, J. F., et al.: Medical versus Surgical Therapy for Coronary Artery Disease—Effect on Symptoms. (Presented at the Annual Meeting of the Association of University Cardiologists, Phoenix, Arizona, January 19, 1978.)

56 Williams, W. O., Aldridge, H., Silver, M.D., et al.: Preinfarction Angina—What Is It?, in J. C. Norman (ed.), "Coronary Artery Medicine and Surgery: Concepts and Controversis," Appleton-Century-Crofts, Inc., New York, 1975, p. 344.

57 Murphy, M. L., Hultgren, H. N., Detre, K., et al.: Treatment of Chronic Stable Angina: A Preliminary Report of Survival Data of the Randomized Veterans Administration Cooperative Study, *N. Engl. J. Med.*, 297:621, 1977.

58 Plotnick, G. D., and Conti, C. R.: Unstable Angina: Angiography, Short- and Long-term Morbidity, Mortality and Symptomatic Status of Medically Treated Patients, *Am. J. Med.*, 63:870, 1977.

59 Hurst, J. W.: Coronary Bypass Surgery: The Evolution of a Personal View, *Primary Cardiol.*, in press.

60 Takaro, T., Hultgren, H. N., Lipton, M. J., et al.: The VA Cooperative Randomized Study of Surgery for Coronary Arterial Occlusive Disease. II. Subgroup with Significant Left Main Lesions, *Circulation,* 54 (suppl. 3):107, 117, 1976.

61 Greene, D. G., Bunnell, I. L., Arani, D. T., et al.: "Long-term Survival after Coronary Bypass Surgery." Buffalo General Hospital, State University of New York (brochure for exhibit at American Heart Association Meeting, Miami, 1977).

62 Lawrie, G. M., Morris, G. C., Jr., Howell, J. F., et al.: Results of Coronary Bypass More than 5 Years after Operation in 434 Patients: Clinical, Treadmill Exercise and Angiographic Correlations, *Am. J. Cardiol.,* 40:665, 1977.

63 Austen, W. G.: Personal communication, April 1978.

64 Kirklin, J. W.: Personal communication, April 1978.

65 Gunnar, R.: Improved Survival following Surgical Therapy in Patients with Chronic Angina Pectoris. A Single Hospital's Experience in a Randomized Trial. (Presented at the Annual Meeting of the Association of University Cardiologists, Phoenix, Arizona, January 19, 1978.)

66 Read, R. C., Murphy, M. L., Huntgren, H. N., et al.: Survival of Men Treated for Chronic Stable Angina Pectoris: A Cooperative Randomized Study, *J. Thorac. Cardiovasc. Surg.,* 75:1, 1978.

67 Hultgren, H. N., Takaro, T., Detre, K. M., et al.: Evaluation of the Efficacy of Coronary Bypass surgery—1, *Am. J. Cardiol.,* 42:157, 1978.

68 Abedin, Z., and Dack, S.: Isolated Left Anterior Descending Coronary Artery Disease: Choice of Therapy, *Am. J. Cardiol.,* 40:654, 1977.

69 Jones, E. L., Douglas, J. S., Jr., Craver, J. M., et al.: Results of Coronary Revascularization in Patients with Myocardial Infarction, *J. Thorac. Cardiovasc. Surg.,* in press.

Coronary Bypass Surgery at Emory University Clinic: Service Organization, Surgical Technique, and Selected Surgical Results*

CHARLES R. HATCHER, JR., M.D.

During the past decade it has become increasingly apparent that myocardial revascularization is of significant benefit to many patients with coronary atherosclerotic heart disease. Bypass surgery can be performed at acceptably low risk.[1-7] This is true even for patients with unstable angina pectoris, although the surgical mortality may be somewhat higher than it is for bypass surgery performed for stable angina.[8,9] Perioperative infarction rates have declined as a result of increased surgical and anesthetic experience and improved techniques for myocardial preservation.[10-17] Symptomatic relief of angina pectoris following bypass surgery has been impressive.[18-20] Improved survival rates for certain subsets of surgical patients treated for coronary atherosclerotic heart disease at a number of centers, including Emory University, have been reported.[20-29]

These facts have encouraged more aggressive surgical management of coronary artery disease to reduce symptoms, prevent myocardial infarction, and preserve maximum ventricular function.

SERVICE ORGANIZATION

As 5-year follow-up reports become available in 1973, the evidence mounted rapidly that bypass surgery had been effective in relieving angina pectoris and in improving the quality of life. Acceptance of these facts placed new demands on existing open heart surgery teams and resulted in the establishment of new cardiac surgical units in many hospitals. The decision was made by Emory University 5 years ago to expand its service facilities in order to accommodate the rapidly increasing number of patients being referred there for bypass surgery. In planning to meet this clinical responsibility, it was assumed that the Emory University service facility would function as the major car-

diac emergency team for that area, providing surgical back up not only for Emory's own cardiovascular laboratories but also for numerous catheterization laboratories springing up in hospitals without cardiac surgical services. Thus, Emory's patient population was to be the elective cases referred to the cardiologists and cardiac surgeons at the clinic and the emergency and urgent cases emanating from the numerous catheterization laboratories in the informal Emory referral network.

This commitment involved other major divisions of the Woodruff Medical Center of Emory University, i.e., Emory University Hospital, the Crawford W. Long Memorial Hospital, and the Emory University School of Medicine.

Two conditions were attached to Emory's expansion plans: (1) resources would be committed as needed to assemble the best personnel and equipment available, and (2) the growth of the cardiovascular services would not be allowed to inhibit the growth and development of other services within the institution. The latter condition made it obvious that all the private hospitals owned or affiliated with Emory University would be involved in the expansion.

As an initial step the cardiovascular services at Emory University Hospital were relocated on a single floor containing approximately 100 beds and consisting of two clinical wings with laboratories (catheterization, exercise, graphics, pulmonary function) located on the connecting corridor. A coronary care unit and cardiac surgical intensive care unit were located on this floor, as were appropriate offices, conference rooms, and a newly established computerized cardiac data center. Previously, coronary angiography had been performed in special procedures rooms by radiologists in the X-ray Department. The catheterization and angiography laboratories were reorganized with a staff of cardiologists who were selected by the Section of Medicine but who held joint appointments in Medicine and Radiology and functioned administratively as a subsection of the Radiology Section. It

* From the Joseph B. Whitehead Department of Surgery, Emory University School of Medicine, Atlanta.

139

is vital that such laboratories be supervised by specially trained cardiologists if they are to realize their full potential value in the management of patients with coronary artery disease. Coincident with the expansion taking place at Emory University Hospital, the Carlyle Fraser Heart Center was established at the Crawford W. Long Memorial Hospital. This center consists of new facilities—catheterization laboratory, computerized medical and surgical intensive care units, and operating suites. Whereas the staff of Emory University Hospital consists almost entirely of the members of Emory University Clinic, the staff of the Crawford W. Long Hospital is "open" as a community hospital. The cardiologists in the catheterization laboratory and the cardiac surgical teams are Emory University Clinic staff, but the cardiology staff also includes physicians in private practice in the community. This unique interface of university and community physicians allows for maximum participation by private cardiologists in the perioperative care of their patients and preserves the expertise of the university's highly experienced cardiac catheterization and surgical teams. The surgical results obtained in the two hospital settings have remained almost identical over a 4-year period.

New or refurbished cardiac surgery operating theaters were occupied in all university hospitals. The four-room unit at Emory University Hospital and the two rooms at the Carlyle Fraser easily permit an elective schedule of 30 to 40 cases per week. Simultaneously, all of our surgery in infants and children was concentrated at the Henrietta Egleston Hospital for Children located on the Emory campus adjacent to Emory University Clinic. New pediatric catheterization laboratories and cardiac surgical facilities at Egleston have improved the care of children with congenital heart disease and freed up the space desperately needed at the adjacent adult hospitals to the mutual advantage of all institutions.

The cardiac surgical staff of Emory University Clinic was increased to five surgeons, for a total of eight thoracic and cardiovascular surgeons in this Division of Surgery. The residency program was purposefully not expanded during this period of clinical growth. It remains at a total of six residents (three trainees in each year of a 2-year program). The surgical staff was augmented by the utilization of ten physicians assistants (PA). These PAs are graduates of approved Allied Health Programs at Duke University and Emory University and function as permanent junior house officers under supervision of the resident and senior staff. Duties are assigned to the PAs in the operating room, on the surgical floors, and in the intensive care units of the hospitals. They are considered to be invaluable members of the surgical team by all who are familiar with their work.

Cardiopulmonary bypass is supervised by a staff of seven perfusion technologists, five of whom are graduates of the program at Ohio State University. This highly professional group functions as a unit, making its own schedules and being responsible for the purchase and maintenance of equipment and supplies.

In many hospitals, cardiac anesthesia is administered by various members of the anesthesiology staff, with some members handling an occasional case to "keep up their expertise" for reasons of professional pride and a more favorable on-call schedule for their group. It is our feeling that the best results are obtained by having a group of cardiac anesthesiologists whose clinical and research interests are limited to open heart surgery. At Emory University Clinic, there is a subsection of cardiac anesthesiology in the Section of Anesthesiology, and the members of the cardiac anesthesiology staff handle all elective and emergency cases. This concentration of anesthesiology talent has not only enhanced patient care in the operating room but also greatly improved the quality of teaching and clinical research at our institution. The opportunity to create a cardiac anesthesiology service is perhaps the greatest advantage we have realized from an expanded volume of open heart cases.

As the volume of work increased for our cardiac surgeons, it became apparent that the traditional postoperative responsibilities for patient care in the intensive care unit would have to be altered. Accordingly, an Intensivist Service was established consisting of four highly trained cardiac anesthesiologists who supervise the cardiac surgical intensive care unit on a continuous basis and are readily available for consultation with the Nursing Service about any acute problem which arises. Cardiologists and cardiac surgeons continue to exercise an appropriate input into the care of patients in the intensive care unit during morning and evening rounds and during certain emergency situations, but routine base-line care in the unit is assumed by the Intensivist Service staff. This specialization is an additional advantage of a large clinical volume.

Prompt evaluation of results is made possible by the Cardiac Data Center, a computer activity supported jointly by medical cardiology and cardiac surgery, cardiac radiology, and cardiac anesthesia. Data are assembled by a staff of research associates and organized and analyzed by computer and statistical experts. Our management plans for various subsets of coronary atherosclerotic heart disease are based on data compiled by the center and presented at weekly staff conferences.

OPERATIVE TECHNIQUE

Once the decision to operate has been made, attention is given to the timing of surgery. Emergency surgery is avoided if circumstances permit. With the use of aggressive medical therapy, most patients can be stabilized and added as need be to the routine operative schedule. In extremely unstable patients the intraaortic balloon is used preoperatively to reduce or terminate ventricular arrhythmia or to manage ischemia. In most patients, similar beneficial results are obtained with intravenous nitroglycerin or nitroprusside by reducing afterload.

In the operating room the staff of cardiac anesthesiologists strives to maintain the delicate balance between myocardial O_2 supply and myocardial O_2 demand. Hypotension, hypoxia, hypocapnia, tachycardia, anemia, or increased blood viscosity is corrected or controlled to avoid decreased O_2 supply. Hypertension (increased afterload), increased cardiac volume (increased preload), tachycardia, and increased contractility are managed as major causes of increased myocardial O_2 demand. Adequate attention to the balance between myocardial O_2 supply and demand is essential to avoid perioperative infarction in patients with ischemic heart disease.

All bypass procedures are performed through a median sternotomy incision under cardiopulmonary bypass and moderate systemic hypothermia. As the heart is being exposed, saphenous vein(s) is removed as needed by a second operator. The arterial flow from the pump is momentarily dropped precipitously while an atraumatic clamp is applied across the ascending aorta just proximal to the arterial cannula. Total electrical arrest of the heart is then achieved by root injection of iced potassium solution. Simultaneously, the heart is immersed in iced saline solution. All distal anastomoses are performed regardless of number before the aortic clamp is released. The proximal anastomoses are then performed within the confines of a partial occlusion clamp, removing buttons of aorta with a surgical punch. Distal anastomoses are performed with a No. 7-0 continuous prolene suture under magnification, and proximal anastomoses are done with Nos. 5-0 and 6-0 continuous prolene sutures under magnification ($\times$ 3.5).

In patients with poor ventricular function, an inotropic agent may be required when cardiopulmonary bypass is being discontinued. Calcium chloride is administered and if the response is inadequate, either dopamine, 5 to 20 μg (kg) (min), or epinephrine, 2 to 8 μg/min, is begun. The choice between these two agents depends upon blood pressure, heart rate, cardiac rhythm, urine output, and peripheral perfusion. If low output persists after cardiopulmonary bypass has been discontinued, an inotropic drug is used in conjunction with a vasodilator (nitroprusside) to decrease left ventricular wall tension. If the intropic/vasodilator drug combination is unsuccessful or if large doses are required for up to 1 h, the intraaortic balloon is employed.

In the early postoperative period, hypertension may be a problem. Ordinarily, nitroglycerin or nitroprusside infusions control such hypertension. In resistant cases, diazoxide, phentolamine, or chlorpromazine may be utilized. Patients are mechanically ventilated overnight via the endotracheal tube, using either assisted ventilation of intermittent mandatory ventilation with positive end-expiratory pressure as required. Patients are extubated using the criteria of normal blood gases and minute ventilation, a vital capacity greater than 15 ml/kg and an inspiratory force greater than 25 cm/H_2O.

RESULTS

In the 5-year period between 1973 and 1978, 1,125 patients underwent direct myocardial revascularization at Emory University Hospital and 379 patients underwent revascularization at the Carlyle Fraser Heart Center of the Crawford W. Long Memorial Hospital (total 1,504). The patient population consisted of 87 percent males and 13 percent females.

The overall hospital mortality was 1.2 percent. Late mortality for the group has been 3 percent. Actuarial survival curves for 30 months for Emory University Hospital patients are presented in Fig. 1 for the overall group and for those patients with single-, double-, and triple-vessel disease (Fig. 2). The most important factor in survival is the state of ventricular function at the time of bypass surgery (Fig. 3). Patients with good ventricular function do well in the long term even with extensive multivessel disease if the significant lesions are effectively bypassed (Fig. 4).

With improvement in cardiac anesthesia and the techniques for myocardial preservation, the perioperative infarction rate of 15 percent in 1973 has been reduced to 4 percent in 1977.

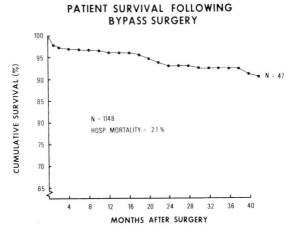

PATIENT SURVIVAL FOLLOWING BYPASS SURGERY

N = 1148
HOSP. MORTALITY = 2.1 %

N = 47

FIGURE 1 Patient survival following bypass surgery.

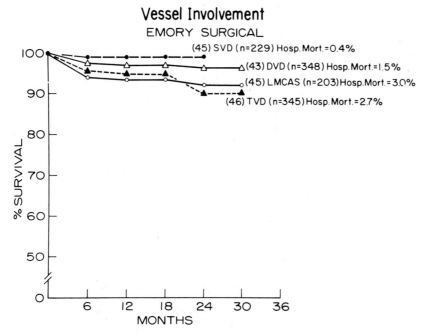

FIGURE 2 Patient survival by extent of coronary artery disease.

Clinical improvement in angina pectoris has been observed in 92 percent of our surgical patients. Angina pectoris was completely relieved in 74 percent of patients and improved in 18 percent. These clinical observations correlate quite closely with the vein graft patency rate at our institution, that is, 90 percent patency of all vein grafts and 92 percent patency of at least one graft in over 250 patients undergoing recatheterization.

Our group has concentrated a major effort on patients with unstable angina pectoris. We include the following clinical subsets under the heading of unstable angina pectoris:[29]

1 Recent angina pectoris without rest pain (occurring for the first time within 60 days).

2 Recent-onset angina pectoris with rest pain.

3 Progressive angina pectoris without rest pain. This indicates that a change has occurred so that pain is occurring with increasing frequency or severity and with less provocation.

4 Progressive angina pectoris with rest pain (not disabling). This indicates that the effort-related pain has not appreciably interfered with the patient's life-style but that episodes of angina are occurring at rest as well.

5 Progressive angina pectoris with rest pain (disabling). The effort-related pain has reached the point of interfering sig-

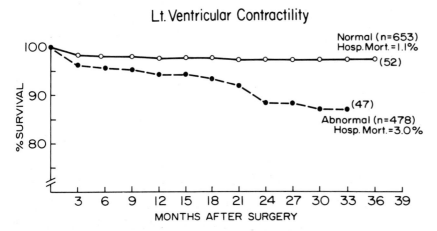

FIGURE 3 Effects of ventricular function on patient survival.

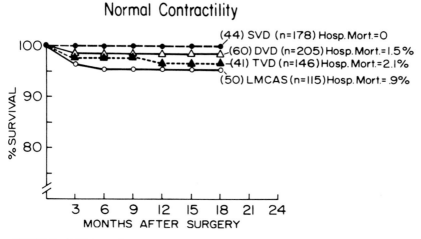

FIGURE 4 Effects of ventricular function and extent of disease on patient survival.

nificantly with the patient's usual life-style. In addition the patient has angina at rest.

6 Prolonged chest discomfort for longer than 20 min attributed to myocardial ischemia without previous angina or objective signs of coronary arterosclerotic heart disease.

7 Prolonged chest discomfort for longer than 20 min attributed to myocardial ischemia with previous angina pectoris or objective signs of coronary artherosclerotic heart disease. (Subsets 6 and 7 are not technically angina pectoris, since the pain is not brief; however, they are classified in the broad category of unstable angina pectoris when they are not associated with objective signs of myocardial necrosis.)

From January 1973 to August 1978, 779 patients with unstable angina pectoris were operated on by our service at Emory Univeristy Hospital. Table 1 shows the distribution of patients by clinical subset. Progressive disabling effort angina plus angina at rest (41 percent) was the most frequent subset encountered. Patients in the unstable angina group were typical of the overall group but did include a higher percentage of patients with 75 percent stenosis of two or three major coronary arteries. The hospital mortality in the

TABLE 1
Clinical subsets of unstable angina

		%
1	Recent onset without rest pain	5.2
2	Recent onset with rest pain	8.4
3	Progressive without rest pain	16.4
4	Progressive (not disabling) with rest pain	8.1
5	Progressive (disabling) with rest pain	42.3
6	Prolonged discomfort without previous discomfort or objective signs	8.4
7	Prolonged discomfort with previous discomfort or objective signs	11.2
	Total	100

unstable group was 2.8 percent, as compared to 1.2 percent of the total surgical group for this period. Mortality could be related to the state of ventricular contractility. The mortality was 1.3 percent in patients with normal or mildly impaired ventricular contractility and unstable angina and 3.8 percent in patients with moderate and severe left ventricular dysfunction. Similarly, mortality was related to the extent of arterial disease, that is, 0.6 percent for single-vessel disease, 2.1 percent for double-vessel disease, 4.0 percent for triple-vessel disease, and 5.6 percent for left main disease.

The clinical subset with the highest mortality (5 percent) was exertional angina plus pain at rest and the lowest (0 percent) occurred in patients with recent-onset angina.

Higher mortality was noted in patients with a history of congestive heart failure and in the presence of anterior Q waves. Sex and previous propranolol therapy had no influence on mortality.

Complete follow-up is available from 1 to 60 months. Angina pectoris was completely relieved in 58 percent and was significantly improved in 33.5 percent. No improvement was found in 8.5 percent of patients. The 91.5 percent improvement (58 + 33.5 percent) for the unstable group is almost identical to the 92 percent improvement in the total bypass group at Emory.

Seventy-nine percent of patients reported that they were active (i.e., able to do housework, play golf, garden, etc.) or very active (able to run, perform manual labor, participate in sports, etc.) at the time of follow-up. Twenty percent were moderately inactive (able to drive, walk, shop), and 1 percent were quite limited in activities. While 50 percent of the total group had returned to work, 95 percent of the self-employed or professional group had resumed working, which im-

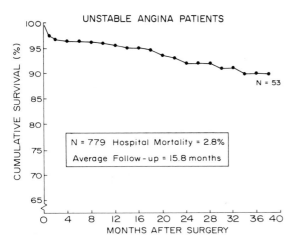

FIGURE 5 Survival of patients with unstable angina pectoris at 36 months.

plies that if motivation and employment opportunities are present, patients can return to work following bypass surgery.

Survival analysis by the actuarial method is available for patients with single-vessel, double-vessel, triple-vessel, and left main disease and for patients with normal and abnormal ventricular contractility. The cumulative survival rate for the total group at 36 months was 91 percent (Fig. 5). Cumulative survival at 18 months for patients with single-vessel disease was 98.1 percent; double-vessel disease, 95.1 percent at 28 months; triple-vessel disease, 89.7 percent at 20 months; and left main disease, 91.6 percent at 16

months. Patients with normal or mildly impaired ventricular contractility had a cumulative survival at 32 months of 97.1 percent. Survival dropped to 85.6 percent at 28 months for patients with significant abnormality in ventricular contractility (Fig. 7).

Although operative mortality in patients with unstable angina pectoris is slightly higher than in stable patients, symptomatic improvement and survival at 24 months is comparable to the total group of bypass patients and compared quite favorably to any reported series of unstable patients treated medically.

SUMMARY

The development of the Cardiovascular Services at Emory University Clinic over the past 5 years has been described, and the institutional commitment of personnel and equipment required by an expanding volume of cardiac surgery has been outlined. With this organizational plan the number of open heart surgery cases at Emory University Clinic has increased from approximately 500 in 1973 to over 1800 in the past year without sacrifice in therapeutic results and without encroachment upon the legitimate activities of other services.

Experience with 1,504 patients undergoing coronary bypass surgery (1973–1978) has been described, and early and late results of surgical treatment of 779 patients with unstable angina pectoris have been presented. The relief of angina pectoris, the increased activity levels, and the improved survival of patients undergoing bypass surgery for coronary artery disease have fully justified the efforts of our institution.

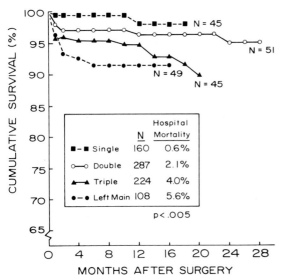

FIGURE 6 Survival of patients with unstable angina by vessels diseased.

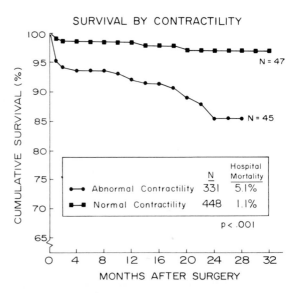

FIGURE 7 Effects of ventricular contractility on survival of patients with unstable angina pectoris.

REFERENCES

1 Greene, D. G., Bunnell, I. L., Arani, D. T., et al.: "Long-term Survival after Coronary Bypass Surgery," Buffalo General Hospital, State University of New York (brochure for exhibit at American Heart Association Meeting, Miami, 1977).

2 Lawrie, G. M., Morris, G. C., Jr., Howell, J. F., et al.: Results of Coronary Bypass More than 5 Years after Operation in 434 Patients: Clinical, Treadmill Exercise, and Angiographic Correlations, *Am. J. Cardiol.,* 40:665, 1977.

3 Miller, D. W., Jr., and Dodge, H. T.: Benefits of Coronary Artery Bypass Surgery. *Arch. Intern. Med.,* 137:1439, 1977.

4 Miller, D. W., Jr.: The Practice of Coronary Artery Bypass Surgery, in E. Sonnenblick and W. W. Parmley (eds.), "Topics in Cardiovascular Disease," Plenum Publishing Corporation, New York, 1977, p. 1.

5 Mundth, E. D., and Austen, W. G.: Surgical Measures for Coronary Heart Disease, *N. Engl. J. Med.,* 293:124, 1975.

6 Sheldon, W. C., Rincon, G., Pichard, A. I., et al.: Surgical Treatment of Coronary Artery Disease. Pure Graft Operations with a Study of 741 Patients Followed 3-7 Years, *Prog. Cardiovasc. Dis.,* 18 (3):237, 1975.

7 Spencer, F. C., Isom, O. W., Glassman, E., et al.: The Long-term Influence of Coronary Bypass Grafts on Myocardial Infarction and Survival, *Ann. Surg.,* 180:439, 1974.

8 Hutter, A. M., Jr., Russell, R. O., Jr., Resnekov, L., et al.: Unstable Angina Pectoris—National Randomized Study of Survival vs. Medical Therapy: Results in 1,2, and 3 Vessel Disease, *Circulation,* 55,56 (suppl. 3):60, 1977.

9 Mundth, E. D., and Austen, W. G.: Surgical Measures for Coronary Heart Disease, *N. Engl. J. Med.,* 293:124, 1975.

10 Bertolasi, C. A., Tronge, J. E., Riccitelli, M. A., Villamayor, R. M., and Zuffardi, E.: Natural History of Unstable Angina with Medical or Surgical Therapy, *Chest,* 70:596, 1976.

11 Cohn, L. H.: "Selection of Patients for Emergency Coronary Revascularization." An International Symposium of Cleveland Clinic Foundation, 1977.

12 Dunbar, R. W., Kaplan, J. A., and King, S. B.: Vasodilator Treatment of Heart Failure after Cardiopulmonary Bypass, *Anesth. Analg.,* 54:842, 1975.

13 Kaplan, J. A., Dunbar, R. W., and Jones, E. L.: Nitroglycerin Infusion during Coronary Artery Surgery, *Anesthesiology,* 45:14, 1976.

14 Kaplan, J. A., and King, S. B.: The Precordial Electrocardiographic Lead (V_5) in Patients Who Have Coronary Artery Disease, *Anesthesiology,* 45:570, 1976.

15 Kaplan, J. A., Dunbar, R. W., et al.: Propranolol and Cardiac Surgery: A Problem for the Anesthesiologist?, *Anesth. Analg.,* 54:571, 1975.

16 Kaplan, J. A., Craver, J. M., Jones, E. L., et al.: The Role of the Intraaortic Balloon in Cardiac Anesthesia, in H. Bolooki (ed.), "Clinical Application of Intraaortic Balloon Pump," Futura Publishing Company, Mt. Kisco, N.Y., 1977.

17 Leonard, A. R., Golding, A. R., Loop, F., Sheldon, W. C., et al.: Emergency Revascularization for Unstable Angina, *Am. J. Cardiol.,* 41:356, 1977.

18 Cohn, L. H., Boyden, C., and Collins, J. J.: Improved Long-term Survival after Aorto-coronary Bypass for Advanced Coronary Artery Disease, *Am. J. Surg.,* 129:380, 1975.

19 Conti, C. R., Hodges, M., Hutter, A., Resenokov, L., Rosati, R., Russell, R., Schroeder, J., and Wolk, M.: Unstable Angina—a National Cooperative Study Comparing Medical and Surgical Therapy, in S. H. Rahimtoola (ed.), "Coronary Bypass Surgery," F. A. Davis Company, Philadelphia, 1977.

20 Hurst, J. W., King, S. B., Logue, R. B., Hatcher, C. R., et al.: Value of Coronary Bypass Surgery, *Am. J. Cardiol.,* 42:308, 1978.

21 Hultgren, H. N.: Medical versus Surgical Treatment of Unstable Angina, *Am. J. Cardiol.,* 38:379, 1976.

22 Hultgren, H. M., Pfeifer, J. F., Angell, W. W., and Lipton, M. J.: Unstable Angina: Comparison of Medical and Surgical Management. *Am. J. Cardiol.,* 39:734, 1977.

23 McNeer, J. F., Starmer, C. F., Bartel, A. G., et al.: The Nature of Treatment Selection in Coronary Artery Disease: Experience with Medical and Surgical Treatment of Chronic Disease, *Circulation,* 49:606, 1974.

24 Read, R. C., Murphy, M. L., Hultgren, H. N., et al.: Survival of Men Treated for Chronic Stable Angina Pectoris: A Cooperative Randomized Study, *J. Thorac. Cardiovasc. Surg.,* 5:1, 1978.

25 McIntosh, H. D., and Garcia, J. A.: The First Decade of Aortocoronary Bypass Graftings, 1967–1977. A Review, *Circulation,* 57:405, 1978.

26 Russell, R. O. et al.: Unstable Angina Pectoris—National Randomized Study of Surgical vs. Medical Therapy: Results in Left Anterior Descending Disease., *Am. J. Cardiol.,* 41:397, 1977. (Abstract.)

27 Swan, H. J. C., and Conti, C. R.: Debate on Coronary Artery Disease, *Adv. Cardiol.,* 17:144, 1976.

28 Takaro, T., Hultgren, H. N., Lipton, J. J., et al.: The VA Cooperative Randomized Study of Surgery for Coronary Arterial Occlusive Disease. II. Subgroup with Significant Left Main Lesions, *Circulation,* 54 (suppl. 3):107, 1976.

29 Hurst, J. W., and King, S. B., III: Definitions and Classification of Coronary Atherosclerotic Heart Disease, in J. W. Hurst (ed.), "The Heart," 4th ed., McGraw-Hill Book Company, New York, 1978, p. 1094.

Myocardial Infarction with Normal Coronary Arteries*

ALBERT E. RAIZNER, M.D., and ROBERT A. CHAHINE, M.D.

And in a few fatal cases no lesions whatever are found; we must accept the fact that angina pectoris may kill without signs of obvious disease in the heart or blood vessels.

SIR WILLIAM OSLER, 1910[1]

The association between fixed atherosclerotic narrowing of the coronary arteries and the clinical manifestation of myocardial ischemia is clearly established. Postmortem studies have shown that patients dying of myocardial infarction almost invariably have critical narrowing of one or more coronary arteries.[2–4] Furthermore, with the development and proliferation of coronary arteriographic studies, the firm etiologic relationship between atheromatous occlusive coronary artery disease and the clinical syndromes of myocardial ischemia has been tightly welded.[5]

Nevertheless, as John F. Kennedy commented, "The greater our knowledge increases, the greater our ignorance unfolds."[6] As information and studies have expanded, individuals who do not fit into the conceptual mold of ischemic cardiac syndromes have been recognized.[7–36] Patients with documented myocardial infarction have been found to have normal coronary arteriograms or mild atheromatous disease with no apparent hemodynamic explanation to account for the myocardial necrosis. Such patients with normal or near normal coronary arteriograms have been described throughout the spectrum of ischemic heart disease, including cases of stable angina, unstable angina, myocardial infarction, and sudden death.[37]

The existence of the entity of myocardial infarction with normal coronary arteries has been questioned.[38] Certainly, evidence for specific pathophysiologic mechanisms has been sparse. Postmortem examinations confirming the myocardial lesion and the patency of the coronary arteries have been infrequent. Nevertheless, enough information is available to affirm the existence of the entity, and it is likely that multiple pathophysiologic mechanisms may be operative.

Since postmortem studies are scarce, most of the available information on this entity is based on the documentation of coronary artery patency by coronary arteriography. As such, any discussion of this group of patients should properly begin with a consideration of the difficulties and limitations in the diagnosis of "myocardial infarction" and "normal coronary arteries."

DIFFICULTIES AND LIMITATIONS IN THE DIAGNOSIS OF MYOCARDIAL INFARCTION

The general criteria for the diagnosis of myocardial infarction include the patients' subjective description of prolonged chest pain and objective evidence of myocardial necrosis. The latter may consist of electrocardiographic changes, cardiac enzyme elevations, contraction abnormalities on angiography, and more recently, abnormalities detected by nuclear scanning techniques. The chest pain description is limited by the patients' ability to describe such discomfort and the clinicians' subjective interpretation of these complaints. Electrocardiographic changes may be nonspecific, such as persistent ST and T wave abnormalities or, more specifically, the development of Q waves or loss of R waves. Despite greater specificity, Q waves can be seen in entities other than myocardial infarction, such as congestive and hypertrophic cardiomyopathy, myocarditis, W-P-W syndrome, etc. Nuclear scanning techniques utilizing 99mTc stannous pyrophosphate are often helpful in the diagnosis but, unfortunately, are also nonspecific.[39]

Nevertheless, most of the cases of myocardial infarction with normal coronary arteriograms which have been reported have demonstrated Q waves or loss of R waves on the electrocardiogram associated with enzymatic evidence of myocardial necrosis. In addition, the diagnosis has generally been supported by the demonstration of correlative contraction abnormalities on ventriculography. Thus, most of the reported cases reliably document myocardial infarction. Since myocardial infarction can sometimes occur without definitive electrocardiographic, enzymatic, or other laboratory abnormalities, the true incidence of infarction with patent coronary arteries may be even higher.

* From the Department of Medicine, Baylor College of Medicine and the Cardiology Section of the Veterans Administration Hospital, Houston.

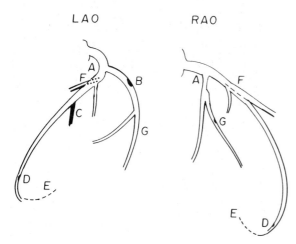

FIGURE 1 A schematic diagram of the left coronary artery in the left anterior oblique (LAO) and right anterior oblique (RAO) projections. A through G illustrate common sources of error in the interpretation of "normal" coronary arteriograms. (See text for description.)

DIFFICULTIES AND LIMITATIONS IN THE DIAGNOSIS OF NORMAL CORONARY ARTERIES

To date, autopsy studies have been scarce. In most reported cases the diagnosis was attained at coronary arteriography. It is generally accepted that in order to produce significant obstruction to flow, a lesion must involve 50 to 75 percent or more of the lumen diameter.[40] Coronary arteries are considered angiographically "normal" when only minimal plaques or irregularities are noted. Such situations will still be considered as representing normal coronary arteries with the understanding that anatomic studies, if possible, might reveal minor abnormalities.

The potential for incorrect interpretation of "normal" coronary arteriograms has been stressed.[41] The following common errors of interpretation (Fig. 1) may result in the incorrect diagnosis of normal coronary arteries:

A Foreshortening of vessels coursing perpendicular to the plane of projection.

B Minor luminal plaques may produce minimal or no angiographic defect. Plaques may not be significant hemodynamically but can be a source of thrombus formation or embolization or may serve to trigger vasospasm.

C Flush occlusion of a branch vessel may not be recognized.

D Occlusive disease of distal segments may not be appreciated because of small lumen caliber.

E A distal segment may be occluded and appear as a congenitally "short but otherwise normal" artery. This

should be considered in patients whose anterior or posterior descending arteries do not reach the apex.

F Overlapping of vessels may hinder accurate interpretation.

G Eccentric lesions may be apparent only in a particular view but appear normal in other views.

Improvements in overall radiologic quality, the obtaining of multiple oblique projections and (when necessary) hemiaxial views, and greater experience of the angiographer have minimized these sources of error. Despite close attention to each of the above details, discrepancies between coronary arteriography and pathological findings exist, an extreme example of which is illustrated by the following case:

C. N., a 31-year-old male in previously good health, suffered severe burns in a fire. On admission his electrocardiogram showed an acute inferior infarction (Fig. 2). One month later, he had an anterior infarction (Fig. 3) complicated by cardiogenic shock and persistent congestive heart failure. He gave a history of smoking one to two packs of cigarettes per day but had no other risk factors.

He was referred to us for further study 6 months later with refractory congestive heart failure. Cardiac catheterization disclosed an enlarged left ventricle with an ejection fraction of 0.15. Coronary arteriograms showed luminal irregularities but no hemodynamically significant lesions in the right (Fig.4*A*) or left (Fig.4*B*) coronary arteries. His case was presented at numerous conferences as an example of myocardial infarction with no significant obstructive coronary artery disease.

Three weeks after the above studies were performed, he died suddenly. Postmortem examination disclosed acute myocardial infarction as the cause of death. The coronary arteries exhibited severe atheromatous narrowing of the proximal segments of the anterior descending and the right coronary arteries (Fig.5). (Autopsy findings courtesy of Dr. Peter L. Lardizabal, Chief Medical Examiner, Tampa, Florida. Prior hospital records courtesy of Dr. Francisco Fuentes, Houston, Texas.)

This case pointedly and painfully illustrates an unfortunate fact: incorrect interpretation of coronary arteriograms remains an important "etiology" of myocardial infarction with normal coronary arteries.

INCIDENCE

Patients who undergo coronary arteriography clearly represent a select group of individuals. Consequently, an exact incidence of the occurrence of normal coronary arteriograms in the broad population of patients with ischemic heart disease cannot be firmly established. In patients undergoing coronary arteriography for evaluation of angina pectoris, the incidence of normal coronary arteriograms may exceed 15 percent.[5]

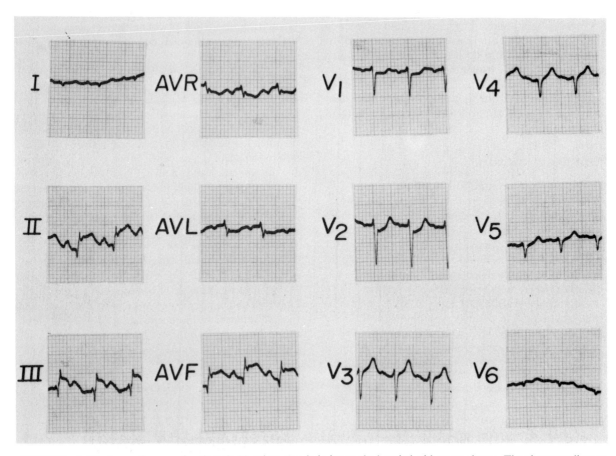

FIGURE 2 Electrocardiogram of patient C. N. taken on admission to the hospital with severe burns. The electrocardiogram shows an acute inferior myocardial infarction.

If one restricts consideration to individuals with objective documentation of myocardial infarction, the incidence of normal coronary arteriograms is smaller. The incidence of normal coronary arteriograms in patients with myocardial infarction ranges from 1[5,38] to 12 percent.[22] In selected groups of individuals, however, the incidence may be considerably higher. For instance, in patients with myocardial infarction under 35 years of age, over 15 percent may have normal coronary arteriograms.[32] Similarly, an incidence of over 20 percent has been observed in women with infarction under age 50.[43] Therefore, the incidence of this entity increases when a younger population of patients are included and the diagnosis is attained by coronary arteriography and decreases when older patients are studied and the diagnosis is based on autopsy material.

CLINICAL CHARACTERISTICS

Most of the cases available for review represent isolated case reports or small series from single institutions. Just as the elephant may be interpreted differently if viewed from the tail or leg or trunk, most authors have viewed the phenomenon of myocardial infarction with normal coronary arteries with necessarily limited observations. Consequently, an accurate clinical profile encompassing the spectrum of patients with myocardial infarction and normal coronary arteries has not been presented. The following clinical profile is based on a review of 110 cases, including those of our own experience.[7–36]

Age

The mean age of patients having myocardial infarction and normal coronary arteries is 36.8 years, with males averaging 36.7 years and females 38.1 years. The youngest patient reported was 14 years old at the time of infarction,[19] and the oldest was 81 years.[21] The age distribution is shown in Fig. 6. Over 65 percent of cases occur in individuals under 40 years of age. There have been more cases reported in teenagers than in individuals over the age of 60. The peak occurrence in males is in the third decade of life, while that of females is in the fourth decade. Thus, patients with myocardial infarction and normal coronary arteries differ considerably from patients with myocardial infarction resulting from occlusive atheromatous coronary artery disease, where the peak occurrence is in the sixth and seventh decades. This difference is most impressive with regard to young females, in whom occlusive coronary artery disease is relatively uncommon.

Sex Distribution

Of the 110 cases being reviewed, 83 are males and 27 females. Thus, males outnumber females in a ratio of approximately 3:1. It is of interest that some authors have considered myocardial infarction with normal coronary arteries to be a disease almost exclusively of males,[30] while others report series containing only females.[31] The explanation for these differences is unclear but may merely reflect patient selection.

Although a male/female ratio of 3:1 is similar to that seen overall in patients with coronary occlusive disease, it is significantly lower than that observed in subjects of comparable young age. This reflects a

greater representation of young females with myocardial infarction and normal coronary arteries.

Risk Factors

The prevalence of coronary artery disease risk factors in patients with myocardial infarction and normal coronary arteries is shown in Fig. 7. Smoking is the most common risk factor and is described in 46 of 110 cases, a prevalence of 42 percent. Other coronary disease risk factors are less common;[30] hypertension is noted in only 5 percent, lipid abnormality in 10 percent, a family history of ischemic heart disease in 7 percent, and diabetes mellitus in 5 percent. It is possible that the actual incidence of coronary disease risk factors is higher than these figures would suggest, since not all case reports provide complete details regarding risk factors. Eslami et al. report a higher incidence of risk factors in their 13 cases: 11 had at least one risk factor (smoking and family history were most common), and 6 of these had 2 or more risk factors.[26] Nevertheless, the incidence of risk factors in patients with myocardial infarction and normal coronary arteries is signif-

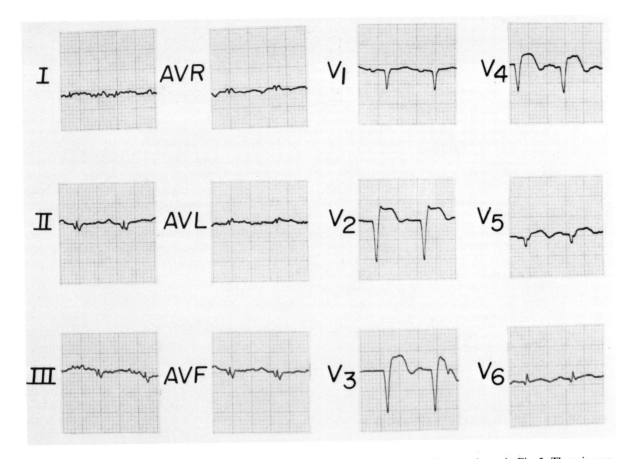

FIGURE 3 Electrocardiogram of patient C. N. obtained 1 month after the electrocardiogram shown in Fig. 2. There is now an acute anterior infarction in addition to the previous inferior infarction.

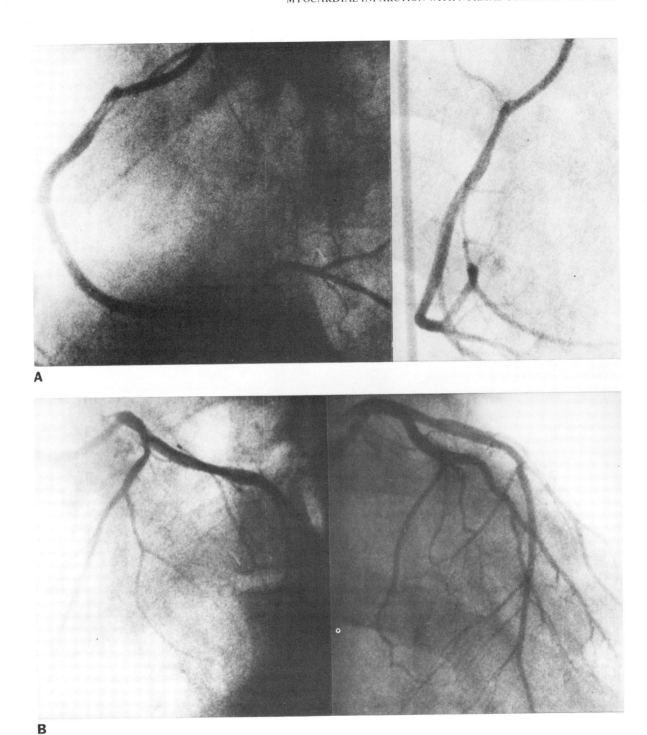

FIGURE 4 The coronary arteriogram of patient C. N. obtained 6 months after the myocardial infarction. *A*. The right coronary artery in the left anterior oblique (left panel) and right anterior oblique (right panel) projections. *B*. The left coronary artery in the left anterior oblique (left panel) and right anterior oblique (right panel) projections. Mild luminal narrowing is seen in the proximal right and left anterior descending coronary arteries, but no hemodynamically significant lesions are noted. Major branches and distal vessels appear patent. (With the assistance of Ms. Marsha Bane.)

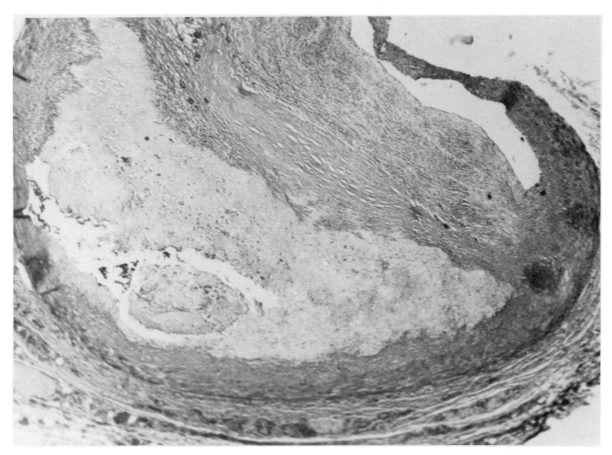

FIGURE 5 A cross section of the proximal anterior descending coronary artery of patient C. N. showing extensive atherosclerotic changes. A major proportion of the cross-sectional area is occluded, and only a small eccentrically displaced lumen (upper right) remains. Similarly severe pathology was seen in the right coronary artery and the distal segments of these vessels showed significant intimal thickening (× 100). (Photograph courtesy of Dr. Ferenc Gyorkey, Baylor College of Medicine, Houston, Texas.)

icantly lower than that found in a comparable population of patients with coronary occlusive disease.[30]

Of particular interest is the possible risk imposed by the use of oral contraceptives. Impressively, one-third (9 of 27) of the women with myocardial infarction and normal coronary arteries were taking oral contraceptives at the time of infarction.[10,14,16,24,31] While a definite cause-and-effect relationship has not been firmly established, the association of oral contraceptives with an increased risk of myocardial infarction has been noted by several authors.[44–46] In addition, the combination of oral contraceptive use and cigarette smoking augments the risk of myocardial infarction.[46] Of the 9 women on oral contraceptives who suffered myocardial infarction despite normal coronaries, 6 (67 percent) were also smokers. It seems apparent that oral contraceptives should be considered a risk factor in patients with myocardial infarction and normal coronary arteries, particularly when other risk factors are present.

Patients have been described with other medical or cardiologic associations, such as pregnancy,[12,23] alcoholism,[25] amphetamine ingestion,[19] hyperthyroidism,[33,36] and mitral valve prolapse.[28] Whether or not these should be considered as risk factors or of etiologic significance remains to be determined.

Clinical Course

It is well known that the majority of patients with myocardial infarction resulting from occlusive coronary artery disease have prodromal anginal symptoms (unstable angina) or other medical complaints preceding the infarction.[47] Such is not the case in patients with myocardial infarction and normal coronary arteries.[30] Only 11 of 110 patients, or 10 percent of reported cases, describe angina preceding the infarction. Most patients are in good health prior to infarction. The infarction pain generally occurs de novo, and precipitating factors are scarce.[30] In some patients, the onset

AGE DISTRIBUTION

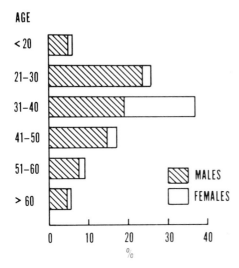

FIGURE 6 The age distribution of 110 cases of myocardial infarction with normal coronary arteries. Note the overwhelming preponderance of individuals between the ages of 20 and 40 years. The peak incidence for males is in the third decade, while that for females, in the fourth decade of life.

of chest pain coincides with extreme physical effort.[26]

The quality and type of chest pain are similar to that which generally occurs with myocardial infarction. Associated symptoms such as nausea, diaphoresis, and lightheadedness are common and not of distinguishing value. There appears to be no predilection for a specific area of infarction.[22,30] An anterior (anteroseptal, anteroapical, anterolateral) site of infarction is most common and is described in 54 percent of cases. An inferoposterior (inferior, diaphragmatic, posterior, inferolateral) location occurs almost as frequently in 43 percent. Both anterior and inferior infarction sites are observed in 3 percent.

Most infarctions in this group of patients are transmural, documented by the appearance of Q waves or loss of R waves on the electrocardiogram. Subendocardial infarction can occur[48] but is not frequently described. This relatively low occurrence of subendocardial infarction and normal coronary arteries probably reflects inconclusiveness of documentation of infarction and, therefore, a hesitancy to report such cases. The true incidence of subendocardial infarction with normal coronary arteries may be higher than currently appreciated.

The clinical course of patients with normal coronary arteries following an episode of infarction is characterized by an impressive infrequency of postinfarction angina. Only 15 of 110 patients (14 percent) had angina after recovery from the acute episode. The paucity of postinfarction angina contrasts sharply with its occurrence in approximately two-thirds of patients

with coronary occlusive disease.[30] In addition, recurrent myocardial infarction is uncommon but can occur in patients with normal coronary arteries.[12,20,24,30] Postinfarction congestive heart failure symptoms can result from left ventricular dysfunction if a sufficiently large infarct develops.[7]

Long-term follow-up studies to assess late mortality of patients with myocardial infarction and normal coronary arteries are not available. It has been suggested that the survival of patients who do not succumb to the initial infarction is better than that expected in patients with coronary occlusive disease[30,49] if severe left ventricular dysfunction is not present.

A comparison of pertinent clinical differences between patients with myocardial infarction and normal coronary arteries and those with occlusive coronary atherosclerosis is shown in Table 1.

ETIOLOGY AND PATHOPHYSIOLOGY OF MYOCARDIAL INFARCTION WITH NORMAL CORONARY ARTERIES

The observation that ischemic heart disease can occur without fixed critical coronary artery narrowing has reawakened cardiologists and cardiac physiologists to the need for an intense search for etiologic and pathophysiologic mechanisms. Much discussion and speculation have arisen.

A classification of the proposed etiologic and pathophysiologic mechanisms of myocardial infarction

PREVALENCE OF REPORTED RISK FACTORS

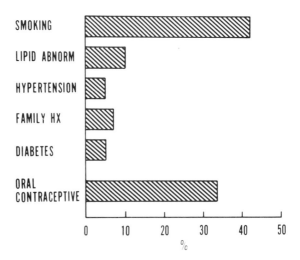

FIGURE 7 The prevalence of reported risk factors in patients with myocardial infarction and normal coronary arteriograms. Of the classical coronary artery disease risk factors, only smoking was highly prevalent. Among females the use of oral contraceptives was common.

TABLE 1

Clinical features of patients with myocardial infarction (MI) and normal coronary arteries compared to patients with occlusive coronary atherosclerosis

Feature	MI with normal coronary arteries	MI with occlusive coronary arteries
1. Age	Mean = 36.8 years	Older
2. Male/female ratio	3:1	Similar, lower percentage of females in young age groups
3. Risk factors	Smoking, oral contraceptives, others uncommon	Multiple risk factors common
4. Prodromal (unstable) angina	Uncommon (10%)	Common (60%–70%)
5. Location of infarction	Anterior, 54% Inferoposterior, 43%	Similar, excluding nontransmural
6. Postinfarction angina	Uncommon (14%)	Common (60%–70%)
7. Recurrent infarction	Uncommon	Common

with normal coronary arteries is shown in Table 2. Each of these entities should be considered in the evaluation of a patient with ischemic heart disease who is found to have normal coronary arteriograms. Conversely, patients known to have one or another of these abnormalities may manifest myocardial ischemia, including myocardial infarction, in the course of their illness.

Transient Mechanical Vascular Obstruction

CORONARY ARTERY SPASM

Since the nineteenth century, coronary artery spasm was considered an important mechanism underlying ischemic heart disease.[50] However, attention justifiably shifted to a fixed-lesion concept because of the strong correlation between coronary atherosclerosis and the clinical syndromes of ischemic heart disease.[2–5] In the early 1970s, interest in coronary spasm was revived by the demonstration that this phenomenon underlies the chest pain in patients with Prinzmetal's variant angina.[51,52]

The pathophysiology of coronary artery spasm remains largely unknown.[53] The autonomic nervous system is strongly implicated.[54] The production of spasm by the injection of methacholine or a combination of epinephrine and propranolol strongly supports this possibility.[55,56] Reflexes and cortical influences also seem to play a role. Coronary artery spasm has been described during REM (rapid eye movement) sleep,[57] and both focal and diffuse coronary constriction have been produced by the cold pressor test.[58,59]

Spasm may occur in apparently normal or diseased

coronary arteries. It may be focal or diffuse and may occur in any of the branches of the coronary tree.[60,61] The best available objective documentation of myocardial ischemia secondary to coronary artery spasm

TABLE 2

Classification of etiologic mechanisms of myocardial infarction and normal coronary arteries

I Transient mechanical vascular obstruction
  A Coronary artery spasm
  B Coronary embolism, in situ thrombosis, and platelet aggregation
  C Myocardial bridge
  D Coronary artery dissection
II Intramyocardial—small vessel disease
  A Diabetes mellitus
  B Collagen vascular diseases
    1 Periarteritis nodosum
    2 Progressive systemic sclerosis
    3 Systemic lupus erhythematosus
    4 Rheumatoid arthritis
    5 Rheumatic fever
  C Infiltrative diseases
    1 Amyloidosis
  D Connective tissue diseases
    1 Marfan's syndrome
    2 Hurler's syndrome
  E Neuromuscular diseases
    1 Friedreich's ataxia
    2 Progressive muscular dystrophy
    3 Progressive myotonic dystrophy
  F Hematologic
    1 Thrombotic thrombocytopenic purpura
    2 Disseminated intravascular coagulation
III Physiologic imbalance of oxygen supply and demand
  A Abnormality of hemoglobin-oxygen affinity
  B Ventricular hypertrophic diseases
IV Trauma

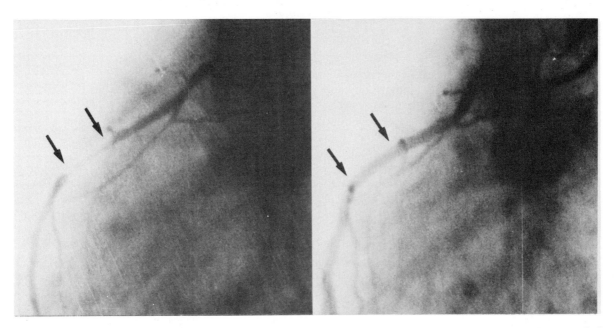

FIGURE 8 Spontaneous coronary artery spasm is seen in the right coronary artery (left panel) before the acute marginal branch. Following nitroglycerin administration (right panel) the spasm is completely relieved and the vessel is fully patent. Coronary artery spasm has been noted in some patients with myocardial infarction whose coronary arteries are otherwise normal.

is found in Prinzmetal's variant angina.[51,52,62,63] This type of angina may occur in patients with normal coronary arteries as well as with atheromatous coronary artery disease.[64-67] In these patients, coronary artery spasm produces or contributes to complete or subtotal occlusion of a major epicardial artery, resulting in transmural ischemia with corresponding ST-segment elevation.[63,68,69] Coronary artery spasm has also been documented in some cases of classic angina pectoris.[70,71] Thus, coronary artery spasm causing transient and reversible myocardial ischemia in patients with normal coronary arteries, as well as in patients with atheromatous disease, is a well-documented phenomenon (Fig.8).

Depending on the severity of the spasm, more severe degrees of myocardial ischemia may result. Several observations suggest that spasm may play a role in the production of myocardial infarction both in patients with normal coronary arteries and in those with atherosclerotic lesions.[53,60,72-74] Oliva studied several patients during the acute phase of myocardial infarction and concluded that spasm contributed to the genesis of infarction.[75] However, each of these patients had severe occlusive coronary atheromatous disease.

The evidence linking coronary artery spasm to the production of myocardial infarction in patients with normal coronary arteries has been more indirect. Engel attributed an acute myocardial infarction occurring during cardiac catheterization to coronary artery spasm induced by the catheter.[27] In other reports of patients studied after recovery from myocardial infarction and

found to have normal coronary arteries, coronary artery spasm was noted and provided a plausible explanation for the infarction.[15,76,77] Coronary vasospasm was also implicated in the production of myocardial infarction in the presence of normal coronaries in cases of withdrawal from chronic industrial exposure to nitrates.[78]

Perhaps the most potent evidence relating coronary artery spasm to myocardial infarction can be gathered from patients with Prinzmetal's variant angina. Spontaneous ischemic episodes in these patients is caused by coronary artery spasm.[51,52] Myocardial infarction may occur in the course of these patients' illness,[66,67,79] including patients with normal coronaries arteries,[15,76,77] as the following case illustrates.

S. M., a 39-year-old male, presented with a 3-month history of intermittent crushing substernal chest discomfort which was unrelated to effort and was most prevalent in the morning hours. His resting electrocardiogram was normal. A treadmill exercise test revealed good exercise tolerance and no evidence of myocardial ischemia. During 24-h electrocardiographic monitoring several episodes of chest pain were associated with ST-segment elevation (Fig.9). Coronary arteriography demonstrated minimal luminal irregularity in the anterior descending coronary artery but no significant occlusive lesions (Fig.10). Three days following the study, he developed prolonged chest pain. Electrocardiograms showed evolution of an acute anterior myocardial infarction (Fig.11A and 11B). (Courtesy of Dr. William R. Gaston, Houston, Texas.)

BEFORE DURING PAIN AFTER

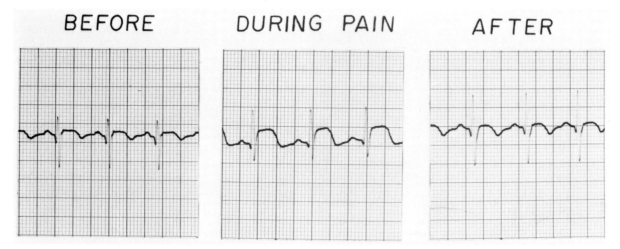

FIGURE 9 Segments of a 24-h electrocardiographic recording of patient S. M. showing ST-segment elevation occurring during episodes of chest pain and resolving after the pain subsides. This is characteristic of Prinzmetal's variant angina and has been shown to be caused by coronary artery spasm.

The extent of the role of spasm in the production of myocardial infarction with normal coronary arteries and, for that matter, in the broad spectrum of ischemic heart disease remains difficult to determine because of diagnostic limitations. The definitive diagnosis of coronary artery spasm can only be established with certainty by coronary angiography, a procedure rarely performed during the acute phase of infarction. Arteriographic studies done before or after infarction may fail to demonstrate this dynamic and transient phenomenon. The utilization of provocative testing with ergonovine maleate[80] or the cold pressor test[58] may increase the likelihood of diagnosis. Radionuclide studies,[62] with further refinements, offer future promise.

Although coronary artery spasm appears to be an extremely attractive etiologic mechanism to explain myocardial infarction with normal coronary arteries in some patients, the assessment of its etiologic role in these cases may have to await the development of more readily applied diagnostic techniques.

CORONARY ARTERY EMBOLISM, IN SITU THROMBOSIS, AND PLATELET AGGREGATION

Coronary artery embolism has long been known to be a cause of myocardial infarction and death.[81] More recent reviews have investigated its clinical and pathologic correlations.[82,83] Common conditions which predispose to coronary embolism include infective endocarditis, prosthetic aortic or mitral valves, noninfective aortic or mitral valve disease, cardiomyopathy with mural thrombus, atrial fibrillation, and coronary artery disease.[82,83] Less common causes of coronary

artery embolism include coronary arteriography, tumor emboli, fat emboli, and paradoxical emboli from peripheral veins.[82,83] Emboli can lodge in any coronary vessel, although the left coronary artery is involved three to four times more often than the right, with the left anterior descending coronary artery being the single most common site.[83] Typically, the embolus lodges distally and usually results in a small transmural infarction[83] which is often not clinically recognized.

Coronary embolism is an important cause of myocardial infarction with normal coronary arteries. Although at the time of embolization the coronary artery is occluded, coronary arteriography performed after the acute episode may reveal patent and apparently "normal" coronary arteries because of (1) distal lodgement of the embolus or (2) recanalization, resulting in a patent artery.

In situ thrombosis of a coronary artery represents another mechanism of myocardial infarction. While in situ thrombosis typically occurs in coronary arteries which already have severe stenotic lesions,[84] it is apparent that thrombosis can also occur in the absence of hemodynamically significant atheromatous disease. Once formed, infarction ensues and subsequent lysis of the thrombus can restore vessel patency. Lysis of thrombus in vivo has been demonstrated by Weisse et al.[85] These investigators electrically induced thrombus formation in the coronary arteries of dogs. After 30 days there was significant or complete resolution of the thrombus which was demonstrated arteriographically and at postmortem examination. That this process can occur in human beings is suggested by the resolution of an occlusive lesion to full patency on serial coronary arteriograms in a patient with myocardial infarction reported by Henderson et al.[16] In situ thrombosis with subsequent clot lysis has been pro-

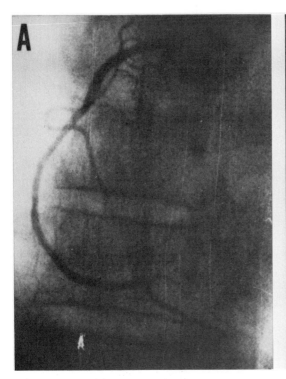
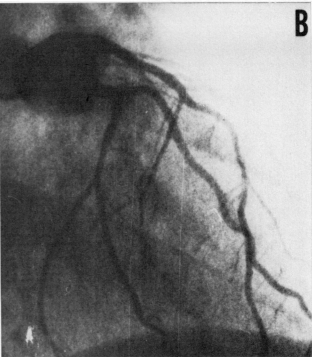

FIGURE 10 Coronary arteriogram of patient S. M. *A.* The right coronary artery in the left anterior oblique view. *B.* The left coronary artery in the right anterior oblique view. No significant occlusive disease is noted in either coronary artery or their major branches.

posed as the cause of myocardial infarction with normal coronary arteries in numerous reports.[7,10-12,14,16,24]

The role of platelet aggregation in the pathogenesis of myocardial ischemia has been the subject of important investigation. Platelet aggregation is involved in the formation of arterial thrombi and occurs in areas of damaged endothelium or turbulent flow.[86] Folts has shown that in normal canine coronary arteries made stenotic by partial banding, platelet aggregates constantly form and disperse, resulting in cyclic reductions in coronary blood flow and myocardial ischemia.[87] Platelet aggregates form even in the presence of an intact and normal endothelium.[87] It would be enticing to speculate that transient stenosis in an otherwise normal coronary artery, such as might occur with coronary artery spasm or a myocardial bridge, could similarly precipitate platelet aggregation, augment ischemia, and perhaps initiate thrombus formation. Furthermore, vasoactive substances such as serotonin, prostaglandin G_2, and thromboxane A_2 are released during platelet aggregation.[88] These substances are potent vasoconstrictors and might enhance or perpetuate the vasospastic process. It is also possible that platelet aggregation at the site of a mild luminal plaque in an arteriographically "normal" artery might initiate the above events.

The role of platelet aggregation in the syndrome of myocardial infarction with normal coronary arteries is speculative. However, it is of interest that factors which have been associated with this syndrome, such as smoking, oral contraceptive use, strenuous exercise, and thrombocytosis,[14] are known to increase platelet aggregation.[89-91]

MYOCARDIAL BRIDGES

Myocardial bridges are bands of heart muscle which overlie a coronary artery segment. They may be recognized clinically by systolic narrowing of the coronary artery during cinearteriography.[92] While their incidence varies between 5 and 85 percent in autopsy specimens,[93,94] myocardial bridges were recognized in 1.6 percent of our coronary arteriograms.[95]

The role of myocardial bridges in the production of myocardial ischemia has been the subject of recent interest. Since coronary artery narrowing secondary to myocardial bridges occurs in systole, a phase in which only about 20 percent of coronary flow occurs,[96] it would seem unlikely that significant ischemia should result. During tachycardia, however, when diastolic time is shortened relative to systolic time, systolic flow may assume greater importance. Under these circumstances, myocardial bridges may adversely affect coronary flow. Noble has shown that myocardial is-

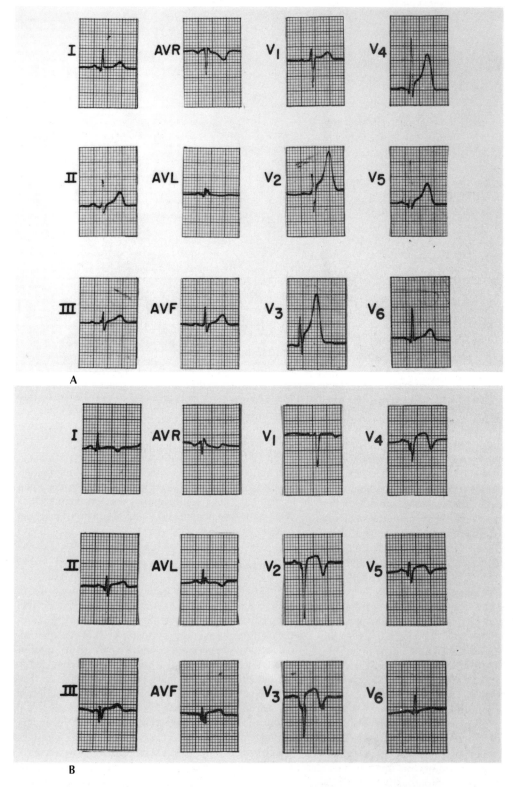

FIGURE 11 A. The electrocardiogram of patient S. M. recorded 3 days after the coronary arteriograms seen in Fig. 10. There was ST-segment elevation and hyperacute T wave abnormalities suggestive of acute infarction. B. The electrocardiogram recorded several days later shows evolution of an acute anterior myocardial infarction. In view of this patient's clinical presentation of Prinzmetal's variant angina and the demonstration of normal coronary arteriograms, the cause of the myocardial infarction is presumed to be coronary artery spasm.

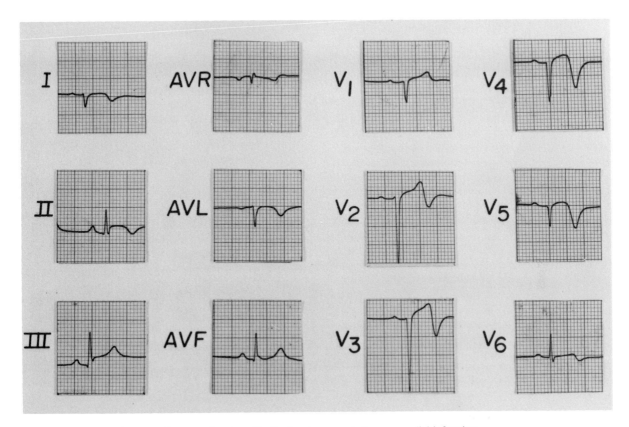

FIGURE 12 The electrocardiogram of patient W. G. showing an anterior myocardial infarction.

chemia, documented by coronary sinus lactate production, can be produced in patients with myocardial bridges by rapid atrial pacing.[97] We have demonstrated that patients with myocardial bridges but otherwise normal coronary arteries can develop myocardial ischemia during exercise manifested by thallium scan defects and segmental contraction abnormalities in the region of the ventricle perfused by the bridged artery. Surgical interruption of the bridge corrected the perfusion and contraction abnormally.[98]

The evidence relating myocardial bridges to myocardial infarction has, to date, been indirect, as the following case illustrates.

W. G., a 33-year-old male, was in good health until February 1978 when he suddenly developed crushing chest pain while strenuously exerting himself in an automobile race. An acute anterior myocardial infarction was documented by electrocardiography (Fig.12) and elevation of cardiac enzymes. He had no risk factors for coronary artery disease.

Cardiac catheterization was performed 4 months later. Left ventriculography disclosed a hypokinetic anteroapical segment (Fig.13). Coronary arteriograms revealed normal coronary arteries except for a 90 percent systolic narrowing of the middle segment of the left anterior descending coronary artery. The vessel was fully patent during diastole (Fig.14).

In the face of mounting evidence that myocardial bridges can produce ischemia, the finding of a bridge in a patient with myocardial infarction but otherwise normal coronary arteries takes on greater significance. Endo reports one such patient with hyperthyroidism who developed a myocardial infarction during an arrhythmia. Coronary arteriography showed a myocardial bridge with systolic coronary artery narrowing. During rapid atrial pacing at 150 beats per minute, the artery was obstructed during diastole as well as systole.[99] Farugui describes another case of myocardial infarction with no coronary abnormality other than a myocardial bridge.[100] This phenomenon must be considered as a possible cause, in some individuals, of myocardial infarction with normal coronary arteries.

CORONARY ARTERY DISSECTION

Ciraulo describes a patient with myocardial infarction resulting from coronary artery dissection. Repeat coronary arteriograms 19 months later showed resolution of the dissection with return of luminal patency.[24] This rare mechanism of myocardial infarction with normally appearing coronary arteries was considered in another case[12] but is, at best, a rare cause of this syndrome.

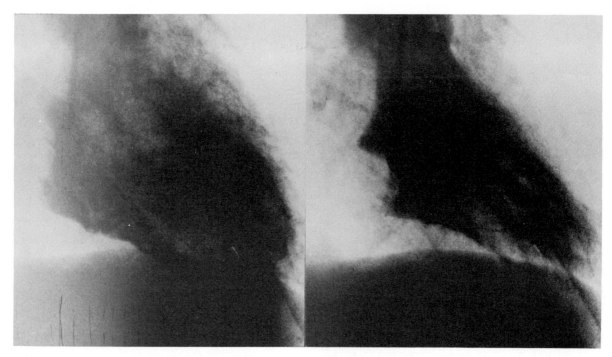

FIGURE 13 The left ventriculogram of patient W. G. There is hypokinesis of the anteroapical segment, but other regions of the left ventricle contract well.

Intramyocardial, Small Vessel Disease

Adequate perfusion of the myocardium requires patency of both the large epicardial coronary arteries and the small intramyocardial vessels. This latter group of vessels penetrates the epicardium in a perpendicular manner and then may terminate as end-arteries in the myocardium or course to the endocardium where they divide, forming a diffuse anastomatic network. These vessels generally range in diameter between 0.1 and 1.0 mm. The smaller of these vessels cannot be visualized angiographically. Some of the larger ones may be seen during coronary arteriography, but details regarding the presence or absence of intraluminal disease cannot be appreciated because of limited resolution capabilities of current cineangiographic equipment. Consequently, diseases which affect these small arteries can produce the clinical syndromes of myocardial ischemia, including myocardial infarction, with coronary arteries which appear normal on arteriograms.

Pathologic studies have documented disease of the small, intramyocardial coronary arteries in a wide variety of disease states (see Table 2).[38,101-113] Many of these diseases may present with a clinical picture of myocardial infarction. Nevertheless, it is not likely that small vessel disease offers a satisfactory explanation for more than a rare patient with myocardial in-

farction with normal coronary arteries for the following reasons: (1) Reports of myocardial infarction with normal large coronary arteries in patients with these disorders are rare. (2) Patients with these diseases generally have involvement of multiple organ systems and a myriad of clinical problems. Multisystem involvement, however, is extremely unusual in patients with myocardial infarction and normal coronary arteries. (3) Some of the diseases with small vessel pathology also have large vessel involvement which is more typical of the disease and more likely to be the cause of myocardial infarction, e.g., diabetes mellitus. (4) Reports of myocardial infarction with normal large coronary arteries in patients with these diseases have not always shown small vessel involvement.[114] Other, more likely mechanisms, such as coronary artery spasm or a coronary Raynaud's phenomenon, have been proposed.[114]

Physiologic Imbalance of Myocardial Oxygen Supply and Demand

ABNORMALITY OF HEMOGLOBIN-OXYGEN DISSOCIATION

Another interesting etiologic factor that has been postulated as a possible mechanism underlying myocardial infarction with normal coronary arteries is an abnormality of the hemoglobin-oxygen dissociation curve which might result in an impaired release of oxygen at the myocardial tissue level. Eliot, Mizukami, and their colleagues have described this abnormality in a variety of patients with myocardial infarction, the anginal syndrome, and normal coronary arteriograms and in some asymptomatic smokers.[19,100-115] They speculated that such abnormalities may account for some cases of myocardial infarction without obstructive coronary disease. However, documentation of an abnormality of hemoglobin-oxygen dissociation in patients with myocardial infarction and normal coronary arteries has been scarce.[19] Other workers have investigated patients with the anginal syndrome and normal coronary arteries and failed to find any hemoglobin abnormality.[116] Therefore, an abnormality of hemoglobin-oxygen dissociation, although interesting, has not been substantiated as a mechanism to explain myocardial infarction in the absence of coronary obstructive disease.

VENTRICULAR HYPERTROPHIC DISEASES

Myocardial ischemia may result from an abnormally large myocardial oxygen demand which exceeds the delivering capacity of the coronary vascular bed. Clinical manifestations of myocardial ischemia can develop in patients with left ventricular hypertrophy associated with hypertrophic cardiomyopathy, hypertensive heart disease, and aortic valve disease.[117] Myocardial infarction may occur under these circumstances but is typically subendocardial. Since most patients with the syndrome of myocardial infarction with normal coronary arteries have transmural infarction and since very few reports have described left ventricular hypertrophy, this mechanism is not likely to be playing an important role.

Trauma

Blunt chest trauma frequently results in myocardial contusion, manifested as nonspecific ST and T wave abnormalities on the electrocardiogram. Several reports describe the development of myocardial necrosis with Q wave formation following chest trauma.[29,118,119] Follow-up coronary arteriograms in young patients have revealed both normal[29] and occluded[119] coronary arteries. It is not clear whether the myocardial necrosis resulted from direct injury to the myocardium per se or to the coronary artery with interruption of blood flow and myocardial infarction.

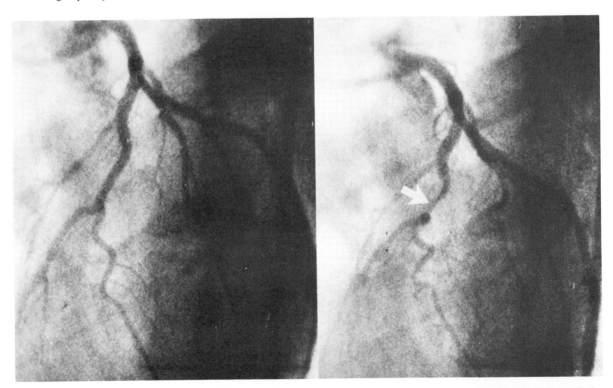

FIGURE 14 The left coronary artery of patient W. G. in the left anterior oblique projection. During diastole (left panel) the coronary artery is fully patent. During systole (right panel) there is severe narrowing of the middle segment of the anterior descending coronary artery. This is the only arteriographic abnormality seen in this patient with otherwise normal coronary arteries and is presumed to be the cause of his anteroapical infarction. (With the assistance of Dr. Robert Berglund, Mrs. Sherry Teeter, and Mr. Tim Peasgood.)

COMMENTS REGARDING ETIOLOGIC MECHANISMS OF MYOCARDIAL INFARCTION WITH NORMAL CORONARY ARTERIES

A multiplicity of etiologic and pathophysiologic mechanisms have been presented. It is unlikely that any single proposed mechanism could be operative in all reported cases of myocardial infarction with normal coronary arteries.

Some of the mechanisms discussed might explain the findings in one or more patients but are not likely to account for a large percentage of cases. Of the pathophysiologic explanations offered, coronary artery spasm and in situ thrombosis or platelet aggregation are the most intriguing and perhaps the most promising. Unfortunately, much of the evidence implicating either or both of these mechanisms is only circumstantial. It should be considered that both phenomena may have a combined role, one presidposing to or triggering the other. The transient nature of these phenomena has hindered their diagnosis and documentation. Additional studies directing attention to these phenomena are needed before the full extent of their role in the genesis of the syndrome can be ascertained.

The knowledge and understanding of the mechanisms involved can have far-reaching consequences. Not only might we learn more about the specific syndrome of myocardial infarction with normal coronary arteries, but the possibility exists that similar mechanisms may be operative in patients with occlusive atheromatous coronary artery disease. "Whatsoever this matter and its power be, it is a thing positive and inexplicable, and must be taken absolutely as it is found, and not be judged by any previous conception."[120]

REFERENCES

1 Osler, W.: The Lumleian Lectures on Angina Pectoris, *Lancet,* 1:839, 1910.

2 Miller, R. D., Burchell, H. B., and Edwards, J. E.: Myocardial Infarction with and without Acute Coronary Occlusion, *Arch. Intern. Med.,* 88:597, 1951.

3 Blumgart, H. L., Schlesinger, M. J., and Davis, D.: Studies on the Relation of the Clinical Manifestations of Angina Pectoris, Coronary Thrombosis and Myocardial Infarction to the Pathologic Findings, *Am. Heart J.,* 19:1, 1940.

4 Roberts, W. C., and Buja, L. M.: Frequency and Significance of Coronary Arterial Thrombi and Other Observations in Fatal Acute Myocardial Infarction: A Study of 107 Necropsy Patients. *Am. J. Med.,* 52:425, 1972.

5 Proudfit, W. L., Shirey, E. K., and Sones, F. M., Jr.: Selective Cine Coronary Arteriography. Correlation with Clinical Findings in 1000 Patients, *Circulation,* 33:901, 1966.

6 Kennedy, J. F.: Address, Rice University, Houston, Texas, Sept. 12, 1962.

7 Campeau, L., Lesperance, J., Bourassa, M. G., and Ashekian, P. B.: Myocardial Infarction without Obstructive Disease at Coronary Arteriography, *J.A.M.A.,* 99:837, 1968.

8 Sidd, J. J., Kemp, H. G., and Gorlin, R.: Acute Myocardial Infarction in a Nineteen-Year-Old Student in the Absence of Coronary Obstructive Disease, *N. Engl. J. Med.,* 282:1306, 1970.

9 Nizet, P. M., and Robertson, L.: Normal Coronary Arteriogram following Myocardial Infarction in a 17-Year-Old Boy, *Am. J. Cardiol.,* 28:715, 1971.

10 Glancy, D. L., Marcus, M. L., and Epstein, S. E.: Myocardial Infarction in Young Women with Normal Coronary Arteriograms, *Circulation,* 44:495, 1971.

11 Dear, D., Ruysell, H. O., Jones. W. B., and Reeves, J.: Myocardial Infarction in the Absence of Coronary Occlusion, *Am. J. Cardiol.,* 28:718, 1971.

12 Bruschke, A. V. G., Bryneel, K. J. J., Bloch, A., and van Herpen, G.: Acute Myocardial Infarction without Obstructive Coronary Artery Disease Demonstrated by Selective Cinearteriography, *Br. Heart J.,* 33:585, 1971.

13 Potts, K. H., Stein, P. D., and Houk, P. C.: Transmural Myocardial Infarction with Arteriographically Normal Appearing Coronary Arteries, *Chest,* 62:549, 1972.

14 Kimbiris, D., Segal, B. L., Munir, M., Katz, M., and Likoff, W.: Myocardial Infarction in Patients with Normal Patent Coronary Arteries as Visualized by Cinearteriography, *Am. J. Cardiol.,* 29:724, 1972.

15 Cheng, T. O., Bashour, T., Singh, B. K., and Kelser, G. A.: Myocardial Infarction in the Absence of Coronary Arteriosclerosis, *Am. J. Cardiol.,* 30:680, 1972.

16 Henderson, R. R., Hansing, C. E., Razavi, M., and Rowe, G. G.: Resolution of an Obstructive Coronary Lesion as Demonstrated by Selective Angiography in a Patient with Transmural Myocardial Infarction, *Am. J. Cardiol.,* 31:785, 1973.

17 Barcala, R. P.: Acute Myocardial Infarction in the Presence of Patent Coronary Arteries, *J. Thorac. Cardiovasc. Surg.,* 65:786, 1973.

18 DePasquale, N. P., and Bruno, M. S.: Normal Coronary Arteriogram in a Patient with Clinical Evidence of Myocardial Infarction, *Chest,* 63:618, 1973.

19 Schatz, I. J., Mizukami, H., Gallagher, J., and Greenslit, F. S.: Myocardial Infarction in a 14-Year-Old Boy with Normal Coronary Arteriograms, *Chest* 63:963, 1973.

20 Brest, A. N., Wiener, L., Kasparian, H., Duca, P., and Rafter, J. J.: Myocardial Infarction without Obstructive Coronary Artery Disease, *Am. Heart J.*, 88:219, 1974.

21 Eliot, R. S., Baroldi, G., and Leone, A.: Necropsy Studies in Myocardial Infarction with Minimal or No Coronary Luminal Reduction Due to Atherosclerosis, *Circulation*, 49:1127, 1974.

22 Khan, A. H., and Haywood, L. J.: Myocardial Infarction in Nine Patients with Radiologically Patent Coronary Arteries, *N. Engl. J. Med.*, 291:427, 1974.

23 Sasse, L., Wagner, R., and Murray, F. E.: Transmural Myocardial Infarction during Pregnancy, *Am. J. Cardiol.*, 35:448, 1975.

24 Ciraulo, D. A.: Recurrent Myocardial Infarction and Angina in a Woman with Normal Coronary Angiograms, *Am. J. Cardiol.*, 35:923, 1975.

25 Regan, T. J., Wu, C. F., Weisse, A. B., Moschos, C. B., Ahmed, S. S., and Lyons, M. M.: Acute Myocardial Infarction in Toxic Cardiomyopathy without Coronary Obstruction, *Circulation*, 51:453, 1975.

26 Eslami, B., Russell, R. O., Bailey, M. T., Oberman, A., Tieszen, R. L., and Rackley, C. E.: Acute Myocardial Infarction in the Absence of Coronary Arterial Obstruction, *Ala. J. Med. Sci.*, 12:322, 1975.

27 Engel, H. J., Page, H. L., and Campbell, W. B.: Coronary Artery Spasm as the Cause of Myocardial Infarction during Coronary Arteriography, *Am. Heart J.*, 91:501, 1976.

28 Chesler, E., Matisonn, R. E., Lakier, J. B., Popcock, W. A., Obel, I. W. P., and Barlow, J. B.: Acute Myocardial Infarction with Normal Coronary Arteries, *Circulation*, 54:203, 1976.

29 Oren, A., Bar-Shlomo, B., and Stern, S.: Acute Coronary Occlusion following Blunt Injury to the Chest in the Absence of Coronary Atherosclerosis, *Am. Heart J.*, 92:501, 1976.

30 Rosenblatt, A., and Selzer, A.: The Nature and Clinical Features of Myocardial Infarction with Normal Coronary Arteriogram, *Circulation*, 55:578, 1977.

31 Engel, H., Hundeshagen, H., and Lichtlen, P.: Transmural Myocardial Infarction in Young Women Taking Oral Contraceptives, *Br. Heart J.*, 39:477, 1977.

32 Thompson, S. I., Vieweg, W. V. R., Alpert, J. S., and Hagan, A. D.: Incidence and Age Distribution of Patients with Myocardial Infarction and Normal Coronary Arteriograms, *Cath. Cardiovasc. Diag.*, 3:1, 1977.

33 Proskey, A. J., Saksena, F., and Towne, W. D.: Myocardial Infarction Associated with Thyrotoxicosis, *Chest*, 72:109, 1977.

34 Nemickas, R., Fishman, D., Killip T., Dalton, W.,

Brynjolfsson, G., Robinson, J., and Gunnar, R. M.: Massive Myocardial Necrosis in a Young Woman, *Am. Heart J.*, 95:766, 1978.

35 Chesler, E., Mitha, A. S., Weir, E. K., Matisonn, R. E., and Hitchcock, P. J.: Myocardial Infarction in the Black Population of South Africa: Coronary Arteriographic Findings, *Am. Heart J.*, 95:691, 1978.

36 Raizner, A. E., Chahine, R. A., Ishimori, T., Luchi, R. J. and Gaston, W. R.: Unpublished data.

37 Bemiller, C. R., Pepine, C. J., and Rogers, A. K.: Long-term Observations in Patients with Angina and Normal Coronary Arteriograms, *Circulation*, 47:36, 1973.

38 Arnett, E. N., and Roberts, W. C.: Acute Myocardial infarction and Angiographically Normal Coronary Arteries. An Unproven Combination, *Circulation*, 53:395, 1976.

39 Willerson, J. T., Parkey, R. W., Bonte, F. J., Meyer, S. L., Atkins, J. M., and Stokely, E. M.: Technetium Stannous Pyrophosphate Myocardial Scintigrams in Patients with Chest Pain of Varying Etiology, *Circulation*, 51:1046, 1975.

40 Hillis, W. S., Faulkner, S. L., Fisher, R. D., Dean, R. M., Friesenger, G. C., and Bender, H. W.: Significance of Severity of Coronary Arterial Stenosis: Metabolic Studies and Correlation with Hyperemic Response, *J. Surg. Res.*, 18:125, 1975.

41 James, T. N.: Angina without Coronary Disease, *Circulation*, 42:189, 1970.

42 Vlodaver, Z., Frech, R., Van Tassel, R. A., and Edwards, J. E.: Correlation of the Antemortem Coronary Arteriogram and the Post-mortem Specimen, *Circulation*, 47:162, 1973.

43 Welch, C. C., Proudfit, W. L., and Sheldon, W. C.: Coronary Arteriographic Findings in 1000 Women under Age 50, *Am. J. Cardiol.*, 35:211, 1975.

44 Mann, J. I., and Inman, W. H. W.: Oral Contraceptives and Death from Myocardial Infarction, *Br. Med. J.*, 2:245, 1975.

45 Arthes, F. G., and Masi, A. T.: Myocardial Infarction in Younger Women. Associated Clinical Features and Relationship to Use of Oral Contraceptive Drugs, *Chest*, 70:574, 1976.

46 Ory, H. W.: Association between Oral Contraceptives and Myocardial Infarction. A Review, *J.A.M.A.*, 237:2619, 1977.

47 Soloman, H. A., Edwards, A. L., and Killip, T.: Prodromata in Acute Myocardial Infarction, *Circulation*, 40:463, 1969.

48 Eliot, R. S., and Bratt, G.: The Paradox of Myocardial Ischemia and Necrosis in Young Women with Normal Coronary Arteriograms. Relation to Abnormal Hemoglobin-Oxygen Dissociation, *Am. J. Cardiol.*, 23:633, 1969.

49 Russell, R. O., Jr., Eslami, B., and Rackley, C. E.:

Acute Myocardial Infarction without Coronary Arteriographic Abnormalities, *Chest,* 72:133, 1977.

50 Latham, P. M.: "Collected Works," Vol. 1, New Sydenham Society, London, 1876, p. 445.

51 Oliva, P. B., Potts, D. E., and Pluss, R. G.: Coronary Arterial Spasm in Prinzmetal Angina: Documentation by Coronary Arteriography, *N. Engl. J. Med.,* 288:745, 1973.

52 Maseri, A., Mimmo, R., Chierchia, S., Marchesi, C., Pesola, A., and L'Abbati, A.: Coronary Artery Spasm as a Cause of Acute Myocardial Ischemia in Man, *Chest,* 68:625, 1975.

53 Chahine, R. A., and Luchi, R. J.: Coronary Arterial Spasm: Culprit or Bystander?, *Am. J. Cardiol.,* 37:936, 1976.

54 Yasue, H., Tonyama, M., Shimamoto, M., Kato, H., Tanaka, S, and Akiyama, F.: Role of Autonomic Nervous System in the Pathogenesis of Prinzmetal's Variant Form of Angina, *Circulation,* 50:535, 1974.

55 Endo, M., Hirosawa, K., Kaneko, N., Hase, K., Inoue, Y., and Konno, S.: Prinzmetal's Variant Angina. Coronary Arteriogram and Left Ventriculogram during Angina Attack Induced by Methacholine, *N. Engl. J. Med.,* 294:252, 1976.

56 Yasue, H., Touyama, M., Kato, H., Tanaka, S., and Akiyama, F.: Prinzmetal's Variant Form of Angina as a Manifestation of Alpha-Adrenergic Receptormediated Coronary Artery Spasm: Documentation by Coronary Arteriography, *Am. Heart J.,* 91:148, 1976.

57 King, M. J., Zir, L. M., Kaltman, A. J., and Fox, A. C.: Variant Angina Associated with Angiographically Demonstrated Coronary Artery Spasm and REM Sleep, *Am. J. Med. Sci.,* 265:419, 1973.

58 Raizner, A. E., Ishimori, T., Chahine, R. A., and Jamal, N.: Provocation of Coronary Spasm by Cold Pressor, *Am. J. Cardiol.,* 41, 358, 1978.

59 Mudge, G. H., Grossman, W., Mills, R. M., Lesch, M., and Braunwald, E.: Reflex Increase in Coronary Vascular Resistance in Patients with Ischemic Heart Disease, *N. Engl. J. Med.,* 295:1333, 1976.

60 Chahine, R. A., Raizner, A. E., Ishimori, T., Luchi, R. J., and McIntosh, H. D.: The Incidence and Clinical Implications of Coronary Artery Spasm, *Circulation,* 52:972, 1975.

61 Wiener, L., Kasparian, H., Duca, P. R., Walinsky, P., Gottlieb, R. S., Hanckel, F., and Brest, A. N.: Spectrum of Coronary Arterial Spasm. Clinical, Angiographic and Myocardial Metabolic Experience in 29 Cases, *Am. J. Cardiol.,* 38:945, 1976.

62 Maseri, A., Parodi, D., Severi, S., and Pesola, A.: Transient Transmural Reduction of Myocardial Blood Flow, Demonstrated by Thallium-201 Scintigraphy, as a Cause of Variant Angina, *Circulation,* 54:280, 1976.

63 Chahine, R. A., Raizner, A. E.: Another Look at Prinzmetal's Variant Angina, *Eur. J. Cardiol.,* 6:71, 1977.

64 MacAlpin, R. M., Kattus, A. A., and Alvaro, A. B.: Angina Pectoris at Rest with Preservation of Exercise Capacity: Prinzmetal's Variant Angina, *Circulation,* 47:946, 1973.

65 Cheng, T. O., Bashour, T., Kelser, G. A., Weiss, L., and Bacos, J.: Variant Angina of Prinzmetal with Normal Coronary Arteriogram: A Variant of the Variant, *Circulation,* 47:476, 1973.

66 Heupler, F. A.: Current Concepts of Prinzmetal's Variant Form of Angina Pectoris, *Cleve. Clin. Q.,* 43:131, 1976.

67 Higgins, C. B., Wexler, L., Silverman, J. F., and Schroeder, J. S.: Clinical and Arteriographic Features of Prinzmetal's Variant Angina: Documentation of Etiologic Factors, *Am. J. Cardiol.,* 37:831, 1976.

68 Maseri, A., Pesola, A., Marzilli, M., Severi, S., Parodi, O., L'Abbati, A., Ballestva, A. M., Maltinti, G., DeNes, D. M., and Biagini, A.: Coronary Vasospasm in Angina Pectoris, *Lancet,* 1:713, 1977.

69 Chahine, R. A.: Prinzmetal's Variant Angina. A Syndrome Apart or Another Presentation of Atheromatous Heart Disease, *Arch. Intern. Med.,* in press.

70 Chahine, R. A., Raizner, A. E., and Luchi, R. J.: Coronary Arterial Spasm in Classic Angina Pectoris, *Cath. Cardiovasc. Diag.,* 1:337, 1975.

71 Levene, D. L., and Freeman, M. R.: Alpha-Adrenoreceptor-mediated Coronary Artery Spasm, *J.A.M.A.,* 236:1018, 1976.

72 Sewell, W. H.: Coronary Spasm as a Primary Cause of Myocardial Infarction, *Angiology,* 17:1, 1966.

73 Hellstrom, H. R.: The Advantages of a Vasospastic Cause of Myocardial Infarction, *Am. Heart J.,* 90:545, 1975.

74 Gensini, G. G.: Coronary Artery Spasm and Angina Pectoris, *Chest,* 68:709, 1975.

75 Oliva, P. B., and Breckinridge, J. C.: Arteriographic Evidence of Coronary Arterial Spasm in Acute Myocardial Infarction, *Circulation,* 56:366, 1977.

76 Oliva, P. B., and Breckinridge, J. C.: Acute Myocardial Infarction with Normal and Near Normal Coronary Arteries. Documentation with Coronary Arteriography within 12½ Hours of the Onset of Symptoms in Two Cases, *Am. J. Cardiol.,* 40:1000, 1977.

77 Johnson, A. D., and Detwiler, J. H.: Coronary Spasm, Variant Angina, and Recurrent Myocardial Infarctions, *Circulation,* 55:947, 1977.

78 Lange, R. L., Reid, M. S., Tresch, D. D., Keelan, M. H., Bernhard, V. M., and Coolidge, G.: Nonatheromatous Ischemic Heart Disease following Withdrawal from Chronic Industrial Nitroglycerin Exposure, *Circulation,* 46:666, 1972.

79 Johnson, A. D., Stroud, H. A., Vieweg, W. V. R., and Ross, J.: Variant Angina Pectoris. Clinical Presentations, Coronary Angiograhic Patterns and the Results of

Medical and Surgical Management in 42 Consecutive Patients, *Chest,* 73:786, 1978.

80 Shroeder, J. S., Bolen, J. L., Quint, R. A., Clark, D. A., Hayden, W. G., Higgins, C. B., and Wexler, L.: Provocation of Coronary Spasm with Ergonovine Maleate, *Am. J. Cardiol.,* 40:487, 1977.

81 Virchow, R.: Ueber Capillare Embolic, *Virchows Arch.* [Pathole Anat.], 9:307, 1856.

82 Wenger, N. K., and Bauer, S.: Coronary Embolism. Review of the Literature and Presentation of Fifteen Cases, *Am. J. Med.,* 25:549, 1958.

83 Prizel, K. R., Hutchins, G. M., and Bulkley, B. H.: Coronary Artery Embolism and Myocardial Infarction. A Clinicopathologic Study of 55 Patients, *Ann. Intern. Med.,* 88:155, 1978.

84 Roberts, W. C.: Relationship between Coronary Thrombosis and Myocardial Infarction, *Mod. Concepts Cardiovasc. Dis.,* 41:7, 1972.

85 Weisse, A. B., Lehan, P. H., Ettinger, P. O., Moschos, C. B., and Regan, T. J.: The Fate of Experimentally Induced Coronary Artery Thrombosis, *Am. J. Cardiol.,* 23:229, 1969.

86 Mitchell, J. R. A., and Phil, D.: The Pathogenesis of Thrombosis, in "Plenary Session Papers," XII Congress, International Society of Hematology, New York, 1968, p. 321.

87 Folts, J. D., Crowell, E. B., and Rowe, G. G.: Platelet Aggregation in Partially Obstructed Vessels and Its Elimination with Aspirin, *Circulation,* 54:365, 1976.

88 Steele, P. P., Weily, H. S., Davies, H., and Genton, E.: Platelet Function Studies in Coronary Artery Disease, *Circulation,* 48:1194, 1973.

89 Levin, P. H.: An Acute Effect of Cigarette Smoking on Platelet Function, *Circulation,* 38:619, 1973.

90 Dugdale, M., and Masi, A. T.: Effects of Oral Contraceptives on Blood Clotting, in "Second Report on Oral Contraceptives," Advisory Committee on Obstetrics and Gynecology, Food and Drug Administration, Washington, D.C., 1969, p. 43.

91 Kumpuris, D., Luchi, R. J., Waddell, C., and Miller, R. R.: Production of Circulatory Platelet Aggregates by Exercise in Coronary Patients, unpublished data.

92 Bloor, C. M., and Lowman, R. M.: Myocardial Bridges in Coronary Angiography, *Am. Heart J.,* 65:195, 1963.

93 Edwards, J. C., Burnsides, C., Swarm, R. L., and Lansing, A. I.: Arteriosclerosis in the Intramural and Extramural positions of Coronary Arteries in the Human Heart, *Circulation,* 13:235, 1956.

94 Polacek, P., and Kralove, H.: Relation of Myocardial Bridges and Loops on the Coronary Arteries to Coronary Occlusions, *Am. Heart J.,* 61:44, 1961.

95 Ishimori, T., Raizner, A. E., Chahine, R. A., Awdeah, M., and Luchi, R. J.: Myocardial Bridges in Man: Clinical Correlation and Angiographic Accentuation with Nitroglycerin, *Cath. Cardiovasc. Diag.,* 3:59, 1977.

96 Gregg, D. E., Khouri, E. M., and Rayfor, C. R.: Systemic and Coronary Energetics in the Resting Unanesthetized Dog, *Circ. Res.,* 16:102, 1965.

97 Noble, J., Bourassa, M. G., Petitclerc, R., and Dyrda, I.: Myocardial Bridging and Milking Effect of the Left Anterior Descending Coronary Artery: Normal Variant or Obstruction?, *Am. J. Cardiol.,* 37:993, 1976.

98 Ishimori, T., Raizner, A. E., Spencer, W., Verani, M. Costin, J., Chahine, R. A., Miller, R. R.: Unpublished data.

99 Endo, M., Lee, Y. W., Hayashi, H., and Wada, J.: Angiographic Evidence of Myocardial Squeeze Accompanying Tachyarrhythmia as a Possible Cause of Myocardial Infarction, *Chest,* 73:3, 1978.

100 Farugui, A. M. A., Maloy, W. C., Felner, J. M., Schlant, R. C., Logan, W. D., and Symbos, P.: Symptomatic Myocardial Bridging of a Coronary Artery, *Am. J. Cardiol.,* 41:1305, 1978.

101 James, T. N.: Pathology of Small Coronary Arteries, *Am. J. Cardiol.,* 20:679, 1967.

102 Wenger, N. K.: Rare Causes of Coronary Artery Disease, in J. W. Hurst (ed.), "The Heart," McGraw-Hill Book Company, New York, 1978, p. 1345.

103 Blumenthal, H. T., Alex, M., and Goldenberg, S.: Study of Lesions of the Intramural Coronary Artery Branches in Diabetes Mellitus, *Arch. Pathol.,* 70:13, 1960.

104 Siperstein, M. D., Cowell, A. R., Sr., and Meyer, K.: "Small Blood Vessel Involvement in Diabetes Mellitus," American Institute of Biological Sciences, Washington, D.C., 1964.

105 Ledet, T.: Histological and Histochemical Changes in the Coronary Arteries of Old Diabetic Patients, *Diabetologia,* 4:268, 1968.

106 Holsinger, D. R., Osmundson, P. J., and Edwards, J. E.: The Heart in Periarteritis Nodosa, *Circulation,* 25:610, 1962.

107 Benisch, B. M., and Pervez, N.: Coronary Artery Vasculitis and Myocardial Infarction with Systemic Lupus Erythematosus, *N. Y. State J. Med.,* 74:873, 1974.

108 James, T. N., Rupe, C. E., and Monto, R. W.: Pathology of the Cardiac Conduction System in Systemic Lupus Erythematosus, *Ann. Intern. Med.,* 63:402, 1965.

109 Cruickshank, B.: The Arteritis of Rheumatoid Arthritis, *Ann. Rheumat. Dis.,* 12:136, 1953.

110 Bor, I.: Myocardial Infarction and Ischemic Heart Disease in Infants and Children: Analysis of 29 Cases and Review of the Literature, *Arch. Dis. Child.,* 44:268, 1969.

111 Barth, R. F., Willerson, J. T., Buja, L. M., Decker, J. L., and Roberts, W. C.: Amylord Coronary Artery

Disease, Primary Systemic Amyloidosis and Paraproteinemia, *Arch. Intern. Med.,* 126:627, 1970.

112 James, T. N.: An Etiologic Concept Concerning the Obscure Myocardiopathics, *Prog. Cardiovasc. Dis.,* 7:43, 1964.

113 Amorosi, E., and Ultmann, J. E.: Thrombotic Thrombocytopenic Purpura: Report of 16 Cases and Review of the Literature, *Medicine,* 45:139, 1966.

114 Bulkley, B. H., Klacsmann, P. G., and Hutchins, G. M.: Angina Pectoris, Myocardial Infarction and Sudden Cardiac Death with Normal Coronary Arteries: A Clinicopathologic Study of 9 Patients with Progressive Systemic Sclerosis, *Am. Heart J.,* 95:563, 1978.

115 Eliot, R. S., and Mizukami, H.: Oxygen Affinity of Hemoglobin in Persons with Acute Myocardial Infarction and in Smokers, *Circulation,* 34:331, 1966.

116 Vokonas, P. S., Cohn, P. F., Klein, M., Laver, M. B., and Gorlin, R.: Hemoglobin Affinity for Oxygen in the Anginal Syndrome with Normal Coronary Arteriogram, *J. Clin. Invest.,* 54:409, 1974.

117 Friedberg, C. K., and Horn, H.: Acute Myocardial Infarction Not Due to Coronary Artery Occlusion, *J.A.M.A.,* 112:1675, 1939.

118 Jones, F. L.: Transmural Myocardial Necrosis after Non-penetrating Cardiac Trauma, *Am. J. Cardiol.,* 26:419, 1970.

119 Jenkins, J. L., and Nishimura, A.: Coronary Artery Òbstruction and Myocardial Infarction Resulting from Non-penetrating Chest Trauma, *Texas Med.,* 71:78, 1975.

120 Bacon, Sir Francis: DePrincipiis atque Originibus, Works, V, p. 291.

Vasodilator Therapy of Congestive Heart Failure*

JAMES F. SPANN, M.D. and J. WILLIS HURST, M.D.

Cases in Which Digitalis Was Given by the Direction of the Author
1775
Case XVI
August 18th. Mrs. B——, Aet. 33.
Pulmonary consumption and dropsy. The Digitalis, and that failing, other diuretics were used, in hopes of gaining some relief from the distress occasioned by the dropsical symptoms, but none of them were effectual. He was then attended by another physician, and died in about two months.

WILLIAM WITHERING, 1785[1]

INTRODUCTION

Congestive heart failure is one of the common end results of many different types of heart disease. It has been estimated that more than 2 million people in the United States have chronic congestive heart failure and that this syndrome causes 30,000 to 60,000 hospitalizations annually at a cost of one-half billion dollars.[2] Older therapy, such as rest, sodium restriction, and digitalis, and newer agents, such as modern diuretics, are available and well established. However, the long-term survival, as well as the quality of life, remains rather limited for many patients, and better treatment has been needed. [2,15] Vasodilators have recently been proposed and studied extensively as important additional therapy in selected patients with heart failure. Vasodilator therapy of congestive heart failure is based on solid principles of altering the pathophysiology of this syndrome. Consequently, it is the opinion of the authors that this class of drugs will evolve to be relatively standard therapy in heart failure. At present, some of the vasodilator drugs require relatively complex regimens, and some have undesirable side effects. Better drugs are likely to become available. The goal of this discussion is to provide information which will allow the most effective selection and use of currently available drugs and to provide a solid background of pathophysiology upon which better drugs, when they appear in the future, can be understood and optimally applied. The pathophysiology underlying the symptoms of heart failure and how this pathophysiology is modified by

vasodilator treatment will be emphasized. The current vasodilator drugs and their pharmacology and clinical use will then be described in detail. Finally, practical treatment plans using currently available agents will be outlined.

PATHOPHYSIOLOGY OF CONGESTIVE HEART FAILURE AND ITS MODIFICATIONS BY VASODILATORS

Cardiac dysfunction implies that the heart cannot perform its function. The clinical counterpart of this altered physiology may be nothing more than a ventricular gallop. Congestive heart failure is a complex of signs and symptoms which comprise a recognizable clinical syndrome of congestion of pulmonary and peripheral tissues with or without the effects of decreased cardiac output at rest. When the word "congestion" is used, it implies that body fluid has either been increased or redistributed. Congestion is caused either by direct damage to heart muscle or by chronic pressure or volume overload on the heart combined with the damage to heart muscle which such an overload may cause. In addition, the congestive and low output symptoms can be brought about by restriction of diastolic filling in mitral stenosis or constrictive pericarditis without extensive damage to the ventricular muscle. The current discussion is limited to patients who have direct myocardial damage and overload damage, since it is in these situations that vasodilators are generally used. The use of vasodilators in the therapy of shock resulting from acute myocardial infarction has been reviewed extensively and will not be discussed.[3,4] Overt, or end-stage, congestive heart failure is that situation in which a severe abnormality of cardiac function causes an inability of the heart to pump blood at the rate needed for the systemic circulation at rest. The multiple factors that lead to salt and water retention act in concert to produce this condition. Compensated congestive heart failure is common and may be described as a condition in which the heart and circulation utilize compensatory mechanisms (mechanisms which frequently result in the signs and symptoms that we recognize as the

* From the Temple University Health Sciences Center, Philadelphia (Dr. Spann) and the Department of Medicine, Emory University School of Medicine, Atlanta (Dr. Hurst).

167

congestive syndrome) to prevent a fall in cardiac output below systemic requirements at rest and to optimally distribute the limited cardiac output during exercise. Much of our therapy of heart failure, including the vasodilators, involves the selective manipulation of some of these compensatory mechanisms. An in-depth understanding of these mechanisms is necessary to have a rational framework for the therapy of heart failure with vasodilators as well as with other drugs. These compensatory mechanisms and associated symptoms will be discussed next, and the effects of the vasodilators will then be described in the context of the pathophysiology.

The basic lesion in this common form of heart failure is a depression of myocardial contractility with or without a continuing overload on the heart.[5-8] The myocardial lesion can result from direct damage, as in cardiomyopathy or coronary heart disease,[9] or can be related to a chronic overload on the heart, such as in valve disease[8] or systemic hypertension.[10,11] The compensatory mechanisms can maintain a relatively normal resting cardiac output even when there is extensive depression of myocardial contractility.[6,8] Therefore, it is not until relatively late in the usual clinical course of congestive failure that the patient's symptoms are caused by a reduced cardiac output at rest. Before the resting cardiac output becomes reduced, the disturbing congestive symptoms of heart failure are unfortunate side effects of the compensatory mechanisms which are striving to maintain the cardiac output. The undesirable secondary effects produced by the compensatory mechanisms them-

selves limit the extent to which they can be utilized.

The Frank-Starling mechanism is vital for the maintenance of cardiac output but is also responsible for many of the congestive symptoms of heart failure.[12] Figure 1 shows this relationship. When the heart muscle is damaged, the systolic muscle function falls from the upper solid curve, at point A, to the lower solid curve, at point B. However, at point B the systolic cardiac output would be too low to support systemic needs, and low output symptoms such as fatigue, weakness, poor renal function, and even confusion and stupor would ensue. This would be incompatible with life. Fortunately, cardiac residual volume increases as a result of the low ejection fraction, venous constriction occurs, and salt and water are retained. All of these events cause an increase in left ventricular volume from point A' to point C' along the dashed curve. At the new ventricular diastolic volume C', a greater systolic cardiac output C occurs as a result of the Frank-Starling principle whereby diastolic cardiac dilatation causes increased force of the subsequent systolic contraction. Now the vital cardiac output has been maintained, at least at rest. As is usual, however, nothing is free, and a price has been paid. The price is dyspnea and other congestive symptoms. As the heart increases its diastolic volume from A' to C', it has moved to the right along the dashed line relating passive ventricular diastolic distension to left ventricular end-diastolic pressure (LVEDP) and LVEDP becomes elevated. The symptoms of pulmonary congestion with dyspnea, orthopnea, and even pulmonary edema are thus the unfortunate side effects

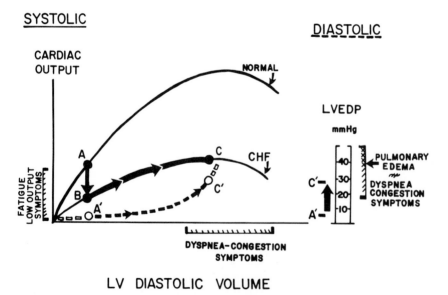

FIGURE 1 Compensated heart failure: Frank-Starling compensation for heart failure and how it causes congestive symptoms. (See text for explanation.) LV, left ventricle. LVEDP, left ventricular end-diastolic pressure.

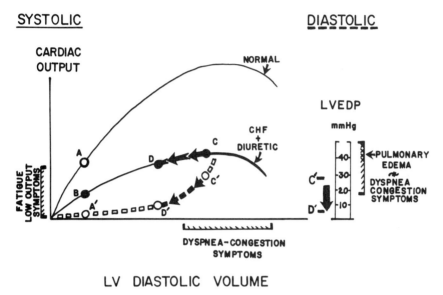

FIGURE 2 Heart failure and diuretic: Effect of diuretics on the Frank-Starling compensation, the cardiac output, and the congestive symptoms of heart failure. (See text for explanation.)

of the Frank-Starling compensation which is maintaining cardiac output. The use of diuretics, salt restriction, digitalis, and rest in the treatment of heart failure can be examined in the above context. As shown in Fig. 2, when diuretics are given and salt and water are excreted, the ventricular end-diastolic volume decreases from C' to D' along the dashed diastolic curve. Simultaneously, because of the Frank-Starling relationship, the systolic cardiac output is reduced from C to D on the solid curve of congestive heart failure (CHF). However, since the movement from C to D on the solid curve of systole is in a relatively flat area of the curve, there is only modest reduction of cardiac output. Conversely, since the same lateral movement from C' to D' on the dashed curve of diastole is on a relatively steep portion of the curve, there is an appreciable reduction in the elevated LVEDP. The patient's congestive symptoms are relieved by the careful removal of a portion of the Frank-Starling compensation but without severe reduction of cardiac output. Salt restriction has a similar effect. Accordingly, diuretics and salt restriction decrease ventricular preload. Conversely, as shown in Fig. 3, when digitalis is given there is an increase in myocardial contractility. The solid lower systolic curve of CHF is increased to the intermediate solid curve of increased contractility with CHF at point F. On this improved curve, the required cardiac output can be achieved at point G. As the ejection fraction increases, cardiac size decreases and the stimulus to retain salt and water decreases. The ventricle then has moved from C' to G' on the dashed diastolic pressure

curve with a resultant low LVEDP, and there is relief of congestive symptoms with maintenance of cardiac output.

As cardiac function continues to deteriorate, a point is reached where low cardiac output and congestive symptoms coexist despite maximum use of the natural compensatory mechanisms, optimum diuresis, and maximum digitalis dosage. Such a situation is shown in Fig. 4. In this severe stage of heart failure, it is clear that additional reduction of preload by more diuretics would only move the patient to a more unfavorable position on the ventricular function curve with even more severe depression of cardiac output.[13,14] Similarly, the toxic arrhythmogenic effects of digitalis prevent the achievement of any further increase in contractility by this drug. Something else is needed.

The next area of compensation to be discussed is the alterations in the peripheral venous and arterial circulation and sympathetic nervous system in heart failure. In congestive heart failure there is an increase in total sympathetic discharge as reflected by an increased urinary excretion of norepinephrine at rest[15] and an abnormal augmentation of the norepinephrine blood level with exercise.[16] The failing heart has improved support of contractility and an increase in heart rate by the increased circulating catecholamines despite a reduction of intrinsic cardiac norepinephrine[15,17] and impairment of direct cardiac sympathetic nerve function.[18] The patient with heart failure has increased venous pressure and venous tone at rest which is due to increased blood volume, venous tone, and tissue pressure.[19,20]

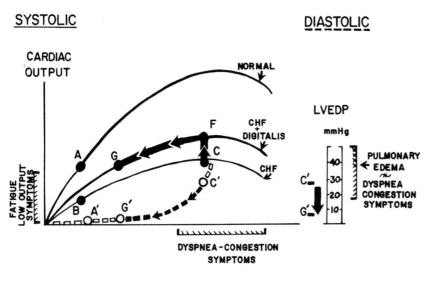

FIGURE 3 Heart failure and digitalis: Effect of digitalis on the Frank-Starling compensation, the cardiac output, and the congestive symptoms of heart failure. (See text for explanation.)

With exercise the venous pressure and tone are further exaggerated by a sympathetically mediate constriction of the veins.[21] This aids the return of blood to the heart when heart failure is present. This increased venous return provides part of the increased preload which is used by the Frank-Starling compensation, but it heightens the congestive symptoms such as dyspnea and edema. The systemic arterial system is also abnormal, with increased resistance and altered flow distribution in heart failure.[22] Two major factors appear to cause the increased peripheral resistance of heart failure. First, there is increased sympathetic tone and circulating catecholamines to the peripheral resistance vessels.[23,24] Second, there is increased local stiffness of resistance vessels that is thought to be caused by increased arterial sodium content and in-

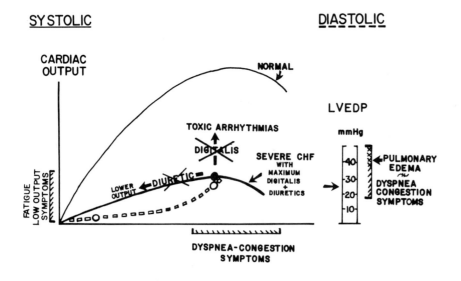

FIGURE 4 End-stage heart failure with maximum digitalis and diuretics: Inability to use more digitalis because of toxic arrhythmias. Inability to use more diuretics because that would further lower the reduced cardiac output. (See text for explanation.)

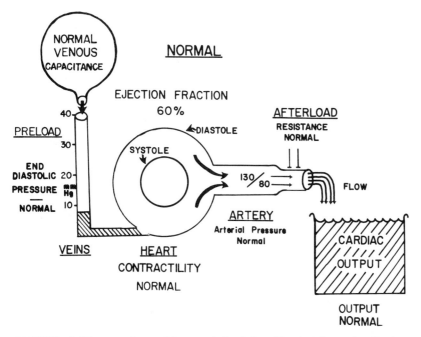

FIGURE 5 Diagram of normal heart and circulation. (See text for explanation.)

creased tissue pressure.[22,25] Furthermore, in heart failure there is a major abnormal response of the resistance vessels to exercise, resulting in intense visceral vasoconstriction and less than normal dilatation of the arterial vessels to muscles.[26,27] In severe failure this redistribution is present even at rest.[26] The ability of the heart to increase cardiac output with exercise and, in late stages, even to maintain output at rest is reduced in congestive failure. The changes in arterial resistance that occur in heart failure will maintain central blood pressure and redistribute the limited blood flow in order to perfuse such vital areas as the brain and heart, reduce the flow to relatively nonessential areas such as the skin, renal system and viscera; and provide an intermediate level of flow to the exercising muscles. Again, the compensation is essential to life but causes adverse symptoms and signs as well. The decreased skin flow is accompanied by an increase of anteriovenous oxygen extraction and produces the cool, bluish extremities and, in advanced situations, impairs the ability of the body to rid itself of heat. The decreased arterial vasodilatation to exercising muscle, while preventing hypotension, also causes fatigue and muscle weakness, which are prominent symptoms in advanced heart failure. The chronic disease in general arteriolar tone represents an increased afterload on the heart which may result in a vicious circle; thus the increased afterload may further decrease the already diminished ejection fraction of the compromised heart.[28] It is against this background of excessively utilized mechanisms of compensation, related to both

preload and afterload and the associated symptoms, that vasodilator therapy should be considered.

Vasodilator therapy of heart failure consists of the selective and controlled reduction of afterload and/or preload by drugs. Certain drugs have a principal effect on the resistance vessels of the systemic arterial system and thereby change afterload. Other drugs affect the venous capacitance vessels and thereby change preload. Some drugs affect both arteries and veins. The Frank-Starling diagrams in Figs. 1 through 4 show the effect of changes in diastolic ventricular volume (preload) on the systolic cardiac output and on the diastolic ventricular pressure. The effects of afterload are not shown in these illustrations. Since vasodilator therapy may involve changes in afterload as well as preload, different types of diagrams are useful. Such diagrams are shown in Figs. 5, 6, and 7. These diagrams depict cardiac output and three of the major factors which determine output: preload, contractility, and afterload. The fourth major variable, heart rate, is not shown and is not of major importance to this discussion. In Fig. 5, which shows the normal circulation, one can see that preload is normal because venous capacitance and diastolic ventricular size are normal. Consequently, ventricular end-diastolic pressure is normal, and there are no congestive symptoms. Cardiac contractility is normal. Therefore, from a normal end-diastolic volume (the outer concentric circle) the heart subsequently contracts to a normal end-systolic volume (the inner concentric circle). The ejection fraction, which is the ratio of end-systolic volume to

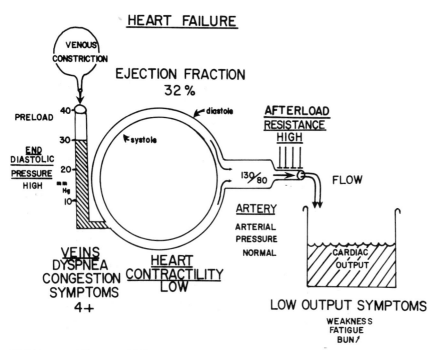

FIGURE 6 Diagram of failing heart and circulation. (See text for explanation.)

end-diastolic volume, is normal at 0.60. The stroke volume, which is the volume of the shell of blood extruded when the outer diastolic circle constricts to the inner systolic circle, is normal. This stroke volume moves, as shown by the arrows, as blood flows into the arteries. The systemic resistance is normal, as is blood pressure, since it is the product of flow times resistance. Cardiac output is normal, and there are no low output symptoms.

Severe overt heart failure is shown in Fig. 6. Cardiac contractility is low.[5-7] Therefore, less systolic contraction occurs from any diastolic volume, and the ejection fraction is low.[29] There is venous constriction to help increase venous return to dilate the heart and allow utilization of Frank-Starling compensation (see Fig. 1).[20,21] The venous constriction, salt and water retention, and increased cardiac residual volume left at the end of systole act in concert to increase the venous pressure and cause congestive symptoms as the increased preload tries to maintain cardiac output.[12] In advanced heart failure, the compensation is inadequate, the stroke volume continues to be low, and less blood flows into the arteries. With a low flow the only way that the vital blood pressure can be maintained is to increase resistance.[22,24] Such an increased peripheral arterial resistance in heart failure is shown in Fig. 6 and represents a high afterload. Cardiac output remains low with resultant low output symptoms.

The effects of both arterial and venous vasodilators on severe heart failure are diagramed in Fig. 7. The arterial vasodilators will be considered first. As a drug

causes a reduction in peripheral arterial resistance, peripheral flow increases.[30,31] If stroke volume did not increase, there would be depletion of central arterial volume, and central blood pressure would fall, with the disastrous consequence of syncope and shock. Fortunately, as resistance falls, the afterload on the heart is reduced. Even though contractility is not improved and remains low, the stroke volume and ejection fraction are increased, since it is easier for the heart to eject blood against a decreased afterload.[28,32,33] Since blood pressure is the product of resistance times flow, the central pressure falls little despite the decreased resistance, since the flow increases simultaneously.[31,34,35] Cardiac output is, of course, increased and low output symptoms are ameliorated. Congestive symptoms are also improved by the arterial vasodilators in the following manner. As the afterload falls and it becomes easier to eject blood from the heart, the end-systolic residual volume and consequently the end-diastolic volume both fall.[36] This effect can be seen by comparing the size of the concentric circles in Fig. 7 with those of Fig. 6. The fall in end-diastolic volume also lowers end-diastolic pressure (also see dashed line of Fig. 1) and relieves congestive symptoms.[31,35]

We now consider the direct venous dilator effects of certain drugs. Some of the drugs cause direct venous dilatation in conjunction with arterial vasodilator, and some drugs act principally as direct venous vasodilators.[34,37,38] Direct venous vasodilatation, either alone or combined with reduction of arterial resistance, causes a fall in peripheral venous pressure. The venous pooling effects, as shown in the left upper corner of Fig. 6, reduce venous return, which in turn reduces ventricular diastolic volume and resultant end-diastolic pressure.[34,37,38] Thus the venous pooling effects further reduce the congestive symptoms which have already been improved by the effects of the decreased afterload. When a drug has only a direct effect to reduced venous tone and thereby increase venous pooling, it only reduces preload.[39] The effect of such a preload reduction can be visualized in Fig. 2. Thus, as venous pooling occurs the diastolic ventricular volume falls from C' to D', with a large reduction in end-diastolic pressure and congestive symptoms. Cardiac output also falls from C to D as preload is reduced; this fall in output may be small or may not be perceived because of the flat curve relating output to ventricular volume in severe heart failure.[40]

Several important therapeutic concepts emerge from the above description of various effects of venous and arterial vasodilators on the pathophysiology of heart failure. It is clear that overuse of a venous vasodilator can cause low output symptoms or even shock in an improperly selected patient. For example, if cardiac output is very low and if end-diastolic pressure is not high, perhaps as a result of previous extensive use of diuretics, then the low output may become worse with venous vasodilatation.[13,14,40] It is therefore important to measure or reliably estimate the

ventricular filling pressure and cardiac output before such therapy. Generally the patient with both a high diastolic ventricular pressure and a low cardiac output is most benefited by vasodilator therapy.[40] Further, one can see that certain patients will require a mixture of venous and arterial vasodilatation.[41–43] A patient with advanced heart failure with weakness on exertion during the day and nocturnal dyspnea may be improved by arterial dilators which may increase the cardiac output during the day and by the addition of venous dilators at bedtime to further reduce preload and resultant nocturnal dyspnea. Full knowledge of the various drugs is necessary to select the best combinations of effects for a given patient.

Vasodilator therapy has additional beneficial effects on patients with mitral or aortic regurgitation.[44,45] Systolic regurgitation of blood across the mitral valve is enhanced by increases in afterload which oppose antegrade ejection from the left ventricle.[45] Therefore, a patient with severe heart failure and severe mitral regurgitation may especially benefit from vasodilator therapy, since the extent of regurgitation is reduced in addition to the usual beneficial effect of the vasodilator. Similarly, the extent of aortic regurgitation is reduced by reduction in the diastolic aortic pressure.[44] Double benefit is gained by vasodilator therapy in such a patient with both severe heart failure and severe aortic regurgitation.

Vasodilator therapy in a patient with heart failure

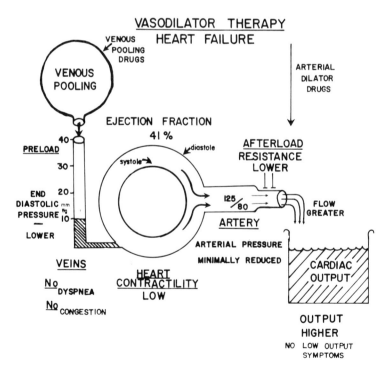

FIGURE 7 Diagram of effects of arterial dilation and venous pooling drugs on the failing heart and circulation. (See text for explanation.)

and ischemic coronary artery disease has unique advantages. Myocardial oxygen consumption is controlled by a number of factors, including heart rate, contractility, mean arterial pressure, left ventricular end-diastolic volume, pressure time per minute, tension-time index, and stress-time index.[46] The pressure time per minute has been shown to fall 16 percent and the stress-time index falls 38 percent following nitroprusside (Nipride) administration.[33,34] This reduction in the determinants of oxygen consumption with no fall in cardiac output nor any increase in heart rate define improvement of ventricular efficiency by this vasodilator. Such an effect is of special benefit to the patient with coronary artery disease and severe heart failure. Angina may be relieved and contractile function of ischemic ventricular muscle improved by an improvement in the relation between myocardial oxygen demand and supply.[3,47-49]

The effects of vasodilator therapy on the heart rate and blood pressure are of special interest. One would expect reflex tachycardia with even moderate decreases in mean arterial pressure. Furthermore, one would expect even greater tachycardia with the use of hydralazine (Apresoline), which has a sympathetically mediated direct effect to increase heart rate.[50] Surprisingly and fortunately, there is no significant change in heart rate when any of the current vasodilators are properly used to treat severe congestive heart failure.[31,35,38,40,41,51] The lack of an increase in heart rate as failure is treated by these vasodilators probably results from withdrawal of the excessive sympathetic discharge of advanced heart failure as the condition is improved.[52] Thus the withdrawal of the excessive sympathetic stimulation to the heart in failure decreases the heart rate and counterbalances any tendency of the therapy to increase heart rate. This is particularly important with hydralazine, where a potentially troublesome side effect is avoided.

SPECIFIC VASODILATOR DRUGS

There are three major categories of vasodilator drugs: those that act principally on the veins to increase venous pooling, those that act principally on the arteries to decrease systemic arterial resistance, and those that have a combined venous pooling and arterial dilatation effect. These drugs also vary in route of administration, onset of action, duration of action, and specific toxic side effects. Table 1 summarizes the action of the major drugs. Each of these drugs will now be described in detail; the venous pooling drugs will be discussed first, then the arterial dilators, and finally the drugs with both actions. It is very likely, however, that this list will soon have to be updated as new drugs are developed.

Venous Pooling Drugs (See Table 1)

The major effect of *nitroglycerin* is a direct relaxation of the smooth muscle in the systemic veins which increases the capacitance of this reservoir.[37,53] As blood pools in the veins, there is a resultant decrease in cardiac size.[54-56] Thus, there is a direct reduction of ventricular preload. Nitroglycerin is usually given sublingually, a route by which it is absorbed rapidly, having a peak hemodynamic effect in 5 min and a duration of action of 30 min. The average sublingual dose in treating chronic heart failure is 0.3 to 0.6 mg. In one very recent report, described below, much larger doses are used as emergency therapy of pulmonary edema. Nitroglycerin is also easily absorbed from the skin with a hemodynamic effect which reaches a peak in 1 h and has a duration of 5 h.[39,57] The average topical dose is 1½ in. of an ointment containing 12.5 mg/in. Taylor and coworkers observed a decrease of pulmonary capillary wedge pressure from an average of 30 to 19 mm Hg when 10 patients with severe chronic congestive heart failure were treated with 1.5 to 4 in. of topical nitroglycerin.[39] Pure nitroglycerin can be given intravenously as well, with a rapid onset and brief duration. Regardless of the route by which nitroglycerin is given to the patient with heart failure, its principal effect is a dramatic decrease in preload.

The effect of nitroglycerin on cardiac output is quite variable and appears to depend on the severity of the heart failure that is present. In general, the higher the initial wedge pressure and the lower the initial cardiac output, the more likely nitroglycerin is to achieve a moderate increase in cardiac output.[39] However, Massie et al. reported no change in an initial cardiac index of 2.1 liters/min (m²), while there was a fall in wedge pressure from 28 to 17 mm Hg with nitroglycerin therapy in an excellent study of 12 patients with refractory heart failure.[41] Accordingly, nitroglycerin can be thought of as a major preload reducing agent which changes points C and C¹ to points D and D¹ on the systolic and diastolic curves of the Frank-Starling relationship in the failing ventricle (see Fig. 2). This change is similar to that produced by diuretics and tourniquets.

Sublingual nitroglycerin has also been used for the treatment of acute pulmonary edema. Gold and coworkers observed a moderate fall of pulmonary wedge pressure in 3 patients treated with 0.3 mg of nitroglycerin administered sublingually.[51] A more recent report by Bussmann and Schupp discussed the use of 1.6 mg of nitroglycerin given sublingually as the sole therapy in 7 patients with severe acute pulmonary edema of diverse causes.[58] No digitalis, diuretics, morphine, or respiratory support were given. Pulmonary artery wedge pressure decreased from 30 to 21 mm Hg within 5 min, and cardiac output increased from 3.3 to 3.7 liters/min. Systemic arterial pressure

TABLE 1
Summary of the action of major vasodilator drugs

Predominant action in heart failure	Drug	Usual route of administration	Peak effect	Duration of action	Average dose	Major side effects and comments	Mechanism of action
Venous pooling	Nitroglycerin	Sublingual	5 min	30 min	0.4–2.4 mg	Occasional headache limited to first weeks of therapy with all nitrates	Direct effect to relax smooth muscle of veins
		Topical	60 min	5 h	1½ in.	Messy	Direct effect to relax smooth muscle of veins
	Isosorbide dinitrate (Isordil)	Sublingual Oral	20 min 60 min	1 h 5 h	10 mg 20 mg		Direct effect to relax smooth muscle of veins
Arterial dilation	Hydralazine (Apresoline)	Oral	60 min	6 h	50–75 mg	Fluid retention, LE-like syndrome, tolerance	Direct effect to relax smooth muscle of arteries
	Minoxidil	Oral	? in CHF	? in CHF	? in CHF	Minimal experience in heart failure, possible salt and water retention, hypertrichosis	Direct effect to relax smooth muscle of arteries
	Phenoxybenzamine (Dibenzyline)	Oral	1 h	3–4 days	10–30 mg	Orthostatic hypotension, sexual impotence, nasal congestion	Alpha-adrenergic blockade
	Phentolamine (Regitine)	I.V.	5 min	12–24 h	1–2 mg/min titrated		Alpha-adrenergic blockade
Mixed venous pooling and arterial dilation	Nitroprusside (Nipride)	I.V.	1 min	5 min	By titration of effect— 40–60 µg/min	Degraded by exposure to light; prolonged infusion produces toxic levels of cyanide	Direct relaxation of smooth muscle of arteries and veins
	Prazosin (Minipress)	Oral	60 min	6 h	2–7 mg	Occasional mild nausea	Blocks phosphodiesterase in vascular smooth muscle and also causes postsynaptic alpha-adrenergic receptor blockade, causing balanced dilation of arteries and veins

was essentially unchanged. A second group of 15 patients with pulmonary edema were given 0.8 to 2.4 mg of nitroglycerin sublingually and repeated at intervals of 5 to 10 min as the only treatment of acute pulmonary edema. Excellent clinical results were observed in 14 of the 15 patients.

Isosorbide dinitrate (Isordil) is the second venous pooling drug which is currently available. The major effect of isosorbide dinitrate, like that of nitroglycerin, is a direct relaxation of the systemic venous smooth muscle, resulting in venous pooling and reduction of ventricular preload. When given sublingually the peak effect occurs in 20 min and the duration of the effect is 1 to 1½ h.[42] The usual sublingual dose is 5 to 10 mg. In 8 patients with chronic congestive failure who received 5 mg of isosorbide dinitrate sublingually, there was a fall in pulmonary artery wedge pressure from 32 to 23 mm Hg in 20 min and a gradual return to 29 mm Hg at 75 min.[42] The relatively short duration of action of sublingual administration of this drug has led to trials of chewable[59] and oral[40,60] preparations. Despite early controversy about hepatic degradation,[61,62] it is now quite clear that the oral route is a proved method of achieving relatively long duration, hemodynamically effective nitrate medication.[40,58] The oral dose of isosorbide dinitrate is 20 mg; the peak effect occurs in 1 h, and a significant effect lasts for 5 h. Figure 8 shows data from the work of Williams et al. in 15 patients with chronic heart failure.[40] The pulmonary

artery wedge pressure fell from an average value of 23 to 14 mm Hg 1 h after swallowing 20 mg of isosorbide dinitrate and was still significantly reduced at a value of 20 mm Hg after 5 h. There was no significant change in the reduced cardiac index of 1.9 liters/min (m²). The excellent study of Kovick et al. shows that the chronic use of isosorbide dinitrate is useful in heart failure.[42] Their conclusions are based on the improvement of the clinical state and catheterization data after 3 to 21 months of sublingual isosorbide dinitrate therapy for preload reduction and arterial vasodilatation combined with oral phenoxybenzamine (Dibenzyline).[42] The pulmonary wedge pressure and cardiac index were 18 mm Hg and 2.9 liters/min (m²), respectively, after an average of 7 months of such therapy, as compared to pretreatment values of 31 mm Hg and 2.2 liters/min (m²). Tolerance to nitrates after long-term use has been questioned but did not seem to be a major problem in Kovick's work. Each patient showed a further reduction in pulmonary wedge pressure when sublingual isosorbide dinitrate was given as a single dose at the time of recatheterization after an average of 7 months of chronic isosorbide nitrate therapy. Side effects of chronic isosorbide dinitrate do not appear to be significant. Williams et al. observed no adverse reactions from nitrates over an average of 7 months.[40] The reduction of preload by any means in improperly selected patients who do not have initially excessive diastolic ventricular volume and pressure can lead to low cardiac output, hypotension, and syncope. A relatively minor side effect of limited duration is the occurrence of headaches in some patients when they first take chronic nitrates. If the patient can tolerate this discomfort for 1 to 2 weeks of continued therapy, the headaches generally resolve and do not give further trouble.

Arterial Dilator Drugs (See Table 1)

There are currently four major arterial dilator drugs: three may be given orally, and one is used intravenously (Table 1). *Hydralazine* (Apresoline), which has been used for a number of years to treat systemic hypertension, is a direct relaxant of the smooth muscle of the arterial wall and has little or no effect on the veins.[35,63,64] It is given orally and has a peak action in 1 h and a duration of 6 h. The usual dosage used in the treatment of congestive heart failure is 50 to 75 mg orally every 6 h, a dosage level that is often less than is needed in the treatment of systemic hypertension. Chatterjee and coworkers studied the acute and chronic effects of hydralazine as the only vasodilator drug in 10 patients with chronic heart failure.[31] They observed a sustained increase of cardiac index from a control of 2 liters/min (m²) to a value of 3 liters/min (m³) as systemic vascular resistance fell from 129 dynes·s·cm²

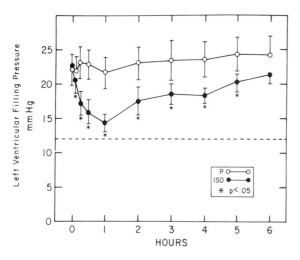

FIGURE 8 Effects of orally administered isosorbide dinitrate (ISO) (closed circles) compared with placebo (P) (open circles) on left ventricular filling pressure measured as pulmonary arterial wedge pressure. (*From D. O. Williams, W. J. Bommer, R. R. Miller, E. A. Amsterdam, and D. T. Mason, Hemodynamic Assessment of Oral Peripheral Vasodilator Therapy in Chronic Congestive Heart Failure: Prolonged Effectiveness of Isosorbide Dinitrate, Am. J. Cardiol., 39:84, 1977.*)

to 115. There was no significant change in pulmonary wedge pressure, systemic arterial pressure, or heart rate. The patients had severe, refractory (New York Heart Association class IV) heart failure prior to hydralazine therapy despite maximum use of diuretics and digitalis. Three to seven months following discharge on hydralazine therapy, 50 to 75 mg every 6 h with continued digitalis and diuretics, 6 of 9 patients were significantly improved to NYHA class II and 2 had returned to work. No patient developed postural hypotension or the lupus erythematosus (LE) syndrome. Similar results in more acute studies have been obtained by others.[35,41] Hydralazine thus acts to reduce afterload and to allow increased cardiac output (Fig. 7) with little or no venous pooling effect. The complication of tachycardia which is seen in use of hydralazine for treatment of hypertension does not occur when this drug is used to treat heart failure (see earlier discussion).[31,35,41] Hydralazine is known to cause a lupus-erythematosus-like syndrome in 2 to 3 percent of hypertensive patients taking 200 to 400 mg of hydralazine per day for prolonged periods.[65] This LE syndrome appears to be dose-related and is totally and rapidly reversed by stopping hydralazine therapy. Antinuclear antibody usually appears in the plasma 3 to 6 months before toxic symptoms develop and therefore provides a valuable screening test which allows the therapy to be discontinued before the LE syndrome occurs. Regular testing for antinuclear antibody is advised for patients taking this drug. Fluid retention is a known side effect of hydralazine use in the treatment of hypertension.

Minoxidil is a new agent which has had moderate trial in treatment of hypertension.[66] It appears to be of potential use in heart failure because it is potent, it is a direct arterial smooth muscle relaxant, less frequent dosage is possible, and it is not associated with a LE-like syndrome.[67,68] It has no effect on venous capacitance. Like hydralazine, minoxidil increases the cardiac output as it drops peripheral resistance in hypertensive patients. Only 1 patient with heart failure who was not hypertensive but was treated with minoxidil has been reported.[67] This patient had advanced heart failure and was dependent on intravenous nitroprusside infusion. With the institution of oral minoxidil, 20 mg three times per day, it was possible to wean him from the nitroprusside. Cardiac index increased from a value of 1.4 liters/min (m²) to 2.2 with minoxidil, but left ventricular filling pressure did not change. Cardiac index was 3.2 liters/min (m²) after 8 weeks of this therapy combined with isosorbide dinitrate, and it fell to 2.0 when minoxidil was withdrawn. Fluid retention is a known side effect of minoxidil therapy in hypertension, and this patient developed peripheral edema.[66] Hypertrichosis is also a known side effect of minoxidil use. The role of minoxidil in heart failure

remains to be determined by future studies once this agent is approved by the Food and Drug Administration (FDA) for clinical trial in heart failure.

Phenoxybenzamine (Dibenzyline) is an alpha-adrenergic blocking agent which has a predominant effect on the arterial resistance vessels.[42,69] It can be given orally, has a peak action in 1 h, and has a duration of action of 3 to 4 days. Phenoxybenzamine, 20 to 80 mg/day given every 8 to 12 h with dosage titrated for each patient, was used in combination with sublingually administered isosorbide dinitrate in chronic therapy of refractory heart failure in 15 patients by Kovick and coworkers.[42] Recatheterization of 9 of these patients was performed an average of 7 months after starting therapy and revealed an increase in cardiac output from 2.2 to 2.9 liters/min (m²), a fall in pulmonary mean wedge pressure from 34 to 18 mm Hg, and a fall in systemic vascular resistance from 1824 to 1165 dynes·s·m². Associated with these hemodynamic changes was a striking clinical benefit. While all patients were classified as NYHA class IV and were refractory to conventional therapy before vasodilator treatment, all improved following therapy and 5 returned to work. Side effects which were attributed to the alpha blockage included 2 patients with sexual impotency, 1 with orthostatic hypotension, and 3 with mild nasal congestion. While it is impossible to tell how much of the beneficial effect seen resulted from the phenoxybenzamine and how much from the isosorbide dinitrate, this study was the first to establish that combined arterial dilators and venous pooling drugs have a sustained, excellent effect in chronic heart failure. The authors state that direct arterial relaxing drugs would be better agents than an alpha blocking drug to combine with venous pooling drugs.

Phentolamine (Regitine), which is an alpha-receptor blocking drug, was used as an intravenous infusion by Majid, Sharma, and Taylor in the first study of vasodilators as a treatment for congestive heart failure.[68] These workers reported an increase in cardiac index from 1.9 to 3.3 liters/min (m²) and a fall in systemic vascular resistance from 4920 to 2290 dynes·s·cm⁻⁵·m². The limitation to intravenous use is the major problem with this drug.

Mixed Venous Pooling and Arterial Dilation (See Table 1)

There are two major drugs that promote both venous pooling and arterial dilation: one can only be given intravenously and the other is given orally. Both of these drugs appear to be of major importance in the current treatment of heart failure by vasodilator therapy. While some patients respond to either selected venous pooling or arterial dilation alone, the best results for the majority of patients can be achieved with a combination of arterial and venous vaso-dilatation.[32,38,41–43,69–71]

Nitroprusside (Nipride) relaxes the smooth muscle of arteries and veins and has no direct effect on non-vascular smooth muscle of the heart.[72] When given intravenously, its peak effect occurs almost instantly, and the effect is gone 5 min after cessation of the drug. Nitroprusside has been widely used as therapy for cardiogenic shock resulting from myocardial infarction,[3,4] but this topic will not be discussed here. More recently, it has been used extensively in the acute therapy of severe refractory congestive heart failure. Guiha and coworkers infused an average dose of 40 μm/min into 18 patients with intractable heart failure.[71] Pulmonary wedge pressure fell from 32 to 17 mm Hg, cardiac output rose from a value of 3 liters/min to 5.2, and systemic vascular resistance fell from 2666 to 1276 dynes·s·cm^{-5}. Miller et al. gave an average dose of 63 μm/min intravenously to 12 patients with chronic congestive heart failure.[32] These workers observed a decrease in left ventricular end-diastolic pressure from 19 to 10 mm Hg, an increase in ejection fraction from 0.47 to 0.55, and a decrease in both systemic vascular resistance and forearm venous tone. The effect on cardiac output was variable and depended on the extent of reduction of left ventricular filling pressure. If the filling pressure fell below 10 mm Hg, there was no change in cardiac output, whereas if the filling pressure did not fall below 10, there was an increase in cardiac output. Kreulen and coworkers have shown similar effects on end-diastolic pressure, cardiac output, and ejection fraction[33] when nitroprusside is given. These workers reported a reduction in major determinants of myocardial oxygen consumption such as stress-time index per beat, end-diastolic volume, and mean arterial pressure but no change in heart rate or cardiac output. Thus the estimated myocardial oxygen consumption per liter of blood pumped by the heart was reduced and myocardial "efficiency" increased. The variable effect of nitroprusside on cardiac output is interesting and represents an interplay between the venous pooling and the arterial dilator effects of this drug (see Fig. 7). The arterial dilation decreases afterload, increases ejection fraction, and tends to increase cardiac output. On the other hand, if venous pooling reduces filling pressure to low levels, this reduced use of the Frank-Starling mechanism (see Fig. 4) either prevents a rise in cardiac output or even causes a net reduction in cardiac output. This is an important point to understand, since treatment of an improperly selected patient with relatively low filling pressure may cause a reduction in cardiac output. It is very important to be sure that left ventricular filling pressure is high before administration of a drug which has venous pooling effects. The metabolic degradation

of nitroprusside produces cyanide. Cyanide toxicity and even death can result from long periods of nitroprusside infusion. To prevent cyanide toxicity, it is recommended that the dose of nitroprusside be limited, and a recent report has shown the usefulness of hydroxocobalamin in the management of this problem.[73]

Prazosin (Minipress) is an oral combined arterial dilator and venous pooling agent which recently has been shown to have great promise in the treatment of heart failure.[34,38,43,70] This quinazoline derivative has a balanced dilator effect on both systemic arteriolar and venous beds.[75] The drug works by blocking phosphodiesterase in vascular smooth muscle and also by producing a postsynaptic, alpha-adrenergic receptor blockade.[75–79] It has a peak effect in 1 h and lasts for 6 h when given orally. Awan and coworkers have compared the effect of oral prazosin with intravenous nitroprusside in patients with refractory heart failure.[34] These workers found that the two drugs have very similar actions. Prazosin, 3 mg, caused a rise in cardiac index from 2 to 3 liters/min (m^2) and a fall in left ventricular filling pressure from 30 to 17 mm Hg. These effects were similar to those produced by nitroprusside, which increased cardiac index from 2.2 to 3 liters/min (m^2) and reduced filling pressure from 28 to 17 mm Hg in these same patients. Neither drug changed the heart rate, and each drug lowered mean arterial pressure 20 percent. The extent of arterial dilation was similar to the extent of venous pooling with each drug. Forearm arterial resistance fell about 50 percent, while forearm venous tone decreased about 65 percent with each drug. Similar results were observed by Mehta and coworkers.[70] More recently, Awan and coworkers have extended these exciting observations to the use of prazosin as ambulatory therapy in 9 patients for an average of 3 months. Excellent results were obtained with 2 to 7 mg of prazosin administered orally every 6 h in addition to continuance of previous digitalis and diuretics. The dose of prazosin in each patient was determined by the effects of the drug on cardiac output, left ventricular filling pressure, and systemic blood pressure, as determined by Swan-Ganz catheterization at the start of therapy. Cardiac output rose from 1.9 to 2.9 liters/min (m^2). Filling pressure decreased from 32 to 19 mm Hg, and mean systemic blood presure was reduced from 100 to 88 by the initial dose of prazosin. After 2 weeks of therapy, there was an increase in maximum treadmill exercise duration to 315, as compared to the pre-prazosin value of 209 s, and there was a decrease in echocardiographic ventricular dimensions. Symptoms of fatigue and dyspnea were improved in all patients over an average follow-up period of 3 months. The average NYHA functional class was 3.7 before prazosin and 2.2 after adding this medication to continued administration of digitalis and diuretics (Fig. 9). Orthostatic hypotension did not occur in any patient. Transient headache and mild nausea were seen in 2 patients. No side effects required the prazosin to be stopped. Five of the 9 patients with angina pectoris noted substantial reduction in its frequency while taking prazosin. This additional beneficial effect is not surprising in view of the reduction of several of the major determinates of myocardial oxygen consumption which were measured in this study.

TREATMENT PLANS

The overall discussion of the therapy of congestive heart failure is presented in Chap. 45 of the fourth edition of *The Heart*.[80] The discussion emphasized the importance of searching for an etiology, decreasing physical activity, the removal of ancillary problems, salt restriction, the use of digitalis, the use of diuretics, and the developing views about vasodilator therapy. Most of these principles of treatment have not changed in the last year, but new data have been gathered in the use of vasodilator therapy. Accordingly, the following comments about the practical application of vasodilators in the treatment of heart failure have been designed to supplement the discussion found in Chap. 45 of *The Heart*. Vasodilator therapy may be used in four major categories of heart failure:

1 Long-term management of severe refractory chronic heart failure

2 Acute, severe heart failure resulting from potentially correctable or transient mechanical problems

3 Emergency treatment of acute pulmonary edema where standard therapy is not available

4 Acute myocardial infarction with pump failure shock

Pump failure shock complicating myocardial infarction has been discussed at length in excellent reviews and will not be described here.[3,4] The major emphasis of this discussion is on the long-term management of severe, chronic heart failure. It is reasonable to propose that a fifth category may be added in the future. In view of the solid physiologic principles underlying vasodilator therapy and the known high frequency of serious complications of digitalis toxicity[81] and over diuresis,[12] it follows that vasodilators might be used routinely in the treatment of moderate heart failure. However, no data on this question are currently available.

First, we will consider vasodilators as an important addition to the oral ambulatory outpatient treatment of severe refractory chronic heart failure. The proper selection of patients is extremely important. Correct-

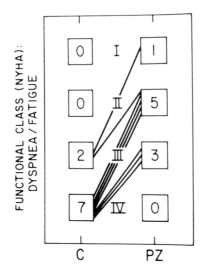

FIGURE 9 Symptomatic evolution of the efficacy of prazosin therapy (2 to 7 mg four times daily) in all 9 chronic heart failure patients during follow-up (mean 94 days) of the agent (PZ) as compared to control symptoms (C). PZ improved New York Heart Association (NYHA) functional class, as indicated by the Roman numerals I through IV and the PZ periods. (*From N. A. Awan, et al., Efficacy of Ambulatory Systemic Vasodilator Therapy with Oral Prazosin in Chronic Refractory Heart Failure, Circulation, 56:346, 1977.*)

able causes and precipitating factors should be removed when possible to do so. The patient should be on a full program of standard therapy, including reduced activity, reduced salt intake, digitalis, and diuretics. If dyspnea or weakness or both persist and especially if toxic complications have attended increased doses of digitalis and diuretics, addition of vasodilators should be considered. The optimum patient for vasodilator therapy is one in whom the cardiac output is low and the filling pressure is quite high. It is very important to be sure that the filling pressure of the left ventricle is elevated about 15 mm Hg prior to starting vasodilator therapy. This is especially true with the venous pooling drugs and also with the drugs having mixed arterial dilator and venous pooling effects. Venous pooling and the consequent decrease in filling pressure can reduce cardiac output and drop systemic blood pressure in the patient with a low left ventricular filling pressure.[3,43] Swan-Ganz catheterization with measurement of pulmonary artery wedge pressure and thermodilution-determined cardiac output is often indicated before starting therapy. If a standard diagnostic cardiac catheterization has been done recently, these data may be used. If such hemodynamic data are not available, clinical and radiologic clues should be used. It a patient has recently had acute pulmonary edema, then one can be reasonably certain that the left ventricular filling pressure is above 15 mm Hg. A strongly positive history of orthopnea, paroxysmal nocturnal dyspnea, and dyspnea on exertion is very suggestive of a high filling pressure. Moist rales, when heard in the absence of lung disease, provide physical findings consistent with a high filling pressure. The upright, posteroanterior chest radiogram is especially useful. In the normal person, an upright chest radiogram reveals relative prominence of the inferior pulmonary veins in relation of the superior veins as a result of the effect of hydrostatic pressure. When there is pulmonary venous hypertension owing to a high left ventricular filling pressure, there is unusual prominence of the superior pulmonary veins in an upright chest radiogram. Kerley B lines, pulmonary artery dilatation, and pleural effusion are other chest radiographic signs of a high left ventricular filling pressure. When there is primary left ventricular failure and no interstitial lung disease, physical findings of pulmonary hypertension and secondary right heart failure strongly suggest an elevated filling pressure of the left ventricle. Once the above factors have been determined, one should then consider which vasodilator drug to start.

It is difficult to make a dogmatic statement in this regard. In such a rapidly developing field, any therapeutic regimen may become outmoded very quickly. However, the following therapeutic plans seems reasonable for oral ambulatory therapy of chronic refractory heart failure at present. If there are both congestive and low output symptoms, prazosin, 2 to 7 mg orally every 6 h, appears to be the drug of choice. If low output symptoms predominate and there are neither congestive symptoms nor hemodynamic, physical, or radiographic evidence of high left ventricular filling pressure, then hydralazine, 50 to 70 mg orally every 6 h, may be best. Such a situation may be seen in the patient who has had extensive diuresis with powerful agents. Particular care should be used in such a patient, since very little informtion has been published on this group. The risk of hypotension and decreased cardiac output is present and could occur if filling pressure is too low. Swan-Ganz catheterization to monitor the effects of the initial therapy appears mandatory in such patients. If filling pressure is very high, if severe dyspnea and congestion predominate, and if low output symptoms are not prominent, then either isosorbide dinitrate, 20 mg orally every 5 to 6 h, or prazosin combined with nitrates may be best. For example, a patient who is dyspneic, fatigued, and weak when up and about during the day but severely troubled by orthopnea and paroxysmal nocturnal dyspnea may be well treated by prazosin, 2 to 7 every 6 h and 1 to 2 in. of topical nitroglycerin ointment at bedtime. The topical nitroglycerin may further lower nocturnal preload and relieve orthopnea and paroxysmal nocturnal dyspnea. The use of sublingually administered nitroglycerin, 0.4 mg, may quickly relieve episodes of nocturnal dyspnea. In hospitalized patients the selection of the best drug or combination of drugs can be accomplished by Swan-Ganz catheterization with measurements of cardiac output and filling pressure and then therapeutic trial of appropriate drugs. Once the best combination of venous pooling and arterial dilation is achieved while hemodynamics are being monitored, this type of therapy is continued. In general the current drug with the most promise for ambulatory therapy in many patients appears to be prazosin. However, one need only review the previous section of this chapter to see how limited our experience is with any of these drugs. Continued research and observations for new side effects are clearly indicated.

The second treatment plan is that for more acute severe failure or end-stage failure complicating more chronic heart failure. Acute ventricular septal defect and acute papillary muscle rupture with mitral regurgitation resulting from myocardial infarction are potentially correctable mechanical problems which cause severe heart failure. Both of these lesions have a very high mortality if surgical correction is undertaken in less than 3 weeks following infarction.[82,83] Intensive medical therapy is needed to tide such patients over until surgery may be done more safely. The use of vasodilators may be a major addition to such medical therapy.[84] Hemodynamic measurements should be made by Swan-Ganz catheter. If the cardiac output is low and the filling pressure high, the patient should be started on intravenous administration of nitroprusside. The dose is titrated to get the desired effect and usually consists of 40 to 60 μm/min. One must remember to protect this solution from light, since it is degraded by light. If the desired effect is achieved by nitroprusside, then the treatment may be changed gradually to an oral vasodilator drug. The appropriate oral drug is selected by review of the hemodynamic data and the effect of nitroprusside on these data. Thus the optimum mix of arterial dilation and/or venous pooling can be selected. As discussed earlier, severe heart failure resulting from mitral regurgitation may be treated with vasodilators which may not only decrease the heart failure but also reduce the degree of regurgitation.[45] Similarly, vasodilator therapy may be of benefit in severe aortic regurgitation with massive heart failure. Again, the regurgitant volume is decreased in addition to the usual effect of the drugs to decrease heart failure. If the severe aortic regurgitation is of the acute variety, it is important to remember that emergency aortic valve replacement is usually necessary for maximum patient salvage.[85] Certain patients with end-stage congestive heart failure complicating chronic heart failure who are only incompletely stabilized by intravenous vasodilators may be helped by a combination of dopamine or dobutamine and nitroprusside.[86–89] Too little experience has been reported to give specific summary recommendations about such combination therapy.

The final treatment plan to be discussed is the emergency treatment of acute pulmonary edema. The standard therapy of morphine, oxygen, rotating tourniquets, and, at times, digitalis and diuretics usually reverses acute pulmonary edema. Gold and coworkers suggested the use of 0.3 mg of sublingual nitroglycerin as an additional medication in refractory pulmonary edema caused by acute myocardial infarction.[51] A very recent report showed good results when large doses of sublingually administered nitroglycerin were used as the sole therapy of acute pulmonary edema.[58] If confirmed, this provocative research finding may

eventually result in modification of the current therapy of pulmonary edema. Since pulmonary edema may be diagnosed where standard therapy is not available and since sublingual nitroglycerin is often carried by the patient with chronic ischemic heart disease, effective emergency therapy may be both needed and available. When pulmonary edema can be clearly recognized and during rapid transport to definitive care, administration of 0.8 to 2.4 mg of nitroglycerin sublingually at intervals of 5 to 10 min, or until pulmonary edema subsides, may be useful. Further data and clinical trials are needed before firm recommendations are possible regarding this treatment plan.

REFERENCES

1 Withering, W.: "An Account of the Foxglove, and Some of Its Medical Uses: With Practical Remarks on Dropsy and Other Diseases," C. G. J. and J. Robinson, London, 1785.

2 National Heart, Blood Vessel, Lung and Blood Program: "Part 1, Report of the Heart and Blood Vessel Disease Panel," April 6, 1973 (DHEW Publication No. (NIH) 73–518), U.S. Government Printing Office, Washington, D.C., 1973, p. 2.

3 Chatterjee, K., and Swan, H. J. C.: Vasodilator Therapy in Acute Myocardial Infarction, *Mod. Concepts Cardiovasc. Dis.*, 43:119, 1974.

4 Chatterjee, K., Swan, H. J. C., Kaushik, V. S., Jobin, G., Magnusson, P., and Forrester, J. S.: Effects of Vasodilator Therapy for Severe Pump Failure in Acute Myocardial Infarction on Short-Term and Later Prognosis, *Circulation*, 53:797, 1976.

5 Spann, J. F., Jr., Bucciono, R. A., Sonnenblick, E. H., and Braunwald, E.: Contractile State of Cardiac Muscle Obtained from Cats with Experimentally Produced Ventricular Hypertrophy and Heart Failure, *Circ. Res.*, 21:341, 1967.

6 Spann, J. F., Jr., Covell, J. W., Eckberg, D. L., Sonnenblick, E. H., Ross, J., Jr., and Braunwald, E.: Contractile Performance of the Hypertrophied and Chronically Failing Cat Ventricle, *Am. J. Physiol.*, 223:1150, 1972.

7 Mason, D. T., Spann, J. F., Zelis, R., and Amsterdam, E. A.: Comparison of the Contractile State of the Normal, Hypertrophied and Failing Heart in Man, in N. R. Alpert (ed.), "Cardiac Hypertrophy," Academic Press, Inc., New York, 1971, p. 433.

8 Spann, J. F., Bove, A. A., Natarajan, G., Kreulen, T.: Ventricular Contractile Performance, Pump Function and Compensatory Mechanisms in Aortic Stenosis in Man, in preparation.

9 Gorlin, R.: "Coronary Artery Disease," W. B. Saunders Company, Philadelphia, 1976.

10 Kannel, W. B., Castelli, W. P., McNarmara, P. M.,

McKee, P. A., and Feinleib, M.: Role of Blood Pressure in the Development of Congestive Heart Failure. The Framingham Study, *N. Engl. J. Med.*, 287:781, 1972.

11 Veterans Administration Cooperative Study Group on Antihypertensive Agents: Effects of Treatment on Morbidity in Hypertension, *J.A.M.A.*, 202:1028, 1967.

12 Spann, J. F., Jr., Mason, D. T., and Zelis, R. F.: Recent Advances in the Understanding of Congestive Heart Failure, Parts I and II, *Mod. Concepts Cardiovasc. Dis.*, 39:73, 1970.

13 Stampfer, M., Epstein, S. E., Beiser, G. D., and Braunwald, E.: Hemodynamic Effects of Diuresis at Rest and during Intense Upright Exercise in Patients with Impaired Cardiac Function, *Circulation*, 37:900, 1968.

14 Plumb, V. J., and James. T. N.: Clinical Hazards of Powerful Diuretics, Furosemide and Etacrynic Acid, *Mod. Concepts Cardiovasc. Dis.*, 47:91, 1978.

15 Chidsey, C. A., Braunwald, E., and Morrow, A. G.: Catecholamine Excretion and Cardiac Stores of Norepinephrine in Congestive Heart Failure, *Am. J. Med.*, 39:442, 1965.

16 Chidsey, C. A., Harrison, D. C., and Braunwald, E.: Augmentation of the Plasma Norepinephrine Response to Exercise in Patients with Congestive Heart Failure, *N. Engl. J. Med.*, 267:650, 1962.

17 Spann, J. F., Chidsey, C. A., Pool, P. E., and Braunwald, E.: Mechanisms of Norephrine Depletion in Experimental Heart Failure Produced by Aortic Constriction in the Guinea Pig, *Circ. Res.*, 17:312, 1965.

18 Covell, J. W., Chidsey, C. A., and Braunwald, E.: Reduction of Cardiac Response to Postganglionic Sympathetic Nerve Stimulation in Experimental Heart Failure, *Circ. Res.*, 19:51, 1966.

19 Wood, J. E., Litter, J., and Wilkins, R. W.: Peripheral Venoconstriction in Human Congestive Heart Failure, *Circulation*, 13:524, 1956.

20 Zelis, R.: The Contribution of Local Factors to the El-

evated Venous Tone of Congestive Heart Failure, *J. Clin. Invest.*, 54:219, 1974.

21 Wood, J. E.: The Mechanism of the Increased Venous Pressure with Exercise in Congestive Heart Failure, *J. Clin. Invest.*, 41:2020, 1962.

22 Zelis, R., and Mason, D. T.: Compensatory Mechanisms in Congestive Heart Failure—the Role of the Peripheral Resistance Vessels, *N. Engl. J. Med.*, 282:962, 1970.

23 Chidsey, C. A., Harrison, D. C., and Braunwald, E.: Augmentation of the Plasma Norepinephrine Response to Exercise in Patients with Congestive Heart Failure, *N. Engl. J. Med.*, 267:650, 1962.

24 Zelis, R., Mason, D. T., and Braunwald, E.: A Comparison of the Effects of Vasodilator Stimuli on Peripheral Resistance Vessels in Normal Subjects and in Patients with Congestive Heart Failure, *J. Clin. Invest.*, 47:960, 1968.

25 Zelis, R., Longhurst, J., Capone, R. J., Lee, G., and Mason, D. T.: Peripheral Circulatory Control Mechanisms in Congestive Heart Failure, in Dean T. Mason (ed.), "Congestive Heart Failure," Yorke Medical Books, New York, 1976, p. 129.

26 Zelis, R., Mason, D. T., and Braunwald, E.: Partition of Blood Flow to the Cutaneous and Muscular Beds of the Forearm at Rest and during Leg Exercise in Normal Subjects and in Patients with Heart Failure, *Circ. Res.*, 24:799, 1969.

27 Higgins, C. B., Vatner, S. F., Franklin, D., and Braunwald, E.: Effects of Experimentally Produced Heart Failure on the Peripheral Vascular Response to Severe Exercise in Conscious Dogs, *Circ. Res.*, 31:186, 1972.

28 Reeve, R., Sakai, F. J., Kennedy, J. W., Hood, W. P., Jr., Rackley, C. E., Alderman, E. L., and Lawson, W.: Ejection Fraction and Varying Afterload, *Am. J. Cardiol.*, 39:284, 1977. (Abstract.)

29 Kruelen, T. H., Bove, A. A., McDonough, M. T., Sands, M. J., and Spann, J. F., Jr.: The Evaluation of Left Ventricular Function in Man. A Comparison of Methods, *Circulation*, 51:677, 1975.

30 Majid, P. A., Sharma, B., and Taylor, S. H.: Phentolamine for Vasodilator Treatment of Severe Heart-Failure, *Lancet*, 2:719, 1971.

31 Chatterjee, K., Parmley, W. W., Massie, B., Greenberg, B., Werner, J., Klausner, S., and Norman, A.: Oral Hydrolazine Therapy for Chronic Refractory Heart Failure, *Circulation*, 54:879, 1976.

32 Miller, R. R., Vismara, L. A., Zelis, R., Amsterdam, E. A., and Mason, D. T.: Clinical Use of Sodium Nitroprusside in Chronic Ischemic Heart Disease, *Circulation*, 51:328, 1975.

33 Kreulen, T. H., Bove, A. A., and Spann, J. F.: Effect of Nitroprusside on Ejection Fraction in Man, in preparation.

34 Awan, N. A., Miller, R. R., and Mason, D. T.: Com-

parison of Effects of Nitroprusside and Prazosin on Left Ventricular Function and the Peripheral Circulation in Chronic Refractory Congestive Heart Failure, *Circulation*, 57:152, 1978.

35 Franciosa, J. A., Pierpont, G., and Cohn, J. N.: Hemodynamic Improvement after Oral Hydralazine in Left Ventricular Failure, *Ann. Intern. Med.*, 86:388, 1977.

36 Cohn, J. M.: Blood Pressure and Cardiac Performance, *Am. J. Med.*, 55:351, 1973.

37 Williams, D. O., Amsterdam, E. A., and Mason, D. T.: Hemodynamic Effects of Nitroglycerin in Acute Myocardial Infarction, *Circulation*, 51:421, 1975.

38 Miller, R. R., Awan, N. A., Maxwell, K. S., and Mason, D. T.: Sustained Reduction of Cardiac Impedance and Preload in Congestive Heart Failure with the Antihypertensive Vasodilator Prazosin, *N. Engl. J. Med.*, 297:303, 1977.

39 Taylor, W. R., Forrester, J. S., Magnusson, P., Chatterjee, K., and Swan, H. J. C.: Hemodynamic Effects of Nitroglycerin Ointment in Congestive Heart Failure, *Am. J. Cardiol.*, 38:469, 1976.

40 Williams, D. O., Bommer, W. J., Miller, R. R., Amsterdam, E. A., and Mason, D. T.: Hemodynamic Assessment of Oral Peripheral Vasodilator Therapy in Chronic Congestive Heart Failure: Prolonged Effectiveness of Isosorbide Dinitrate, *Am. J. Cardiol.*, 39:84, 1977.

41 Massie, B., Chatterjee, K., Werner, J., Greenberg, B., Hart, R., and Parmley, W. W.: Hemodynamic Advantage of Combined Administration of Hydralazine Orally and Nitrates Nonparenterally in the Vasodilator Therapy of Chronic Heart Failure, *Am. J. Cardiol.*, 40:794, 1977.

42 Kovick, R. B., Tillisch, J. H., Berens, S. C., Bramowitz, A. D., and Shine, K. I.: Vasodilator Therapy for Chronic Left Ventricular Failure, *Circulation*, 53:322, 1976.

43 Awan, N. A., Miller, R. R., DeMaria, A. N., Maxwell, K. S., Neumann, A., and Mason, D. T.: Efficacy of Ambulatory Systemic Vasodilator Therapy with Oral Prazosin in Chronic Refractory Heart Failure, *Circulation*, 56:346, 1977.

44 Miller, R. R., Vismara, L. A., DeMaria, A. N., Salel, A. F., and Mason, D. T.: Afterload Reduction Therapy with Nitroprusside in Severe Aortic Regurgitation: Improved Cardiac Performance and Reduced Regurgitation Volume, *Am. J. Cardiol.*, 38:564, 1976.

45 Chatterjee, K., Parmley, W. W., Swan, H. J. C., Berman, G., Forrester, J., and Marcus, H. S.: Beneficial Effects of Vasodilator Agents in Severe Mitral Regurgitation Due to Dysfunction of Subvalvar Apparatus, *Circulation*, 48:684, 1973.

46 Braunwald, E.: Control of Myocardial Oxygen Consumption, *Am. J. Cardiol.*, 27:416, 1971.

47 Cohn, P. F., and Gorlin, R.: Abnormalities of Left Ventricular Function Associated with the Anginal State, *Circulation*, 46:1065, 1972.

48 McAnulty, J. H., Hattenhauer, M. T., Rosch, J., Kloster, F. E., and Rahimtoola, S. H.: Improvement in Left Ventricular Wall Motion following Nitroglycerin, *Circulation*, 51:140, 1975.

49 Dumesnil, J. G., Ritman, E. L., David, G. D., Gau, G. T., Rutherford, B. D., and Frye, R. L.: Regional Left Ventricular Wall Dynamics before and after Sublingual Administration of Nitroglycerin, *Am. J. Cardiol.*, 36:419, 1975.

50 Moyer, J. H.: Hydralazine (Apresoline) Hydrochloride, *Arch. Intern. Med.*, 91:419, 1953.

51 Gold, H. K., Leinbach, R. C., and Sanders, C. A.: Use of Sublingual Nitroglycerin in Congestive Failure following Acute Myocardial Infarction, *Circulation*, 46:839, 1972.

52 Rutenberg, H. L., and Spann, J. F.: Alterations of Sympathetic Neurotransmitter Activity in Heart Failure, *Am. J. Cardiol.*, 32:472, 1973.

53 Mason, D. T., and Braunwald, E.: The Effects of Nitroglycerin and Amyl Nitrite on Arteriolar and Venous Tone in the Human Forearm, *Circulation*, 32:755, 1965.

54 DeMaria, A. N., Vismara, L. A., Auditore, K., Amsterdam, E. A., Zelis, R., and Mason, D. T.: Effects of Nitroglycerin on Left Ventricular Cavitary Size and Cardiac Performance Determined by Ultrasound in Man, *Am. J. Med.*, 57:754, 1974.

55 Williams, J. F., Glick, G., and Braunwald, E.: Studies of Cardiac Dimensions in Intact Unanesthetized Man: Effects of Nitroglycerin, *Circulation*, 32:767, 1967.

56 Burggraf, G. W., and Parker, J. O.: Left Ventricular Volume Changes after Amyl Nitrite and Nitroglycerin in Man as Measured by Ultrasound, *Circulation*, 49:136, 1974.

57 Armstrong, P. W., Mathew, M. T., Boroomand, K., and Parker, J. O.: Nitroglycerin Ointment in Acute Myocardial Infarction, *Am. J. Cardiol.*, 38:474, 1976.

58 Bussman, W. D., and Schupp, D.: Effect of Sublingual Nitroglycerin in Emergency Treatment of Severe Pulmonary Edema, *Am. J. Cardiol.*, 41:931, 1978.

59 Mikulic, E., Franciosa, J. A., and Cohn, J. N.: Comparative Hemodynamic Effects of Chewable Isosorbide Dinitrate and Nitroglycerin in Patients with Congestive Heart Failure, *Circulation*, 52:477, 1975.

60 Franciosa, J. A., Mikulic, E., Cohn, J. N., Jose, E., and Fabie, A.: Hemodynamic Effects of Orally Administered Isosorbide Dinitrate in Patients with Congestive Heart Failure, *Circulation*, 50:1020, 1974.

61 Needleman, P.: Oral Nitrates: Efficacious?, *Ann. Intern. Med.*, 78:458, 1973.

62 Krantz, J. C., and Leake, C.D.:: The Gastrointestinal Absorption of Organic Nitrates, *Am. J. Cardiol.*, 36:407, 1975.

63 Stunkard, A., Wertheimer, L., and Redisch, W.: Studies on Hydralazine; Evidence for a Peripheral Site of Action, *J. Clin. Invest.*, 33:1047, 1954.

64 Ablad, B.: A Study of the Mechanisms of the Hemodynamic Effects of Hydralazine in Man, *Acta Pharmacol. Toxicol.*, 20 (suppl 1):1, 1963.

65 Perry, H. M.: Late Toxicity to Hydralazine Resembling Systemic Lupus Erythematosus or Rheumatoid Arthritis, *Am. J. Med.*, 54:58, 1973.

66 Gilmore, E., Weil, J., and Chidsey, C.: Treatment of Essential Hypertension with a New Vasodilator in Combination with Beta-Adrenergic Blockade, *N. Engl. J. Med.*, 282:521, 1970.

67 Chatterjee, K., Drew, D., Parmley, W. W., Klausner, S. C., Polansky, J., and Zacherle, B.: Combination Vasodilator Therapy for Severe Chronic Congestive Heart Failure, *Ann Intern. Med.*, 85:467, 1976.

68 Klotman, P. E., Grim, C. E., Weinberger, M. H., and Judson, W. E.: The Effects of Minoxidil on Pulmonary and Systemic Hemodynamics in Hypertensive Man, *Circulation*, 55:394, 1977.

69 Braunwald, E.: Vasodilator Therapy—a Physiologic Aproach to the Treatment of Heart Failure, *N. Engl. J. Med.*, 297:331, 1977.

70 Mehta, J., Iacona, M., Feldman, R. L., Pepine, C. J., and Conti, C. R.: Comparative Hemodynamic Effects of Intravenous Nitroprusside and Oral Prazosin in Refractory Heart Failure, *Am. J. Cardiol.*, 41:925, 1978.

71 Guiha, N. H., Cohn, J. N., Mikulic, E., Franciosa, J. A., and Limas, C. J.: Treatment of Refractory Heart Failure with Infusion of Nitroprusside, *N. Engl. J. Med.*, 291:587, 1974.

72 Palmer, R. F., and Lasseter, K. C.: Drug Therapy: Sodium Nitroprusside, *N. Engl. J. Med.*, 292:294, 1975.

73 Cottrell, J. E., Casthely, P., Brodie, J. D., Patel, K., Klein, A., and Turndorf, H.: Prevention of Nitroprusside-induced Cyanide Toxicity with Hydroxocobalmin, *N. Engl. J. Med.*, 298:809, 1978.

74 Awan, N. A., Miller, R. R., Maxwell, K., and Mason, D. T.: Comparative Clinical Effects of Oral Prazosin on the Forearm Resistance and Capacitance Vessels, *Clin. Pharmacol. Ther.* 22:79, 1977.

75 Cohen, B. M.: Prazosin Hydrochloride (CP-12, 299-1) and Oral Antihypertensive Agent: Preliminary Clinical Observations in Ambulatory Patients, *J. Clin. Pharmacol.*, 10:408, 1970.

76 Constantine, J. W., McShane, W. K., Scriabine, A., and Hess, H. J.: Analysis of the Hypotensive Action of Prazosin, in G. Onesti, K. E. Kim, and J. H. Moyer (eds.), "Hypertension: Mechanisms and Management," Grune & Stratton, Inc., New York, 1973, p. 429.

77 Constantine, J. W., McShane, W. K., Scriabine, A., and Hess, H. J.: Analysis of Hypertensive Action of Prazosin, *Postgrad. Med.*, Spec. No. 18-35, November 1975.

78 Hess, H. J.: Prazosin: Biochemistry and Structure-Activity Studies, *Postgrad. Med.,* Spec. No. 9-17, November 1975.

79 Davey, M. J., and Massingham, R.: Review of the Biological Effects of Prazosin, Including Recent Pharmacological Findings, *Curr. Med. Res.* Opin., 4 (suppl 2):47, 1977.

80 Spann, J. F., Jr., and Hurst, J. W.: Treatment of Heart Failure, in J. Hurst (ed.), "The Heart," 4th ed., McGraw-Hill Book Company, New York, 1978, p. 580.

81 Mason, D. T., Zelis, R., Lee, G., Hughes, J. L., Spann, J. F., and Amsterdam, E. A.: Current Concepts and Treatment of Digitalis Toxicity, *Am. J. Cardiol.,* 27:546, 1971.

82 Daggett, W. M., Guyton, R. A., Mundth, E. D., Buckley, M. J., McEnancy, M. T., Gold, H. K, Leinbach, R. C., and Austen, W. G.: Surgery for Postmyocardial Infarct Ventricular Septal Defect, *Ann. Surg.,* 186:260, 1977.

83 Vlodaver; Z., and Edwards, J. E.: Rupture of Ventricular Septum or Papillary Muscle Complicating Myocardial Infarction, *Circulation,* 55:815, 1977.

84 Tecklenberg, P. L., Fitzgerald, J., Allaire, B. I., Alderman, E. L. and Harrison, D. C.: Afterload Reduction in the Management of Postinfarction Ventricular Septal Defect, *Am. J. Cardiol.,* 38:956, 1976.

85 Morganroth, J., Perloff, J. K., Zeldis, S. M., and Dunkman, W. B.: Acute Severe Aortic Regurgitation, *Ann. Intern. Med.,* 87:223, 1977.

86 Miller, R. R., Awan, N. A., Joye, J. A., Maxwell, K. S, DeMaria, A. N., Amsterdam, E. A., and Mason, D. T.: Combined Dopamine and Nitroprusside Therapy in Congestive Heart Failure, *Circulation,* 55:881, 1977.

87 Mikulic E., Cohn, J. N., and Franciosa, J. A.: Comparative Hemodynamic Effects of Inotropic and Vasodilator Drugs in Severe Heart Failure, *Circulation,* 56:528, 1977.

88 Goldberg, L. I., Hsieh, Y. Y., and Resnekov, L.: Newer Catecholamines for Treatment of Heart Failure and Shock: An Update of Dopamine and a First Look at Dobutamine, *Prog. Cardiovasc. Dis.,* 19:327, 1977.

Cardiovascular Manifestations of Sickle-Cell Anemia*

JOSEPH E. HARDISON, M.D. and C. MILFORD ROGERS, M.D.

This case is reported because of the unusual blood findings, no duplicate of which I have ever seen described. Whether the blood picture represents merely a freakish poikilocytosis or is dependent on some peculiar physical or chemical condition of the blood or is characteristic of some particular disease, I cannot at present answer....†

JAMES B. HERRICK, 1910[1]

INTRODUCTION

Normal adult hemoglobin (Hgb A) is composed of four heme molecules and four amino acid chains, two alpha and two beta. Sickle hemoglobin (Hgb S) results from the mutation of one of the genes governing the production of hemoglobin. In hemoglobin S, valine replaces glutamine at the number six position of the beta chain. This change gives hemoglobin S its different physical and chemical properties.[2]

Sickle-cell anemia occurs when a sickle-cell gene is transmitted from each parent. The majority of hemoglobin is then S-S. Sickle-cell trait occurs when only one gene for sickle hemoglobin is inherited. Approximately 40 percent of the hemoglobin is Hgb S and the rest is Hgb A. Combinations of Hgb S with Hgb C, Hgb D, and thalassemia occur.[3]

Sickle-gene inheritance is found almost entirely in people of African descent. It rarely occurs in Caucasians or in individuals of Mediterranean origin.[2,3]

In the United States 1 of every 12 blacks has sickle-cell trait, and 1 in 500 has sickle-cell anemia.[3] Sickle-cell trait has little clinical significance, while sickle-cell anemia has serious morbidity and mortality.[4]

Pathology Resulting from Sickle-Cell Anemia

When hemoglobin S-S is deoxygenated, it forms linear aggregates that force the red cell into a crescent or sickle shape. The sickled red blood cell has a shortened survival owing to increased mechanical fragility. The average life-span of a sickle cell is 15 days, as compared to that of a normal cell, which is 120 days. This results in a hemoglobin concentration of 6 to 9 g/dl.[3]

Sickled erythrocytes are stiff and do not pass freely through the microcirculation. These abnormal erythrocytes often jam up at sharp turns in the capillaries and cause aggregation of platelet thrombi, resulting in occlusion. Tissue hypoxia occurs, and the lactic acid produced during the ensuing anaerobic metabolism promotes more sickling. Microinfarction and macroinfarction can occur depending upon the size of the vessel obstructed. Infarction is common in the lungs, spleen, kidney, liver, and bone marrow.[5,6] In these organs, combinations of low oxygen tension, acidosis, high osmolarity, or stasis cause sickling and obstruction. The heart is spared from infarction even though its oxygen extraction is high.[7,8] The rapid flow rate may pass the deoxygenated red blood cells through the myocardium before sickling has time to occur.[9,10]

At autopsy the heart is diffusely hypertrophied and dilated.[11] The small vessels within the myocardium contain clumps of sickled red cells. This probably represents postmortem sickling, since infarction is not found in the myocardium.[7,8,12,13] In fact the coronary arteries in patients with sickle-cell anemia may be larger than normal, as demonstrated by postmortem angiography.[13] The myocardium contains only occasional foci of fibrosis and scattered areas of degeneration, manifested by vacuolization of the sarcoplasm, disappearance of muscle striations, and separation of muscle fibers by edema. The endocardium and heart valves are normal.[13–15]

The lungs, unlike the heart, are not spared from infarction. At postmortem examination, thrombus-in-situ or thromboembolism is present in up to two-thirds of cases. Pulmonary infarction is often detected. Fat emboli from infarcted bone marrow are not rare. Pneumonitis or bronchitis is commonly found. Morphologic evidence of pulmonary hypertension and corpulmonale has been documented by autopsy in a few cases.[13,16,17]

Abnormal Physiology Resulting from Sickle-Cell Anemia

Tissue oxygenation is governed by the oxygen content of arterial blood, the distribution of blood flow, and the diffusion of oxygen from hemoglobin to tissue.

* From the Department of Medicine (Drs. Hardison and Rogers), Emory University School of Medicine and the Veterans Administration Hospital (Drs. Hardison and Rogers), Atlanta.

† James Herrick made many contributions to medicine. Two of the most important were the description of sickle cells in 1910 and the correlation of the pathologic finding of coronary atherosclerosis with the clinical syndrome of angina pectoris in 1912.

The total oxygen supply available to meet the metabolic needs of the body depends upon the amount of oxygen carried in arterial blood and the cardiac output. The amount of oxygen carried by the blood in turn depends upon the hemoglobin concentration and the ability of the lungs to oxygenate it.[18]

The decreased oxygen delivery to the tissues in sickle-cell anemia results primarily from hypoxemia secondary to pulmonary infarction, diminished diffusion capacity of the alveolar membranes, decreased vital capacity, decreased maximal breathing capacity, venoarterial shunts, and ventilation-perfusion mismatch.[16,19–21] In addition, the ability of sickle hemoglobin to pick up oxygen in the lungs is decreased. Once oxygen is bound to sickle hemoglobin, however, the bond is stronger than normal, and the release of oxygen to the tissues is decreased.[22] The end result of these two properties of S-S hemoglobin is a lower hemoglobin oxygen saturation for a given Pa_{O_2} than normal (see Fig. 1).[16,21] These properties of S-S hemoglobin are probably not detrimental to the patient unless the hemoglobin concentration is very low.[22]

An increased cardiac output is the major compensation for a reduced oxygen supply. Cardiac output is increased at rest and during exercise in patients with sickle-cell anemia. The resting cardiac output begins to increase at a hemoglobin of 10 g/dl. In other chronic anemias, the resting cardiac output does not increase until the hemoglobin is reduced to 7 g.[23–25] The difference is explained by the hypoxemia resulting from pulmonary disease and the abnormal affinity of the S-S hemoglobin for oxygen.[21]

The elevated cardiac output in chronic anemia results from increased myocardial contractility and reduced afterload.[26] Increased preload and heart rate are

not compensatory mechanisms in sickle-cell anemia or in any chronic anemia.[27] Myocardial fiber tension and contractility is increased in anemic dogs.[28]

Afterload is determined by arteriolar tone and blood viscosity. Since blood viscosity is not reduced in sickle-cell anemia, vasodilatation is the major factor in afterload reduction.[12,28]

Coronary artery blood flow increases proportionately to the cardiac output in anemia, but the myocardial oxygen extraction decreases. The very high cardiac outputs attained and the reduction in myocardial oxygen extraction prove that the heart operates efficiently in anemia.[22,23,28,29] However, a small percentage of patients with long-standing anemia do lose the ability to compensate. At very low hemoglobin concentrations, under 5 g, the right atrial and systemic venous pressures rise. The patient develops signs compatible with congestive heart failure. In severe anemia there is a shift of peripheral blood volume centrally resulting in S_3 gallop, jugular venous distension, and hepatomegaly. This may occur without an increase in the total blood volume. Edema and an increased blood volume may result from the effect of anemia on the kidney.[28] Other features of chronic pump failure are absent. The circulation time is decreased, and the resting cardiac output is increased. However, the percentage increase in cardiac output during exercise is less in patients with hemoglobins under 4 g than in those not so anemic. The decompensation is reversed by correction of the anemia, not by digitalization. This ill-defined state is called circulatory congestion to distinguish it from congestive heart failure.[12,28,30]

Distribution of blood flow depends on arteriolar resistance within the different organs. Tissue hypoxia decreases local arteriolar resistance, thereby increasing blood flow to areas of high metabolism such as the kidneys and muscles.[18]

The final step in tissue oxygenation is diffusion of oxygen from hemoglobin to cells. The pressure gradient between arterial blood and tissue and the affinity of hemoglobin for oxygen determine the rate of oxygen release. In sickle-cell anemia the hemoglobin dissociation curve is shifted to the right, enhancing oxygen release to the tissue[18,31] (Fig. 1) Increased 2,3-diphosphoglycerate (2,3 DPG) within the red blood cell causes the right shift of the oxyhemoglobin dissociation curve. 2,3 DPG preferentially binds to deoxyhemoglobin and reduces its affinity for oxygen. Increased 2,3 DPG lowers the pH within the red cell, further reducing hemoglobin affinity for oxygen.[22,31]

In summary, ventricular hypertrophy is the major structural change in sickle-cell anemia. Increased stroke volume, reduced afterload, and elevated cardiac output are significant hemodynamic changes. The lack of consistent pathologic evidence for intrinsic heart disease leads to the conclusion that the cardiac

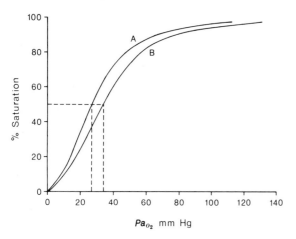

FIGURE 1 A. The standard oxyhemoglobin dissociation curve. Hemoglobin is 50 percent saturated at PA_{O_2} of 27 mm Hg. B. A right-shifted oxyhemoglobin dissociation curve such as occurs in sickle-cell anemia. Hemoglobin is 50 percent saturated at 34 mm Hg.

changes found are compensatory for the chronic increased stroke volume necessary to meet the demand for tissue oxygenation. The heart, in patients with sickle-cell anemia, performs well for long periods of time. When decompensation does occur, it results from additional stress caused by alterations in other organ systems.[12,13,32]

SICKLE-CELL TRAIT

Patients with sickle-cell trait are not anemic and do not have disease arising from abnormal red blood cell shape except in unusual circumstances. They have no significant increase in morbidity or mortality. Sickling occurs in areas of stasis, hypertonicity, and acidosis. The only well-documented complications are hyposthenuria, hematuria, and papillary necrosis secondary to sickling in the renal medulla. Splenic infarction rarely occurs at high altitudes or during anesthesia.[4] Many of the case reports of sudden death or vascular occlusive phenomena attributed to the sickle trait do not satisfactorily document the absence of other abnormal hemoglobins. The finding of sickled erythrocytes at autopsy is considered evidence for a casual relationship between the terminal event and sickle-cell trait. However, postmortem anoxia adequately explains sickling of the red blood cells.[4,12] Patients with sickle-cell trait can be reassured that neither their health nor their life expectancy is seriously impaired.[3]

Clinical Manifestations
of Sickle-Cell Anemia

Exertional dyspnea and palpitations are the most common cardiovascular symptoms experienced by patients with sickle-cell anemia. Dyspnea at rest is less common and can often be attributed to pulmonary infarction or infection rather than left ventricular failure. Angina, orthopnea, paroxysmal nocturnal dyspnea, and chronic cough are unusual.[11,14]

The cardiovascular examination is always abnormal. A widened pulse pressure results from lowered diastolic blood pressure. The arterial pulse is brisk and full. Capillary pulsations and pistol shot sounds over arteries are common.[11] Jugular venous pulsations are usually normal. The precordium is active. The apex impulse is sustained, enlarged, and laterally displaced. Parasternal lifts are common, and a systolic impulse in the left second intercostal space from increased pulmonary artery flow is not unusual. An apical systolic thrill may be present. The heart sounds are increased, and the second sound is often widely split with accentuation of the pulmonic component. All patients have a systolic murmur. The murmur is usually of the ejec-

tion type and is maximal along the left sternal border with radiation over the entire precordium. Less frequently there is a holosystolic murmur. Patients with very low hemoglobins may have a middiastolic apical rumble as a result of increased flow across the mitral valve during ventricular filling. S_3 gallops are the rule, but S_4 gallops occur infrequently. Hepatomegaly and edema occur.[11,12,14,15,33]

The chest x-ray shows generalized cardiomegaly in 95 percent of patients with sickle-cell anemia.[14] Pulmonary artery enlargement and straightening of the border on the left side of the heart are often present. Disproportionate left atrial enlargement is not seen in sickle-cell anemia.[11,15] The pulmonary vascular pattern may be increased as seen in left-to-right shunts (Fig. 2). These x-ray findings are not specific for sickle-cell disease. However, biconcavity of the vertebrae (fish vertebrae) on the lateral chest x-ray is indicative of Hgb S-S or Hgb S-C (Fig. 3).[34]

Electrocardiographic changes are frequent and nonspecific. Abnormalities include left ventricular hypertrophy, first-degree AV block, and nonspecific T wave changes. Signs of biventricular hypertrophy are occasionally seen. Isolated right ventricular hypertrophy resulting from cor pulmonale, abnormal QRS axis, or changes of myocardial ischemia may occur but are quite rare.[14,15,35]

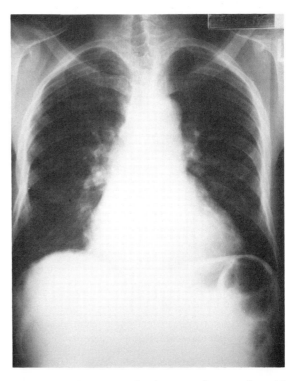

FIGURE 2 Posteroanterior chest x-ray from a patient with sickle-cell anemia showing generalized cardiomegaly and prominence of the upper lobe vasculature.

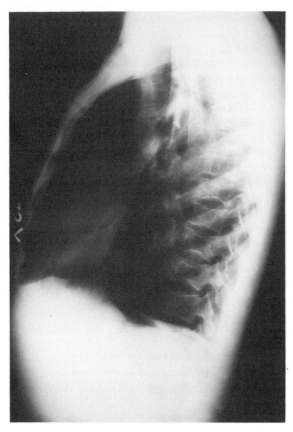

FIGURE 3 Lateral chest x-ray of a patient with sickle-cell anemia showing biconcave deformity of the vertebral bodies which is attributed to local inhibition of bone growth caused by obstruction of the nutrient artery.[33]

Echocardiographic findings include vigorous left ventricular contraction, generalized chamber enlargement, and increased stroke volume. Velocity of circumferential fiber shortening, ejection fractions, and systolic time intervals are normal.[12,31]

Resting pulmonary artery and wedge pressures studied by catheterization of the right side of the heart are normal.[22,23,29] During exercise there may be a mild increase in pulmonary artery pressure reflecting loss of pulmonary vasculature from infarction or infection.[19]

Differential Diagnosis

Cardiovascular findings in sickle-cell anemia mimic rheumatic fever, mitral stenosis, congenital heart disease, bacterial endocarditis, and congestive heart failure.

A patient in sickle-cell crisis from microvascular occlusion may present with fever, anemia, joint pain, leukocytosis, heart murmur, and first-degree AV block simulating acute rheumatic fever and carditis. Whether rheumatic fever occurs less often than expected in sickle-cell anemia remains controversial. However, the coexistence of the two diseases is definitely infrequent.[36,37]

The following features help distinguish sickle-cell crisis from acute rheumatic fever:

1 In crisis there is pain over long bones as well as joints.

2 Subcutaneous nodules and erythema marginata are sometimes present in rheumatic fever but not in sickle-cell anemia.

3 Sickle-cell crisis does not respond to salicylates.[11,38]

An apical systolic murmur, a diastolic rumble, and a chest x-ray showing prominent pulmonary vasculature are findings that are easily confused with those of mitral stenosis. However, patients with sickle-cell anemia lack the left atrial enlargement and right axis deviation characteristic of mitral stenosis.[11,12]

Congenital heart disease occurs in patients with sickle-cell anemia, but cardiac catheterization is required for proof.[38,39] A systolic murmur in the left second intercostal space, a widely split second heart sound, and a pattern of increased vasculature on chest x-ray suggest an atrial septal defect. In sickle-cell anemia, however, right ventricular hypertrophy is rarely present.[14]

Anemia, leukocytosis, fever, arthralgias, and murmur, compatible with bacterial endocarditis, occur in patients in sickle-cell crisis. Blood cultures are necessary to rule out this possibility.[7,11,14]

Exertional dyspnea, rales, S_3 gallop, hepatomegaly, and edema occur in patients with sickle-cell anemia without congestive heart failure.[12] These findings may result from the severe anemia.[28] In spite of dyspnea, pulmonary capillary wedge pressure which is normal at rest usually does not rise during exercise in sickle-cell anemia.[22] The absence of orthopnea and paroxysmal nocturnal dyspnea in sickle-cell disease is helpful in ruling out congestive heart failure. Rales in sickle-cell patients may be caused by pulmonary infection or infarction rather than by pulmonary edema.[12]

TREATMENT

There is no treatment that will reverse the abnormal properties of sickle hemoglobin. The patient with sickle-cell anemia is similar to the patient with the anemia of chronic renal failure in that the degree of anemia is almost always at a symptomatic level. Any further compromise of the chronic anemia must be avoided if possible. The rate of hemolysis in sickle-cell anemia is constant unless there is glucose 6-phosphate dehydrogenase (G-6-PD) deficiency, and any drop in hemoglobin is usually the result of blood loss, folic acid deficiency, infection, or spontaneous aplasia of the marrow.[2] Transfusions with packed red blood cells should be reserved for those situations in which the symptoms precipitated by the anemia and the physiologic deficits demand it. Digitalis and diuretics are rarely indicated.

SUMMARY

In sickle-cell anemia the genetically controlled exchange of valine for glutamine produces Hgb S. Red blood cells containing Hgb S-S are rigid when sickled.

Hemolysis from increased mechanical fragility results in a chronic severe anemia. Capillary obstruction causes tissue hypoxia and infarction. The heart compensates for the blood's reduced oxygen-carrying capacity by an increased stroke volume. Eventually cardiac dilatation and hypertrophy develop, but congestive heart failure is a late complication. The hemoglobin desaturation seen in sickle-cell anemia is caused by alterations in pulmonary function and a shift in the oxyhemoglobin dissociation curve to the right. The findings associated with sickle-cell anemia mimic atrial septal defect, rheumatic heart disease, bacterial endocarditis, and congestive heart failure. Clues are often present to lead one to the correct diagnosis.

REFERENCES

1 Herrick, J. B.: Peculiar Elongated Sickle-shaped Red Blood Corpulses in a Case of Severe Anemia, *Arch. Intern. Med.,* 6:517, 1910.

2 Jacobs, J.: Family History of Sickle Cell Gene Inheritance, in H. K. Walker et al. (eds.), "Clinical Methods, the History, Physical and Laboratory Examinations," Butterworth & Co, (Publishers), Ltd., London, 1976, p. 339.

3 Desforges, J. F., Milner, P., Wethers, D. L., and Whitten, C. F.: Tell the Facts, Quell the Fables, *Patient Care,* June 1978, p. 164.

4 Sears, D. A.: The Morbidity of Sickle Cell Trait, *Am. J. Med.,* 64:1021, 1978.

5 Murphy, R. C., Jr., and Shapiro, S.: The Pathology of Sickle Cell Disease, *Ann. Intern. Med.,* 23:376, 1945.

6 Rimmelstiel, Paul: Vascular Occlusion and Ischemic Infarction in Sickle Cell Disease, *Am. J. Med. Sci.,* 216:11, 1948.

7 Baroldi, G.: High Resistance of the Human Myocardium to Shock and Red Blood Cell Aggregation, *Cardiology,* 54:271, 1969.

8 Baroldi, G.: Revelance of Thrombosis to Infarction, *Adv. Cardiol.,* 9:15, 1973.

9 Finch, C. A.: Pathophysiologic Aspects of Sickle Cell Anemia, *Am. J. Med.,* 53:1, 1972.

10 Desforges, J. F., and Wang, May: Sickle Cell Anemia, *Med. Clin. North Am.,* 50:1519, 1966.

11 Klinefelter, H. F.: The Heart in Sickle Cell Anemia, *Am. J. Med. Sci.,* 203:34, 1942.

12 Lindsey, J., Meshel, J. C., and Patterson, R. H.: The Cardiovascular Manifestations of Sickle Cell Disease, *Arch. Intern. Med.,* 133:643, 1974.

13 Gerry, J. L., Buckley, B. H., and Hutchins, G. M.: Clinicopathologic Analysis of Cardiac Dysfunction in 52 Patients with Sickle Cell Anemia, *Am. J. Cardiol.,* 42:211, 1978.

14 Winson, T., and Burch, G. E.: The Electrocardiogram and Cardiac State in Active Sickle Cell Anemia, *Am. Heart J.,* 29:685, 1945.

15 Uzsoy, N. K.: Cardiovascular Findings in Patients with Sickle Cell Anemia, *Am. J. Cardiol.,* 13:320, 1964.

16 Bromberg, P. A.: Pulmonary Aspects of Sickle Cell Disease, *Arc. Intern. Med.,* 133:652, 1974.

17 Oppenheimer, E. H., and Esterly, J. R.: Pulmonary Changes in Sickle Cell Disease, *Am. Rev. Respir. Dis.,* 103:858, 1971.

18 Thomase, H. M., Lefrak, S. S., Irwin, R. S., Fritts, H. W., and Caldwell, P. R. B.: The Oxyhemoglobin Dissociation Curve in Health and Disease, *Am. J. Med.,* 57:331, 1974.

19 Moser, R. M., Luchsinger, P. C., and Katz, S.: Pulmonary and Cardiac Function in Sickle Cell Lung Disease. Preliminary Report, *Chest,* 37:637, 1960.

20 Miller, G. J., Serjeant, G. B., Sivaprabasam, S., and Petch, M.D.: Cardio-pulmonary Responses and Gas Exchange during Exercise in Adults with Homozygous Sickle Cell Disease, *Clin. Sci.,* 44:113, 1973.

21 Bromberg, P. A., and Jensen, W. N.: Arterial Oxygen Unsaturation in Sickle Cell Disease, *Am. Rev. Respir. Dis.,* 96:400, 1967.

22 Guy, C. R., Salhany, J. M., and Eliot, R. S.: Disorders of Hemoglobin-Oxygen Release in Ischemic Heart Disease, *Am. Heart J.,* 82:824, 1971.

23 Leight, L., Snider, T. H., Clifford, G. O., and Hellems, H. K.: Hemodynamic Studies in Sickle Cell Anemia, *Circulation,* 10:653, 1954.

24 Duke, M., and Abelmann, W. H.: The Hemodynamic Response to Chronic Anemia, *Circulation,* 39:503, 1969.

25 Brannon, E. S., Merrill, A. J., Warren, J. V., and Stead, E. A., Jr.: The Cardiac Output in Patients with Chronic Anemia as Measured by the Technique of Right Atrial Catheterization, *J. Clin. Invest.* 24:332, 1945.

26 Roy, S. B., Bhatia, M. L., Mathur, V. S., and Virmani, S.: Hemodynamic Effects of Chronic Severe Anemia, *Circulation,* 28:346, 1963.

27 Fowler, N. O., Franch, R. H., and Bloom, W. L.: Hemodynamic Effects of Anemia with and without Plasma Volume Expansion, *Circ. Res.,* 4:319, 1956.

28 Varat, M. A., Adolph, R. J., and Fowler, N. O.: Cardiovascular Effects of Anemia, *Am. Heart J.,* 83:415, 1972.

29 Sproule, B. J., Halden, E. R., and Miller, W. F.: A Study of Cardio-pulmonary Alterations in Patients with Sickle Cell Disease and Its Variants, *J. Clin. Invest.,* 37:486, 1958.

30 Graettinger, J. S., Parsons, R. L., and Campbell, J. A.: A Correlation of Clinical and Hemodynamic Studies in Patients with Mild and Severe Anemia with and without Congestive Failure, *Ann. Intern. Med.,* 58:617, 1963.

31 Rodman, T., Close, H. P., Cathcart, R., and Purcell, M. K.: The Oxyhemoglobin Dissociation Curve in the Common Hemoglobinopathies, *Am. J. Med.,* 27:558, 1959.

32 Gerry, J. L., Baird, M. G., and Fortiun, N. J.: Evaluation of Left Ventricular Function in Patients with Sickle Cell Anemia, *Am. J. Med.,* 60:968, 1976.

33 Manual, L., and Liebmann, J.: Cardiovascular Findings in Children with Sickle Cell Anemia, *Dis. Chest,* 52:788, 1967.

34 Greenfield, G. B.: "Radiology of Bone Disease", 2d ed., J. B. Lippincott Company, Philadelphia, 1972, p. 50.

35 Jones, H. L., Wetzel, F. E., and Black, B. K.: Sickle Cell Anemia with Striking Electrocardiographic Abnormalities and Other Unusual Features with Autopsy, *Ann. Intern. Med.,* 29:928, 1948.

36 Wiernik, P. H.: Rheumatic Heart Disease Occurring in Sickle Cell Disease and Trait, *South. Med. J.* 61:404, 1968.

37 D'Arbela, P. G., Kyobe, J., and Tumwesigye, C. R.: Sickle Cell and Foetal Haemoglobins in Rheumatic Heart Disease, *East Afr. Med. J.,* 51:141, 1974.

38 West, J. H.: Sickle Cell Heart Disease, *J. Med. Assoc. Ga.,* 61:120, 1972.

39 Maurer, H. M.: Hematologic Effects of Cardiac Disease, *Pediatr. Clin. North Am.,* 19 (4):1083, 1972.

The Heart in Protein-Calorie Undernutrition*

STEVEN B. HEYMSFIELD, M.D., and DONALD O. NUTTER, M.D.

There is a widespread belief, supported by the textbooks of physiology and cardiology, that the heart is resistant to undernutrition and, unlike other tissues of the body, does not undergo important degeneration or functional changes in starvation. The prevalence of this erroneous concept may explain the fact that, except in beriberi, cardiologic research and practice has shown a remarkable indifference to questions of nutritional status.

The widespread famines produced by World War II have forced attention to a few of these questions. It should be realized, however, that undernutrition occurs in normal times and that, in fact, a large proportion of seriously ill patients are semistarved. The results of alteration in the caloric nutritional status have much relevance to ordinary cardiovascular problems in the United States.

ANCEL KEYS, PH.D.[86]

INTRODUCTION AND BACKGROUND

A nutritional etiology is known or suspected in coronary artery disease, obesity-heart syndrome, beriberi, hypertension, and cobalt cardiomyopathy, each of which have previously been reviewed in the fourth edition of *The Heart* (Chaps. 62H, 81C, 89, and 91). Another diet-heart interaction is deficient intake of protein and calories. Previously considered a rarity on the hospital wards of industrialized nations, protein-calorie undernutrition (PCU) is now being recognized and treated with increasing frequency in medical and surgical patients. This rekindled interest has led us to present this review of the heart in PCU.

Although mass starvation has been reduced by improving agricultural technology, famine remains endemic and sometimes epidemic in developing nations. PCU is the leading cause of morbidity and mortality in children from these deprived regions. Furthermore, societies with advanced technology are now experiencing a rising prevalence of PCU in the chronically ill,[1-4] even though undernutrition has become infrequent in their general populations. Each noncurative therapeutic advance (e.g., hemodialysis for uremia, chemotherapy for metastatic cancer) is associated with an increased prevalence of cachexia. The response of the cardiovascular system to prolonged negative nitrogen balance with resorption of lean body mass has been of considerable interest to several generations of investigators.

Voit is generally credited with the first investigations on cardiac mass in starvation.[5] In a small series of acutely starved cats, this pioneer investigator noted that heart mass was relatively preserved, while other tissues atrophied. This study strongly influenced teaching over the next several decades, to the extent that Vaquez, in his authoritative cardiology monograph of 1924, stated that "inanition has no harmful effect on the heart."[6] Three events in world history and medicine caused this conclusion to be questioned and shaped the subsequent direction for investigation into the cardiovascular events during starvation. The first was the mass starvation of millions of unfortunate World War II victims. Reports of congestive failure and sudden death in undernourished prison camp inmates led Keys and his coworkers to evaluate prospectively cardiovascular and metabolic derangements in adult volunteers subjected to semistarvation.[7] The next era of investigation (1960s) stemmed largely from the recognition during the 1930s of widespread PCU in African infants.[8-10] Sudden death or congestive heart failure during recovery again suggested that starvation adversely affected the heart.[11-15] The third and most recent event in nutritional epidemiology and therapeutics was the recognition of a high prevalence of PCU in hospitalized medical[1,3] and surgical patients[2,4] and the potential for complete reversal of the undernourished state by modern nutritional methods such as intravenous hyperalimentation.

The purpose of this chapter is to review the epidemiology and pathogenesis of PCU and to discuss the cardiovascular changes associated with infantile and adult undernutrition in human beings and experimental animals.

NUTRIENT REQUIREMENTS IN HEALTH AND DISEASE

In order to understand the pathogenesis of PCU and to evaluate the validity of experimental animal models of undernutrition, it is necessary to review the nutrient requirements in health and disease.

---

* From the Department of Medicine, Emory University School of Medicine, Atlanta.

Essential and Nonessential Nutrients

Although the adult human body is composed of many thousands of species of organic molecules, only 20 organic compounds and a source of calories are required for maintenance of health: eight essential amino acids, one fatty acid, 11 vitamins, and water. The remaining organic molecules ingested in the diet are "nonessential" in that their deletion from the diet does not cause disease. In addition to the organic nutrients, there are 15 essential inorganic compounds: calcium, phosphorus, iodine, iron, magnesium, zinc, copper, potassium, sodium, chloride, cobalt, chromium, manganese, molybdenum, and selenium.

The Minimal Daily Requirement

The minimal daily requirement (MDR) of an essential nutrient is the smallest quantity which maintains normal composition and physiologic function of the various tissues and which prevents any clinical or biochemical sign of the corresponding deficiency state.

The cardiovascular syndromes which develop when the daily intake of a nutrient is persistently below the MDR are presented in Table 1.

The Recommended Daily Allowance

The recommended daily allowance (RDA) was introduced to provide a margin of safety for ingestion of each nutrient. It ranges from 1.5 to 10 times the minimal daily requirement.

The Maximal Daily Tolerance

Just as chronic ingestion of less than the minimal daily requirement of a specified nutrient eventually causes disease, intake exceeding the maximal daily tolerance for many nutrients (essential and nonessential) will cause disturbances in tissue structure and function. The cardiovascular syndromes which develop when the maximal daily tolerance of essential nutrients is exceeded are presented in Table 2.

Inadequate intake of protein and calories is by far the most common abnormality of the essential nu-

TABLE 1

Cardiovascular syndromes which develop when the daily intake of a nutrient is persistently below the minimal daily requirement

Essential nutrient	Species	Cardiac abnormalities	Reference
Energy, protein	Human	See "Cardiovascular System in PCU"	
Essential amino acids	Human,* rat	Endomyocardial and interstitial fibrosis, cardiomegaly, and congestive failure secondary to dietary tryptophan deficiency	16–19
Ascorbic acid	Human	Hemorrhagic pericardium; electrocardiographic abnormalities	20 20
Thiamine	Human, rat	Cardiac beriberi; high output heart failure, depressed myocardial contractility	21, 22
Niacin	Human	Electrocardiographic abnormalities	22
Vitamin E	Rabbit	Necrosis of cardiac muscle fibers and fibrosis	22
Calcium	Human, rat	Depression of myocardial contractility, myofibrillar degeneration, and irreversible depression of contractility and excitability	23
Phosphorus	Human,* dog	Congestive cardiomyopathy	24, 25
Magnesium	Human, dog, rat	Predisposition to sudden death in soft water areas; focal necrosis and myocardial calcification, vascular degenerative lesions, vacuolation, and swelling of sarcosomes and mitochondria.	26, 27, 28
Copper	Swine	Myocardial fibrosis and hypertrophy	29
Potassium	Human,* rat	Loss of myofiber striation, vacuolation and fragmentation, interstitial cellular infiltrate, myocardial necrosis, and fibroblastic proliferation	30, 31
Selenium and vitamin E	Pig	Hydropericardium, patchy necrosis of myocardium, myofibrillar degeneration and lysis, mitochondrial swelling and disruption; mild fibrosis and scattered macrophage	32

* Suspected relationship.

TABLE 2
Cardiovascular syndromes which develop when the daily intake of a nutrient is persistently above the maximal daily tolerance

Essential nutrient	Species	Cardiac abnormalities	Reference
Energy	Human	Obesity-heart disease	33
Calcium	Human	Increased myocardial contractility and decreased myocardial automaticity	34
Iron	Human	Conduction disturbances and congestive cardiac failure	35
Magnesium	Human	Vasodilation, electrocardiographic abnormalities, myocardial depression	36
Potassium	Human	Conduction abnormalities and arrhythmias	37
Cobalt	Human, rat	Congestive cardiomyopathy, hyaline necrosis, and dystrophic vacuolar degeneration of cardiac muscle cells	38
Vitamin D	Human	Metastatic calcifications	38

trients and causes development of the protein-calorie undernutrition syndromes. The remainder of this chapter will focus on PCU.

PROTEIN-CALORIE UNDERNUTRITION

Definition and Pathogenesis

Protein and caloric undernutrition in children occurs in two recognizable patterns termed marasmus and kwashiorkor. Although these broad clinical prototypes have been defined, it is common to find a gradation of one type to the other creating a clinical spectrum of disease. Marasmus and kwashiorkor are often complicated by deficiencies of other essential nutrients, including vitamins, minerals, and trace elements.[39] The terminal state of these nutritional diseases is often characterized by intercurrent infection and/or circulatory collapse and shock.[40]

The child with marasmus (Fig. 1) shows marked emaciation with wasting of adipose and muscle tissue, stunting of growth, a weight deficit (<60 percent of expected for age), and hypothermia. The skin and hair appear normal, and edema is usually absent. The serum albumin level is either normal or only modestly reduced. The clinical pattern emerges in infancy after severe dietary inadequacy. The typical patient has had inadequate breast-feeding and intercurrent infections. Although numerous pathogenic factors have been considered, the primary cause is inadequate intake of calories (energy) and protein.[39]

The child with kwashiorkor (Fig. 1) is usually somewhat older than the marasmic infant; is listless, apathetic, and irritable; and has a protuberant abdomen as a result of ascites and hepatomegaly (30 percent).[40a] The latter is caused by fatty infiltration,

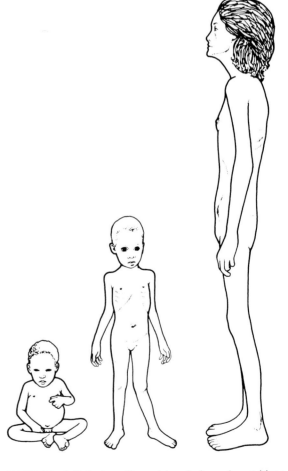

FIGURE 1 Patients with protein-calorie undernutrition; child with kwashiorkor (left), child with marasmus (middle), and adult with marasmus-like state secondary to anorexia nervosa (right).

which may account for up to 80 percent of liver mass. Growth is retarded, and weight is usually 60 to 80 percent of that expected for age. Anorexia, hypothermia, skin lesions, and hair changes are common.[39] There may be surprising preservation of subcutaneous adipose tissue, which masks the invariable atrophy of muscle. Anemia and hypoalbuminemia are notable components of the syndrome and may be accompanied by varying degrees of diarrhea, hypokalemia, and infection.[39] The clinical pattern usually emerges in children who, after prolonged breast-feeding, are weaned on starchy and sugary foods. Kwashiorkor is thus primarily a deficiency of protein accompanied by an adequate intake of calories (energy).

The pathways leading to adult PCU are usually more variable than those in childhood, but it is convenient for pathophysiologic and therapeutic reasons to consider a similar spectrum of disease ranging from marasmus (Fig. 1), with depletion of skeletal muscle and adipose stores but normal or near normal levels of serum albumin, to kwashiorkor, with preservation of adipose tissue, hypoalbuminemia, and edema.[41] Typical adult types who develop PCU include individuals with anorexia nervosa, advanced cardiac disease (cardiac cachexia), chronic lung disease (pulmonary cachexia), cancer (cancer cachexia), uremia, and advanced cirrhosis. Patients with severe cases of PCU, regardless of etiology, characteristically have multiple mineral and vitamin deficiencies, anemia, impaired cell-mediated immunity, infections, fever, and bed sores.[42]

EXTRACARDIAC DETERMINANTS OF VENTRICULAR OUTPUT IN PROTEIN-CALORIE UNDERNUTRITION

The control of cardiac performance and output is determined by four principal factors: (1) ventricular end-diastolic volume (preload), (2) the inotropic state of the myocardium (myocardial contractility), (3) the tension the heart muscle, which develops during contraction (the afterload), and (4) the heart rate.[43] In the remaining sections, selected cardiac and extracardiac physiologic processes which influence each of these four determinants of ventricular function will be reviewed. Our goal is to present an integrated view of the circulatory state in starvation and subsequent recovery.

Metabolic State in Protein-Calorie Undernutrition

One of the key determinants of ventricular output is the level of metabolic activity, fluctuations in which are reflected primarily by changes in heart rate. In PCU, a metabolic adaptation occurs which aids in conserving limited tissue protein and energy stores; total-body oxygen consumption and metabolic rate decline in the undernourished individual, and the decrements are more than would be expected from the reduction in body size.[44,44a] This results in a characteristic bradycardia, which is discussed in more detail below. Hypothermia (<35°C) develops in 15 to 20 percent of undernourished children and adults and results from a combination of hypometabolism and increased heat loss secondary to depletion of the insulating adipose layer.[44]

Consideration of thyroid and sympathetic activity is important because of the numerous direct and indirect effects these hormones have on the heart. The starvation-induced curtailment in oxidative metabolism is accompanied and in part caused by a depression in thyroid and sympathetic stimuli.[45,46] The decline in thyroid activity is mediated by a reduction in serum T_3 [45] (free tri-iodothyroxine) and in the T_3 nuclear receptor.[47] Serum levels of T_4 (free thyroxin) and TSH (thyrotropin) remain normal. Apart from an important role in regulating metabolic rate, catecholamines have a direct inotropic effect on the myocardium.[43] The cardiac metabolism of these compounds has been examined during short-term starvation in the rat.[46] The rate of myocardial norepinephrine synthesis and turnover is depressed, with a parallel reduction in the catecholamine content of the nerve terminal.[46,48] An expected consequence of the slowing of sympathetic nerve impulse traffic would be a reduction in the inotropic state of the myocardium. This important possibility will be discussed again in the section "Cardiovascular Function and Myocardial Mechanics."

Blood Volume in Protein-Calorie Undernutrition

One of the major determinants of end-diastolic volume and preload is total blood volume.[43] This compartment and its two principal components, plasma and red blood cell volumes, were examined by Keys and colleagues in adult men after 6 months of voluntary semi-starvation.[49] Results indicated that the loss of body weight and lean body mass was not accompanied by a proportional depletion of plasma volume. Absolute plasma volume had changed little during food restriction at a time when body weight was reduced by one-fourth, resulting in an elevated plasma volume index. Consequently, these individuals were relatively over-hydrated. The distribution of this "enlarged" plasma volume between intrathoracic and extrathoracic compartments is unknown, making it difficult to evaluate the influence of this "relative" hypervolemia on ventricular end-diastolic volume and cardiac output. In PCU complicated by severe diarrhea, sepsis, and fluid shifts, as is often the case in the undernourished child, plasma volume may, in fact, be markedly reduced.[50-53] In contrast to plasma volume, red blood cell volume declines at the same rate as lean body mass. The result is a gradual decline in hematocrit values and development of anemia, the latter often complicated by additional deficiencies, including those of folate and iron.[54]

THE CARDIOVASCULAR SYSTEM IN PROTEIN-CALORIE UNDERNUTRITION

Clinical Observations

The undernourished subject often experiences fatigue, lethargy, and swelling of the extremities and abdomen. Specific cardiovascular symptoms are uncommon if underlying heart disease is absent.[55] The undernourished patient rarely complains of dyspnea, palpitations, or precordial chest pain.

Heart sounds are distant or muffled and the precordium is quiet,[55] in keeping with the hypokinetic circulatory state and occasional pericardial effusion.[56] Gallop rhythms or pericardial rubs are not features of undernutrition unless the patient is in a state of congestive heart failure. Systolic flow murmurs have been reported, especially in the undernourished child.[11,12,15,39] These murmurs are usually considered functional, especially since most starved patients are anemic.

Physical examination often reveals a slow pulse,[57,58] sometimes less than 35 beats per minute, unless PCU is complicated by fever or sepsis, in which case a tachycardia may be present.[11,12,15,59] Both systolic and diastolic blood pressures are lowered, and preexisting hypertension may be ameliorated.[55] The extremities are cool, with cyanosis of the nailbeds, decreased peripheral pulses, and prolonged circulation time.[7] Neck vein distension is rare, and central venous pressure is low.[7]

Electrocardiographic abnormalities are common in PCU, but often underlying metabolic (e.g., hypokalemia, etc.) and infectious complications influence the observed pattern.

Heart rate is frequently subnormal, with a sinus mechanism as the predominant rhythm.[60] Arrhythmias are occasionally present in the cachectic child and adult and have often been cited as a possible cause of sudden death in advanced PCU. The abnormalities in rhythm include atrial fibrillation,[11] nodal rhythm,[60] exercise-induced ventricular tachycardia,[61] and frequent nodal escape beats and premature ventricular contractions.[61,61a] A possible anatomic basis for these abnormalities has been suggested by Sims, who detected varying degrees myolysis in the AV node and bundle branches in 5 of 7 kwashiorkor cases,[14] with lesser or no involvement in nonconducting tissue. This interesting observation, however, has not been regularly confirmed in other autopsy series.[62-67]

The QRS axis shifts to the right and may become vertical.[60] One of the most characteristic electrocardiographic accompaniments of progressive cachexia is a reduction in QRS amplitude, which returns to normal following recovery. Possible explanations for a declining QRS amplitude include loss of cardiac tissue, rotation of axis, pericardial effusion, and hypometabolism.[60]

Abnormalities in ventricular repolarization in PCU have been frequently described, but the interpretation and significance of these findings remain controversial. Regarding the Q-T interval, Smythe, Swanepoel, and Campbell found one-half of their kwashiorkor patients had a prolonged Q-T_c interval (Q-T/$\sqrt{RR}$).[11] However, these infants frequently suffered from diarrhea, profound hypokalemia, and hypocalcemia; electrolyte supplements improved the Q-T abnormality in some but not all children. Wharton's infants with kwashiorkor rarely had Q-T_c intervals outside the range of normal,[62] but little information on electrolyte status is provided in the report. In adult PCU, the anorectic subjects studied by Gottdiener and associates rarely had prolonged Q-T intervals (1/11) adjusted for heart rate.[61] In a similar group of 9 patients with anorexia nervosa, however, Thurston and Marks reported that 5 had slightly prolonged Q-T intervals for heart rate.[62] In these latter two studies, serum electrolytes were normal in all subjects investigated. A partial explanation for these discrepancies in the length of the Q-T interval may be found in the report of Keys and colleagues concerning the adult male volunteers of the Minnesota experiment who lost 24 percent of their initial body weight during 6 months of semistarvation.[60] The absolute Q-T interval lengthened by 25.9 percent over base-line, but the Q-T_c was shorter by 1.9 percent. During the recovery phase of the experiment, however, the absolute Q-T remained unusually long, the Q-T_c actually lengthened; after 8 months of rehabilitation, when body weight had been fully restored, Q-T and Q-T_c were respectively 10.2 and 4.5 percent longer than base line. This prospective study clearly underlines the importance of specifying in which phase of PCU, starvation or recovery, the electrocardiographic tracing is made. We can conclude the following: (1) Electrolyte disorders are a frequent and reversible cause of a prolonged Q-T interval in PCU. (2) When serum electrolytes are normal in semistarvation, the absolute Q-T interval may lengthen; the Q-T corrected for heart rate (i.e., Q-T_c), however, is normal or only slightly prolonged. (3) During recovery from PCU, body weight and heart rate correct more rapidly than does the lengthened absolute Q-T, and therefore, the Q-T_c may become prolonged. The significance and pathophysiology of Q-T abnormalities is unknown.

Depression of the ST segment and flattened or inverted T waves without apparent ischemic heart disease have been noted in both human[11,14,59,63] and animal forms of PCU.[64,65]

Cardiac Size

HEART MUSCLE MASS

In the starving individual, the heart atrophies along with the other components of lean body mass, and this reduction is evident both at autopsy and during life in the shrunken radiographic cardiac silhouette. Is the erosion of cardiac mass in proportion to or less than loss of body weight? The latter would imply ''sparing'' of the heart in starvation. Before examining this important question, we should consider the factors influencing heat size[68] in the undernourished subject. A smaller myocardium in PCU would be favored by the reduced workload imposed by a smaller lean body mass, reduced thyroid and sympathetic activities, and lowered systemic arterial pressure. Factors tending to preserve myocardial mass would be increased cardiac demands resulting from severe anemia, fever, or defective contractility. The latter abnormality could theoretically develop if PCU per se caused a weakening of the heart muscle, thus requiring a larger total cardiac mass per unit body weight to maintain cardiac output consistent with metabolic requirements.

Most workers now agree that in uncomplicated cases of human or animal undernutrition, the heart atrophies in proportion to or slightly less than body weight,[60,69,70] and therefore the heart weight/body weight ratio remains relatively constant. The myocardium of all four chambers is proportionately reduced in mass.[71] However, when PCU is complicated by hypermetabolism (e.g., fever, sepsis, trauma),[70] preexisting hypertension, ischemic heart disease, cardiomyopathy (e.g., endomyocardial fibrosis),[72] or profound anemia, the heart weight/body weight ratio is often increased. Thus the degree of cardiac atrophy in starvation might therefore be the net result of factors diminishing or augmenting cardiac work (i.e., reduced blood pressure, hypometabolism, and depressed sympathetic stimulation versus anemia and hypermetabolism).

The reduced cardiac mass at autopsy is paralleled by a shrinking of muscle fibers evident under the light microscope. Abel found a 20 percent reduction in myofiber diameter following a 42 percent weight loss in protein-deficient beagles.[73] When rhesus monkeys were similarly subjected to a kwashiorkor-like protein-deficient diet, myofiber diameter decreased by 33 percent from base line, with a body weight loss of 20 percent.[64] The atrophied fibers became tightly packed, camera lucida drawings revealing a 33 percent increase in the number of fibers per square inch.

INTRACARDIAC CHAMBER VOLUMES

The effect of undernutrition on cardiac chamber volumes and dimensions has been studied in living human subjects by echocardiography. Left ventricular volumes were examined in adult patients with PCU secondary to diverse chronic diseases by Heymsfield et al.[70] These investigators found an absolute reduction in left ventricular end-diastolic and end-systolic volume for height, but normal or near normal values per unit body weight. Gottdiener and coworkers[61] found normal or slightly subnormal left ventricular, left atrial, and aortic dimensions per square meter in young women with anorexia nervosa. Thus, intracardiac volumes in PCU respond in the same manner as heart mass and decline approximately in proportion to body size.

The kinetics of the reduction in heart size was examined by Keys and associates in adult men subjected to 6 months of a famine-like diet.[57] Using chest radiographs, these workers calculated heart volume, which represents the composite of mass plus intracardiac chamber volumes. During the first 3 months of restricted dietary intake, heart volume declined parallel to body weight. During the next 3 months, however, body weight decreased more rapidly than heart volume, so that at the end of 6 months of semistarvation the heart volume/body weight ratio had increased by 7 percent over base line.

Cardiac Structure and Pathology

In gross appearance, the PCU heart is small and, in some cases, flabby and pale. Epicardial fat is absent, and pericardial effusions are often present in patients with generalized edema.[57,70,74] The coronary arteries, valves, and endocardium are usually normal.[75]

Microscopically, the principal feature is atrophy of the myocardial fibers.[64,73] More advanced lesions within the myofibril have been reported, but the occurrence of these abnormalities varies with species and with the type of PCU studied (Table 3). The lesions observed include fragmentation of the myofibril, loss of striations, vacuolation, and patchy necrosis of fibers. Possible explanations for this diversity of lesions with unpredictable occurrence include variable presence of severe anemia and infections, differing ages and species investigated, and differences in relative deficiency of protein and calories.

The interstitium is edematous in approximately one-fourth of autopsy cases[59,63,74,] and is most evident in subjects receiving intravenous fluids high in sodium and in those with marked preterminal dependent edema or ascites.[59,74] An occasional finding is an interstitial lymphocytic infiltrate (Table 3), most often surrounding foci of patchy necrosis.

Light microscopy of skeletal muscle in PCU often

TABLE 3
Light microscopy of the heart in protein-calorie undernutrition

Species and type of PCU	Myofiber					Interstitium		Comments	References
	Atrophy	Fragmentation of myofibril	Loss of striations	Vacuolation	Patchy necrosis	Edema	Lymphocytic infiltrate		
Human									
Infantile kwashiorkor and marasmus	+	+	+	+		+	−	Infection (bronchopneumonia, sepsis, measles, etc.) most common (85%) cause of death	63
Kwashiorkor	+			+		+ (4/24)		Infection common cause of death	11
Kwashiorkor			+	+	+	+ (2/6)	+	Children dying from non-PCU-related diseases showed a similar degree of necrosis and edema but less vacuolation; authors concluded findings did not support a specific cardiomyopathy of protein deficiency	12
Adult prisoners of war (Japanese)	+	+	+				+		59
Adult prisoners of war (American)			+			+			74
Animal models									
Protein-deficient rhesus monkey (infant)	+	+	+		+	+	+		66
Protein-deficient rhesus monkey (juvenile)	+	−	−	−	−	−	−	Rhesus monkeys in this study were slightly older than those above, perhaps accounting for the differences in pathologic findings.	65
Protein-deficient beagle	+	−	−	−	−	+	−		73
Protein-calorie-deficient rat	+	−	−	−	−	−	−		67

shows pathology similar to the heart (Table 3), but the lesions are usually more advanced than in cardiac tissue.

Electron-microscopic studies of cardiac tissue have been performed in both human beings and animals with PCU. Common features include scattered foci of atrophy with loss of myofibrils and glycogen.[67] Mitochondria are decreased in number, with occasional swelling of the matrix and disruption of the cristae.[63,66,67] The sarcoplasmic reticulum and plasma membrane are usually normal, but the former may show some occasional distension.[63,66,67]

Myocardial Biochemistry in Protein-Calorie Undernutrition

Relatively few studies have examined the structural and functional biochemistry of the chronically undernourished heart. A detailed discussion of how the cardiac electrophysiologic, pathologic, and functional alterations of PCU reviewed in this chapter relate to biochemical processes must await further activity in these areas. In this section, we review recent work in two areas, structural biochemistry and metabolic pathways.

STRUCTURAL BIOCHEMISTRY

Microscopic examination of the PCU heart (see ''Cardiac Structure and Pathology,'' above) often shows a tight packing of shrunken myofibers surrounded by an apparent increase in connective tissue.[64] By analyzing the left ventricular concentration of DNA, protein, collagen, and actomyosin in a marasmic-like rat model,[69] Nutter and coworkers provide us with the biochemical counterpart of these histologic findings. Following 6 weeks of caloric and protein deprivation, the body weight and cardiac mass of these animals were reduced by 52 and 43 percent, respectively, as compared to controls. DNA, enclosed mainly in the nucleus, has traditionally been used as an index of cell number.[76] In fact the myocardial concentration of DNA was larger by 45 percent in undernourished than in control hearts, suggesting that the atrophic PCU myocardium has a greater cellular density. However, this study leaves unanswered two important questions: (a) Is there irreversible loss, and therefore, fewer *total* number of myofibers (i.e., ''fiber dropout'') in the PCU heart? (2) Is the increased concentration of left ventricular DNA in PCU partially attributable to proliferation of nonmyocardial elements (e.g., fibroblasts)? Further studies will be required to answer these questions. Next, by measuring total cardiac protein, these investigators were able to estimate cell size by the left ventricular protein/DNA ratio.[72] The latter was smaller

by 30 percent in the PCU myocardium as compared to controls, which is the same order of magnitude as microscopically measured fiber diameter reduction in the animal studies discussed earlier, i.e., 20 to 33 percent. Two specific proteins, collagen and actomyosin, were examined further. Left ventricular collagen concentration was increased 95 percent over control, but it is unknown if this represents a failure to reabsorb connective tissue during the wasting state or a pathologic infiltration of myocardium by new collagen. The investigators also examined the functional impact of this increased connective tissue on myocardial stiffness. Passive length-tension curves from isolated papillary muscles demonstrated no abnormality. In contrast to collagen, actomyosin concentration was identical in patients with PCU and in controls, implying that contractile protein per unit of tissue is unchanged in the starving heart. Viewed collectively, these findings tend to confirm the microscopic impression of small, tightly packed fibers surrounded by an abundance of connective tissue.[64]

METABOLISM

Relatively little is known regarding the flux of substrates through the metabolic pathways of the chronically undernourished myocardium. Recent workers have, however, examined these processes following 1[77] to 7 days[78] of total starvation in the rat.

Glycolysis This metabolic pathway is most active in the immediate postprandial state, when the heart uses glucose as the main source of energy. As the duration of fasting lengthens from several hours to 1 week, progressive inhibition of the key regulatory enzyme phosphofructokinase (PFK) blocks glycolytic flux.[77,78] PFK is inhibited during the first day of fasting by rising levels of intracellular citrate, a by-product of fatty acid metabolism. The mechanism of late inhibition (7 days) of PFK is unclear, because at this point citrate levels are only slightly elevated.[78]

Lipid metabolism Free fatty acids, transported to the heart from adipose tissue by serum albumin and, to a lesser degree, by acetoacetate and 3-hydroxybutyrate, supply about two-thirds of myocardial energy requirements in the postabsorbtive state.[79] After 1 day of fasting the heart levels of these latter two metabolites are elevated fourfold.[77] In contrast, 7 days of total starvation results in only a modest increase in heart ketone bodies at a time when plasma levels of these compounds remain high. This may reflect a shift in ketone body utilization from the heart to other tissues, most notably brain tissue.[78]

Citric acid cycle and ATP In the studies of Gold and Yaffe, 7 days of total starvation produced little evidence to suggest any major alterations in the control of myocardial citric acid cycle activity.[78] The tissue level of ATP in the starved rat heart was increased, but the authors did not determine if this reflected an increased production or reduced utilization of chemical energy. The authors did conclude, however, that an ample supply of ATP was available.

Amino acid metabolism Alanine yields pyruvate directly on transamination with α-ketoglutarate, and in turn, pyruvate may either be converted to glucose or be oxidized in the citric acid cycle.[79] That these latter two processes are occurring after 1 week in the starving rat heart is suggested by the low cardiac tissue level of alanine and a fall in the alanine/pyruvate equilibrium ratio.[78]

Glutamate, which enters the citric acid cycle directly at the α-ketoglutarate step, similarly declines with a fall in the glutamate/α-ketoglutarate ratio. The shift in amino acid metabolism from an anabolic flux to oxidative pathways suggests that free amino acids may become important fuels in late starvation. The various species of protein in the heart are a most likely reservoir of these oxidizable amino acids.

Cardiac Function and Myocardial Mechanics

The occurrence of significant cardiac atrophy during PCU has been well documented by radiographic and pathologic data, as presented in preceding sections. Controversy persists as to whether the atrophic PCU heart functions normally or demonstrates ventricular dysfunction and congestive heart failure. In review, physicians treating marasmus and kwashiorkor in children living in developing countries have observed hypotension, a hypodynamic circulatory state, and congestive manifestations in a number of these patients.[11,62,63,72] They have concluded that heart failure is a frequent complication of PCU and that the heart may be responsible for the occasional case of sudden death in these nutritional diseases.[14] The autopsy findings of myocardial edema and myofiber damage presented above tend to support these conclusions. Other authors have postulated that severe undernutrition may be an important etiologic factor in many cases of congestive or restrictive cardiomyopathy encountered in African or Asian countries.[16,80,81] The circumstantial evidence for this theory includes: (1) a higher incidence of idiopathic cardiomyopathy in the lower socioeconomic segments of these populations; (2) a high prevalence of malnutrition in patients with these cardiomyopathies; and (3) demonstrations that the indigenous diet can produce myocardial fibrosis, dilatation, and failure in experimental animals.[18,19]

A number of investigators have studied the changes in hemodynamics and ventricular function that occur during starvation or chronic PCU in human beings. Cardiac output has been shown by Alleyne to be reduced in proportion to the body weight deficit in malnourished Jamaican children;[82] cardiac output recovered with nutritional therapy. Viart performed a comprehensive hemodynamic evaluation of protein-calorie undernourished children in Zaire. He found bradycardia, hypotension in the pulmonary and systemic circulations, and a depression of cardiac output and concluded that these children showed an adaptive hypocirculatory state in the presence of body wasting and lowered metabolic requirements.[58] A few children in this study were severely malnourished (serum albumin <1.5 g /dl) and appeared to be in hypovolemic shock with circulatory failure. The presence of small hearts and low cardiac filling pressures did not suggest the presence of typical heart failure.

Keys and associates measured cardiac output by an indirect radiographic technique in adult men voluntarily subsisting on a semistarvation regime. A significant reduction in heart rate, stroke volume, and cardiac output developed in these cachectic subjects, although cardiac output did not appear to decline out of proportion to their lowered metabolic requirements.[57] Two recent studies in protein-calorie undernourished adults have utilized echocardiography to directly measure left ventricular function. Heymsfield and associates,[70] studying patients with PCU secondary to diverse chronic diseases, found that absolute values for stroke volume and cardiac output were depressed, but when cardiac output was adjusted for body weight the resultant indices were equivalent to those of normal height-matched adult controls. The cachectic patients in this investigation demonstrated normal or slightly enhanced left ventricular function (e.g., ejection fraction or circumferential fiber shortening velocity). In the study of Gottdiener et al., patients with anorexia nervosa were studied as a prototype of uncomplicated adult marasmus,[61] and in that sense, they resembled the emaciated men studied by Keys and colleagues. Systolic ejection phase indexes of ventricular function (e.g., percentage of fractional shortening) were normal in all patients. Furthermore, these women with anorexia nervosa were able to augment left ventricular ejection fraction in a normal fashion in response to exercise stress. There was no evidence of congestive heart failure or ventricular dysfunction in these undernourished adults.

In summary, hemodynamic studies in malnourished children and adults suggest that the bradycardia, hypotension, and low cardiac output are secondary to the general depression in metabolic rate and oxygen consumption.[7,44] These metabolic and circulatory adjustments in PCU may, in turn, be mediated by a central depression of sympathetic nervous activity[46,49] and a relative state of hypothyroidism resulting from depressed levels of active thyroid hormone.[45,47]

Several studies of cardiac function have been performed in animal models of PCU. Total blood volume, red blood cell volume, and cardiac output declined progressively in proportion to body weight in undernourished dogs.[83] Abel and colleagues found that severe PCU in dogs was associated with myofiber atrophy and marked myocardial intestitial edema.[73] In these animals, left ventricular function was evaluated in an isovolumic preparation during cardiopulmonary bypass. Ventricular compliance was decreased, and calculated force-velocity data suggested a depression of left ventricular contractility. A kwashiorkor-like state resulting in cardiac atrophy without evidence of myocardial edema was produced by Kyger and associates in rats fed an isocaloric, protein-free diet.[84] When left ventricular function curves were prepared from hemodynamic measurements in the isolated perfused hearts of these animals, ventricular contractility appeared normal at physiologic ventricular filling pressures. Although ventricular contractility was depressed at unphysiologically high filling pressures, the methods employed did not allow preload (end-diastolic volume) to be matched between the atrophic hearts of experimental animals and the normal-sized hearts of control animals. Nutter et al. produced chronic PCU in rats whose atrophic hearts did not exhibit either edema or histologic abnormalities.[69] When hemodynamics were measured on the in situ hearts of these rats, bradycardia, systemic hypotension, and depressed cardiac output were found. However, when cardiac output was adjusted for body weight, the resultant index was normal. Preparation of ventricular function curves that employed stroke-work index did not demonstrate a loss of functional reserve capacity in these hearts.

The possible effects of undernutrition on myocardial stiffness and contractility have been investigated in isolated myocardium from PCU rats. Cohen et al.[21] and Nutter et al.[69] produced chronic PCU in rats of 6 to 7 weeks' duration without significant vitamin or mineral deprivation. Neither of these studies demonstrated an alteration in passive myocardial stiffness. Myocardial contractility measured in the left ventricular papillary muscle of these undernourished rats was augmented, and the duration of contraction was prolonged. The primary purpose of Cohen's study was to determine the effect of thiamine deficiency on myocardial mechanics. In contrast to PCU, thiamine deficiency depressed myocardial contractility and shortened the duration of contraction.[21] Myocardial contractility was also enhanced in rats starved for periods of 1 to 7 days when the isometric mechanics of atrial[85] and left ventricular papillary muscle[69] were studied.

The present information concerning the effects of undernutrition on the heart leads to the following conclusions: (1) When the chronic marasmic state in human beings or animals is not complicated by myocardial damage or edema, passive and active myocardial mechanics are normal and myocardial contractility may even be enhanced. At the same time a hypodynamic circulatory state develops that is characterized by bradycardia, hypotension, and low cardiac output. This represents an adaptation to the general state of hypometabolism present in marasmic subjects. Ventricular pump function adjusted for body mass is normal under these conditions. (2) The presence of interstitial edema or myofiber damage secondary to severe protein deprivation, or complicating factors such as thiamine deficiency or severe chronic anemia, may result in decreased myocardial compliance, decreased contractility, and true cardiac failure. In addition, circulatory collapse may occur in the advanced stage of chronic undernutrition or starvation.

CARDIOVASCULAR EVENTS DURING RECOVERY FROM PROTEIN-CALORIE UNDERNUTRITION

Starvation is generally characterized by a "quiescent" cardiovascular system: angina and hypertension may resolve, the pulse is slow, heart sounds are reduced, and congestive heart failure is rare.[86] This situation is reversed during early recovery, when the circulation must respond to the augmented requirements of intercurrent infections, new tissue deposition, and sudden increases in dietary sodium, nitrogen and calories. It is not surprising, therefore, that the first few weeks of recovery are occasionally punctuated by bouts of congestive heart failure or arrhythmias.[4,6,7,11,13,57,61a,72,74] Because the repletion process itself is so variable, and the number of cardiovascular investigations during realimentation so few, the following discussion examines three specific recovery patterns: (1) slow recovery in the adult by gradually increasing oral feedings, (2) rapid nutritional repletion of the adult by enteral or parenteral hyperalimentation, and (3) recovery of the child with PCU.

Slow Recovery in the Adult

EPIDEMIOLOGY

Cardiac abnormalities rarely develop in the adult recovering gradually from prolonged semistarvation. One case, however, is worthy of mention, as it is often cited as an example of recovery heart failure. The individual was one of Keys' 32 volunteers recuperating from 6 months of a famine-like diet.[7] This man at first consumed gradually increasing quantities of food; however, upon release after 12 weeks of recovery, he began to gorge himself and maintained a caloric intake of 7,000 to 10,000 cal per day for a week. A state resembling congestive heart failure developed, which was easily managed by salt restriction and diuretics. This case actually resembles the occasional heart failure seen during the rapid recovery of undernourished adults undergoing hyperalimentation, which will be discussed in more detail below.

CLINICAL OBSERVATIONS

As the chronically undernourished adult patient responds to increasing caloric intake, a general feeling of well-being is restored. Physical examination now reveals moisture and warmth of the extremities and resolving starvation edema.[57,70] Fluctuating edema in previously nonedematous subjects is not rare and is usually noncardiac in origin.[70] Pulse, blood pressure, and body temperature are restored to normal at approximately the same rate as body weight.[57] These findings are exemplified by the patient recovering from near-fatal PCU secondary to anorexia nervosa, as shown in Fig. 2.

Most electrocardiographic abnormalities have resolved by the time body weight is restored;[60] QRS and T axes move toward the left, QRS and T voltages enlarge, and T wave abnormalities resolve. The notable exception is the Q-T interval. The typical electrocardiographic changes observed in a patient with anorexia nervosa during starvation and recovery from PCU are presented in Fig. 3.

METABOLIC CHANGES

Important metabolic and compartmental adjustments parallel the increased dietary intake. The metabolic rate rises more rapidly than the body weight because there is increased oxygen consumption per unit of tissue and because the total cell mass is enlarging.[39,44] The depressed serum T_3 returns rapidly to prestarvation levels.[45] No information is available on sympathetic activity during recovery of cachectic human beings, but the depressed norepinephrine turnover in the rat heart following a short period of total starvation increases rapidly to or above base-line values when eating is resumed.[46]

It will be recalled that the PCU subject is relatively overhydrated. As recovery in the adult progresses, absolute plasma volume (and extracellular fluid) remains unchanged or expands slightly, and thus increasing body weight is accomplished by a falling plasma volume index.[49] Red blood cell mass is restored at the same rate as lean body mass, and thus hematocrit values rise.

CARDIAC SIZE

The reduced cardiac mass and chamber volumes of PCU subjects gradually enlarge in proportion to increases in body weight. Gottdiener and associates, studying patients recovering from anorexia nervosa, found echocardiographic aortic, left atrial, and ventricular end-diastolic dimensions, and left ventricular mass increased at the same rate as body weight.[61] The enlarging cardiac mass and chamber dimensions are apparent clinically as an enlarging radiographic cardiac silhouette (Fig. 4).

CARDIAC FUNCTION

Evaluation of hemodynamics and ventricular function during recovery has been a subject of considerable interest, because it has been proposed that the "stress" of refeeding unmasks latent left ventricular pump dysfunction, resulting in heart failure.[60] Keys and coworkers examined cardiac output and stroke volume by a radiographic method in human volunteers subjected to 6 months of semistarvation followed by an equal period of gradual recuperation.[60] When body weight had been fully restored, cardiac output remained below prestarvation levels by about 10 percent. This was caused by a reduction in calculated stroke volume (and stroke work), since heart rate was above base-line levels. The authors interpreted these findings as an impairment in cardiac function and proposed that "the heart was closer to failure during early rehabilitation than in starvation." In a more recent study, Gottdiener and coworkers used echocardiography to examine left ventricular function (percentage of fractional shortening) in patients recovering from anorexia nervosa.[61] All subjects had values within normal limits, and these authors concluded that systolic left ventricular ejection performance was unimpaired. Figure 5 demonstrates, by echocardiography, the enlarging cardiac mass, increasing cardiac output, and normal systolic ejection function of a patient recovering from severe undernutrition.

From these two investigations we can conclude that (1) during slow recovery from uncomplicated adult PCU, congestive failure is rare, and (2) noninvasive radiographic and echocardiographic evaluation of cardiac function is normal or near normal.

Rapid Recovery in the Adult Undergoing Enteral or Parenteral Hyperalimentation

EPIDEMIOLOGY

Modern nutritional methods now permit the rapid repletion of the emaciated individual, who usually has

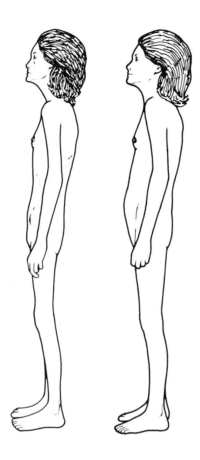

	Baseline Starvation	Partial Recovery	Normal
Caloric Intake (Kcal/day)	340	1950	1700-2000 *
Body Weight (Kg)	30	41.3	50*
Basal Temperature (°C)	34.4	36.8	35-37
Heart Rate (beats/min)	40	68	> 60
Blood Pressure (mmHg)	72/58	90/58	115/75
Basal Oxygen Consumption (cc/min)	103	143	185 *
Serum T$_3$ (ng/dl)	<32	126	60-170

*normal value expected for ideal body weight

FIGURE 2 Patient with marasmus-like condition resulting from anorexia nervosa. On admission (left), this 16-year-old girl suffered from near fatal starvation characterized by pallor, bradycardia, hypotension, hypothermia, and subnormal serum T$_3$ level. Despite these profound abnormalities, the patient continued to obsessively perform many hours of calisthenic exercises daily, without apparent difficulty. A short course of subclavian hyperalimentation and psychotherapy resulted in an improved outlook. Partial recovery (right) with improvement of clinical findings was evident 4 months following admission. The electrocardiogram, chest x-ray, and echocardiogram from this patient are presented in Figs. 3 through 5.

PCU secondary to underlying disease, by enteral or parenteral hyperalimentation.[87-90] This technique is capable of providing anywhere from one to six times the recommended daily allowance for all essential nutrients, depending on the therapeutic goal. Congestive heart failure during hyperalimentation is relatively infrequent, occurring in less than 1 percent of patients overall. However, when rates of repletion are rapid, when emaciation is particularly severe, when underlying heart disease is present, or when the treatment diet contains excessive sodium, heart failure becomes unpredictably more frequent.[70]

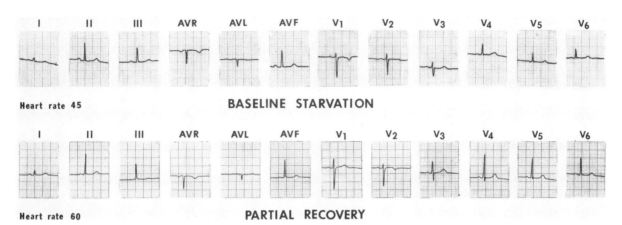

FIGURE 3 Electrocardiographic tracings prepared during the base-line starvation state (top) and following partial recovery (bottom) in the patient with anorexia presented in Fig. 2. Note the following: during recovery the sinus bradycardia of starvation has resolved, the QRS and T amplitudes have increased, the Q-T interval remains unchanged at 0.4 s (normal < 0.42), and the Q-T$_c$ (Q-T/$\sqrt{RR}$) has lengthened from 0.35 to 0.4 s (normal < 0.43). (See text for further discussion.)

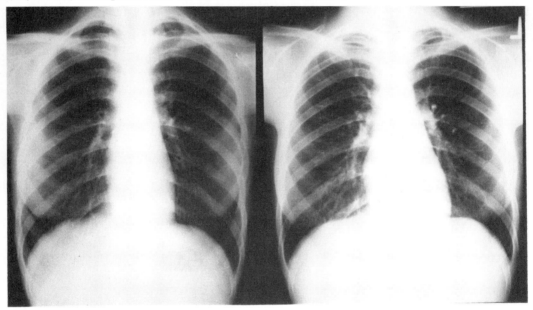

	Baseline Starvation	Partial Recovery	Normal *
Radiographic[†] Heart Volume (cc)	350	430	500

[†] Keats TE and Enge I. P.:   Radiology 85: 850, 1965
*Normal Value expected for ideal body weight

FIGURE 4 Chest roentgenogram during baseline starvation and partial recovery in the patient with anorexia nervosa presented in Figure 2. Note the increase in the cardiac silhouette and radiographic heart volume with partial recovery. Both enlarging chamber volumes and myocardial mass contribute to the expanding heart shadow, as shown in the echocardiogram presented in Figure 5.

204

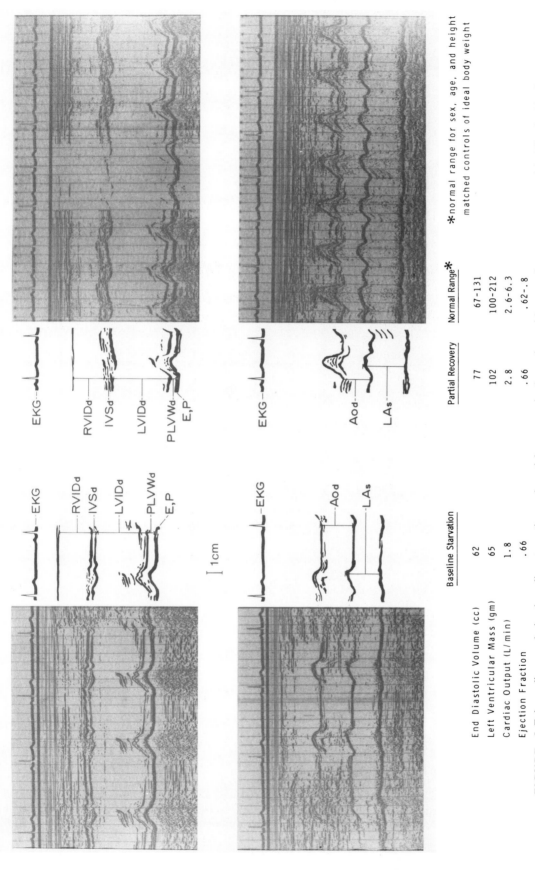

	Baseline Starvation	Partial Recovery	Normal Range*
End Diastolic Volume (cc)	62	77	67-131
Left Ventricular Mass (gm)	65	102	100-212
Cardiac Output (L/min)	1.8	2.8	2.6-6.3
Ejection Fraction	.66	.66	.62-.8

*normal range for sex, age, and height matched controls of ideal body weight

FIGURE 5 Echocardiogram during base-line starvation and partial recovery in the patient with anorexia nervosa presented in Fig. 2. Absolute end-diastolic volume, left ventricular mass, and cardiac output are depressed (for height) in the starving state (left), but all increase into the normal range with partial recovery (right). Left ventricular systolic ejection function, as represented by ejection fraction, is normal in both examinations. Aod, aortic diastolic dimension. E, epicardium. EKG, electrocardiogram. IVSd, interventricular septal diastolic dimension. LAs, left atrial systolic dimension. LVIDd, left ventricular diastolic dimension. P, pericardium. PLVWd, posterior left ventricular wall diastolic dimension.

CLINICAL OBSERVATIONS

Symptomatically, the undernourished medical or surgical patient undergoing hyperalimentation responds much in the same manner as do those who are recuperating more slowly. On physical examination, however, pulse rate recovers more rapidly than body weight, and in some cases the characteristic bradycardia is quickly supplanted by a tachycardia. This is discussed in more detail below. Hypothermia, if present, resolves rapidly, but blood pressure remains low.[70]

METABOLIC CHANGES

Abrupt changes in metabolic activity and plasma volume occur during rapid rates of hyperalimentation, unlike the more gradual normalization seen with slow recovery. Heymsfield and coworkers found a dose-related augmentation of basal metabolic rate, as measured by total-body oxygen consumption, in patients undergoing subclavian hyperalimentation.[70,91] At high daily doses of the standard 1,800 mOsm solution[87,89] (50 to 60 kcal/kg) infused over 24h, metabolic rate rose 75 to 100 percent over base-line levels. This hypermetabolic state is quickly reversible with termination of therapy. These investigators also detected a modest enlargement of plasma volume by 10 to 15 percent during the first 2 weeks of therapy, perhaps related to the high sodium content of the infusate (2 to 4 g/day).

CARDIAC SIZE

The size of the heart increases rapidly under these conditions, primarily as a result of an expansion of chamber volumes; left ventricular mass continues to replete at the same rate as body weight.[70]

CARDIAC FUNCTION

Cardiac output (approximated by echocardiography) closely parallels the rise in metabolic rate and may return to or exceed the normal range before body weight is restored. Indexes of systolic ejection function, e.g., ejection fraction, remain normal. Under the conditions of rapid repletion, 2 of the 5 patients studied developed a state resembling congestive heart failure characterized by hypermetabolism, ventricular gallop, augmented cardiac output, and normal ejection fraction. Rapid resolution followed diuretic therapy, a slower rate of hyperalimentation, and a reduction in the daily intake of sodium.

From this study, we can conclude that (1) rapid refeeding of the cachectic patient with high doses of hyperalimentation may result in a rapid 50 to 100 percent increase in total-body oxygen consumption and cardiac output, and a 10 to 15 percent enlargement of plasma volume before recovery of cardiac mass and body weight; (2) despite this augmented metabolic load on the heart, systolic ejection function remains normal; and (3) some patients develop a state resembling congestive heart failure of unknown mechanism.

Recovery of the Child with Protein-Calorie Undernutrition

EPIDEMIOLOGY

Most cases of heart failure or sudden death during recovery from PCU have been reported in children with marasmus or kwashiorkor.[11–13,15,92] The congestive symptoms usually appear during the first week of therapy, at a time when fever, infections, sepsis, anemia, and severe electrolyte and fluid disturbances are common. In some cases, sudden death may occur during an otherwise uneventful course, possibly as a result of arrhythmias.[11] The exact frequency of cardiac complications during nutritional rehabilitation varies among geographic regions and treatment centers. In Smythe's series, 13 of 98 PCU infants died, and the authors speculate that hypervolemia caused by mobilization of edema fluid and severe anemia imposed an excessive burden on the atrophic myocardium.[11] A similar mechanism has been proposed by Wharton's group in Uganda[12,15] who detected 32 cases of heart failure in children recuperating from kwashiorkor. When the high sodium intake (6 mEq/kg daily) was lowered (1 mEq/kg daily), the incidence of heart failure was significanty reduced. In Edozien's series, 20 percent of Nigerian children with PCU fed high doses of milk protein developed heart failure.[92] When the daily protein intake was lowered, or when the child received a high protein diet with low sodium content or diuretics, heart failure became rare.

CLINICAL OBSERVATIONS

The child recovering from PCU is frequently beset with a wide range of infectious[11–13,15,92] and metabolic complications during the first few weeks of hospitalization. Otherwise the pattern of recovery resembles that in the adult.

METABOLIC CHANGES

The basal metabolic rate during the first year of recovery of the undernourished child is increased when compared to normally nourished children of the same age.[44] This is to be expected, since the child who is recovering from PCU is growing at a rate much above the normal child of similar age.

In contrast to the adult, a marked increase in plasma volume may occur during the early phase of recovery from marasmus or kwashiorkor.[11,53,92] Dietary sodium restriction limits, but does not prevent the plasma volume from expanding.

CARDIAC SIZE

The only information available on heart size during recovery of the child with PCU is the radiographic cardiothoracic (CT) ratio. In both Wharton's[11] and Smyth's[12] series, the CT ratio rapidly increased, especially during the first week of therapy.

CARDIAC FUNCTION

Alleyne, studying severely undernourished Jamaican children, found that dye dilution cardiac output actually exceeded expected normal age-matched values following recovery.[82] The author speculates that this may be related to the increased metabolic rate and "catch-up" growth observed in these children. Using a flow-guided catheter technique, Viart studied ventricular function and hemodynamics for up to 2 months after admission of severely undernourished African children.[93] The recovered state (2 months) was characterized by a short circulation time, low vascular resistance, and narrow arteriovenous differences in blood oxygen content. Absolute cardiac output and cardiac index were both increased over base-line values. The author concluded that a relative "hyperkinetic" circulatory state replaces the hypokinetic circulation of starvation. Although no mechanism was proposed, these children may be entering the "catch-up" growth phase, with consequent increased metabolic and cardiac demands.

In summary, the child recovering from PCU appears to be at high risk for developing cardiac abnormalities during the repletion process. The studies reviewed permit four general conclusions: (1) Hypervolemia, which is potentially reversible by restricting dietary sodium, is a probable cause of congestive heart failure in the early recovery period. (2) Fever, sepsis, pneumonia, and electrolyte imbalance may all contribute to or aggravate circulatory abnormalities. (3) Late recovery (months) is characterized by a "hyperkinetic" circulatory state. (4) The mechanism of occasional sudden death during treatment, although possibly resulting from arrhythmia, is unknown.

REFERENCES

1 Leevy, C. M., Cardi, L., Frank, O., et al.: Incidence and Significance of Hypovitaminemia in a Randomly Selected Municipal Hospital Population, *Am. J. Clin. Nutr.,* 17:259, 1965.

2 Bistrian, B. R., Blackburn, G. L., Hallowell, E., et al.: Protein Status of General Surgical Patients, *J.A.M.A.,* 230:858, 1974.

3 Bistrian, B. R.,Blackburn, G. L., Vitale, J., Cochran, D., and Naylor, J.: Prevalence of Malnutrition in General Medical Patients, *J.A.M.A.,* 235:1567, 1976.

4 Hill, G. L., Pickford, I., Young, G. A., Schorah, C. J., Blackett, R. L., Burkinshaw, L., Warren, J. V., and Morgan, D. B.: Malnutrition in Surgical Patients. An Unrecognized Problem, *Lancet,* 2:689, 1977.

5 Voit, C.: Ube die Verschiedenheiten der Erweisszersetzung being Hungern, *Z. Biol.,* 2:309, 1866.

6 Keys, A., Brozak, J., Wenschel, A., et al.: In "The Biology of Human Starvation," University of Minnesota Press, Minneapolis, 1950, p. 202.

7 Keys, A., Henschel, A., and Taylor, H. L.: The Size and Function of the Human Heart at Rest in Semi-starvation and in Subsequent Rehabilitation, *Am. J. Physiol.,* 50:153, 1947.

8 Scrimshaw, N. S., and Behar, M.: Malnutrition in Underdeveloped Countries, *N. Engl. J. Med.,* 272:137, 1965.

9 Williams, C. D.: A Nutritional Disease of Childhood Associated with a Maize Diet, *Arch. Dis. Child.,* 8:423, 1933.

10 Williams, C. D.: Kwashiorkor, *Lancet,* 2:1151, 1935.

11 Smythe, P. M., Swanepoel, A., and Campbell, J. A. H.: The Heart in Kwashiorkor, *Br. Med. J.,* 7:67, 1962.

12 Wharton, B. A., Balmer, S. E., Somers, K., and Templeton, A. C.: The Myocardium in Kwashiorkor, *Q. J. Med.,* 38:107, 1969.

13 Piza, J., Troper, L., Cespedes, R., Miller, J. H., and Berenson, G. S.: Myocardial Lesions and Heart Failure in Infantile Malnutrition, *Am. J. Trop. Med. Hyg.,* 20:343, 1971.

14 Sims, B. A.: Conducting Tissue of the Heart in Kwashiorkor, *Br. Heart J.,* 34:828, 1972.

15 Wharton, B. A., Howels, G. R., and McCance, R. A.: Cardiac Failure in Kwashiorkor, *Lancet,* 2:384, 1967.

16 Crawford, M. A.: Endomyocardial Fibrosis and Carcinoidoses. A Common Denominator? *Am. Heart J.,* 66:273, 1963.

17 Crawford, M. A., Gale, M. M, Somers, K., and Han-

sen, I. L.: Studies on Plasma Amino Acids in East African Adults in Relation to Endomyocardial Fibrosis, *Br. J. Nutr.,* 24:393, 1970.

18 Reid, J. V. O., and Berjak, P.: Dietary Production of Myocardial Fibrosis in the Rat, *Am. Heart J.,* 71:240, 1966.

19 McKinney, B., and Crawford, M. A.: Fibrosis in Guineapig Heart Produced by Plantain Diet, *Lancet,* 2:880, 1965.

20 Samen, S.: Cardiac Disorders in Scurvy, *N. Engl. J. Med.,* 282:282, 1970.

20a Shafar, J.: Rapid Reversion of Electrocardiographic Abnormalities after Treatment in Two Cases of Scurvy, *Lancet,* 2:176, 1967.

21 Cohen, E. M., Abelmann, W. H., Messer, J. V., and Bing, O. H. L.: Mechanical Properties of Rat Cardiac Muscle During Experimental Thiamine Deficiency, *Am. J. Physiol.,* 231:1390, 1976.

22 Akbarian, M., Yankopoulos, N. A., and Abelmann, W H.: Hemodynamic Studies in Beriberi Heart Disease, *Am. J. Med.,* 41:197, 1966.

22a Rachmilewitz, M., and Braun, K.: Electrocardiographic Changes and the Effect of Niacin Therapy in Pellagra, *Br. Heart J.,* 7:72, 1945.

22b Bragdon, J. H., and Levine, H. D.: Myocarditis in Vitamin E Deficient Rabbits, *Am. J. Pathol.,* 25:265, 1949.

23 Weiss, D. L., Surawicz, B., and Rubenstein, I.: Myocardial Lesions of Calcium Deficiency Causing Irreversible Myocardial Failure, *Am. J Pathol.,* 48:653, 1966.

24 O'Connor, L. R., Wheeler, W. S., and Bethune, J. E.: Effect of Hypophosphatemia on Myocardial Performance in Man, *N. Engl. J. Med.,* 297:901, 1977.

25 Fuller, T. J., Nichols, W. W., Brenner, B. J., and Petersen, J. C.: Reversible Depression in Myocardial Contractility in the Dog with Experiments Phosphorous Deficiency, *Clin. Res.,* 26:33A, 1978.

26 Chipperfield, B., and Chipperfield, J. R.: Magnesium Content of Normal Heart Muscle in Areas of Hard and Soft Water, *Lancet,* 1;121, 1976.

27 Wacker, W. E. C., and Parisi, A. F.: Magnesium Metabolism, *N. Engl. J. Med.* 278:658, 1968.

28 Wener, J., Pintar, K., Simon, M. A., Motala, R., Friedman, R., Mayman, A., and Schucher, R.: The Effects of Prolonged Hypomagnesemia on the Cardiovascular System in Young Dogs, *Am. Heart J.,* 67:221, 1964.

29 Shields, G. S., Coulson, W. F., Kimball, D. A., Carnes, N. H., Cartwright, G. E., and Wintrobe, M. M.: Cardiovascular Lesions in Copper Deficient Swine, *Am. J. Pathol.,* 41:603, 1962.

30 Voni, N. K.: The Myocardium in Periodic Paralysis, *Postgrad. Med. J.,* 45:691,1969.

31 Weaver, W. F., and Burchell, H. B.: Serum Potassium and the Electrocardiogram in Hypokalemia, *Circulation,* 21:505, 1960.

31a Follis, R. H., Orent, K. E., McCollum, E. V.: The Production of Cardiac and Renal Lesions in Rats by a Diet Extremely Deficient in Potassium, *Am. J. Pathol.,* 18:29–39, 1942.

31b Molnar, Z., Larsen, K., Spargo, B.: Cardiac Changes in the Potassium Depleted Rat, *Arch. Path.,* 74:339–347, 1962.

31c Perkins, J. G., Petersen, A. B., Riley, J. A.: Renal and Cardiac Lesions in Potassium Deficiency Due to Chronic Diarrhea, *Am. J. Med.,* 8:115–123, 1950.

31d Rodriguez, C. E., Wolfe, A. L., Bergstrom, V. W.: Hypokalemic Myocarditis: Report of Two Cases, *Am. J. Clin. Path.,* 20:1050–1055, 1950.

31e Keye, J. D.: Death in Potassium Deficiency: Report of a Case Including Morphologic Findings, *Circulation,* 5:766–770, 1952.

31f McAllen, P. M.: Myocardial Changes Occurring in Potassium Deficiency, *Brit. Heart J.* 17:5–14, 1955.

32 VanFleet, J. F., Ferrans, V. J., and Ruth, G. R.: Ultrastructural Alterations in Nutritional Cardiomyopathy of Selenium-Vitamin E Deficient Swime, *Lab. Invest.,* 37:188, 1977.

33 Alexander, J. K.: Obesity and the Circulation, *Mod. Concepts Cardiovasc. Dis.,* 32:799, 1963.

34 Harrison, D. C., and Nelson, D.: The Effects of Calcium on Isometric Tension in Isolated Heart Muscle During Coupled Pacing, *Am. Heart J.,* 74:663, 1967.

35 Skinner, C., and Kenmure, A. C. F.: Haemochromatosis Presenting as Congestive Cardiomyopathy and Responding to Venesection, *Br. Heart J.,* 35:466, 1973.

36 Wacker, W. E. C., and Parisi, A. F.: Magnesium Metabolism, *N. Engl. J. Med.,* 278:712, 1978.

37 Surawicz, B.: Relationship between Electrocardiogram and Electrolytes, *Am. Heart. J.,* 73:814, 1967.

38 Rona, G.,: Experimental Aspects of Cobalt Cardiomyopathy, *Br. Heart J.,* 33 (suppl.):171, 1971.

38a Boner, J. M., and Freyberg, R. H.,: Vitamin D Intoxication with Metastatic Calcification, *J.A.M.A.,* 130, 1208, 1946.

39 Alleyne, G. A. O., Hay, R. W., Picou, D. I., Stanfeld, J. P. and Whitehead, R. G.: ''Protein-Energy Malnutrition,'' Butler and Tanner Ltd., London, 1977, p. 26.

40 Whitehead, R. G., and Alleyne, G. A. O.: Pathophysiological Factors of Importance in Protein-Calorie Malnutrition, *Br. Med. J,* 28:72, 1972.

40a MacDonald, I.: Hepatic Lipid of Malnourished Children, *Metabolism,* 9:838, 1960.

41 Bistrian, B. R.: Interaction of Nutrition and Infection in the Hospital Setting, *Am. J. Clin. Nutr.,* 30:1228, 1977.

42 Butterworth, C. E., and Blackburn, G. L.: "Hospital Malnutrition and How to Assess the Nutritional Status of a Patient," Nutrition Today, Inc., Annapolis, 1974.

43 Braunwald, E.: "Mechanisms of Contraction of the Normal and Failing Heart," Little, Brown and Company, Boston, 1968.

44 Montgomery, R. D.: Changes in the Basal Metabolic Rate of the Malnourished Infant and their Relation to Body Composition, *J. Clin. Invest.,* 41:1653, 1962.

44a Keys, A., Brozak, J., Wenschel, A., et al.: In "The Biology of Human Starvation," University of Minnesota Press, Minneapolis, 1950, p. 303.

45 Schimmel, M., and Utiger, R. D.: Thyroidal and Peripheral Production of Thyroid Hormones, *Ann. Intern. Med.,* 87:760, 1977.

46 Landsberg, L., and Young, J. B.: Fasting, Feeding and Regulation of the Sympathetic Nervous System, *N. Engl. J. Med.,* 298:1295, 1978.

47 Schussler, G. C., and Orlando, J.: Fasting Decreases Triiodothyronine Receptor Capacity, *Science,* 199:686, 1978.

48 Balasubramanian, V., and Dhalla, N. S.: Biochemical Basis of Heart Function. V. Effect of Starvation on Storage, Transport, and Synthesis of Cardiac Norepinephrine in Rats, *Can. J. Physiol. Pharmacol.,* 50:238, 1972.

49 Henschel, A., Mickelsen, O., Taylor, H. L., and Keys, A.: Plasma Volume and Thiocynate Space in Famine Edema and Recovery, *Am. J. Physiol.,* 50:170, 1947.

50 Brinkman, G. L., Bowie, M. D., Friis-Hansen, B. J., and Hansen, J. D. L.: Body Water Composition in Kwashiorkor before and after Loss of Edema, *Pediatrics,* 36:94, 1965.

51 Alleyne, G. A. O.: Plasma and Blood Volumes in Severely Malnourished Jamaican Children, *Arch. Dis. Child.,* 41:313, 1960.

52 Zoumboulakis, D., Anagnostakis, D., Kossoglou, K., Agathopoulos, A., and Tsenghi, C.: Plasma and Blood Volumes in Severely Malnourished Infants, *Acta Paediatr. Scand.,* 63:507, 1974.

53 Viart, P.: Blood Volume Changes during Treatment of Protein-Calorie Malnutrition, *Am. J. Clin. Nutr.,* 30:349, 1977.

54 Alleyne, G. A. O., Hay, R. W., Picou, D. I., Stanfield, J. P., and Whitehead, R. G.: "Protein-Energy Malnutrition," Butler and Tanner Ltd., London, 1977, p. 41.

55 Brozek, J., Chapman, C. B., and Keys, A.: Drastic Food Restriction, *J.A.M.A.,* 137:1569, 1948.

56 McKiney, B.: "Pathology of the Cardiomyopathies. XIV. Metabolic Disease," Butterworth and Co. (Publishers) Ltd., London, 1974, p. 362.

57 Keys, A., Brozak, J., Wehschel, A., et al.: In "The Biology of Human Starvation," University of Minnesota Press, Minneapolis, 1950, p. 607.

58 Viart, P.: Hemodynamic Findings in Severe Protein-Calorie Malnutrition, *Am. J. Clin. Nutr.,* 30:334, 1977.

59 Schnitker, M. A., Mattmen, P. E., and Bliss, T. L.: A Clinical Study of Malnutrition in Japanese Prisoners of War, *Ann. Intern. Med.,* 35:69, 1951.

60 Simonson, E., Henschel, A. J., and Keys, A. The Electrocardiogram of Man in Semi-starvation and Subsequent Rehabilitation, *Am. Heart J.,* 35:584, 1948.

61 Gottdiener, J. S., Gross, H. A., Henry, W. L., Borer, J. S., and Ebert, M. H.: Effects of Self-induced Starvation on Cardiac Size and Function in Anorexia Nervosa, *Circulation,* 58:425, 1978.

62 Thurston, J., and Marks, P.: Electrocardiographic Abnormalities in Patients with Anorexia Nervosa, *Br. Heart J.,* 36:719, 1974.

63 Piza, J., Troper, L., Cespedes, R., Miller, J. H., and Berenson, G. S.: Myocardial Lesions and Heart Failure in Infantile Malnutrition, *Am. J. Trop. Med. Hyg.,* 20:343, 1970.

64 Chauhan, S., Nayak, N. C., and Ramalingaswami, V.: The Heart and Skeletal Muscle in Experimental Protein Malnutrition in Rhesus Monkeys, *J. Pathol. Bacteriol.,* 90:301, 1965.

65 Deo, M. G., Sood, S. K., and Ramalingaswami, V.: Experimental Protein Deficiency, *Arch. Pathol.,* 80:14, 1965.

66 Racela, A. S., Jr., Grady, H. J., Higginson, J., and Svoboda, D. J.: Protein Deficiency in Rhesus Monkeys, *Am. J. Pathol.,* 49:419, 1966.

67 Svoboda, D., Grady, H., and Higginson, J.: The Effects of Chronic Protein Deficiency in Rats, *Lab. Invest.,* 15:731, 1966.

68 Ford, L. E.: Heart Size, *Circ. Res.,* 39:297, 1976.

69 Nutter, D. O., Heymsfield, S. R., Murray, T. G., and Fuller, E. O.: Cardiac Dynamics and Myocardial Contractility in Chronic Protein-Calorie Undernutition, *Clin. Res.,* 26:256A, 1978.

70 Heymsfield, S. B., Bethel, R. A., Ansley, J. D., Gibbs, D. M., Felner, J. M., and Nutter, D. O.: Cardiac Abnormalities in Cachectic Patients before and during Nutritional Repletion, *Am. Heart J.,* 95:584, 1978.

71 Beznak, M.: The Behavior of the Weight of the Heart and the Blood Pressure of Albino Rats Under Different Conditions, *J. Physiol.,* 124:44, 1954.

72 Thomas, J., Josserand, C., Chastel, C., Sagnet, H., Lassalle, Y., and LeVourche, C.: Les Manifestations Cardiovasculaires au Cours de la Malnutrition Protidique, *Med. Trop.,* 32:505, 1972.

73 Abel, R. M., Grimes, J. B., Alonso, D., Alonso, M. L., and Gay, W. H. L., Jr.: Adverse Hemodynamic and Ultrastructural Changes in Dog Hearts Subjected to

Protein-Calorie Malnutrition, *Circulation,* (suppl. 3): 55, 1977.

74 Ellis, L. B.: Electrocardiographc Abnormalities in Severe Malnutrition, *Br. Heart J.,* 8:53, 1946.

75 Keys, A., Brozak, J., Wenschel, A., et al.: In "The Biology of Human Starvation," University of Minnesota Press, Minneapolis, 1950, p. 206.

76 Winick, M., and Nobel, A.: Quantitative Changes in DNA, RNA, and Protein during Prenatal and Postnatal Growth, *Dev. Biol.,* 12:451, 1965.

77 Kraupp, O., Adler-Kastner, L., Neisser, H., and Plank, B.: The Effects of Starvation and of Acute and Chronic Alloxan Diabetes on Myocardial Substrate Levels and on Liver Glycogen in the Rat in Vivo, *Eur.J. Biochem.,* 2:197, 1967.

78 Gold, A. M., and Yaffe, S. R.: Effects of Prolonged Starvation on Cardiac Energy Metabolism in the Rat, *J. Nutr.,* 108:410, 1978.

79 Lehninger, A. L.: "Biochemistry, XXX. Organ Interrelationships in the Metabolism of Mammals," Worth Publishers, Inc., New York, 1975, p. 839.

80 Obeyesekere, I.: Idiopathic Cardiomegaly in Ceylon, *Br. Heart J.,* 3:226, 1968.

81 Higginson, J., Gillanders, A. D., and Murray, J. F.: The Heart in Chronic Malnutrition, *Br. Heart J.,* 14:213, 1952.

82 Alleyne, G. A. O.: Cardiac Function in Severely Malnourished Jamaican Children, *Clin. Sci.,* 30:553, 1966.

83 Haxhe, J. J.: Experimental Undernutrition, I. Its Effects on Cardiac Output, *Metabolism,* 16:1036, 1967.

84 Kyger, E. R., Block, W. J., Roach, G., and Dudrick, S. J.: Adverse Effects of Protein Malnutrition on Myocardial Function, *Surgery,* 84:147, 1978.

85 Ko, K. C., and Paradise, R. P.: Effect of Prolonged Starvation on the Functional Status of the Isolated Rat Atria, *Proc. Soc. Exp. Biol. Med.,* 141:310, 1972.

86 Keys, A.: Cardiovascular Effects of Undernutrition and Starvation, *Mod. Concepts Cardiovasc. Dis.,* 17:21, 1948.

87 Dudrick, S. J., Wilmore, D. W., Vars, H. M., et al.: Long-term Parenteral Nutrition with Growth Development, and Positive Nitrogen Balance, *Surgery,* 64:134, 1968.

88 Isaacs, J., Millikan, J., Stackhouse, J., et al.: Parenteral Nutrition of Adults with a 900 Milliosmolar Solution via Peripheral Veins, *Am. J. Clin. Nutr.,* 30:552, 1977.

89 Rudman, D., Millikan, J., Richardson, R. J., et al.: Elemental Balances during Intravenous Hyperalimentation of Underweight Adult Subjects, *J. Clin. Invest.,* 55:94, 1975.

90 Rhea, J. W., Ghazzawi, O., and Weidman, W.: Nasojejunal Feeding: An Improved Device and Intubation Technique, *J. Pediatr.,* 82:931, 1973.

91 Heymsfield, S., Chandler, J., and Nutter, D.: Hyperalimentation Causes a Hyperdynamic Hypermetabolic State, *Clin. Res.,* 26:284A, 1978.

92 Edozien, J. C., and Rahim-Khan, M. A.: Anaemia in Protein Malnutrition, *Clin. Sci.,* 34:315, 1968.

93 Viart, P.: Hemodynamic Findings during Treatment of Protein-Calorie Malnutrition, *Am. J. Clin. Nutr.,* 31:911, 1978.

Heart Disease in the Elderly (Geriatric Cardiology)*

R. JOE NOBLE, M.D., F.A.C.C., and
DONALD A. ROTHBAUM, M.D., F.A.C.C.

When the physician said to him, "You have lived to be an old man," he said, "that is because I never employed you as my physician."

PAUSANIAS (fl. 479 B.C.), quoted by Plutarch in Moralia

The principle of minimal interference is paramount in the management of the elderly. The older a patient, the less his way of life should be disturbed.... The older, more rigid personality is like a crystal, easily shattered by unwise impacts.

DAVID SEEGAL[1]

INTRODUCTION

Nearly one-half the population over 65 years of age will present some evidence of heart abnormality, such as previous myocardial infarction, angina pectoris, murmurs, or electrocardiographic abnormalities, and cardiovascular disease is the principal cause of death in the elderly.[1a] Although this sort of epidemiologic data is important in defining population risks and frequency of disease, the information is no help to the clinician in determining whether a specific, elderly patient has cardiac disease, particularly an abnormality which is clinically significant in eliciting symptoms or in requiring therapy or an alteration in life-style. Furthermore, the knowledge that cardiac disease is so common in this group of patients might discourage the physician from recommending an active life for the fit elderly patient, when, in fact, inactivity and deconditioning might actually be the *cause,* not the result, of much cardiac disability.

Thus, this chapter does not consider geriatric cardiology in terms of population studies of epidemiology or pathology; instead, it approaches the elderly patient with possible cardiac disease much as the physician would—by considering symptoms of heart disease (*cardiac pain, heart failure, syncope*); physical findings (*murmurs* or *hypertension*); or *electrocardiographic* abnormalities.

As a general rule, cardiac disease in the elderly differs only quantitatively, not qualitatively, from that in younger patients. The same diseases occur in the elderly, but do so with greater frequency and, in some instances, with greater severity because of the longer period over which the pathologic state has developed. Certain disease states are peculiar to the geriatric population, but these are the distinct minority. Physicians must approach geriatric *patients* a bit differently than they would younger patients, since the old patients may respond differently to various diagnostic or therapeutic maneuvers. However, clinicians approach the *disease* the same as they would approach it in a younger patient, since the pathophysiology is basically the same.

CHEST PAIN: CORONARY ARTERY DISEASE

Coronary artery disease accounts for over 70 percent of the cardiac deaths in the elderly.[2,3] However, the clinical features of acute myocardial infarction in the elderly are often quite subtle: sudden dyspnea or exacerbation of heart failure, acute confusion, stroke or other evidence of systemic embolization, syncope, or profound weakness.[4]

Older patients admitted to a coronary care unit with proved myocardial infarction develop heart block and conduction defects, cardiogenic shock, pulmonary edema, and right-sided heart failure significantly more often than do younger patients. Mortality, both in the coronary care unit and later in the hospitalization, approaches 40 percent in patients over 70 years of age, a rate twice that of younger patients.[5] Even though, in comparison with younger patients, the older patients' infarctions are often larger, their complications more frequent and severe, their hospital stay longer, and their mortality greater, many elderly patients derive the same benefits from the coronary care units as do their younger counterparts.[6,7] The therapy for arrhythmias and for cardiac failure is the same as for younger patients. Caution is indicated in the use of drugs, however, since elderly patients are more likely to develop toxic effects as a result of their low cardiac output and impaired renal, hepatic, and central nervous system function.

* From St. Vincent Hospital and Health Care Center and the Indiana School of Medicine, Indianapolis.

211

Two aspects of myocardial infarction merit special attention in the elderly: painless subendocardial infarction and cardiac rupture. Painless subendocardial infarction is commonly seen in the elderly patient as a result of profound hypotension, anemia, or hypoxemia. In a setting such as septic shock or hemorrhage, the subendocardial damage may be overlooked until malignant ventricular arrhythmias appear. Fortunately, with correction of the precipitating factor, the clinician may avoid extensive, irreversible myocardial damage. Cardiac rupture, an uncommon but catastrophic complication of myocardial infarction, is found most frequently in the elderly.[8] Rupture usually occurs 3 to 12 days after myocardial infarction, is frequently preceded by postinfarction hypotension, is often heralded by the reappearance of chest pain, and is associated with sinus rhythm at the onset of hypotension, i.e., electromechanical dissociation. In an attempt to minimize the possibility of cardiac rupture in the elderly, extreme postinfarction hypertension should be treated and excessive physical activity, such as prolonged forceful straining on the commode, should be avoided.[9]

The diagnosis of angina pectoris may be difficult to establish in the older patient, since the patient's relative inactivity may preclude a convincing history of effort-related discomfort. Furthermore, deconditioning, arthritis or leg claudication may preclude stress testing. However, angina at rest, postprandial angina, or increasing angina with minor activity has the same poor prognostic implication as does unstable angina in a younger patient. Hospitalization, with the recording of ischemic electrocardiographic changes during spontaneous pain, will often prove the diagnosis. The more fit the patient, the more extensive should be the evaluation to determine the presence of coronary disease: stress testing, radionuclide imaging, and coronary cineangiography when the symptoms significantly limit the patient's life-style and activity.

Medical therapy is similar to that in younger patients, although older patients are more sensitive to the side effects of vasodilator and betablocking drugs owing to the greater incidence of compromised baroreceptor reflexes, intrinsic sinus node or atrioventricular node dysfunction, and orthostatic hypotension. Angina at rest, not preceded by tachycardia or hypertension, is unlikely to respond to betablockade. Instead, vasodilators and management of any underlying heart failure are indicated. Effort-related angina or angina associated with hypertension or tachycardia does require beta blockade. Although the prognosis of coronary artery disease is clearly dependent upon the extent of vessel involvement and ventricular function in younger patients, it is not clear that the same prognostic implications hold true in the geriatric population. Elderly patients derive the same symptomatic benefits from coronary artery bypass grafts as do younger patients. Hence, surgical revascularization is justified for the otherwise fit and reasonably active older patient whose angina interferes with his or her life-style despite medical therapy.[10] However, the mortality is higher in the elderly, and a beneficial effect on longevity has not been demonstrated. Until proven otherwise, coronary revascularization does not seem justified in an effort to prolong the life of elderly patients. For such complications of myocardial infarction as ventricular septal perforation, papillary muscle dysfunction, or left ventricular aneurysm, surgery may be indicated for refractory heart failure. However, the geriatric mortality is quite high, and the long-term survival still low.

HEART FAILURE

Physiology

The hemodynamic manifestations of heart failure are a depression of cardiac output and an elevation in left ventricular filling pressure. Aging, per se, seems to be accompanied by the same hemodynamic changes,[11] at least with exercise; yet these changes do not infer that all elderly patients have heart failure.

The degree of depression in cardiac output with age is extremely variable but may approximate 1 percent per year.[11–14] As diagrammed in Fig. 1, cardiac output is the product of heart rate and stroke volume. Although sinus bradycardia is common in the elderly, hemodynamic studies have indicated that the fall in cardiac output with age is the consequence of a decrease in stroke volume rather than in heart rate.[11–14]

The determinants of stroke volume are preload, afterload, and contractile state. Preload, or left ventricular filling pressure, is normal at rest in elderly patients. Contractility is much more difficult to assess. In studies on the senescent animal heart, contractility, as measured by peak tension development and rate of development, was not depressed with age.[15] In animals, however, the duration of isometric contraction was prolonged, and in human beings, the duration of the phase of isovolumic relaxation lengthened with age. In other words, an abnormality in relaxation, or increased "stiffness," of the elderly heart may account for observed abnormalities of muscle function, without inferring a significant abnormality in contractile state.[15] The next consideration is afterload. The increased rigidity or the larger arteries with age increases the impedance or resistance to left ventricular emptying. Increased afterload, therefore, may result in a decrease in stroke volume and hence cardiac output, particularly if there is any subtle abnormality in contractile state.

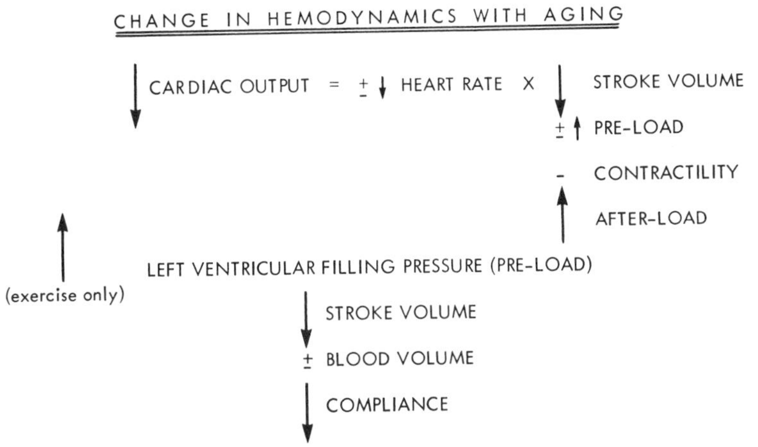

CHANGE IN HEMODYNAMICS WITH AGING

FIGURE 1 Normal hemodynamics of aging. The arrows indicate the changes expected with advancing age; the size of the arrow is proportional to the change.

Finally, with age there is a progressive decrease in body muscle mass and basal metabolic rate. Since cardiac output is generally related to metabolic demands, autoregulatory mechanisms would be expected to decrease cardiac output as a normal, physiologic response to age.[14]

Left ventricular filling pressure is normal at rest in the elderly patient and yet increases abnormally with exercise. This increase is not caused by "heart failure" but by reduced compliance of increased stiffness.[13] Left ventricular filling pressure is also a function of stroke volume, since as stroke volume diminishes, end-systolic volume increases.

Cardiac mass increases with age. By echocardiography, the thickness of the left ventricular posterior wall increases. However, left ventricular cavity size does not change. The E to F slope of the mitral valve also decreases with advanced age; this decrease presumably represents a diminished filling rate owing to increased stiffness of the left ventricle. No change in contractility is seen in a normal, elderly patient.[16] The reason for the increase in ventricular mass and decrease in compliance with age is not entirely clear, but, again, an increase in aortic impedance as a result of increased stiffness of the peripheral vascular tree would provide a reasonable explanation.

If the decrease in cardiac output with age is, in fact, simply a response to the body's need for blood flow, it would be of considerable interest to analyze cardiac output in healthy, conditioned elderly patients. Such studies are not available, but in a limited number of elderly patients undergoing rather intense physical training, there was a distinct increase in maximal oxygen uptake, stroke volume, and cardiac output, with some decrease in heart rate.[14] From limited experimental studies and clinical observations, one may conclude that the abnormal hemodynamics recorded in

elderly patients are, at least in part, the result of deconditioning. In other words, physical inactivity may result in subnormal cardiac performance rather than heart failure leading to a restriction in physical capability. We conclude that an effort should be made not to sentence the elderly patient to a life of inactivity because of "heart failure" with age.

Etiology

The same diseases which produce heart failure in younger patients produce heart failure in the elderly patient—coronary artery disease, valvular heart disease, hypertensive cardiovascular disease, and the cardiomyopathies. Whether or not a "geriatric cardiomyopathy" exists remains debatable. "Presbycardia" has been hypothesized when elderly patients were found to have heart failure without obvious explanation.[17] However, careful clinical and pathologic studies rarely document a specific, clinically significant "presbycardia" of the aged. Senile cardiac amyloidosis is a common pathologic finding; however, the amyloid is usually limited to sparse amounts in atria only, not in the ventricle.[18] Rarely is the pathologic finding of any clinical significance. Similarly, there is an increase in lipofuscin in the elderly heart which is responsible for "brown atrophy."[19] However, this is also of no clinical significance, and atrophic hearts are found only in those elderly patients who have suffered from chronic wasting diseases. Idiopathic sclerosis of the cardiac skeleton resulting in conduction disturbances and valvular abnormalities is seen more commonly in the elderly patient, but this is by no means a universal finding. From the clinical standpoint, it would seem inappropriate to attribute an elderly patient's symptoms of heart failure to "presbycardia." Instead,

TABLE 1
An approach to heart failure

I Determine the pathophysiologic mechanism of heart failure. Is the mechanism *mechanical, myocardial, or pericardial?*
II Eliminate extracardiac factors
  A Hypoxemia
  B Hypertension
  C Anemia and polycythemia
  D Fever and tachycardia
  E Thyrotoxicosis
  F Alcohol
  G Excess sodium
III Rest, digitalis, and diuretics
IV Exclude bradycardia (or other arrhythmia) as a contributory factor
V Vasodilator therapy
VI Consider pulmonary embolization

SOURCE: Based on data of Noble[20] with permission of author and publisher.

the clinician should hunt diligently for evidence of other, more common types of heart disease in an effort to diagnose a treatable condition.

Clinical Approach

The symptoms of heart failure in the elderly patient are the same as those experienced by younger patients: (1) weakness and fatigability (resulting from decreased cardiac output), (2) dyspnea (from pulmonary congestion), and (3) edema. The therapeutic goal is to relieve these symptoms by augmenting cardiac output and alleviating pulmonary congestion and edema.

Table 1 lists a step-by-step approach to the management of heart failure in the elderly.[20] The first step is to determine the mechanism of the heart failure. In general terms, heart failure is caused by one of three mechanisms: a mechanical defect, myocardial failure, or pericardial disease (Table 2). Mechanical defects include intracardiac or extracardiac pressure or volume overload, such as systemic hypertension or valvular lesions. The importance of identifying mechanical defects is that they may be definitely treated either surgically or medically. A careful examination, electrocardiogram, and chest x-ray will usually lead to the proper recognition of the mechanical defect. Although most mechanical defects are relatively easily recognized, a few should be listed, both because they may be overlooked and because they are remediable causes of heart failure in the elderly: atrial septal defect, idiopathic hypertrophic subaortic stenosis, valvular aortic stenosis, and ventricular aneurysm. Myocardial failure is identified by cardiomegaly, the auscultation of gallops, and the radiographic demonstration of car-

diomegaly without specific chamber enlargement but with pulmonary venous congestion. Pericardial effusion is suggested by the combination of venous hypertension, systemic arterial hypotension with or without pulsus paradoxus, a large cardiac silhouette on chest radiogram, but a quiet cardiac apex on examination. Pericardial constriction is more difficult to diagnose. A relatively small and quiet heart with venous hypertension, hepatomegaly, and ascites should always suggest this diagnosis. Less evident, but just as important in pericardial constriction, is the venous hypertension without other obvious cause, particularly in the absence of ventricular gallops. Pericardial calcification on chest x-ray is strongly supportive of this diagnosis (Fig. 2).

It is mandatory to determine which of these three mechanisms is responsible for the heart failure, since therapy differs, depending upon which mechanism is present. While effective for myocardial failure, digitalis and diuretics would be of little help or even contraindicated for the patient with pericardial tamponade. Failure to identify the mechanism responsible for the heart failure often leads to unsuccessful, even deleterious therapy.

The second step in managing heart failure in the elderly is to eliminate any extracardiac factor that could be contributing. These factors are listed in Table 1. When the arterial oxygen saturation decreases to less than 90 percent, when the hemoglobin level is less than 8 or greater than 17 g/dl, when the blood pressure is elevated, when the temperature is elevated with resultant tachycardia, when thyrotoxicosis is present, or when the patient consumes excessive amounts of alcohol or salt, conventional therapy for heart failure will be unsuccessful until these factors are identified and corrected. "Apathetic thyrotoxicosis" may be particularly hard to diagnose in the elderly. The patient seems depressed and sluggish rather than hyper-

TABLE 2
Pathophysiologic mechanism of "heart failure"

I Mechanical: A pressure or volume overload

	Pressure overload	Volume overload
Intracardiac:	Aortic stenosis	Aortic regurgitation
	Mitral stenosis	Mitral regurgitation
Extracardiac:	Hypertension	Arteriovenous fistula
		Anemia

II "Muscle": Myocardial failure
  Coronary artery disease
  Primary myocardial process
  Secondary to mechanical defect
III Pericardial
  Pericardial effusion
  Pericardial tamponade

SOURCE: Based on data of Noble,[20] with permission of author and

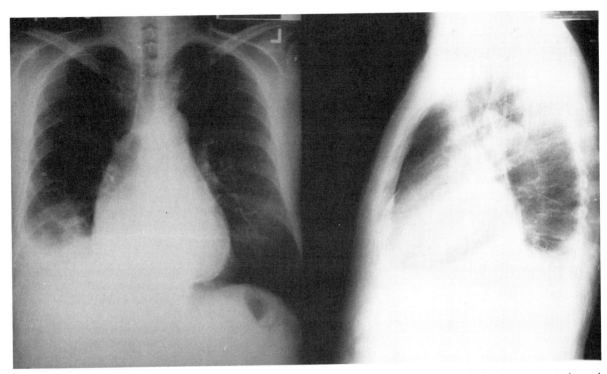

FIGURE 2 Constrictive pericarditis. The calcified pericardium is best visualized at the apex on both the posteroanterior and lateral chest radiograms.

metabolic. Such patients demonstrate atrial fibrillation with a rapid ventricular response, heart failure, and weight loss and may show a sunken facies. Thyroid function tests will confirm the diagnosis and only therapy appropriate for this metabolic state, specifically propranolol, will ameliorate the heart failure.

Rest is even more important in the elderly patient with heart disease than it is in younger patients. The failing heart must be put to rest, and this involves both physical and emotional rest on the part of the patient. Paul Dudley White has said: "The patient may need saturation with rest at first and then rations of it daily or weekly thereafter; dosage with digitalis should follow the same pattern. . . . The skill of the physician can often be judged by the way he prescribes rest and digitalis."[21]

Digitalis is indicated in the elderly patient with myocardial failure. Optimal digitalization in the elderly patient is a challenge. On the one hand, doses of digitalis adequate to augment the contractile state are necessary; on the other hand, elderly patients are particularly susceptible to the toxic effects of digitalis glycosides.[22]

Two preparations are generally used: digoxin and digitoxin. Creatinine clearance is always reduced in the elderly; consequently, a standard dose of digoxin is often excessive for an elderly patient, since digoxin elimination is dependent upon renal function.[23]

It is well to recall that digitalis is administered for two clinical purposes: to augment contractile state and to slow the ventricular response to a supraventricular tachyarrhythmia, such as atrial fibrillation. The dose and serum level of digitalis needed to realize each of these two goals are quite different.[24] Whereas relatively large doses and high serum levels of digitalis are necessary to slow the ventricular response to rapid supraventricular tachyarrhythmias, more moderate doses and serum levels of digitalis are sufficient to augment contractile state. In the elderly patient, the measurement of serum digitalis levels may be helpful in an effort achieve optimal digitalization while avoiding toxicity. Since serum digoxin levels of 2 ng/ml and serum digitoxin levels of 25 ng/ml are often associated with toxic manifestations, serum levels approaching but not reaching these measurements are desirable. Thus, a serum digoxin level of 1 to 1.5 ng/ml or a serum digitoxin level of 15 to 18 ng/ml should augment contractile state without eliciting toxicity.[25] Digitalis intoxication is manifested in the elderly, as it is in the young, by anorexia, vomiting, or cardiac arrhythmias. In addition, the senescent patient is susceptible to lethargy or even psychosis or coma as a manifestation of digitalis intoxication.

Diuretics are indicated for pulmonary congestion. However, before prescribing diuretics for the elderly patient, it is well to consider the hemodynamic manifestations of failure. The clinician should determine if there is principally a depression in cardiac output (weakness, easy fatigability, depressed urinary output), or an elevation in left ventricular filling pressure (dyspnea and radiographic evidence of pulmonary congestion). Diuretics are clearly indicated for the latter. However, by reducing blood volume and hence preload, diuretics may also reduce cardiac output (Fig. 1). Thus, improperly or excessively prescribed diuretics may have disastrous consequences in an old patient. Azotemia, oliguria, hypotension, confusion, coma, or even a cerebrovascular accident or myocardial infarction may result from volume depletion. Consequently, mild diuretics should be prescribed in small amounts initially and titrated as required to control volume overload.

Potassium balance is also a problem in the elderly. Hypokalemia from thiazide diuretics or furosemide may produce weakness or precipitate digitoxic rhythm disturbances. Hyperkalemia from potassium-sparing diuretics, such as triamterene, or the aldosterone-blocking agents may be life-threatening. Thus, serum potassium levels are a prerequisite in treating the elderly patient with any diuretic. Potassium supplementation in the form of KC1 is generally required with a thiazide diuretic. The combination of a thiazide and a potassium-sparing diuretic may be particularly effi-

cacious in the elderly patient, but serial potassium levels need to be followed. The same considerations apply to salt and fluid restriction in the elderly. Vigorous restriction is generally contraindicated in this age group, since impaired renal function, further depression of cardiac output, and hypotension may occur.

Arrhythmias will be discussed subsequently, but in the elderly patient bradycardia may aggravate heart failure. Consider the hemodynamic response to pacing illustrated in Fig. 3. Certainly, bradycardia, per se, is not an indication for pacing in the elderly patient. However, when a patient has heart failure which does not respond to conventional therapy, then a trial of temporary pacing would test the hypothesis that the hemodynamics and symptoms of heart failure improve with an accelerated rate. If so, permanent pacing would be indicated.

In recent years, it has become apparent that vasodilator therapy is particularly efficacious in the management of patients with heart failure.[26] The long-acting oral nitrates, such as isosorbide dinitrate, are quite effective in reducing pulmonary congestion. Afterload-reducing agents, such as prazosin, are quite effective in increasing the cardiac output and improving the symptoms of weakness and fatigue. The precise role of vasodilating agents in the management of heart failure in the elderly has not as yet been well defined. Without doubt, these agents should be considered in the management of the patient whose symptoms of heart failure do not respond to conventional therapy. As experience accumulates, it is likely that these agents will be used earlier in the management of the older patient's heart failure. As with other agents, the elderly patient is particularly susceptible to the toxic effects of vasodilator therapy. Particularly when the patient is relatively hypovolemic, vasodilator therapy may cause unacceptable hypotension, or even shock. Thus, these agents may be prescribed only in limited dosage and under careful monitoring. When oral agents are employed, hemodynamic monitoring is not required; however, careful clinical monitoring, preferably in the hospital, is essential (Fig. 4).

Pulmonary embolization may be a contributory cause, if not the primary cause, of heart failure in the elderly patient, particularly the patient who is bedridden from other medical or surgical disease or from preexisting heart failure. Periodic oppressive chest discomfort with dyspnea, tachycardia, hypoxemia, and atrial rhythm disturbances or a rightward shift in QRS axis strongly suggest this possibility. A negative lung scan is helpful in excluding this diagnosis. A positive lung scan supports but does not prove the diagnosis of pulmonary embolization. When the condition is strongly suspected clinically and a lung scan supports that impression, then anticoagulation with heparin is indicated. Pulmonary angiography would confirm the diagnosis but is not essential in the patient in

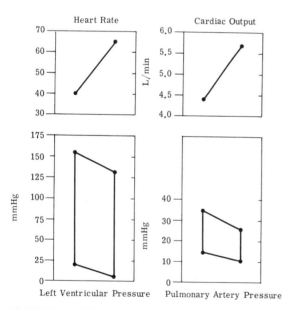

FIGURE 3 Effect of pacing on hemodynamics of heart failure with bradycardia. In this patient with aortic regurgitation, the cardiac output increases from 4.3 to 5.7 liters/min and left ventricular diastolic pressure decreases from 22 to 4 mm Hg as the heart rate is accelerated from 40 to 67 beats per minute. Symptoms of heart failure promptly resolved. (Reproduced from R. J. Noble, An Approach to Refractory Heart Failure, Am. Fam. Physician, 15:138, 1977, with permission of the publisher.)

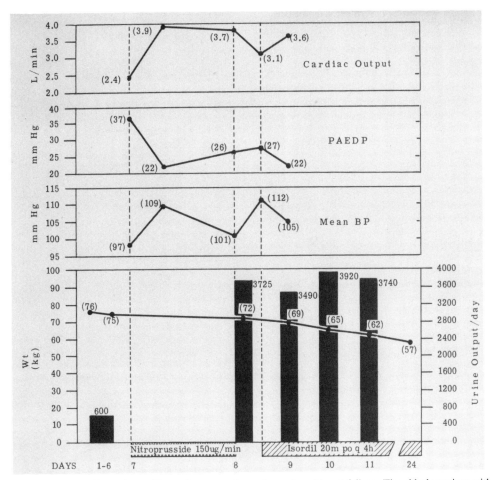

FIGURE 4 Effect of vasodilator therapy on hemodynamics of heart failure. The elderly patient with chronic coronary artery disease and severe heart failure (marked anasarca, pulmonary congestion, impaired mentation, oliguria) unresponsive to conventional therapy responded to parenteral and oral afterload-reducing therapy with a distinct improvement in cardiac output, decrease in pulmonary diastolic pressure, and effective diuresis. Clinical improvement paralleled the hemodynamic changes. PAEDP, pulmonary arterial end-diastolic pressure.

whom the diagnosis is strongly suspected clinically. A continuous intravenous infusion of heparin (adjusted to prolong the partial thromboplastin time to two and one-half times normal) is preferable to intermittent administration, since the latter results in intensive anticoagulation after each bolus injection.

SYNCOPE

Syncope may result from one of four causes (Fig. 5): (1) intrinsic cerebral circulatory insufficiency, (2) cardiogenic syncope, (3) hypotension, or (4) deficit in the essential energy substrates contained in the blood delivered to the brain.[27-30]

Physiology

While cerebrovascular disease is common in the elderly, syncope uncommonly results from a plaque or clot unless the anatomic process is particularly extensive. More commonly, fainting results from a combination of some other mechanism of diminished perfusion, such as postural hypotension, superimposed upon occlusive cerebrovascular disease. Coughing or hyperventilation may produce syncope as a result of an increase in cerebrovascular resistance, causing physiologic obstruction to flow.

Considering cardiogenic mechanisms, any tachycardia or bradycardia, if it is of sufficient degree to diminish cardiac output, may provoke syncope, particularly in the elderly patient with an already compromised cerebral circulation. Stokes-Adams syndrome resulting from heart block is generally preceded by ECG evidence of bifascicular or trifascicular block, such as the combination of right bundle branch block and left anterior hemiblock[31] (Fig. 6). However, since only about 10 percent of patients with this pattern progress to complete heart block, the ECG alone does

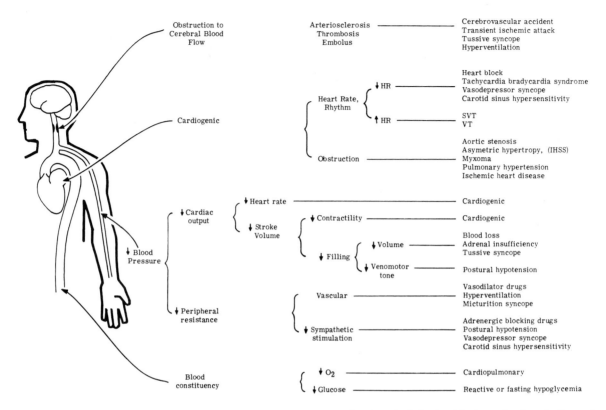

FIGURE 5 Mechanisms of syncope. The four causes of syncope are listed on the left, physiologic mechanisms in the center, clinical syndromes on the right. (*Reproduced from R.J. Noble, The Patient with Syncope, J.A.M.A., 237:1372, 1977, with permission of the publisher.*)

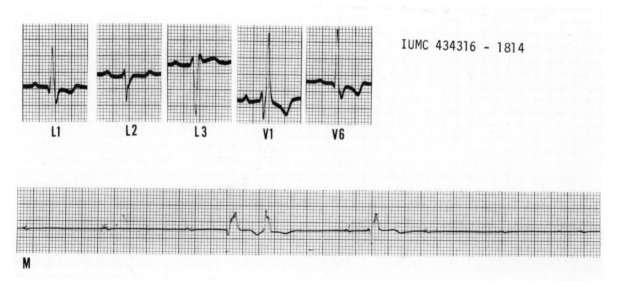

IUMC 434316 - 1814

FIGURE 6 Bifascicular block progressing to complete heart block. Prior to the recording of complete heart block (monitor, M) right bundle branch block (V₁) and left anterior hemiblock (L₂ and L₃) were recorded. (This informative tracing was kindly provided by Dr. Charles Fisch.)

not justify the implantation of a pacemaker.[31] Furthermore, in most elderly patients with syncope and ECG evidence of bifascicular block, it may be shown that there is a cause other than heart block for the syncope.[32] A complete evaluation for all causes of syncope is mandatory, including prolonged monitoring. The demonstration of delayed conduction in the distal conducting system (prolonged H-V interval) by intracardiac electrophysiologic studies (His bundle electrocardiography) may aid in the selection of those patients with bifascicular disease who are most likely to benefit from pacing,[33] although the prognostic implications of prolonged H-V conduction are not established.[34]

Syncope, transient cerebral ischemic attacks, or other central nervous system dysfunction resulting from marked sinus slowing or arrest, often in associ-

ation with a tachycardia, constitutes the tachycardia-bradycardia (or "sick sinus") syndrome.[35] Figure 7 illustrates one of the most common mechanisms: atrial fibrillation with a rapid ventricular response; when the supraventricular tachyarrhythmia terminates, atrial arrest occurs, probably as a result of inappropriate suppression of an abnormal sinus mechanism. A less common mechanism of syncope in the elderly is sinus exit block (Fig. 8).

Carotid sinus hypersensitivity may be manifested as (1) a cardioinhibitory type with profound bradycardia (Fig. 9), (2) a vasodepressor type of hypotensive response to carotid sinus massage, or (3) a central type of syncope without bradycardia or hypotension.[36] The most common anatomic cause for cardiogenic syncope in the elderly is aortic valvular stenosis.

Hypotension results from either a decreased car-

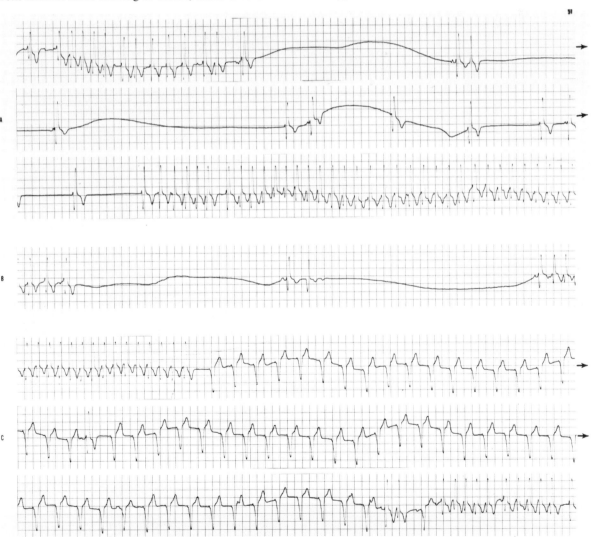

FIGURE 7 Tachycardia-bradycardia syndrome. In panels A and B, abnormal sinus suppression follows the atrial fibrillation with rapid ventricular response. A demand inhibited pacemaker has been activated in panel C.

diac output or a decreased peripheral resistance. The decrease in cardiac output can result from any of the cardiogenic mechanisms listed above or from decreased ventricular filling. In the elderly, one of the most common causes of decreased cardiac filling is the hypovolemia which results from sodium and water deprivation owing to diuretics or salt restriction prescribed for mild heart failure.

When hypotension results from decreased peripheral resistance in the elderly, the most common ex-

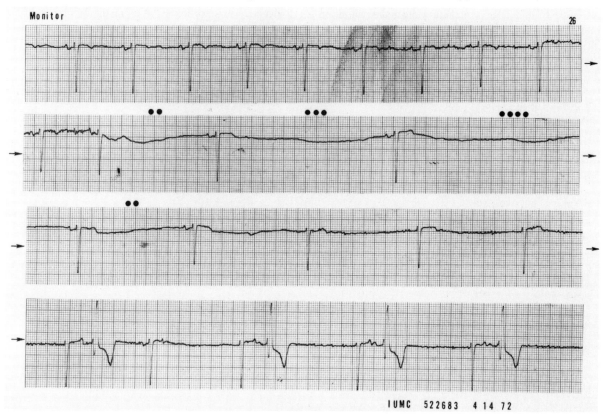

FIGURE 8 Sinus exit block. 2:1 (two dots); 3:1 (three dots); and 4:1 (four dots) exit blocks are demonstrated by the p-p intervals of the pauses measuring two, three, and four normal sinus intervals.

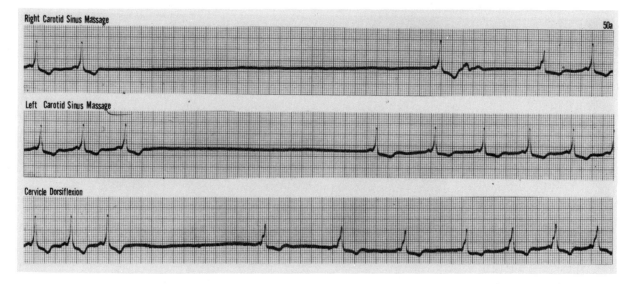

FIGURE 9 Carotid sinus hypersensitivity. Prolonged sinus arrest follows left or right carotid sinus massage or dorseflexion of the neck (to reproduce the clinical syndrome) in this patient with Wolff-Parkinson-White electrocardiographic pattern.

planations are drugs, such as antihypertensive medications, or idiopathic postural hypotension.[30,37]

With respect to deficiency of energy substrates, hypoglycemia and hypoxemia are uncommon causes of syncope in the elderly.

Clinical Evaluation

Table 3 lists the historical questions which should be posed in an effort to determine the clinical syndrome

responsible for syncope, the physical findings which should be elicited, and the ECG abnormalities which should be sought.

HISTORY

Most syncope occurs when the elderly patient is upright; this posture is a prerequisite for the diagnosis of postural hypotension. Exercise precipitates syncope resulting from aortic stenosis or ventricular tachycar-

TABLE 3
Clinical approach to syncope

		Clinical syndrome	Second-order evaluations
History			
Provocation	Upright position	Postural hypotension (and most others)	
	Recumbent position	Hysteria, hyperventilation, hypoglycemia	
	Exercise	Aortic stenosis, tachycardia	
	Emotional stress	Vasodepressor, hyperventilation	
	Food intake	Fasting or reactive hypoglycemia	Blood sugar, fasting and postprandial
	Drugs	Iatrogenic	
Duration	Prolonged – several seconds	Aortic stenosis, hypoglycemia, hysteria, cerebrovascular disease	
Premonitory symptoms	None	Arrhythmia, postural hypotension	
	Palpitations	Arrhythmia	
	"Vagal"	Vasodepressor	
	Dyspnea, lightheadedness, "numbness"	Hyperventilation	
	Neurologic symptoms	Cerebrovascular disease	EEG
Physical examination			
Blood pressure:			Tests for adrenal insufficiency, volume loss
Orthostatic hypotension			
With ↑ HR		Volume	
Without ↑ HR		Autonomic postural hypotension	Tests for integrity of autonomic and voluntary nervous systems (tabes, diabetes)
Carotid pulse, Cardiac Murmur		LV outflow obstruction, localized vascular disease	Radiogram, echocardiogram, ECG, catheterization
Carotid sinus massage		Carotid sinus hypersensitivity	
Voluntary hyperventilation		Hyperventilation, vasodepressor	
Electrocardiogram			
Heart block, bilateral bundle branch block		Heart block	
Sinus bradycardia, block, arrest		Bradycardia	Prolonged monitoring, rest or ambulatory, stress, with monitoring pacing and His studies
Supraventricular tachycardia, W-P-W syndrome		Tachycardia	
PVCs or ventricular tachycardia			

SOURCE: Based on data of Noble,[27] with permission of author and publisher.

dia. The drug history is extraordinarily important; antihypertensives, tranquilizers, nitroglycerin, diuretics, quinidine, and digitalis may all cause syncope. If the syncope persists for longer than a few seconds, aortic stenosis, hypoglycemia, or hysteria should be considered. The absence of any premonitory symptoms suggests an arrhythmia or postural hypotension. The common faint is suggested by a feeling of warmth over the head, yawning, faintness, epigastric distress, and diaphoresis. Cerebrovascular disease is likely if the syncope is preceded by confusion, alteration in personality, expressive aphasia, or unilateral weakness.

PHYSICAL EXAMINATION

The presence of orthostatic hypotension and a heart rate that increases to the degree expected for hypotension are probably indications of volume depletion secondary to salt and water deprivation, diuretics, blood loss, or adrenal insufficiency. In contrast, if the heart rate fails to accelerate, then idiopathic orthostatic hypotension owing to dysfunction of the autonomic nervous system should be suspected.

Palpation of the carotid pulse and ascultation for a heart murmur may suggest aortic stenosis.

Carotid massage may confirm the diagnosis of carotid sinus hypersensitivity, particularly if symptoms are reproduced. However, the examination must be conducted most carefully with ECG monitoring in an elderly patient, and only after having excluded significant occlusive carotid disease if a carotid bruit is present.

Voluntary hyperventilation may prove this to be the mechanism for the elderly patient's syncope.

ELECTROCARDIOGRAM

Bilateral bundle branch block should be sought. Prolonged ambulatory monitoring may be required to prove the tachycardia-bradycardia syndrome. Training the patient's family to measure the pulse rate during an episode of near syncope is informative in determining the relationship of syncope to a rhythm disturbance.

ADDITIONAL EVALUATIONS

Electroencephalography or computed tomography of the head may be required when neurologic abnormalities are suspected. Hemoglobin determination and tests for renal function and electrolyte balance are always required when volume disturbances are suggested. A chest x-ray, echocardiogram, or cardiac catheterization may be indicated to confirm aortic stenosis. When suspected rhythm disturbances are not apparent, exercise stress testing or prolonged ambulatory monitoring may be helpful. A less expensive and equally productive method of documenting rhythm disturbance may be transtelephonic transmission of the ECG, using the same sort of device made available in pacemaker surveillance clinics. His bundle electrocardiography is occasionally indicated with suspected heart block;[33] however, the prognostic implications of an abnormal conduction time are not as yet sufficiently well clarified to permit therapeutic decisions based solely on the abnormal evaluation.[34]

With a perceptive history, a targeted physical examination, and an ECG, clinicians can diagnose syncope in the majority of their elderly patients. The common causes of syncope in the elderly—heart block, tachycardia-bradycardia syndrome, and hypovolemia—are readily responsive to proper therapy. Whether or not elderly patients with syncope resulting from aortic stenosis should undergo aortic valve replacement depends upon age and concomitant medical history; the authors would tend to be aggressive because of the quite acceptable surgical risk in the elderly patient in comparison with the dire prognosis without surgery. Idiopathic postural hypotension responds much less satisfactorily to therapy; measures such as elevation of the head of the bed at night; tight, constricting garments below the waist; increased salt and fluid intake, and salt-retaining steroids are indicated. The reader is referred to a more complete review of the pathophysiologic mechanisms, clinical evaluation, and therapy of the patient with syncope.[27]

HEART MURMURS

Systolic murmurs are common in the elderly; their frequency increases from 30 percent in patients 65 years of age to almost 60 percent by 80 years of age.[38–40] The typical benign murmur is a short, early peaking, grade 1-2/6 diamond-shaped systolic murmur located at the base and radiating poorly to the carotids.[41] The second sound is physiologically split unless congestive heart failure or left bundle branch block (LBBB) causes reverse splitting. Carotid upstroke is brisk. Most of these systolic murmurs originate from the aortic area and may be attributed to dilatation of the aortic annulus[42] and ascending aorta[43] or to thickening, deformity, and calcification of the aortic cusps without hemodynamic stenosis, i.e., aortic sclerosis.[44]

Aortic Stenosis

Clinically significant aortic stenosis is present in approximately 5 percent of elderly patients with a systolic murmur. Etiologically, in the absence of mitral valve disease, congenitally bicuspid valves are frequently the explanation for aortic stenosis in the 60- to 75-year-old age group; degenerative calcification of an otherwise normal tricuspid valve is unusual before 75 years of age but is the most frequent cause of stenosis in patients 85 years old.[45] The predominant symptom is congestive heart failure, but angina and syncope are frequent.[46] Pertinent physical findings include a grade 2-5/6 late peaking and long-lasting systolic ejection murmur, a slowly rising carotid pulse, and a diminished or absent aortic component of the second heart sound. Often the murmur is loudest at the apex and can be misinterpreted as originating from the mitral valve.[47] Left ventricular hypertrophy is usually seen on ECG. Chest x-ray confirms this and may also display calcification of the aortic valve and dilatation of the ascending aorta. The accurate diagnosis of aortic stenosis is frequently overlooked in the geriatric patient for several reasons: presentation with congestive failure, absence of a history of a heart murmur, elevated systolic blood pressure, deceptively brisk carotid upstroke in a noncompliant artery, typical location of the murmur at the apex, and frequent findings of left ventricular hypertrophy (LVH) by ECG and chest x-ray in the elderly.[47,48] Instead, these abnormalities are attributed to hypertension, coronary artery disease, or cardiomyopathy with papillary muscle dysfunction.

Graphic recordings are often invaluable in the elderly (Fig. 10). Echocardiography is helpful in determining not only the presence but also the severity of aortic stenosis. M-mode echocardiography is often useful in excluding significant aortic stenosis in the elderly when normal aortic valve opening is demonstrated; however, the finding of dense or calcified valve leaflets does not permit estimation of the severity of the stenosis. With cross-sectional echocardiography, it is possible not only to establish the presence or absence of the disease but also to estimate its severity by measuring the degree of systolic cusp separation (Fig. 11).[49] Thus, these noninvasive techniques usually permit separation of those patients with "innocent" systolic murmurs from those with hemodynamically significant aortic stenosis. However, if doubt exists and the patient is symptomatic, cardiac catheterization is indicated.

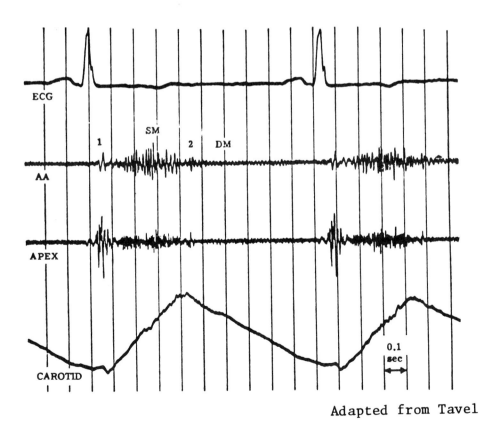

Adapted from Tavel

FIGURE 10 Carotid pulse and phonocardiographic tracing of patient with aortic stenosis. The upstroke of the carotid pulse is markedly delayed with a shudder, and simultaneously, a long, late-peaking systolic murmur and single S_2 are recorded, to confirm aortic stenosis. (*Reproduced from R. J. Noble, An Approach to Refractory Heart Failure, Am. Fam. Physician, 15:138, 1977, with permission of the publisher.*) (Dr. Morton Tavel provided the initial illustration.)

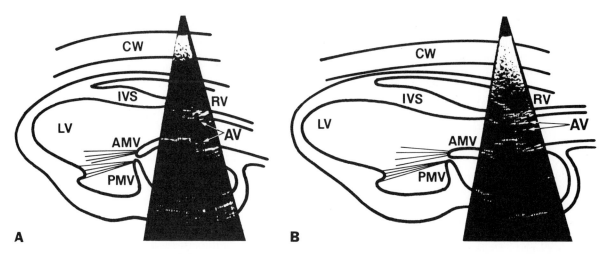

FIGURE 11 Cross-sectional echocardiogram of aortic stenosis. Long-axis views of the aortic valve are contrasted in two elderly patients with systolic ejection murmurs. *A*. The aortic cusps separate widely during systole to exclude significant stenosis. *B*. The aortic cusp separation is less than 1 cm, confirming critical aortic stenosis. The dense, immobile echoes within the aortic root represent fibrosis and calcification of the leaflets.

Mitral Regurgiation

Many systolic murmurs in the aged, even those of ejection timing, are associated with abnormalities of the mitral valve, its annulus, or papillary muscles. Such lesions as papillary muscle dysfunction,[50] mitral valve prolapse,[51] and idiopathic hypertrophic subaortic stenosis[52] may present mid- or late systolic murmurs mimicking aortic stenosis or sclerosis in the elderly. Even with the more classical holosystolic mitral murmur, the etiology is often difficult to establish.

The predominant complaint with chronic mitral insufficiency, most commonly of rheumatic origin, is easy fatigability as a result of low cardiac output. Symptoms of low output failure usually occur after the onset of atrial fibrillation. On the other hand, with papillary muscle insufficiency, the low cardiac output is often caused by severe left ventricular dysfunction rather than by the volume of regurgitant flow, and the rhythm is usually a sinus rhythm.

Mitral valve prolapse may also cause significant hemodynamic problems in the elderly. The valve may undergo progressive degeneration with worsening mitral insufficiency and low output failure,[51] or the chordae tendineae may rupture to produce sudden pulmonary edema.[53] This entity may be easily mistaken for coronary artery disease with papillary muscle dysfunction because of chest pain, an abnormal ECG often suggesting inferior myocardial infarction, and the frequent ventricular ectopy.[54]

Calcification of the mitral valve annulus is a degenerative process in the fibrous mitral annulus that is probably similar to degenerative calcific aortic stenosis.[55,56] Although the murmur is often harsh and well transmitted to the base and there is calcium in the

cardiac silhouette which may suggest calcific aortic stenosis, an overpenetrated chest x-ray or fluoroscopic examination will usually demonstrate the characteristic u- or j-shaped calcification of the mitral annulus.[56]

Idiopathic Hypertrophic Subaortic Stenosis

Idiopathic hypertrophic subaortic stenosis (IHSS) may imitate aortic stenosis, mitral regurgitation, or coronary artery disease with papillary muscle dysfunction. In some series, approximately 30 percent of patients with IHSS were older than 60, but in most of these elderly patients, the diagnosis was overlooked prior to echocardiography (Fig. 12) or catheterization.[52,57] The clinical symptoms of dyspnea, chest pain, and palpitations are similar to those experienced by younger patients, but these symptoms in addition to ECG findings of LVH or pathologic Q waves result in misdiagnosis. Even more misleading is the rare occurrence of a diastolic murmur or aortic valve calcification with IHSS,[52] two findings which are usually highly specific for aortic valvular disease.

Echocardiography (both M-mode and cross-sectional) is usually capable of differentiating the various causes of the pansystolic murmur in the elderly and is also useful in estimating the hemodynamic severity of a lesion.[58] Characteristic mitral valve motion is seen with mitral valve prolapse, flail mitral leaflet, IHSS, low cardiac output, and elevated left ventricular end-diastolic pressure. Dense echoes are recorded in the region of the mitral valve annulus with calcification. Evaluation of left ventricular wall motion can differentiate the murmur of hemodynamically significant mitral regurgitation with left ventricular volume overload from papillary muscle insufficiency resulting either from cardiomyopathy (generalized wall motion abnormality) or from coronary artery disease (segmental abnormality). The presence of IHSS illustrates the necessity for a correct diagnosis. In this instance, the conventional therapy for heart failure (digitalis and diuretics) may be ineffective or even deleterious, while the correct therapy (propranolol) would be contraindicated in other causes of heart failure.

Table 4 outlines the clinical diagnosis of systolic murmurs in the elderly.

Diastolic Murmurs

Statistically, diastolic murmurs are much less common than systolic murmurs in the elderly. The most frequent diastolic murmur, aortic insufficiency, is normally associated with dilatation of the aorta and is rarely of hemodynamic significance.[59] While distinctly less common, aortic regurgitation may also result from either calcific[60] or syphilitic aortic valve disease.[61] Mitral stenosis is an uncommon diagnosis. Because diastolic murmurs have the same significance in the elderly as in younger patients, the evaluation of hemodynamic significance is identical.

Infectious Endocarditis

Closely related to valvular heart disease in the elderly is the problem of bacterial endocarditis. The incidence of bacterial endocarditis is highest in the elderly; approximately 30 percent of all cases occur in patients over the age of 60.[62] Left-sided valvular involvement is most common, with the aortic valve involved slightly more frequently than the mitral valve. However, no underlying valvular disease is found pathologically in approximately 40 percent of patients.[62,63] Because innocent murmurs are common in the elderly, because a murmur is not always present early in the disease, and because elderly patients may remain afebrile, the diagnosis of bacterial endocarditis is often overlooked. Left-sided endocarditis often presents with neurologic signs such as coma or hemiplegia, unexplained anemia, or renal failure; right-sided endocarditis usually presents with pulmonary infection in the presence of a murmur. Even with the correct diagnosis, the disease is extremely virulent in the elderly, with mortality varying from 30 to 70 percent.[64,65]

Valvular Surgery

With clearer recognition of the prognosis of valvular lesions in the elderly and with the general reduction in operative morbidity and mortality, an ever-increasing number of elderly patients are undergoing valve replacement. Despite the presence of heart failure in almost all patients with aortic stenosis, the left ventricle is capable of generating a systolic pressure commonly in excess of 200 mm Hg. Since left ventricular function is usually well preserved, the operative risk of aortic valve replacement may be held to 10 to 20 percent, with the expectation of significant postoperative improvement.[66,67]

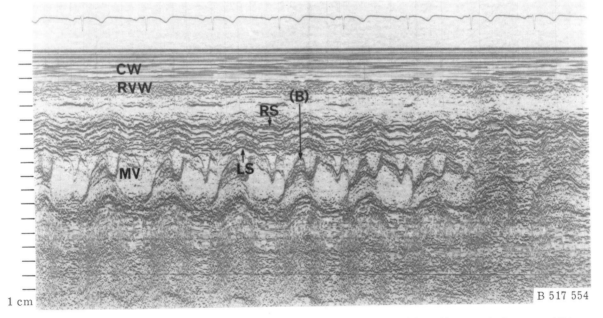

FIGURE 12 M-mode echocardiogram of IHSS. The characteristic features are the thickened interventricular septum (distance between left septum [LS] and right septum [RS]) and systolic anterior motion (B) of the mitral valve (MV).

With mitral regurgitation, patients may be divided into two categories: acute and chronic. In acute lesions, the prognosis is influenced by the etiology. With papillary muscle dysfunction the underlying ventricular function is usually severely compromised. With ruptured chordae tendineae resulting from myxomatous degeneration of the chordae, ventricular function may be well preserved. Severe, irreversible ventricular dilatation and depression of contractility may accompany chronic lesions. Consequently, the mortality

TABLE 4
Differential diagnosis of systolic murmur

	Aortic sclerosis	Aortic stenosis	Rheumatic mitral regurgitation	Mitral regurgitation (papillary muscle dysfunction)
Symptoms	None	Failure, angina, syncope	Chronic failure	Failure with previous angina or prior infarction
Physical findings				
Murmur	Basal, ejection → carotids	Basal, ejection → carotids → apex	Apical, holosystolic → axilla	Apical, mid-, late or holosystolic
Sounds	Normal	Single S_2, S_4	S_1, widely split S_2, S_3	S_4 and/or S_3 common
Precordial palpation	Normal	LVH	LV volume overload	? Aneurysm
Carotid pulse	Normal	Slow upstroke	Normal to brisk	Normal
ECG				
Rhythm	Sinus	Sinus	Atrial fibrillation	Sinus
Pattern	Normal	LVH	LV dilatation	± infarction
X-ray	Normal or dilated ascending aorta	LVH, calcium in aortic valve, poststenotic aortic root dilatation	↑ LA, ↑ LV	Normal, to ↑ LV
Echocardiogram				
M-mode	Normal or dense aortic echoes	Dense aortic echoes	↑ LA, ↑LV	Segmental LV wall motion abnormality
Cross-sectional	Normal aortic cusp separation	Reduced aortic cusp separation	↑ LA, ↑ LV, hyperdynamic LV, mitral leaflets abnormal	Segmental LV wall motion abnormality

Ruptured chordae tendineae	Calcified mitral annulus	IHSS
Acute failure	None or chronic failure	Angina, syncope, failure
Apical, holosystolic, → axilla, back, or base (mimic aortic stenosis)	Apical, holosystolic, or mid-systolic	Lower left sternal border, ejection, → apex and base (mimic stenosis or mitral regurgitation
S_4 and S_3	± S_3	S_4
Normal, acutely	Normal or LV volume overload	LVH
Normal	Normal	Brisk initial upstroke; secondary "dome": bisferians
Sinus	Sinus; atrial fibrillation	Sinus
Normal	Normal; LV volume overload	LVH
Normal heart Pulmonary venous distension	u- or j-shaped calcium ring	Normal to LVH
Hyperdynamic LV; flail mitral leaflet	Dense mitral annulus	Asymmetric septal hypertrophy, systolic anterior motion of mitral valve
Hyperdynamic LV; flail leaflet	Dense mitral annulus	Systolic anterior motion of mitral valve; LV shape abnormality

Key: S, heart sound; LVH, left ventricular hypertrophy; LA, left atrium.

associated with mitral valve replacement in the elderly is quite high (40 to 50 percent), and symptomatic improvement is less dramatic than with aortic valve replacement.[67]

In the elderly, increased morbidity and mortality are related to several factors. Coronary artery disease is frequently present, necessitating a combined procedure of valve replacement and revascularization. Many elderly patients are malnourished or debilitated preoperatively.[68] In others, the aorta or other major vessels may present severe atherosclerotic changes which can complicate the insertion of cannulas or bypass grafts and increase the risk of dissection. Elderly patients have a high incidence of postoperative renal, neurologic, and pulmonary complications. Finally, they are more prone to develop complications from anticoagulation, which is required with most prosthetic valves.

HYPERTENSION

Hypertension, particularly systolic hypertension, is so prevalent in the elderly that it is often considered a part of the aging process rather than a pathologic entity. While diastolic blood pressure plateaus at around age 55, systolic blood pressure continues to rise even into the eighth and ninth decades.[69] The progressive rise in systolic pressure is attributed to the increasing rigidity of the major blood vessels with age.

Hypertension has been shown to increase the risk of sudden death, myocardial infarction, congestive heart failure, and stroke and has been directly implicated in the development of aortic dissection, intracranial hemorrhage, and nephrosclerosis.[70–72] While hypertension is accepted as a significant risk factor for cardiovascular morbidity and mortality in younger patients, it is not generally appreciated that hypertension is just as significant a risk factor in the elderly. The incidence of coronary artery disease, cerebral infarction, and congestive heart failure are all substantially greater in elderly hypertensives than in their normotensive counterparts. In fact, approximately 70 percent of the morbidity and over 50 percent of the mortality in the elderly is attributable to hypertension.[73]

While hypertension confers an increased risk of cardiovascular disease in the elderly, there is no uniformity of opinion as to what level of blood pressure constitutes an indication for therapy. In one study of patients 65 years of age and older, 21 percent had a blood pressure above 180/110, and over 50 percent of this subgroup had hypertensive changes on ECG or cardiomegaly on x-ray.[73] In the elderly hypertensive with evidence of cardiac end-organ damage, the prognosis is ominous, with a 40 to 60 percent 5-year mortality from a cardiovascular event.[73] Under these circumstances, aggressive antihypertensive therapy may be warranted in those patients with a blood pressure above 160/95.

On the other hand, in the totally asymptomatic elderly patient with no evidence of end-organ damage, recommendations for treatment vary.[74,74] At present, there is no available evidence proving the efficacy of antihypertensive therapy in the *asymptomatic* elderly patient; therefore, the clinical decision to treat hypertension in the old must be individualized, weighing the potential benefits of therapy against the increased risk of adverse drug reactions. In the authors' experience, the majority of elderly patients whose blood pressure exceeds 180/100 will require antihypertensive therapy.

Also, in the authors' experience, the most effective and least toxic antihypertensive therapy in the elderly includes (1) mild diuretics which combine both potassium-sparing and potassium-losing properties (with serial determination of serum potassium levels); (2) low doses of reserpine; (3) low doses of propranolol, particularly when systolic hypertension is paramount; and (4) low doses of vasodilators such as prazosin, particularly when heart failure, cardiomegaly, or aortic regurgitation coexist.

Certain problems associated with antihypertensive therapy in the elderly should be considered. Baroreceptor and other postural reflexes are attenuated in the elderly;[76] these patients are more susceptible to orthostatic hypotension resulting from the volume depletion caused by sodium restriction or diuretics, to the loss of vascular tone with certain peripheral vasodilators and autonomic blocking drugs, and to unacceptable bradycardia and a decrease in cardiac output with β-adrenergic blockade.

With the decreased renal function in the elderly, toxicity is more likely. Moreover, with those drugs that have central nervous system side effects (such as α-methyldopa, clonidine, reserpine, and propranolol), adverse reactions are more likely. Probably of even greater importance, the elderly patient often has diminished mental acuity and is easily confused; consequently, errors in following a drug regimen, particularly a complicated one, are frequent. For this reason, antihypertensive therapy should be kept as simple as possible, and if multiple drugs are required, combination compounds may be utilized. In addition, drug interactions are common, as many elderly patients often take several medications in addition to their antihypertensive therapy.

ELECTROCARDIOGRAM

The incidence of ECG abnormalities in the aged varies, of course, depending on whether the geriatric population assayed is institutionalized or apparently well and living at home.[77] Because the frequency of most

TABLE 5
Electrocardiographic abnormalities in the elderly

	Frequency	Statistical association with heart disease
Myocardial infarction patterns	6–10%[77,79]	Yes[77]
LVH	3–4%[77,78]	Yes[78]
Nonspecific ST and T abnormalities	10-30-40%[77–80]	Yes[78]
LBBB	1.2%[81]	Yes[81]
RBBB 7 (L)	2.5%[81]	No[81]
LAD	2-11-20%[78–80]	No[78]
RBBB + LAD	1.2%[81]	Yes[81]
First-degree AV block	1-4%[78,82]	No[83]
Atrial fibrillation	2% (age 65-75)[79]	
	5% (age 75)[79]	Yes[78]
	15% (hospitalized)[79]	
PACs and PVCs	10–11%[78]	No[78]

Key: LVH, left ventricular hypertrophy; LBBB, left bundle branch block; RBBB, right bundle branch block; LAD, left axis deviation; PAC, PVC, premature atrial and ventricular contraction, respectively.

ECG abnormalities increases with age, one may infer that the abnormalities are acquired.[78] Mihalick and Fisch found a similar incidence of clinical evidence of cardiac disease and ECG abnormalities, suggesting that an abnormal ECG constitutes reasonable, objective evidence of an underlying cardiac abnormality. However, these same authors found that about one-third of their elderly patients with abnormal ECGs had no clinical evidence of heart disease.[78] Also, Campbell demonstrated an ECG abnormality in about one-half of his apparently healthy elderly patients.[79]

The ECG abnormalities listed in Table 5 occur with increased frequency in the elderly, and with sufficient frequency to permit analysis of prognostic implications.[77] Some of these abnormalities infer a statistical likelihood of associated heart disease, namely Q-S patterns in leads V_{1-3}, LVH, LBBB, right bundle branch block (RBBB) and left axis deviation (LAD), ST-segment depression and T wave inversion in leads other than III and V_1, and atrial fibrillation. However, these abnormalities are only statistical associations, not proof of cardiac abnormalities. More importantly, most of the ECG abnormalities in the aged are of no prognostic significance.[78]

Abnormal ECG Patterns

Pathologic Q waves occur more frequently in males than in females, corresponding to the higher incidence of coronary disease in the American male population.[80] Studies have indicated the association between pathologic Q waves and previous myocardial infarction.[84]

Similarly, ECG evidence of LVH correlates with clinical evidence of heart disease. LVH is seen more frequently in females, perhaps reflecting a higher incidence of hypertension in elderly females than in males. ST-T wave abnormalities are nonspecific, and only two-thirds of elderly patients with these abnormalities will have clinically evidence heart disease.[78] T wave inversion is also a nonspecific finding often associated with coronary artery disease.[80]

RBBB occurs about twice as frequently as LBBB in the elderly. Isolated RBBB is not associated with any clinical evidence of heart disease unless coupled with LAD, in which case coronary artery disease, hypertension, and cardiomegaly are often documented.[81] LAD is often associated with clinical evidence of coronary artery disease and hypertensive cardiovascular disease, and yet isolated LAD is not associated with an increase in morbidity or mortality.[80,81] LBBB is more frequently associated with heart disease. However, any of these patterns may be found in an asymptomatic, apparently healthy elderly subject.[81] (See "Syncope" and "Arrhythmias.")

Arrhythmias

With regard to the frequency of rhythm and conduction disturbances in the elderly, one should note that the population studies are interpretations of standard 12-lead ECGs, recording only about 1 min of information. Prolonged ambulatory monitoring of a geriatric population has not been recorded, so that an accurate analysis of arrhythmias in the aged is not available nor is their prognosis determined. Of the potential conduction and rhythm disturbances, only first-degree AV block,[83] premature atrial complexes, premature ventricular complexes, and atrial fibrillation occur with sufficient frequency in the aged to be included in Table 5. Of these abnormalities, only atrial fibrillation implies heart disease; it is frequently associated with other clinical findings such as murmurs, cardiomegaly, or heart failure. As with younger age groups, this arrhythmia may result from coronary artery disease or hypertensive cardiovascular disease. In contrast to younger patients, the rhythm is less frequently the result of rheumatic heart disease and more frequently a part of the tachycardia-bradycardia syndrome or apathetic hyperthyroidism.[85]

Several other conduction and rhythm disturbances must be considered, not because of their frequency, but because of their clinical significance. Sinus bradycardia may occur in the elderly as an isolated finding. In such patients, cardiac output is maintained by a compensatory increase in stroke volume, and these patients may be totally asymptomatic. Only if the bradycardia is associated with paroxysmal tachycardia or with symptoms of heart failure or cerebral dysfunction is it of any clinical significance.[86] The demonstration of asymptomatic sinus bradycardiac does not justify therapy.

Second- and third-degree AV block is more common in the elderly than in younger populations and is always abnormal. The cause and prognosis of the conduction disturbances depends upon the location of the block in the conduction system, whether above the bundle of His (supra-His) or below it (infra-His).[87] Supra-His block is generally characterized by a QRS of normal duration and either Wenckebach periodicity (second degree), or complete AV dissociation with a regular escape rhythm at a rate of 40 to 55 per minute. Causes of supra-His block include augmented vagal tone, drugs (particularly digitalis excess), and inferior myocardial infarction.[88,89] Therapy with atropine, isoproterenol, or a pacemaker is indicated only when the heart rate is sufficiently slow to compromise the hemodynamic state. The block is almost always transient. Infra-His block is almost always associated with a QRS duration of greater than 120 ms, with bundle branch block configuration. Mobitz type II second-degree block and complete heart block with a slow ventricular escape focus require a pacemaker, generally permanent (Fig. 13). Acute anterior wall myocar-

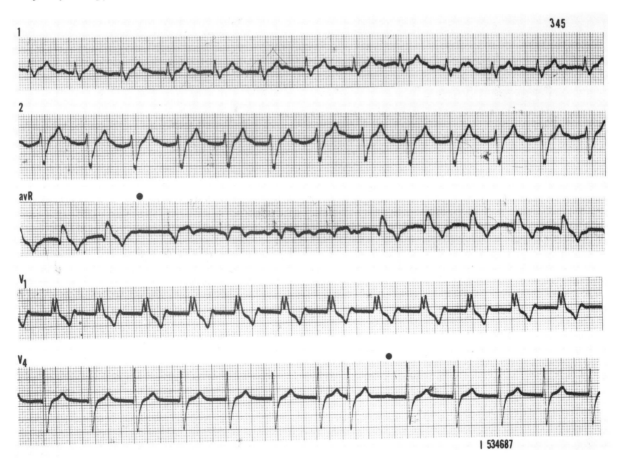

FIGURE 13 Trifascicular block. RBBB and left anterior hemiblock are confirmed in leads V_1 and II. The P-R interval is prolonged in all leads. In lead aV_R, Mobitz type II second-degree block develops under the dot, and aystole is prevented by a demand, ventricular inhibited pacemaker.

dial infarction may cause infra-His block; the condition is highly lethal. However, in the elderly, the most common cause of Stokes-Adams syndrome due to complete heart block is not coronary artery disease but idiopathic, degenerative sclerosis of the cardiac skeleton, i.e., fibrosis and calcification of the mitral and aortic annuli and intervening central fibrous body and ventricular septum.[90,91] The block is recurrent or permanent, and the patient is benefited by permanent pacing. Pacemakers are being perfected which either pace the atrium or sense atrial activation prior to ventricular activation; hence they preserve the "atrial kick" and optimize cardiac output. Such pacemakers may be of value in the active, elderly patient with heart block or in the patient with heart failure and bradycardia.

The tachycardia-bradycardia syndrome has been previously mentioned as a common cause of syncope in the aged.

Ventricular tachycardia, while uncommon, is an important rhythm disturbance both because it may cause syncope or sudden death and because it is generally treatable. As the cardiac output falls consequent to the accelerated ventricular rate and loss of atrial kick, the elderly patient with preexisting cerebrovascular disease is usually symptomatic (Fig. 14). Heart disease is always present, including acute myocardial infarction or chronic coronary disease, mitral valve prolapse, heart failure of any cause or cardiomyopa-

thy. Acutely the episode should respond to cardioversion at low power (even 5 ws) or xylocaine. Prevention of the recurrence of ventricular tachycardia in the aged is particularly challenging because of the patients' intolerance to most available antiarrhythmic medications. Before using such agents the physician must try to identify and correct any precipitating factors: ischemia (with nitrates or propranolol), hypoxemia, chronic bradycardia (with pacemaker), electrolyte imbalance, or heart failure (with digitalis and diuretics). When the disturbance results from coronary artery disease or mitral valve prolapse, or is precipitated by exertion or emotion, propranolol is the preferable agent. The dosage should be titrated to effect a moderate degree of beta blockade, as judged by a resting heart rate of about 60 beats per minute without appreciable acceleration in response to moderate exertion. Quinidine may be helpful; however, serial measurements of QRS and Q-T duration and serum quinidine levels are essential, even with low dosages, to avoid the high incidence of serious toxicity expected in the aged. Nausea and diarrhea often preclude its use. The half-life of procainamide is so short (necessitating such frequent doses) and the incidence of gastrointestinal toxicity so high that the drug is rarely prescribed for an older patient. In the authors' experience, diphenylhydantoin is ineffective except for digitoxic arrhythmias. Disopyramide is at least as effective as quinidine, yet the atropine-like side effects

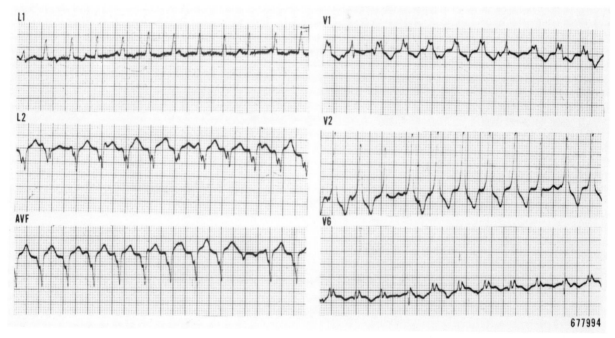

677994

FIGURE 14 Ventricular tachycardia. P waves may be identified in lead V_1 at a rate of 120, dissociated from the ventricular rate of 150 per minute. Captures and fusions (complexes 2 and 8 in V_1; 3 and 9 in V_2; and 4 and 10 in V_6) prove the tachycardia to be ventricular in origin.

of dry mouth and urinary retention may limit its use in the elderly; confusion, psychosis, and heart failure have also occurred in some older patients. Several newer preparations are currently under investigation and when available should prove quite helpful in suppressing malignant ventricular arrhythmias in the aged.

Atrial arrhythmias other than atrial fibrillation and the tachycardia-bradycardia syndrome (paroxysmal supraventricular tachycardia or atrial flutter) are uncommon in the elderly. Digitalis is generally the ideal agent to slow a rapid ventricular response, and yet elderly patients with atrial flutter and 2:1 block with a resultant ventricular rate of 150 beats per minute often respond belatedly or not at all, requiring cardioversion or the addition of propranolol.

The foregoing comments may be summarized as follows: (1) Physicians should anticipate recording an abnormal ECG in about one-half of their geriatric patients; most of these ECG abnormalities are acquired. (2) There is a statistically significant correlation between abnormal ECG and heart disease in the elderly *population*. (3) In an *individual* geriatric patient, most abnormal ECGs per se do not prove clinical heart disease. Some abnormalities strongly suggest heart disease: Q-S in lead V_{1-3}, LVH, LBBB, RBBB and LAD, and atrial fibrillation. Of course, abnormalities such as acute myocardial infarction patterns, high-grade heart block, and ventricular tachycardia indicate unequivocal heart disease. (4) With the exception of the latter abnormalities, an abnormal ECG alone does not justify specific therapy nor indicate prognosis. The prognosis is dependent upon the natural history of the underlying heart disease, not the abnormality in the ECG.

REFERENCES

1 Seegal, D.: Some Comments on the Medical Management of the Older Person, *J. Chronic Dis.*, 3:101, 1956.

1a Caird, F. I., and Kennedy, R. D.: Epidemiology of Heart Disease in Old Age, in F. I. Caird, J. L. C. Dall, and R. D. Kennedy (eds.), "Cardiology in Old Age," Plenum Press, Plenum Publishing Corporation, New York, 1976, p. 1.

2 The President's Commission: National Program to Conquer Heart Disease, Cancer and Stroke, U.S. Government Printing Office, Washington, D.C., 1964.

3 Biorck, G.: The Biology of Myocardial Infarction, *Circulation,* 37:1071, 1968.

4 Pathy, M. S.: Clinical Presentation of Myocardial Infarction in the Elderly, *Bri. Heart J.,* 29:190, 1967.

5 Williams, B. O., Begg, T. B., Semple, T., and McGuinnes, J. B.: The Elderly in a Coronary Care Unit, *Br. Med. J.,* 2:451, 1976.

6 Linn, B. S., and Yurt, R. W.: Cardiac Arrest among Geriatric Patients, *Br. Med. J.,* 2:25, 1970.

7 Chaturvedi, N. C., Shivalingappa, G., Shanks, B., McKay, A., Cumming, K., Walsh, M. J., Scaria, K., Lynas, P., Courtney, D., Barber, J. M., and McC. Boyle, D.: Myocardial Infarction in the Elderly, *Lancet,* 1:280, 1972.

8 Zerman, F. D., and Rodstein, M.: Cardiac Rupture Complicating Myocardial Infarction in the Aged, *Arch. Intern. Med.,* 105:431, 1960.

9 Friedman, H. S., Kuhn, L. A., and Katz, A. M.: Clinical and Electrocardiographic Features of Cardiac Rupture following Acute Myocardial Infarction, *Am. J. Med.,* 50:709, 1971.

10 Hurst, J. W., King, S. B., III, Logue, R. B., Hatcher, C. R., Jr., Jones, E. L., Craver, J. M., Douglas, J. S., Jr., Franch, R. H., Dorney, E. R., Cobbs, B. W., Jr., Robinson, P. H., Clements, S. D., Jr., Kaplan, J. A., and Bradford, J. M.: Value of Coronary Bypass Surgery, *Am. J. Cardiol.,* 42:308, 1978.

11 Rothbaum, D. A., Shaw, D. J., Angell, C. S., and Shock, N. W.: Cardiac Performance in the Unanesthetized Senescent Male Rat, *J. Gerontol.,* 28:287, 1973.

12 Brandfonbrener, M., Landowne, M., and Shock, N. W.: Changes in Cardiac Output with Age, *Circulation,* 12:557, 1955.

13 Granath, A., Jonsson, B., and Strandell, T.: Circulation in Healthy Old Men, Studied by Right Heart Catheterization at Rest and during Exercise in Supine and Sitting Position, *Acta Med. Scand.,* 176:425, 1964.

14 Strandell, T.: Cardiac Output in Old Age, in F. L. Caird, J. L. C. Dall, and R. D. Kennedy (eds.), "Cardiology in Old Age," Plenum Press, Plenum Publishing Corporation, New York, 1976, p. 81.

15 Lakatta, E. G.: Perspectives on the Aged Myocardium, in J. Roberts, R. C. Adelman, and V. T. Cristofalo (eds.), "Pharmacological Intervention in the Aging Process," Plenum Publishing Company, New York, 1978, p. 147.

16 Gerstenblith, G., Frederiksen, J., Yin, F. C. P., Fortuin, N. J., Lakatta, E. G., and Weisfeldt, M. L.: Echocardiographic Assessment of a Normal Adult Aging Population, *Circulation,* 56:274, 1977.

17 Dock, W.: Presbycardia, or Aging of the Myocardium, *N.Y. State J. Med.,* 45:983, 1945.

18 Pomerance, A., Slavin, G., and McWatt, J.: Experience in the Sodium Sulfate-Alcian Blue Stain for Amyloid in Cardiac Pathology, *J. Clin. Pathol.,* 29:22, 1976.

19 Pomerance, A.: Pathology of the Myocardium and Valves, in F. L. Caird, J. L. C. Dall, and R. D. Kennedy (eds.), "Cardiology in Old Age," Plenum Press, Plenum Publishing Corporation, New York, 1976, p. 11.

20 Noble, R. J.: An Approach to Refractory Heart Failure, *Am. Fam. Physician,* 15:138, 1977.

21 White, P. D.: Cardiovascular Disorders, in E. V. Cowdry and F. U. Steinberg (eds.), "The Care of the Geriatric Patient," 4th ed., The C. V. Mosby Company, St. Louis, 1971, p. 51.

22 Smith, T. W., and Haber, E.: Digitalis, *N. Engl. J. Med.,* 289:945, 1973.

23 Bloom, P. M., and Nelp, W. B.: Relationship of the Excretion of Tritiated Digoxin in Renal Function, *Am. J. Med. Sci.,* 251:133, 1966.

24 Kim, Y. I., Noble, R. J., and Zipes, D. P.: Dissociation of the Inotropic Effect of Digitalis from Its Effect on Atrioventricular Conduction (AVC), *Am. J. Cardiol.,* 36:459, 1975.

25 Noble, R. J., Rothbaum, D. A., Wantanabe, A. M., Besch, H. R., and Fisch, C.: Limitations of Serum Digitalis Levels, *Cardiovasc. Clin.,* 6:299, 1974.

26 Mason, D. T.: Symposium on Vasodilator and Inotropic Therapy of Heart Failure, *Am. J. Med.,* 65:101, 1978.

27 Noble, R. J.: The Patient with Syncope, *J.A.M.A.,* 237:1372, 1977.

28 Weissler, A. M., and Warren, J. V.: Syncope and Shock, in J. W. Hurst (ed.), "The Heart," 3rd ed., McGraw-Hill Book Company, New York, 1974, p. 570.

29 Wright, K. E., Jr., and McIntosh, H. D.: Syncope: A Review of Pathophysiological Mechanisms, *Prog. Cardiovasc. Dis.,* 13:580, 1971.

30 Stead, E. A., Jr., and Ebert, R. V.: Postural Hypotension: A Disease of the Sympathetic Nervous System, *Arch. Intern. Med.,* 67:546, 1941.

31 Lasser, R. R., Haft, J. I., and Friedburg, C. K.: Relationship of RBBB and Marked Left Axis Deviation to Complete Heart Block and Syncope, *Circulation,* 37:429, 1968.

32 Dhingra, R. C., Denes, P., Wu, D., Chuquimia, R., Amat-y-Leon, S., Wyndham, C., and Rosen, K. M.: Syncope in Patients with Chronic Bifascicular Block, *Ann. Intern. Med.,* 81:302, 1974.

33 Narula, O. J., Gann, D., and Sanet, P.: Prognostic Value of H-V Intervals, in O. J. Narula (ed.), "His Bundle Electrocardiography and Clinical Electrophysiology," F. A. Davis Company, Philadelphia, 1975, p. 437.

34 McAnulty, J. H., Rahimtoola, S. H., Murphy, E. S., Kauffman, S., Ritzman, L. W., Kanarer, P., and DeMots, H.: A Prospective Study of Sudden Death in "High Risk" Bundle Branch Block, *N. Engl. J. Med.,* 299:209, 1978.

35 Walter, P. F., Reid, S. D., and Wenger, N. K.: Transient Cerebral Ischemia Due to Arrhythmias, *Ann. Intern. Med.,* 72:471, 1970.

36 Weiss, S.: Syncope and Related Syndromes, *Oxford Med.,* 2:250, 1935.

37 Bradbury, S., and Eggleston, C.: Postural Hypotension, *Am. Heart J.,* 1:73, 1925.

38 Bethel, C. S., and Crow, E. W.: Heart Sounds in the Aged, *Am. J. Cardiol.,* 11:763, 1963.

39 Griffithe, R. A., and Sheldon, M. G.: The Clinical Significance of Systolic Murmurs in the Elderly, *Age Aging* 4:99, 1975.

40 Perez, G., Jacob, M., Bhat, P. K., Rao, D. B., and Luisada, A. A.: Incidence of Murmurs in the Aging Heart, *J. Am. Geriatr. Soc.,* 14:29, 1976.

41 Aravanis, C., and Luisada, A. A.: Obstructive and Relative Aortic Stenosis, *Am. Heart J.,* S4:32, 1957.

42 Krovetz, L. J.: Age-related Changes in Size of the Aortic Valve Annulus in Man, *Am. Heart J.,* 90:569, 1975.

43 Vittal, S. B., Luisada, A. A., and Rao, D. B.: Importance of Aortic Dilatation in the Genesis of the Innocent Systolic Ejection Murmur of the Aged, *J. Am. Geriatr. Soc.,* 14:366, 1976.

44 Pomerance, A.: Ageing Changes in Human Heart Valves, *Br. Heart J.,* 29:222, 1967.

45 Pomerance, A.: Pathogenesis of Aortic Stenosis and Its Relation to Age, *Br. Heart J.,* 34:569, 1972.

46 Finegan, R. E., Gianelly, R. E., and Harrison, D. C.: Aortic Stenosis in the Elderly, *N. Engl. J. Med.,* 281:1261, 1969.

47 Davison, E. T., and Friedman, S. A.: Significance of Systolic Murmurs in the Aged, *N. Engl. J. Med.,* 279:225, 1968.

48 Andersen, J. A., Hansen, B. F., and Lyngborg, K.: Isolated Valvular Aortic Stenosis, *Acta Med. Scand.,* 197:61, 1975.

49 Weyman, A. E., Feigenbaum, H., Dillon, J. C., and Chang, S.: Cross-sectional Echocardiography in Assessing the Severity of Valvular Aortic Stenosis, *Circulation,* 52:828, 1975.

50 Burch, G. E., DePasquale, N. P., and Phillips, J. H.: Clinical Manifestations of Papillary Muscle Dysfunction, *Arch. Intern. Med.,* 112:112, 1963.

51 Higgins, C. B., Reinke, R. T., Gosink, B. B., and Leopold, G. R.: The Significance of Mitral Valve Prolapse in Middle-aged and Elderly Men, *Am. Heart J.,* 91:292, 1976.

52 Whiting, R. B., Powell, W. J., Dinsmore, R. E., and Sanders, C. A.: Idiopathic Hypertrophic Subaortic Stenosis in the Elderly, *N. Engl. J. Med.,* 285:196, 1971.

53 Singh, R., Schrank, J. P., Nolan, S. P., and McGuire, L. B.: Spontaneous Rupture of Mitral Chordae Tendineae, *J.A.M.A.,* 219:189, 1972.

54 Barlow, J. B., Bosman, C. K., Pocock, W. A., and Marchand, P.: Late Systolic Murmurs and Non-ejection ("Mid-Late") Systolic Clicks, *Br. Heart J.,* 30:203, 1968.

55 Pomerance, A.: Pathological and Clinical Study of Calcification of the Mitral Valve Ring, *J. Clin. Pathol.,* 23:354, 1971.

56 Korn, D., DeSangtis, R. W., and Sell, S.: Massive Calcification of the Mitral Annulus, *N. Engl. J. Med.,* 267:900, 1962.

57 Hamby, R. I., and Aintablian, A.: Hypertrophic Subaortic Stenosis is not Rare in the Eighth Decade, *Geriatrics,* 31:71, 1976.

58 Feigenbaum, H.: Mitral Valve, in H. Feigenbaum (ed.), "Echocardiography," 2d ed., Lea Febiger, Philadelphia, 1976, p. 87.

59 Caird, F. I.: Valvular Heart Disease, in F. I. Caird, J. L. C. Dall, and R. D. Kennedy (eds.), "Cardiology in Old Age," Plenum Press, Plenum Publishing Corporation, New York 1976, p. 231.

60 Ben, Zvi, J., Hildner, F. J., Javier, R. P., Fester, A., and Samet, P.: Calcific Aortic Insufficiency—a Reivew of 26 Patients, *Am. Heart J.,* 89:278, 1978.

61 Prewitt, T. A.: Syphilitic Aortic Insufficiency—Its Increased Incidence in the Elderly, *J.A.M.A.,* 211:647, 1970.

62 Lerner, P. I., and Weinstein, C.: Invective Endocarditis in the Antibiotic Era, *N. Engl. J. Med.,* 274:259, 1966.

63 Thell, R., Franklin, H. M., and Edwards, J. E.: Bacterial Endocarditis in Subjects 60 Years of Age and Older, *Circulation,* 51:174, 1975.

64 Lerner, P. I., and Weinstein, C.: Invective Endocarditis in the Antibiotics, *N. Engl. J. Med.,* 274:388, 1966.

65 Applefeld, M. M., and Hornick, R. B.: Infective Endocarditis in Patients over Age 60, *Am. Heart J.,* 88:90, 1974.

66 Austen, W. G., DeSanctis, R. W., Buckley, M. J., Mundth, E. D., and Scannell, J. G.: Surgical Management of Aortic Valve Disease in the Elderly, *J.A.M.A.,* 211:624, 1970.

67 Stephenson, L. W., MacVaugh, H., III, and Edmunds, L. H., Jr.: Surgery Using Cardiopulmonary Bypass in the Elderly, *Circulation,* 58:250, 1978.

68 Harken, D. E.: Malnutrition: A Poorly Understood Surgical Risk Factor in Aged Cardiac Patients, *Geriatrics* 32:83, 1977.

69 Hamilton, M., Pickering, G. W., Roberts, J. A. F., and Sowry, G. S. C.: Aetiology of Essential Hypertension, *Clin. Sci.,* 13:11, 1954.

70 Kannel, W. B.: Blood Pressure and Risk of Coronary Artery Disease, Framingham, *Dis. Chest,* 56:43, 1969.

71 Kannel, W. B., Wolf, P. A., Verter, J., and McNamara, P.: Epidemiologic Assessment of the Role of Blood Pressure in Stroke, *J.A.M.A.,* 214:301, 1970.

72 Kannel, W. B., Castelli, W. P., McNamara, P. M., McKee, P. A., and Feinleib, M.: Role of Blood Pressure in the Development of Congestive Heart Failure, The Framingham Study, *N. Engl. J. Med.,* 287:781, 1972.

73 Kannel, W. B.: Blood Pressure and the Development of Cardiovascular Disease in the Aged, in F. I. Caird, J. L. C. Dall, and R. D. Kennedy (eds.) "Cardiology in Old Age," Plenum Press, New York, 1976, p. 143.

74 Kennedy, R. D.: High Blood Pressure and Its Management, in F. I. Caird, J. L. C. Dall, and R. D. Kennedy (eds.), "Cardiology in Old Age," Plenum Press, Plenum Publishing Corporation, New York, 1976, p. 177.

75 Stewart, I. M. G.: Long-term Observations on High Blood Pressure Presenting in Fit Young Men, *Lancet,* 1:671, 1971.

76 Gribbin, B., Pickering, T. G., Sleight, P., and Peto, R.: Effect of Age and High Blood Pressure on Baroreflex Sensitivity in Man, *Circ. Res.,* 29:424, 1971.

77 Caird, F. I., and Kennedy, R. D.: Epidemiology of Heart Disease in Old Age, in F. I. Caird, J. L. C. Dall, and R. D. Kennedy (eds.), "Cardiology in Old Age," Plenum Press, Plenum Publishing Corporation, New York, 1976, p. 1.

78 Mihalick, M. J., and Fisch, C.: Electrocardiographic Findings in the Aged, *Am. Heart J.,* 87:117, 1974.

79 Campbell, A., Caird, F. I., and Jackson, T. F. M.: Prevalence of Abnormalities of Electrocardiogram in Old People, *Br. Heart J.,* 36:1055, 1975.

80 Ostrander, L. D., Brandt, R. L., Kjelsberg, M. O., and Epstein, F. H.: Electrocardiographic Findings among the Adult Population of a Total Natural Community, Tecumseh, Michigan, *Circulation,* 31:888, 1965.

81 Edmands, R. E.: An Epidemiological Assessment of Bundle Branch Block, *Circulation,* 34:1081, 1966.

82 Kitchin, A. H., Lowther, C. P., and Milne, J. S.: Prevalence of Clinical and Electrocardiographic Evidence of Ishcémic Heart Disease in the Older Population, *Br. Heart J.,* 35:946, 1973.

83 Rodstein, M., Brown, M., and Wolloch, L.: First Degree Atrioventricular Block in the Aged, *Geriatrics,* 23:159, 1968.

84 Horan, L. G., Flowers, N. C., and Johnson, J. C.: Significance of Diagnostic Q-Wave of Myocardial Infarction, *Circulation,* 43:428, 1971.

85 Noble, R. J., and Fisch, C.: Factors in the Genesis of Atrial Fibrillation in Rheumatic Valvular Disease, *Cardiovasc. Clin.,* 5:98, 1973.

86 Agruss, N. D., Rosin, E. Y., Adolph, R. J., and Fowler, N. O.: Significance of Chronic Sinus Bradycardia in Elderly People, *Circulation,* 46:924, 1972.

87 Langendorf, R. M., and Pick, A.: Atrioventricular Block Type 2, *Circulation,* 38,819, 1968.

88 James, T. N.: Arrhythmias and Conduction Disturbances in Acute Myocardial Infarction, *Am. Heart J.,* 64:416, 1962.

89 Rotman, M., Wagner, G. S., and Waugh, R. A.: Significance of High Degree Atrioventricular Block in Acute Posterior Myocardial Infarction, *Circulation,* 47:257, 1973.

90 Lenegre, J.: Etiology and Pathology of Bilateral Bundle Branch Block in Relation to Complete Heart Block, *Prog. Cardiovasc. Dis.,* 6:409, 1964.

91 Lev, M.: Anatomic Basis for Atrioventricular Block, *Am. J. Med.,* 37:742, 1964.

Exercise and the Heart*

DONALD O. NUTTER, M.D.

The performance of muscular work (exercise) constitutes the most common and at times the most severe physiologic stress to which the human cardiovascular system must respond. Interest in exercise physiology and sports medicine has grown rapidly as increasing numbers of men and women have begun to participate in recreational and therapeutic exercise, and widespread use of cardiovascular exercise testing, exercise rehabilitation programs, and physical training in the area of preventive cardiology has occurred. The goal of this chapter is to review current concepts of the cardiovascular system and exercise. After a brief summary of the physical and metabolic characteristics of exercise the acute cardiovascular response to the dynamic and static forms of exercise is discussed, with emphasis on the integrated control mechanisms that permit appropriate circulatory responses; this is followed by a review of exercise training and its effect on cardiac structure and function, with commentary on the role of training in the therapy and prevention of heart disease. The cardiovascular physiology of exercise has been the subject of a number of comprehensive reviews during the last decade, and these can provide additional understanding of this rapidly evolving field.[1-6]

PHYSICAL AND METABOLIC ASPECTS OF EXERCISE

Muscular Contraction

The active contraction of muscle results in the development of force, and when developed force exceeds the resistance offered by an external load, shortening of the muscle occurs. Contractions may be voluntary or involuntary, may be under cortical or reflex neural control, and usually involve an integrated pattern of action between various muscle groups. A muscle is comprised of many motor units, each representing a single motor nerve fiber that innervates several muscle fibers. There are two basic types of these fibers in each muscle, although a single motor unit is homogeneous with respect to its fiber type. The contribution of each fiber type to a contraction is de-

termined by the nature and duration of the work. Slow-twitch (type 1) fibers are used for work that involves repetitive or sustained contractile activity, and as such, they contribute the bulk of muscle work during most forms of exercise. The metabolism of slow-twitch fibers is aerobic; i.e., they have a high oxidative and low glycolytic capacity, with numerous mitochondria and a high lipid content.[7] These fibers demand a high level of blood flow when active and consequently have a higher capillary/fiber ratio. Fast-twitch (type 2) fibers produce rapid, nonsustained muscular activity, e.g., rapid ocular movements, and demonstrate an anaerobic metabolic pattern. Fast-twitch fibers are recruited in increasing number for work that exceeds 50 to 60 percent of maximum aerobic capacity. These fibers are subdivided into type 2b fibers, which have a low oxidative capacity, a high glycolytic capacity, and a lower lipid content, and type 2a fibers, which are intermediate with respect to their metabolic characteristics between slow-twitch fibers and type 2b fibers. Type 1 and type 2 fibers are found in roughly equal numbers in most major muscle groups in the human. Muscular work that lasts for more than a few seconds results in local vasodilatation, and if the involved muscle mass is sizable, a number of systemic cardiovascular adjustments occur in order to provide blood flow that is in proportion to the energy expenditure of the working muscle.

Basic Types of Muscular Work

Two distinct types of exercise, determined by the loading conditions applied to the involved muscles, can occur, and both are involved to some extent in most daily activities. (1) Isotonic or dynamic exercise is the repetitive, rhythmic contraction of muscle groups in work tasks that permit muscle shortening and bodily movement. Examples of dynamic exercise include running, swimming, and bicycling. (2) Isometric or static exercise is the sustained contraction of muscle groups against a fixed resistance and is most often performed by pulling or pushing against an immovable object, e.g., maneuvers in weight lifting or wrestling, or in the laboratory, by squeezing a handgrip dynamometer.

Most dynamic exercise in the submaximal range is aerobic, and the primary hemodynamic response is an increase in cardiac output that is in direct proportion

* From the Department of Medicine, Emory University School of Medicine, Atlanta.

to the oxygen consumption of the working muscle. The increased cardiac output is required to adequately perfuse the dilated vascular bed of large muscle groups involved in the exercise. A maximal aerobic task in the untrained subject may elevate cardiac output to 25 liters/min (five times the resting level), and in trained subjects, maximal responses may reach 35 to 40 liters/min. Physical training that utilizes dynamic exercise produces metabolic adaptations (increased oxidative capacity) with little evidence of hypertrophy in the involved skeletal muscles and important conditioning effects on the circulation that are usually associated with modest degrees of cardiac hypertrophy. Submaximal dynamic exercise ("aerobics"), therefore, is used to provide cardiovascular training in normal subjects and for the rehabilitation of cardiac patients. Although dynamic exercise can be quantitated in physical work units, this presents technical difficulties, since it requires knowledge of body mass and the workload, e.g., speed, grade, and the mass of objects moved. In practice, steady-state aerobic work can be quantitated in terms of absolute oxygen comsumption (milliliters of O_2 per minute or milliliters of O_2 per minute per kilogram of body weight) or in relative terms using multiples of the MET. A MET represents the resting oxygen consumption of the subject and in a normal adult is approximately 3.5 ml O_2(min) (kg) or 250 ml O_2/min in a 70-kg individual. The methodology, application, and interpretation of dynamic exercise testing has been extensively reviewed and will not be discussed in this chapter.[8–10]

Isometric work also causes vasodilatation in the contracting muscle and may be aerobic when the force of contraction is less than 25 percent of the muscle's maximal voluntary contractile force. Sustained contractions above 50 to 75 percent of the muscle's maximal voluntary force mechanically restrict local blood flow despite vasodilatation and result in anaerobic work and rapid fatigue. Although cardiac output increases during isometrics the major hemodynamic response to this type of exercise is an elevation of the systemic blood pressure.[11,12] The isometric pressor response is roughly proportional to the contraction intensity and appears to be necessary for adequate perfusion of the contracted muscle. Diastolic arterial pressures, during high-intensity isometric contractions in normal subjects, may reach 130 to 140 mm Hg. Training with isometric tasks will build muscle mass and strength, but when unaccompanied by aerobic endurance training, it will not produce training effects on skeletal muscle metabolism or cardiovascular dynamics.

Metabolic Aspects of Exercise

Oxygen consumption ($\dot{V}O_2$) increases rapidly following the onset of a constant level of dynamic work and plateaus at the level of energy expenditure or oxygen demand, as illustrated in Fig. 1. The delay in $\dot{V}O_2$ response is the time required for the heart, lungs, and vasculature to adapt and shift respiration and cardiac output to a new level adequate for substrate and oxygen delivery. The plateau phase of $\dot{V}O_2$ is termed

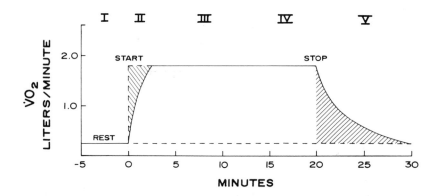

FIGURE 1 Total oxygen uptake (solid line) is shown at rest and during 20 min of exercise at a constant workload. The shaded area at the start of exercise represents the difference between oxygen uptake by working muscle and oxygen demand or energy expenditure (i.e., anaerobic work). The shaded area after cessation of exercise represents excess VO_2 ("oxygen debt"). Note that this area is greater than the initial anaerobic work (see text). Cardiovascular phases: (I) anticipatory, (II) initial or adaptive, (III) steady state, (IV) fine adjustment or drift, (V) recovery.

steady-state work and represents aerobic metabolism. Similar responses with increasingly rapid rates of adjustment occur as the workload is increased up to a point where oxygen consumption fails to increase further despite increased amounts of work. This point is termed the maximal aerobic capacity (MAC). Work levels exceeding the MAC are performed with a significant component of anaerobic metabolism, resulting in lactate production and other deleterious metabolic factors that cause fatigue and limit the duration of work.[13] The maximal aerobic capacity for a given type of exercise is dependent on the involved muscle mass, the metabolic capacity of this muscle mass, and the integrity of the oxygen transport system. The duration over which steady-state work can be sustained falls rapidly when $\dot{V}O_2$ exceeds 40 to 50 percent of the MAC in untrained individuals. Prolonged periods (many hours) of steady-state work can be achieved even up to levels of 60 to 70 percent MAC depending on the degree of physical training and other less well defined factors in individual subjects.

The delivery of substrates and oxygen to fuel aerobic metabolism and the removal of metabolites, carbon dioxide, and heat from the working muscle depends on the integrated function of a multiorgan system. In this system the respiratory apparatus must provide adequate gas exchange; the heart must pump increased volumes of blood to the lungs and working muscles (including the myocardium and respiratory muscles); the blood volume and red blood cell mass must be appropriate to support a high-flow oxygen delivery system; and the peripheral vascular bed must respond with an appropriate degree of vasodilatation in the active muscles and vasoconstriction in certain other vascular beds. In the normal individual the limiting component in the system for MAC appears to be the heart's ability to increase cardiac output beyond a certain point. Other factors being equal, MAC is also determined by the type of exercise performed, sex (MAC is lower for a given task in women), age (MAC decreases with increasing age), and environmental factors, most notably temperature and altitude.[13] A number of disease processes, particularly those that impair muscle mass and function, pulmonary function, cardiovascular function, and red cell mass, will depress MAC.

The profile of $\dot{V}O_2$ during a submaximal dynamic task is illustrated in Fig. 1. The initial phase shows a decreasing anaerobic component (the shaded area below the line for tissue energy expenditure) and is followed by a prolonged steady-state period where $\dot{V}O_2$ matches tissue requirements. Following the cessation of work, a gradual decline in $\dot{V}O_2$ is observed. The terminal shaded area representing "oxygen debt" is a period of augmented oxygen consumption and tissue perfusion necessary to replenish tissue oxygen and

adenosine triphosphate (ATP) stores and metabolize accumulated lactate acid through aerobic pathways or to resynthesize glycogen. In addition, the $\dot{V}O_2$ level of this phase is caused by an elevated temperature, increased levels of circulating catecholamines, and a persistent elevation of cardiac and respiratory work.

A number of studies in recent years have clarified the changing pattern of energy sources that are employed to support exercise over a sustained period. Muscle glycogen is the major substrate utilized for the generation of ATP in the muscle fiber during the onset (first 5 to 10 min) of exercise. The utilization of glycogen progressively declines beyond this point in mild to moderate submaximal work, although it may serve as the major fuel source in high-intensity submaximal or maximal exercise. During the first hour after the onset of steady-state submaximal exercise, circulating free fatty acids (FFA) released from the lipolysis of adipose tissue, blood glucose from hepatic glycogenolysis, and muscle glycogen and lipid stores contribute equally to the substrate pool for muscle metabolism.[14] The percentage of blood glucose utilized progressively increases from 45 to 90 min until it becomes the major substrate (contributing 40 to 50 percent of energy requirements). Blood glucose levels are maintained during this period by hepatic glycogenolysis and hepatic gluconeogenesis that utilizes lactate, pyruvate, glycerol and alanine released from skeletal muscle as substrates. Glucose utilization slowly but progressively declines beyond 90 to 120 min of sustained work, while FFAs become the major fuel source and may provide 60 to 70 percent of the energy requirements by 4 to 5 h.[15] The serum glucose level is well maintained until 1 to 1½ h of exercise, whereupon a slow decline may be observed. The pattern of blood hormonal levels suggests a control system for the metabolic pattern of sustained exercise, i.e., lipolysis, glycogenolysis, and glyconeogenesis without hypoglycemia. Serum insulin levels fall almost immediately upon physical activity, and catecholamines rise. After a lag of 30 to 45 min, serum levels of glucagon, growth hormone, and cortisol progressively increase.[16] At the conclusion of exercise the glycogen stores are replenished in liver and muscle. The performance of repetitive exercise stimulates protein synthesis in muscle and increases the total stores of glycogen in skeletal muscle and liver and of triglycerides (a source of FFA) in muscle.

The cardiovascular adjustments to steady-state dynamic exercise can also be grouped into recognizable phases that parallel the pattern of oxygen consumption as shown in Fig. 1: (1) Shortly before the onset of voluntary exercise the central nervous system (CNS) initiates neural- and hormonal-mediated changes of an anticipatory nature in the heart and vasculature (e.g., an increase in heart rate) that prepare the circulation for the upcoming work. (2) With the onset of exercise, there is a brief adaptive phase, representing the integration of CNS and reflex neural behavior with local mechanical events, that rapidly produces a circulatory state to support the metabolic requirements of exercise. (3) A steady-state phase of cardiovascular function matches the steady state in $\dot{V}O_2$ but is further characterized by fine tuning adjustments in cardiac performance and the regional control of blood flow in order to achieve temperature regulation and support metabolic function in the numerous tissues not involved in exercise. If the workload exceeds the limits that permit a steady state, body temperature will rise excessively, metabolic by-products will accumulate, and substrate levels may not match tissue requirements. Under these circumstances the circulatory parameters will drift or become non-steady state while fatigue ensues and work performance deteriorates. (4) Finally, there is a recovery phase in which neural, hormonal, and mechanical factors interact to slowly readjust the circulation to a resting state.

CARDIOVASCULAR RESPONSES TO ACUTE EXERCISE

During a period of either maximal or prolonged work by skeletal muscle, total oxygen consumption may reach 5 liters/min and body temperature may rise by as much as 3° or 4° C. The circulation must be able to respond in an integrated fashion to support metabolic stress of this magnitude. Stimuli from working muscles arise almost immediately with the onset of exercise and effect two important responses: (1) intense, locally mediated vasodilatation occurs in the vascular bed of muscle to provide an optimal volume and distribution of blood flow in the contracting muscle; and (2) neural reflexes are triggered that evoke an increase in cardiac output and other circulatory adjustments in various regional vascular beds, which together enable muscle blood flow to increase by as much as twenty times the resting level. This hyperemic response in active muscle is necessary to provide substrates and oxygen for contraction, to remove metabolic by-products including carbon dioxide, and to transfer heat to the cutaneous circulation in order for cooling and temperature regulation to take place.

A comprehensive view of exercise hemodynamics has been difficult to obtain because of the dynamic nature of the process and the many variables (e.g., age, sex, environmental temperature, type of work, posture, etc.) that influence the physiologic response to work. Studies of exercise physiology in unanesthetized animals have been compromised by the difficulty of performing quantitated work tasks, by species differences in posture and circulatory control, and by the

need to employ complex implanted instrumentation to directly measure cardiac function. Human studies of hemodynamics and ventricular function during exercise have been limited by ethical and technical constraints on the performance of invasive studies in normal human subjects or in trained athletes undergoing vigorous exercise in both the upright and supine positions. Most human studies have therefore employed relatively simple measurements performed during short periods of steady-state work on the treadmill or with the bicycle ergometer. The recent development of reliable and direct noninvasive measurements of cardiac structure and function, e.g., echocardiography and radionuclide imaging, promises to significantly extend our knowledge of the circulatory response to exercise in normal human beings.

Hemodynamics of Dynamic Exercise

The hemodynamic response to acute exercise revolves around the direct, linear relationship between cardiac output and $\dot{V}O_2$ (Fig. 2). This phenomenon is not influenced appreciably by age, sex, posture, or type of dynamic work performed. Cardiac output in the simplest terms is a function of stroke volume and heart

HEMODYNAMICS: UPRIGHT EXERCISE

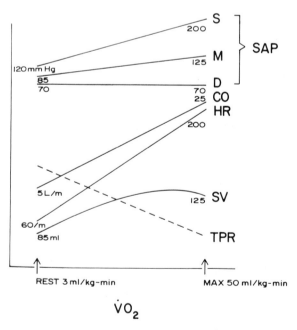

FIGURE 2 Schematic of hemodynamics from rest to maximal work during upright, dynamic exercise. SAP, systemic arterial pressure; S, systolic; M, mean; D, diastolic; CO, cardiac output; HR, heart rate; SV, stroke volume; TPR, total peripheral resistance.

rate, and these variables interact in a manner that is determined by the type of exercise[5] and the posture in which this exercise is performed. Heart rate also demonstrates a direct, linear relationship to $\dot{V}O_2$ and can reach 200 to 220 beats per minute in a young subject at maximal work. The slope of the heart-rate $\dot{V}O_2$ relationship is an inverse function of stroke volume, and the maximal exercise heart rate is also inversely related to age.[17] Relatively small adjustments in stroke volume occur during exercise in normal subjects, and these are significantly influenced by posture. When exercise is performed in the supine position, the initial stroke volume response may be quite variable, with both increases and decreases from the resting level having been described.[18] During steady-state work in the supine position, stroke volume may be unchanged from the resting level or show a modest increase (<10 percent rise). In the upright position, where peripheral blood pooling occurs, causing smaller ventricular and stroke volumes at rest, stroke volume in human beings increases with increasing workloads until $\dot{V}O_2$ reaches 40 to 50 percent of maximum.[18,19] The maximal values obtained for stroke volume during upright exercise, however, usually do not exceed the resting value of stroke volume in the supine subject. Studies performed during running in the human and the dog suggest that stroke volume seldom rises more than 50 percent above the resting level for an upright posture and that stroke volume plateaus or may decline slightly above a $\dot{V}O_2$ of 50 percent maximum.[5,20,21] The cardiac output response to work is therefore a direct function of heart rate in the supine position and is beyond 50 to 60 percent of maximum $\dot{V}O_2$ in the upright position.

The flexibility of cardiac output control during exercise is illustrated by the fact that large increments in stroke volume occur to provide the required level of cardiac output in circumstances when heart-rate responses are blocked or attentuated; e.g., in subjects with complete heart block or where the pre-exercise heart rates are elevated.[22] Studies comparing different work tasks in normal human beings have demonstrated that the stroke-volume-heart-rate interaction is influenced by the type of exercise and the muscle mass involved. Submaximal tasks involving relatively smaller muscle masses, e.g., arm cranking versus running, are associated with higher heart rates and systolic blood pressures and lower stroke volumes or stroke volume increments.[19,23] Bicycling has also been shown to evoke higher rates and lower stroke volume responses than running at a comparable submaximal $\dot{V}O_2$.[24] The explanation of this latter phenomena may not involve a significant difference in the working muscle mass but rather a greater contribution of isometric work in the bicycle task, with a consequent hybrid pattern of hemodynamic response.

Systemic systolic blood pressure increases in direct proportion to $\dot{V}O_2$ and cardiac output, although the slope of this response is an inverse function of working muscle mass.[5,17] Pressures at maximal exercise may easily reach 200 to 220 mm Hg in normal subjects. Diastolic pressure remains constant or declines slightly during most dynamic work, and therefore pulse pressure and mean arterial pressure increase to a modest degree. Since cardiac output is disproportionately augmented with respect to mean blood pressure the calculated value for total systemic resistance is decreased. Peripheral vascular resistance is the net effect of vasoconstriction in several beds (resting muscle, gut, kidney) and vasodilatation in other beds (working muscle and coronary). Pulmonary arterial pressures (PAP) behave in much the same fashion as do systemic pressures, i.e., a linear increase of systolic and mean pressure in relation to $\dot{V}O_2$, with a steeper slope for systolic pressure.[17] Maximal values for systolic PAP may reach 35 to 40 mm Hg at moderate to severe levels of dynamic exercise, and the mean PAP can reach 20 to 25 mm Hg. Dynamic exercise in children evokes hemodynamic responses that are similar qualitatively and in magnitude to those recorded in young to middle-aged adults, although considerably more individual variation has been described in children.[25] The hemodynamic pattern of dynamic exercise is illustrated in Fig. 2.

These initial and steady-state hemodynamic responses to exercise undergo subtle modification when submaximal exercise is prolonged beyond 20 to 30 min, and a "drift" occurs in certain variables. Under these conditions venous return slowly falls and causes a decrease in stroke volume. A slow, progressive increase in heart rate occurs in order to maintain cardiac output nearly constant and in balance with a steady-state $\dot{V}O_2$.[26] These changes are probably the result of several factors, including a slight decline in plasma volume (see below) and redistribution of blood flow to the skin in order to compensate for a gradually rising body temperature. Venous pooling occurs in the skin, and this may reflect changes occurring in the neural vasomotor tone of several capacitance beds. The oxygen uptake by muscle increases slightly during this phase, probably as a result of the gradual shift from carbohydrate to fat as the primary fuel source.

The exercise adjustments of central hemodynamics are closely linked through the central nervous system with the respiratory responses to exercise. A marked increase in minute ventilation results as respiratory rate and tidal volume increase in proportion to $\dot{V}O_2$. The maximal changes in tidal volume approach five to six times base-line values (e.g., from 0.5 to 3.0 liters/min) and are associated with a tripling of rate (e.g., from 15 to 45 breaths per minute).[27] These respiratory adaptations to the metabolic consequences of muscular work produce a progressive rise in systemic venous P_{CO_2} and a fall in P_{O_2}. Systemic arterial P_{CO_2} is relatively stable up to approximately 75 percent maximum $\dot{V}O_2$ and then declines gradually, while arterial P_{O_2} declines very slightly above 50 percent $\dot{V}O_2$.[28] Arterial pH is relatively constant until $\dot{V}O_2$ exceeds 50 percent of maximum, and then pH exponentially declines as the blood lactate level increases. These shifts in arterial P_{O_2} and pH at high work levels may trigger the exponential increase in pulmonary ventilation in this non-steady-state phase of exercise. The systemic arteriovenous oxygen difference progressively widens with increasing $\dot{V}O_2$ and may reach 15 ml/dl of blood from resting levels of 4 to 5 ml/dl. Plasma volume can decrease by 10 to 15 percent during sustained moderate to severe exercise, since fluid is lost by sweating and during respiratory exchange and since a small shift of intravascular volume to the interstitial space takes place.[4] The latter phenomena is caused by a marked fall in the precapillary/postcapillary resistance ratio in the vascular bed of skeletal muscle, with a resultant increase in capillary hydrostatic pressure that favors filtration. The total red blood cell volume does not appear to change during exercise in human beings, but hemoconcentration results from the loss of plasma volume.

Hemodynamics of Static Exercise

Although many of the metabolic and cardiovascular features of static exercise are similar to those of dynamic exercise, certain factors are present during static work that account for important differences in the hemodynamic response. Isometric contractions produce a significant mechanical obstruction to muscle blood flow that is not present in dynamic exercise, where the intermittent contraction pattern may actually favor local flow.[29] This obstruction is minimal when the contraction is below 15 to 20 percent of the muscle's maximal voluntary capacity (MVC) and flow is able to match the metabolic requirements of work that is primarily performed by slow-twitch aerobic fibers. These contractions can be sustained indefinitely, and the hemodynamic responses are characterized by small steady-state increases in heart rate, cardiac output, and systemic arterial pressure. Beyond 15 to 20 percent MVC, muscle blood flow cannot be increased to a level that will match metabolic needs. Blood flow may be totally occluded in calf muscles undergoing isometric contractions of 20 to 30 percent MVC and the same may occur when forearm contractions reach 50 to 60 percent MVC. Contractions above 25 percent MVC are predominantly performed by fast-twitch anaerobic fibers.[30] Contractions of this intensity rapidly

fatigue and manifest an unstable hemodynamic pattern. A marked postcontraction reactive hyperemia is characteristic of isometric work.

The primary hemodynamic response to isometrics is a marked increase in systolic, diastolic, and mean arterial blood pressure that occurs in order to perfuse the high-resistance vascular bed of contracting muscle.[11,12] The pressor response accompanied by a rise in heart rate and cardiac output is immediate with the onset of contraction.[31] Pressure, rate, and output rise progressively during high-intensity contractions (>25 percent MVC) until fatigue interrupts the work.[32] The maximal values for heart rate and cardiac output are considerably lower than those obtained during moderate to severe submaximal levels of dynamic work. Although the increment in cardiac output is modest (peak responses may reach 8 to 12 liters/min), the slope of the output/$\dot{V}O_2$ relationship is steeper with isometric than with dynamic work. The contrasting hemodynamic patterns of isometric and dynamic exercise are illustrated in Fig. 3.

The "excess" cardiac output with isometrics may be more uniformly distributed to the regional circulations by the high arterial pressure head. Alterations in stroke volume during static exercise are small and appear to be related to contraction intensity, since a modest increase (<10 percent) may occur below 50 percent MVC, whereas the marked increase of pressure and heart rate may actually decrease stroke volume at higher contraction intensities. Calculated systemic resistance is not significantly altered by isometrics, unlike the consistent and important decrease in resistance that occurs during dynamic work. Isometrics also have little effect on pulmonary arterial pressures or pulmonary resistance.[31] When isometric work is performed simultaneously with dynamic exercise (i.e., handgrip during treadmill walking), the hemodynamic responses are additive, i.e., a larger pressor response is observed.[33]

The magnitude of the hemodynamic response to static exercise in human beings seems to be primarily a function of relative contraction intensity (percentage of MVC) and remains independent of the muscle mass involved. For example, bilateral handgrip exercise of comparable intensity evokes the same hemodynamic response as a unilateral task. Several investigators have produced involuntary, high-intensity static contractions in the limbs of anesthetized animals by stimulation of motor nerve trunks, and the resultant cardiopulmonary responses (increased ventilation, marked pressor responses, and increased heart rate and cardiac output) have the same pattern as those observed with voluntary isometrics in human beings.[34–36] However, in the anesthetized animal the pressor response appears to be influenced by both contraction intensity and muscle mass, suggesting that when CNS control

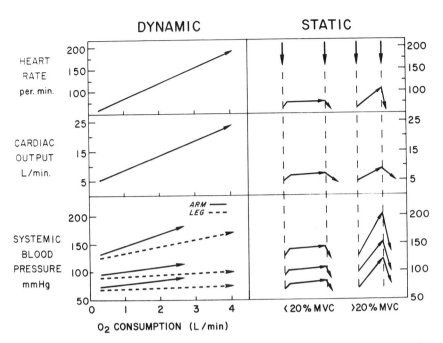

FIGURE 3 Hemodynamic responses to dynamic exercise (running, solid line); cranking arm ergometer, dotted line) and to static (handgrip) exercise, MCV, maximal voluntary contraction.

is absent,[36] reflex stimulation of the cardiovascular adaptation to isometrics is proportional to muscle mass.

Ventricular Function during Dynamic Exercise

The circulatory response to exercise is governed by events in the working muscle; i.e., vasodilatation and reflex signals that indicate to the CNS a need for increased muscle blood flow. The response to these signals is focused on the control of left ventricular function and the cardiac output response. There are four basic determinants of ventricular function: heart rate, preload (end-diastolic volume or fiber length), myocardial contractility or the inherent inotropic state of ventricular muscle, and afterload or the level of wall stress during ventricular ejection as governed by the impedance to ventricular ejection and ventricular chamber dimensions. Augmentation of the first three determinants will increase cardiac output, whereas output is inversely related to afterload. Controversy has persisted for years concerning the relative contribution to the cardiac exercise response of tachycardia, the Frank-Starling effect (i.e., an increased stroke volume in response to elevated preload), and augmented cardiac contractility. A recent series of studies in animal and human subjects performing dynamic exercise has clarified this issue.[20,21,37,38] The anticipatory pre-

exercise increase in heart rate and the progressive elevation of rate that accompanies increasing $\dot{V}O_2$ decreases the diastolic filling period and, to a lesser degree, decreases the duration of ventricular systole. At the same time, a variety of factors, including increased forward flow, vasodilatation with decreased flow resistance in the muscle beds, venoconstriction and decreased venous pooling, rhythmic mechanical venous compression by contracting muscle, and augmented respiratory excursions, act in concert to progressively increase venous return. The net result of an increased venous return and tachycardia is to maintain ventricular end-diastolic volume constant or to permit small increases in volume, depending on the severity of exercise and the body position. A slight fall in end-diastolic volume has sometimes been observed with the onset of exertion or during mild supine exercise, probably reflecting an imbalance between the rapid increase in heart rate and the level of venous return.[37] However, other studies have demonstrated either a constant LVED volume during supine exercise[38] or a small but progressive increase in LVED dimensions and volume during mild to severe levels of upright exercise.[20,21] Maximal ventricular dimensions during vigorous exercise usually do not exceed the LVED volume present in the supine, resting heart. These findings seem to indicate a masked contribution of the Frank-Starling effect to the control of exercise-related cardiac output, since the expected response of end-diastolic volume to tachycardia without acute volume loading is a sizable decrease in ventricular volumes and stroke volume.[39] Conversely, if heart rate is held constant during exercise stress, a marked increase in LVED volume and stroke volume occurs and the cardiac output/$\dot{V}O_2$ relationship is maintained at submaximal work levels.[21,22] The Frank-Starling effect also becomes apparent in the period immediately following exercise, when heart rate falls rapidly, venous return remains augmented, and ventricular end-diastolic volume increases to a significant degree.[38,40] Afterload is increased during exercise, since ventricular dimensions are maintained and mean arterial pressure is elevated, but this factor probably exerts a minimal restraint on the velocity and extent of cardiac contraction. The major exercise effect on ventricular dynamics is a significant increase in myocardial contractility resulting from sympathetic stimulation of the ventricular myocardium and probably enhanced by the tachycardia (Treppe effect). Augmented contractility increases the rate of ventricular pressure development (maximal dp/dt) and the extent and rate of ventricular shortening as manifested by increases in ejection fraction and circumferential or segmental shortening velocity. As a result, ventricular end-systolic dimensions are reduced from the resting level. The effect of exercise on ventricular dimensions and cardiac contractility is shown in Fig. 4, and the cumulative results of these studies indicate that heart rate, preload, and myocardial contractility all have a positive interaction to permit high levels of cardiac output during exercise.

Ventricular Function during Static Exercise

The effect of sustained isometric handgrip (15 to 50 percent MVC) on left ventricular dynamics has been studied with a variety of direct and indirect techniques. In normal subjects, isometrics have been reported to either decrease LV end-diastolic dimensions and volume[41,42] or to have little effect on dimensions.[43] LVED pressure in the normal heart is unchanged or shows a small decline during static exercise.[31,42,44,45] Although ventricular function is augmented in response to isometrics; (i.e., an increased cardiac output and stroke work in the face of increased systemic pressure and ventricular afterload), it is not clear if this results primarily from an increase in heart rate or whether an increase in myocardial contractility also plays a significant role. Left ventricular maximal dp/dt is increased by isometrics,[36,44,46] and ventricular V_{max} calculated from pressure data was elevated during handgrip,[46] but the extent and velocity of LV wall motion and the LV ejection fraction were unchanged

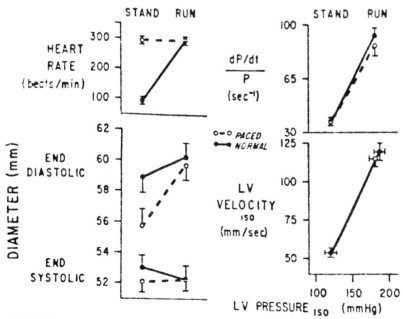

FIGURE 4 Left ventricular dynamics, including internal diameter and its velocity, at rest (standing) and during severe exercise (running) in chronically instrumented, telemetered dogs. The data are presented at spontaneous heart rates and also during fixed rate atrial pacing. (From Vatner et al.: Left Ventricular Response to Severe Exertion in Untethered Dogs, J. Clin. Invest., 51:3057, 1972.)

or depressed during static work.[41,42] These results probably reflect net effects from the opposing influences of increased afterload, heart rate, and myocardial contractility and a decreased preload.

Control of the Circulation during Exercise

The exercise response is a remarkable example of an acute integrated systemic reaction to stress. Central nervous system command, continuously modified by a variety of informational inputs, produces a coordinated neural outflow to the major effector organs, which include skeletal muscle, heart, lungs, and peripheral vascular beds. The principal functional adaptations to exercise include (1) locally controlled vasodilatation in working skeletal muscle, and (2) centrally controlled alteration in ventricular function, hemodynamics, and ventilation (discussed previously), as well as changes in vascular resistance and blood flow in a number of regional beds.

Vasodilatation in contracting muscle occurs immediately with the onset of work, and the subsequent magnitude of the dilator response is directly proportional to the tissues' oxygen demand. The local metabolic factor(s) that mediate this response have not been defined, but the candidates include K^+, pH, lactate, osmolality, and adenosine.[29] This muscle dilator response is an example of local autoregulation overriding systemic neural control, since a local sympatholytic effect has been documented that prevents the generalized sympathetic vasoconstrictor effect of exercise from reducing blood flow in working muscle.[47-49]

The autonomic nervous system provides the efferent limb for circulatory control during exercise. Withdrawal of vagal (parasympathetic) tone from the sinus node is a major factor responsible for both the anticipatory and initial phase tachycardia. Sympathetic stimulation of the sinus node mediates the progressive heart rate increase seen with increasing levels and duration of exertion and also mediates the enhanced cardiac contractility that allows an optimal cardiac output response to result from the increased heart rate and venous return.[3,39,50] Heart-rate regulation during exercise is a complex phenomena that involves circulating catecholamines as well as an intrinsic cardiac control mechanism that has been demonstrated after cardiac denervation and adrenalectomy.[50] A similar pattern of cardiac autonomic control has been delineated for isometric exercise.[51] Sympathetic stimulation of vascular receptors produces constriction in the small arteries, arterioles, and veins in a number of vascular beds. Generalized vasoconstriction of inactive vascular beds elevates arterial blood pressure and promotes the perfusion of working muscle while shift-

ing the distribution of cardiac output from nonessential beds to muscle. Sympathetic-mediated venoconstriction also occurs and displaces blood from the venous reservoirs into the effective circulating blood volume for rapid delivery to muscle. The increase in venous resistance which accompanies venoconstriction does not significantly impair venous return, since an increased peripheral venous pressure, coupled with muscular compression of veins and the cyclic decrease of intrathoracic pressure with increased respiratory activity, actually elevates the driving pressure (peripheral venous pressure minus right atrial pressure) for venous return.[4]

Considerable data have been accumulated on the regional distribution of cardiac output during dynamic exercise. Neurally mediated vasoconstriction with an increased resistance to blood flow occurs during exercise in the vascular beds of inactive skeletal muscle,[52,53] gut, and kidney.[2-4] These vasoconstrictor responses lead to a reduced mesenteric and renal blood flow in exercising human subjects.[54-56] In the dog, however, blood flow to the gut and kidneys is maintained at resting levels even during severe steady-state workloads.[57-60] The reasons for this species difference in flow responses are not fully explained at present, although in the awake, intact dog, neural vasoconstrictor activity appears to be minimized during steady-state exercise.[3] In several essential vascular beds there is little evidence of increase resistance or decreased flow with exercise in either human beings or animals. The pulmonary bed responds to dynamic exercise with passive distension and recruitment of the capillary bed in order to accommodate the increased blood flow, and pulmonary vascular resistance has been shown to fall.[17,61] Cerebral blood flow changes very little during even moderate to severe exercise in human beings[62,63] or in the experimental animal.[64] The coronary vascular bed can be thought of in simple terms as serving another working muscle group during exercise, and coronary flow may increase to four or five times the base-line level during exercise.[65-67] Coronary flow responses to exercise have been described as a linear function of heart rate in both the right and left ventricles. Coronary flow has also shown an equal pattern of distribution to the endocardial and epicardial layers of the left ventricle.[68,69] There is no evidence that myocardial ischemia is associated with severe exercise in the normal heart, and coronary flow does not appear to be the limiting factor in maximal aerobic capacity. The most complex adjustments in regional blood flow occur in the cutaneous beds, where neural vasomotor responses reflect the competition between the demands of working muscle and thermal regulation. Vasoconstriction and decreased skin blood flow occur initially and during mild levels of steady-state work, but when body temperature increases with higher workloads, reflex vasodilatation and increased skin flow occurs. When $\dot{V}O_2$ exceeds 50 to 60 percent of maximum, flow again declines and intense vasoconstriction may occur at maximal exercise.[2,70] This condition can lead to severe hyperthermia and heart stroke when prolonged heavy work is performed in a hot, humid environment.

Limited observations on the regional distribution of blood flow during static exercise have revealed a pattern similar to that occurring with dynamic work. Blood flow to inactive muscle groups in human beings performing static exercise shows little change or a modest increase. This response appears to represent the net effect of an increasing systemic perfusion pressure and an elevated vascular resistance.[32,71] Stimulation of the afferent nerves from the limb muscles of anesthetized dogs has produced vasoconstriction of the isolated vascular beds of muscle, skin, gut, and kidney and vasodilatation in the coronary circulation.[72,73] However, blood flow increased to the intact vascular bed of muscle and kidney, again demonstrating the net effect when regional vasoconstriction occurs with a marked increase in systemic pressure.

The key element in circulatory control during exercise appears to be what Smith and associates have termed a "hydrodynamic feedback control system," which in turn is closely linked with a complex, integrated neural control system.[4] Hydrodynamic feedback refers to the autoregulatory increase in blood flow to working muscle that leads to increased venous return and the mechanical adaptation of cardiac output to match blood flow with muscle $\dot{V}O_2$. Studies of the cardiovascular response to exercise after total cardiac denervation in dogs have demonstrated the fundamental importance of intrinsic mechanical regulation of the heart, as adjustments in cardiac dimensions and stroke volume have, in many cases, permitted nearly maximal exercise in these cardiac-denervated animals.[50] It is equally clear, however, that moderate to maximal exercise in the presence of a denervated heart is dependent on circulating catecholamines (perhaps with augmented cardiac responsiveness) and on the autonomic innervation of the lung.[50,74,75] The central nervous system superimposes neural control on the hydrodynamic feedback system in order both to provide the most efficient cardiovascular adaptation and to extend maximal aerobic capacity. The contributions of neural control include the rapid and optimal responses in heart rate and cardiac contractility as well as selective regional vasoconstriction with redistribution of blood flow and augmentation of perfusion pressure.[76,77]

There are two major interacting components to neural control: (1) Cortical irradiations to the neuronal pools of the hypothalamus and brain stem provide autonomic outflow to respiratory and cardiovascular effectors.[78,79] This cortical activity is probably interrelated with the cortical initiation and subsequent regulation of voluntary muscular activity through the somatic nervous system. (2) Somatic afferent signals from receptors in exercising muscle are integrated under cortical control at the spinal, brain stem, and hypothalamic levels with the autonomic reflex inputs from carotid-aortic chemoreceptors and baroreceptors, as well as numerous cardiac and pulmonary mechanoreceptors.[80,81] A number of investigators working with both human beings and animals have shown that metabolic stimuli in contracting muscle can evoke immediate reflex increases of heart rate, cardiac output, and blood pressure.[34,35,80,82-86] The afferent pathways for these reflex adjustments are small, types 3 and 4, myelinated and unmyelinated somatic fibers. This exercise reflex is potentially in conflict with certain other cardiovascular reflexes, since the venous return, stroke volume, and pressor responses of exercise should activate aorto-carotid and cardiopulmonary mechanoreceptors that reflexly depress heart rate and lower blood pressure. These reflexes, therefore, could interfere with the desired heart rate, blood pressure, and regional blood flow adaptations to exercise. Studies directed to this question have indicated that aorto-carotid baroreflex sensitivity is significantly depressed during exercise.[87-89] It therefore seems likely that the integrated CNS exercise response favors the somatosympathetic cardiovascular reflex from working muscle and suppresses other central, vagally mediated reflexes operating in the negative-feedback mode. The role of more recently described, positive-feedback, sympathetically mediated cardio-cardiovascular reflexes in the cardiovascular response to exercise is unclear at present.[90-92]

Effect of Sex, Age, and Cardiovascular Disease on Responses to Acute Exercise

Aerobic work capacity is similar in boys and girls before puberty, but the maximal exercise capacity in adult women is limited at approximately 70 to 75 percent of that found in men of the same age.[93,94] This appears to be the case even after differences in body mass are taken into account, and the difference occurs despite the fact that there does not appear to be a sex-related difference in the aerobic demand at common submaximal work levels.[95] It is not clear whether this difference in maximal aerobic capacity represents an inherent physiologic difference in the cardiorespiratory system of women or is the result of differing lifestyles and physical training.

Maximal aerobic capacity declines with age in a nearly linear fashion after the age of 18 to 20 years in normal subjects.[13] Maximal workloads are associated with a lower heart rate, stroke volume, cardiac output, and arteriovenous oxygen difference in older subjects.[96,97] The mechanism responsible for the decline in maximal aerobic capacity and cardiovascular performance has not yet been determined, but a number of age-related changes in cardiovascular function have been identified. Two such alterations that might explain age-related limitations in exercise capacity are (1) an increased peripheral vascular resistance, both at rest and during exercise, that increases the impedance to left ventricular ejection; and (2) a decrease in the cardiac responsiveness to catecholamines.[98]

Environmental factors such as high ambient temperature and humidity or a decrease in atmospheric oxygen tension, as might be encountered at high altitudes, will obviously limit maximal aerobic capacity, since oxygen delivery to skeletal muscle at high stress levels would be impaired under these conditions. In a similar fashion, moderate to severe anemia or diseases that impair pulmonary function would allow these factors to replace cardiac pump function as the limiting factor for aerobic work. The presence of cardiovascular disease frequently requires the heart to utilize its functional reserve capacity, normally available to meet stress situations, in order to maintain normal levels of resting performance. This limits maximal aerobic capacity, with the restriction on physical performance clearly being related to the magnitude of the underlying, pathologic dysfunction. Heart-rate responses to exercise are not altered by heart failure, although the resting rate required to sustain a normal cardiac output may be elevated, thus limiting the scope of the work-induced rate response. The ability to increase the extent of cardiac shortening and ejection is impaired during heart failure with the result that stroke volume cannot increase and may fall with progressive exercise loads.[3] Cardiac output and $\dot{V}O_2$ are limited under these conditions. Peripheral vascular responses to exercise are also modified by heart failure or circulatory impairment. A marked reduction in blood flow secondary to intense vasoconstriction in mesenteric, renal, cutaneous, and inactive muscle beds occurs during exercise in the animal or patient with heart failure in order to distribute a limited cardiac output to the exercising muscle groups.[53,99,100] Temperature regulation is impaired under these circumstances and may also limit the individual's exercise capacity. In some patients with coronary artery disease, underlying myocardial damage and latent heart failure may limit maximal $\dot{V}O_2$ in the manner noted above. In other coronary patients with normal ventricles at rest, sudden cardiac failure may result at workloads producing myocardial $\dot{V}O_2$ in excess of the coronary flow capability. This has been noted to decrease stroke volume and cardiac output, leading to a non-steady state at a point where heart rate and the

$A\dot{V}O_2$ difference are still on the rise.[5] Dynamic work capacity in the patient with coronary artery disease may therefore be limited by (1) chronic heart failure that is increased by exercise stress, (2) acute heart failure during stress that places maximal $\dot{V}O_2$ at subnormal levels, or (3) the development of angina pectoris where the maximal myocardial $\dot{V}O_2$ is limited by coronary obstruction.

PHYSICAL TRAINING AND THE CARDIOVASCULAR SYSTEM

Physical training is an adaptive response or conditioning effect observed primarily in skeletal muscle and the cardiovascular system. Training occurs in response to a chronic increase in muscular work and allows an individual to perform a given task with less effort and greater efficiency for a longer duration, as well as increasing the maximal workload that can be performed. Training programs refer to the type, intensity, frequency, and total duration of muscular work that is employed to produce a training effect. Training effects can be measured in skeletal muscle or the circulation and involve structural, metabolic, and physiologic alterations in response to training. Various aspects of physical training have received extensive and recent review.[5,6,101]

The amount or degree of training that can be achieved is controlled by many factors; some of the more important include age, sex, type of training program, initial state of training, and general health status of the individual.[6] The type of training effects that can be expected depend primarily on the type of exercise employed in the training program. Training with dynamic exercise has relatively little effect on skeletal muscle mass but can produce profound alterations in muscle metabolism, whereas it generally has little effect on myocardial metabolism or biochemistry but can produce mild to moderate cardiac hypertrophy and significant changes in both resting and exercise hemodynamics. On the other hand, training that primarily involves isometric work can result in a significant degree of skeletal muscle and myocardial hypertrophy, with little metabolic alteration in either organ, and no change in resting hemodynamics or the circulatory response to either dynamic or static exercise.

The most consistently evoked and sensitive training effect that can be readily measured in human subjects is aerobic capacity or maximum $\dot{V}O_2$ (Fig. 5). This parameter can be significantly increased by endurance training with dynamic exercise when the initial level of training is relatively low (i.e., sedentary subjects or those involved in mild daily work stress). The level of $\dot{V}O_2$ can be used as an indicator of training in the general population when age and sex are taken

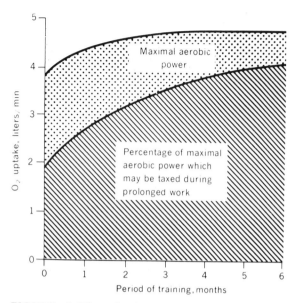

FIGURE 5 Effect of endurance training on maximal oxygen uptake and the percentage of maximal oxygen uptake that can be utilized for long duration work without fatigue. (*From P.-O. Astrand, and K. Rodahl, "Textbook of Work Physiology," 1st ed., McGraw-Hill Book Company, New York, 1970.*)

into account. $\dot{V}O_2$ ranges from 35 to 45 ml O_2 (kg) (min) in sedentary young men (age 20 to 30 years) to 75 to 80 ml (kg) (min) in elite or world-class male long-distance runners of comparable age.[102] The spectrum of training effects or fitness has been further extended by the studies of Saltin, et al., in which normal young men were placed at complete bed rest for 3 weeks and average maximal $\dot{V}O_2$ fell from 43 to 32 ml (kg) (min).[103] A relatively low intensity training program performed for several weeks can increase maximal $\dot{V}O_2$ by 5 to 15 percent and high-intensity, long-duration programs in young, healthy individuals may evoke increases of 90 to 95 percent.

The critical element behind most training effects seems to be the metabolic conditioning of skeletal muscle groups involved in the training exercise. When training is induced by selectively using one group of muscles (e.g., legs versus arms or one leg versus the other) neither maximal $\dot{V}O_2$ nor the hemodynamic responses to exercise are altered when exercise is performed with other, untrained muscle groups.[5,6,19] In addition, the magnitude of the training effect (Δ maximal $\dot{V}O_2$) appears to be a function of trained muscle mass (e.g., arms < legs). These observations suggest that metabolic factors induced by conditioning in the trained muscle groups provide a signal for the appropriate cardiovascular response (decreased Δ heart rate and increased Δ stroke volume) during submaximal

and maximal work. Furthermore, the enhanced maximal $\dot{V}O_2$ present during exercise with trained muscle groups is the result of these metabolically triggered hemodynamic responses and the augmented oxidative capacity of the trained muscle and is not a primary training effect on the heart.

The widespread use of physical training for the therapy and alleged prevention of cardiovascular disease must involve dynamic exercise, since this approach results in metabolic and hemodynamic training effects. Isometric training is ineffective in this regard and poses considerable danger to the cardiac patient or elderly subject because of the abrupt and dramatic pressor response that accompanies static work. For these reasons the remainder of this section will deal with the effects and application of training that employs dynamic exercise.

The Physiology of Training

SKELETAL MUSCLE

Endurance training has no demonstrable effect on muscle contractility and produces only a modest increase in fiber size or muscle mass when the training program is of high intensity and long duration.[104] The adaptive responses to endurance training are designed to improve the aerobic performance of muscle. These responses include increases in capillary number per muscle fiber, myoglobin concentration, the size and number of mitochondria, and the level of mitochondrial respiratory enzymes.[6,101,105] The oxidative capacity of all three fiber types increases to some extent, but a significant augmentation of intramitochondrial respiratory enzymes (as much as twofold) is seen only in type 1 (slow-twitch) or type 2a (fast-twitch) fibers.[104] These fibers also increase their glycolytic capacity (e.g., increased hexokinase activity) and their ability to convert pyruvate into alanine, which may be released from muscle during prolonged activity and utilized by the liver in gluconeogenesis.[104] Fast-twitch fibers, however, are not converted into slow-twitch fibers, so that the fiber populations in a muscle group remain constant.[104,106,107] The net effect of endurance training is to shift the metabolic pattern of skeletal muscle toward the aerobic pattern of myocardium, with an increased dependence on pyruvate and fatty acids for the generation of ATP, less glycogen depletion and lactate production at a given submaximal workload, and a lower blood flow per unit of muscle with an increased oxygen extraction. These factors enable the trained individual to have a higher maximal $\dot{V}O_2$ and to sustain a higher submaximal $\dot{V}O_2$ for longer duration without the onset of fatigue (Fig. 5).

HEMODYNAMICS

The single most consistent training effect on the resting circulation is a lower heart rate with a secondary increase in stroke volume. Training bradycardia has been observed in comparative studies of trained and sedentary human populations as well as in serial studies of training adaptations in both human and animal subjects. The mechanism is still uncertain and is probably multifactorial, including increased parasympathetic and decreased sympathetic influence in the sinus node with uncertain contributions from decreased circulating catecholamine levels and a resetting of intrinsic sinoatrial node control.[6,108,109] Cardiac output is little changed by training, although in some cases the resting level has declined slightly.[19,103,110] Training also has little effect on resting blood pressure in young, normal subjects but may lower the systolic and diastolic levels in older subjects[111] or in hypertensive patients.[6,112] Total blood volume may increase during endurance training as a result of expansion of the plasma volume with little change in red cell volume, an increase in hemoglobin, and a rightward shift of the oxyhemoglobin dissociation curve.

Endurance training modifies the hemodynamic response to submaximal exercise in a characteristic manner with lower heart rates and larger stroke volumes for any $\dot{V}O_2$. Heart rate is the independent variable in this adaptation.[5] Although cardiac output usually remains constant at a given submaximal $\dot{V}O_2$, a slight decrease may be observed in some cases.[110] This phenomenon is particularly common in patients with coronary artery disease and a limited cardiac functional reserve and may be explained by the increased oxygen extraction present during exercise with trained muscles that reduces the requirements for muscle blood flow.[113,114] The ability of trained muscles to extract more oxygen, as well as the altered reflex control of heart rate, at submaximal $\dot{V}O_2$ is based on the metabolic and structural adaptations discussed in the previous section. At maximal $\dot{V}O_2$ the heart rate in trained subjects is the same or somewhat lower than in the untrained state, while the maximal cardiac output is significantly increased in the trained subject in order to match the augmented maximal $\dot{V}O_2$. An increase in stroke volume therefore is necessary to provide the additional cardiac output at maximal $\dot{V}O_2$. In normal subjects, ventilatory responses do not limit maximal $\dot{V}O_2$ and the enhanced $\dot{V}O_2$ maximal after endurance training appears to be made possible by equal contributions from increased cardiac output and muscle blood flow and an increased oxygen extraction from that flow. Training in normal subjects has little effect on blood pressure during submaximal exercise,[110] but mean pressure at submaximal $\dot{V}O_2$ may be lower after

training in patients with hypertension or coronary artery disease.[6,112,113,115] The blood pressure at maximal $\dot{V}O_2$ may be lower, unchanged, or elevated after training. Training shifts the regional distribution of blood flow at submaximal $\dot{V}O_2$ so that there is a relatively greater perfusion of nonworking organs and a decreased flow to exercising muscle.

CARDIAC DIMENSIONS

Endurance training of at least moderate intensity and duration has been shown to produce cardiac enlargement involving both hypertrophy and chamber dilatation in human beings, and this training effect may persist after detraining regression occurs in other variables, e.g., bradycardia.[116] When the cardiac chamber size and mass in highly trained athletes has been measured by echocardiography and compared with measurements in sedentary control subjects, the athletes have shown mild to moderate degrees of right and left ventricular dilatation with eccentric hypertrophy (Fig. 6).[117-120] The study by Morganroth and associates also compared endurance training with strength or isometric training, and athletes trained with isometrics had normal ventricular volumes but increased ventricular wall thickness and a significant degree of concentric hypertrophy.[117] When serial echocardiographic measurements of left ventricular dimensions and mass have been made during a 2- to 3-month endurance training program in young men, a progressive increase in these variables and a subsequent rapid decrease with detraining were observed.[121,122] Cardiac hypertrophy in response to training has been more difficult to produce in animal models.[6] In small animals (rodents) the assessment of hypertrophy is usually based on absolute heart weight and ventricular fiber diameters, as compared to values from body-weight-matched controls, or on heart weight/body weight ratios. Studies utilizing these techniques have shown cardiac hypertrophy in rats exposed to moderate or severe running and swimming training programs.[123] Postmortem heart weights and fiber diameters, as well as measurements of left ventricular dimensions in the awake animal, have also demonstrated chamber enlargement and hypertrophy in trained as compared to control dogs[124] and the development of mild hypertrophy in response to a training program.[125] Training-induced cardiac dilatation and hypertrophy are probably the result of increased cardiac volume loading, both at rest with training bradycardia and during upright exercise stress, and systolic pressure loading during exercise stress. Altered levels of mechanical and/or metabolic wall stress in response to chronic loading conditions could serve to trigger myofiber hypertrophy.

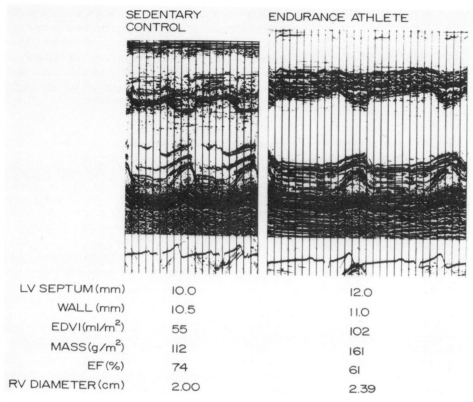

	SEDENTARY CONTROL	ENDURANCE ATHLETE
LV SEPTUM (mm)	10.0	12.0
WALL (mm)	10.5	11.0
EDVI (ml/m²)	55	102
MASS (g/m²)	112	161
EF (%)	74	61
RV DIAMETER (cm)	2.00	2.39

FIGURE 6 Left ventricular echocardiograms from a highly trained young male long-distance runner and an age- and sex-matched sedentary subject. The values for septal and LV posterior wall thickness and LV end-diastolic volume internal diameter are shown.

CARDIAC ULTRASTRUCTURE, CORONARY VASCULATURE, AND METABOLISM

There is evidence to suggest that cardiac mitochondrial mass and concentration are increased by training in the rat, but little information is otherwise available concerning training effects on myocardial ultrastructure.[126] Studies also performed in the rat have indicated that training increases epicardial coronary artery area, the capillary/myocardial fiber ratio, and the relative mass of the coronary vasculature.[127–129] There are no controlled data on coronary vascular responses to training in human beings, partly because of the ethical and technical constraints on such studies. Growth of the coronary vascular bed during training appears to be related to increases in heart size and work, and regression of the coronary mass with detraining is slow, as in the case for exercise hypertrophy.

Few significant training effects on myocardial metabolism have been noted, which is not unexpected, since the capacity for aerobic metabolism in normal myocardium exceeds that present in trained skeletal muscle.[6,123] Although no consistent changes in the respiratory enzymes of myocardial mitochondria are reported after training, there is evidence that cardiac glycogen stores are increased, while triglycerides decline and certain of the glycolytic enzymes are increased.[6,126,130] This change in substrate availability and glycolytic capacity might represent a reserve mechanism to meet or ward off stress-induced myocardial hypoxia during severe exercise. The characteristics of energy utilization in trained hearts are discussed in the following section.

Several studies have indicated that myocardial catecholamine concentration and binding sites are decreased by training, although conflicting data have been reported in this area.[126,131,132] Those observations may be related to indirect data suggesting that the augmented levels of cardiac sympathetic stimulation and circulating catecholamines present during exercise may be decreased by training.[6] Considerable further investigation appears to be necessary before the effects of training on neural and hormonal cardiac control are clarified.

CARDIAC FUNCTION AND MYOCARDIAL CONTRACTILITY

The hemodynamic changes at rest and during stress that are induced by endurance training are well rec-

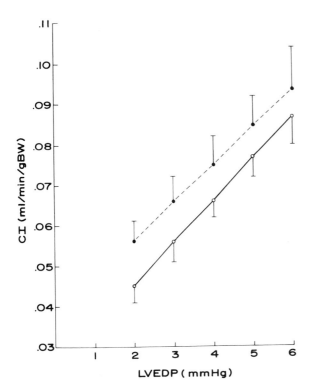

FIGURE 7 Left ventricular function curves generated in the in situ hearts of adult male rats endurance trained by running (*N* = 8, dotted line) and from sedentary control rats (*N* = 11, solid line). CI, cardiac index calculated on the basis of body weight; LVEDP, left ventricular end-diastolic pressure. Vertical bars = standard error. (*From D. O. Nutter and E. O. Fuller, unpublished data.*)

ognized (see above). There is less data and more controversy on the subject of how training affects cardiac function and myocardial contractility. Since cardiac output at rest and for any level of $\dot{V}O_2$ is unchanged after training, an evaluation of altered contractile capacity must rely on measurements of ventricular function that utilize isovolumic phase indices (*dp/dt*) or ejection phase indices involving the velocity and extent of ventricular shortening. Echocardiographic studies of trained athletes and control subjects have failed to show a difference in the resting cardiac function of these groups when variables such as ejection fraction and circumferential shortening velocity are calculated.[118–120,122] Similar comparative studies of ventricular function during exercise stress have been technically impossible in human beings.

A recent study comparing chronically instrumented dogs trained for racing with a group of normal dogs failed to demonstrate any difference in either isovolumic or ejection phase indices of ventricular performance at rest or during a volume loading stress.[124] The trained animals did manifest significantly greater increases in heart rate during volume loading. A similar

study of dogs trained on the treadmill found no difference in resting LV maximal *dp/dt*, but an elevated level of *dp/dt* was present at comparable heart rates during submaximal work.[133] Previous measurements of isometric and isovolumic tension and pressure indices in rats trained by swimming have indicated that ventricular contractility of the in situ heart increased after training.[134,135] On the other hand, resting function of the nonhypertrophied, in situ left ventricle of female rats trained by treadmill running did not differ from that measured in sedentary control animals.[136] In response to a sustained pressure overload stress, however, the trained rats maintained pre-stress levels of contractility, whereas contractility was depressed in the control rats. We have performed similar studies on the hypertrophied, in situ heart of treadmill-trained male rats and have failed to show significant differences in left ventricular function when trained and sedentary hearts were compared. This study examined resting contractility and functional reserve capacity as evaluated with volume loading (Fig. 7). In conclusion, the bulk of studies examining resting and stressed function of the intact endurance-trained heart, subject to neural and humoral control mechanisms, do not indicate that ventricular function is altered aside from the more efficient work pattern provided by a slower rate and a large stroke volume.

A somewhat different conclusion is suggested by the extensive studies of Scheuer and associates on the isolated, perfused hearts of rats trained by swimming. These investigators have shown enhanced external work of the nonhypertrophied left ventricle from trained rats, particularly at higher preload levels and under both normal and hypoxic conditions. The enhanced mechanical performance of trained hearts under nonstressed conditions was associated with a greater aerobic capacity and could be attributed to improved coronary flow and oxygen delivery.[137] The functional improvement of trained hearts seen during hypoxia was not related to differences in myocardial substrate availability, intermediary metabolism, energy stores, or oxygen delivery but did suggest a more efficient pattern of energy utilization.[138] Recent studies have extended these observations and demonstrated an increased level of left ventricular contractility under conditions where the basic determinants of ventricular function (heart rate, afterload, and preload) were held constant.[139] These results, expressed in terms of ventricular force-velocity data, are illustrated in Fig. 8. We have recently employed the isolated, perfused rat heart preparation to study the cardiac function of rats trained by treadmill running and have been unable to show a difference in left ventricular external work or maximal *dp/dt* with training in these animals.

Biochemical support for an elevated myocardial

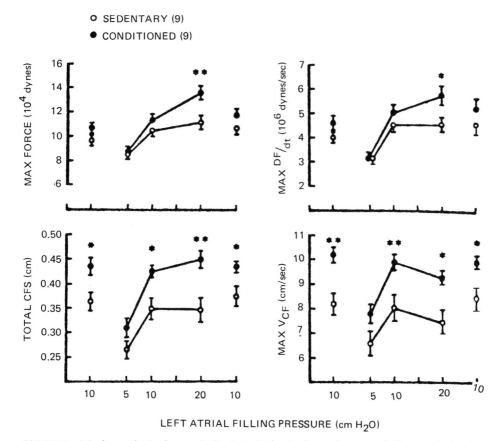

FIGURE 8 Left ventricular force-velocity data obtained at increasing preloads from the isolated, perfused, working heart of rats endurance trained by swimming and their sedentary controls. (*From M. M. Bersohn and J. Scheuer, Effects of Physical Training on End-Diastolic Volume and Myocardial Performance of Isolated Rat Hearts, Circ. Res., 40:514, 1977.*)

contractile state in the trained heart has been provided by several investigators, but the correlation of these observations with the various studies of mechanical function and their reproducibility is not clear at present. Increased cardiac actomyosin ATPase activity has been described in myocardial preparations from rats trained by swimming protocols of varying intensity.[140,141] Calcium transport by the ventricular sarcoplasmic reticulum has also been shown to increase in rats trained by swimming.[142] Conversely, when dogs and rats have been trained on the treadmill, no changes were detectable in ventricular myofibrillar ATPase activity.[133,143]

Several investigators have examined the effect of endurance training on myocardial contractility using the isolated right or left ventricular papillary muscle preparation. The results are in agreement that the passive length-tension (stiffness) properties of ventricular myocardium are unaffected by training. However, divergent results have been obtained from the study of

active length-tension and force-velocity mechanics. Rats and cats trained by running have demonstrated an unchanged or slightly depressed state of myocardial contractility,[144,145] whereas rats trained by swimming manifest enhanced contractility.[146] Our own studies of papillary muscle mechanics in treadmill-trained young and adult rats also demonstrate an unchanged or depressed state of myocardial contractility, with no difference in the contractile response to calcium, norepinephrine, or hypoxic stress (Fig. 9).

The inconclusive results of these studies on the responses of myocardial contractility, biochemistry, and ventricular function to endurance training may be the result of differences in species, training intensity, or experimental methods employed for the study of cardiac function. The intriguing possibility that a different training response in biochemistry, contractility, and pump function may arise depending on whether swimming and running provides the training stress must be pursued further.

Clinical Observations in Trained Subjects

Certain features of the physical examination, chest x-ray, and electrocardiogram are frequently present in the highly trained athlete and may suggest either a hyperdynamic circulation or organic heart disease. These findings have been termed the athlete's heart syndrome and are discussed in more detail in Chap. 9 of *The Heart*.

Clinical Applications of Cardiovascular Endurance Training

REHABILITATION OF PATIENTS WITH HEART DISEASE

Endurance training offers several benefits to selected groups of cardiac patients, including some with regurgitant valvular lesions, certain congenital defects, hypertension, and subgroups of the coronary artery disease population. The importance of a complete cardiovascular evaluation, continuing primary therapy of the underlying disease, and exercise testing in order to prescribe a suitable training program cannot be overemphasized in these patients. Patients with moderate to severe valvular obstruction (e.g., aortic stenosis) and progressive heart muscle disease (e.g., congestive and hypertrophic cardiomyopathies) should not participate in physical stress beyond ordinary sedentary daily activities, since a considerable risk of syncope, serious arrhythmias, and progression of the underlying cardiac muscle disease or heart failure exists. Many aspects of physical rehabilitation for patients with coronary artery disease and myocardial infarction have been reviewed in recent publications[147-149] and in Chap. 62, Section G, of *The Heart*.

General benefits of cardiac rehabilitation with physical training include those of both a psychological and a physiological nature. The psychological benefits of endurance training should not be underestimated, for enormous good may result from the sense of accomplishment, personal satisfaction, and the altered approach to social and work responsibilities that physical fitness can produce in selected patients. The most important physiologic benefit is an increase in work capacity, in terms both of intensity and duration, before the cardiac patient becomes limited by symptoms. Physical training can lower both resting and stress-related blood pressure in hypertensive patients[6,112] and is a synergistic factor in weight reduction programs.

Endurance training as a therapeutic modality for patients with coronary disease and angina pectoris has been widely applied and shown to increase work ca-

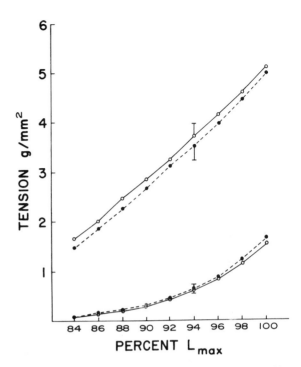

FIGURE 9 Active (upper) and passive (lower) pairs of isometric length-tension curves from trained (*N* = 14, dotted line) and sedentary (*N* = 18, solid line) rats. Vertical bar = standard error. (*From D. O. Nutter and E. O. Fuller, unpublished data.*)

pacity in the majority of cases.[5,18] Therapeutic success seems to be inversely related to the severity of coronary obstruction and to the anginal pattern with better results provided in those patients who manifest typical exertional angina as opposed to those with rest pain and unstable patterns.[150] Training effects in patients with angina include (1) an increase in the minimal workload necessary to provoke angina, and (2) an extended duration of work at lower loads before the onset of pain.[115,151,152] Angina develops in response to myocardial ischemia, and this process reflects an imbalance between oxygen supply to the myocardium and oxygen consumption or demand by the myocardium. In order to increase work capacity in the coronary patient, training must either (1) allow a given workload to be performed at a lower myocardial $\dot{V}O_2$, or (2) adapt the heart so that a higher myocardial workload can be reached by aerobic or anaerobic means before angina develops. The first of these mechanisms is a documented result of training, as shown by a reduction in the heart rate and blood pressure, and hence a lowered ventricular wall stress and minute oxygen consumption at which a given workload can be sustained. This adaptation is explained by the training effect that increases muscular aerobic capacity and the oxygen extraction of working muscle and in turn permits the same work to be performed with a lower muscle blood flow and a decreased cardiac output. The metabolic reflex demand from muscle to heart is therefore decreased, resulting in lower heart rate and blood pressure. Although it is possible that training might also lower myocardial $\dot{V}O_2$ during work by reducing ventricular end-diastolic volume or contractile state, there are few data to support this mechanism. The second mechanism, namely an increase in the cardiac work or $\dot{V}O_2$ necessary to precipitate angina, has been demonstrated in some coronary patients.[153] Several adaptive processes might produce this result, and they include increased coronary flow to potentially ischemic areas or an increased myocardial anaerobic capacity that could provide the required contractile energy (ATP) for brief periods of pain-free work that would ordinarily demand a high myocardial $\dot{V}O_2$. The latter possibility is of interest in view of the increased cardiac glycogen stores and altered glycolytic enzyme activities induced by training (see previous section), as well as the better ventricular performance during hypoxia shown by trained hearts.[138] Proof that these metabolic adaptations function in coronary disease patients is lacking at present.[153] It seems quite likely that training may provide increased collateral coronary flow to ischemic myocardium, since recurrent ischemic stress on the myocardium during training has the potential for stimulating collateral development. This phenomenon has not been demonstrated in human beings, but studies of ischemic heart disease in animal models has provided supportive evidence for an increased collateral flow.[154,155] In addition, a recent study in rats has shown that the increased coronary vascularity after training was associated with a decreased size of myocardial infarction produced by coronary ligation.[156] These and related observations suggest that training in patients with coronary disease may also impede the disease process or limit the extent of complications.[157]

PREVENTION OF CORONARY ATHEROSCLEROTIC HEART DISEASE

The relationship between casual daily recreational and vocational activity levels or chronic exercise training programs and the incidence of coronary atherosclerotic heart disease in the general population remains one of the most controversial medical topics of our time. A definitive answer to the question of whether long-term training prevents coronary heart disease and its complications is not possible at present. Indeed, the issue has been confused by extremists whose viewpoints range from claims for coronary immunity after training to an ultraconservative statistical denial of any relationship or indeed any possibility of further proof of such a relationship. Two aspects of this prob-

lem deserve comment: (1) The role of training can be assessed in terms of known training effects on widely accepted coronary "risk factors"; i.e., it may be possible to establish a place for physical activity with respect to the modification of coronary disease risk even if we cannot prove with rigorous scientific method that exercise has a primary role in prevention. (2) A voluminous body of epidemiologic data can be evaluated, in lieu of what may prove to be technically impossible prospective scientific studies, to establish the place of training in coronary prevention.

Several coronary "risk factors" are reduced or modified by training in a manner that suggests that certain population subgroups may have the incidence of coronary disease reduced. As previously discussed, training can lower hypertensive blood pressures at rest and during stress.[112,158,159] Acute exercise will lower serum triglyceride levels for several days, and although there is little or no change in cholesterol level, a significant elevation of the high-density lipoprotein cholesterol level has been reported.[160,161] Serum high-density lipoprotein levels have shown an inverse correlation with the incidence of coronary disease. A reduction in stressful emotions and beneficial psychological adjustments appear to result from long-term physical conditioning, and these factors have been indirectly linked to the development of coronary disease, (see Chap. 96 in *The Heart*). Finally, exercise regimens may be a useful component of weight reduction programs.

Many epidemiologic studies have shown an inverse correlation between the amount of physical activity in selected vocations, races, countries, and other population divisions and the prevalence of coronary heart disease in these groups. These studies have often been flawed by a failure to account for "selection," i.e., the occurrence of other factors in the populations under study that might explain the lower prevalence of coronary disease.[162] In other instances the statistical analyses or the definitions of physical activity levels have been unacceptable. A review of these problems is beyond the scope of this discussion, but as a prototype of a well-designed and thoughtfully interpreted study, one might consider the work of Paffenburger.[163] This survey of the long-term relationship between daily energy expenditure and coronary disease in longshoremen concluded that high energy expenditure was associated with a significantly lower mortality for coronary disease. Finally, it must be kept in mind that it is often risky to apply the results of a study that examines a specific sex, age, or population subgroup or that involves a specific intermittent form of training activity to the population at large. Despite these many problems, our present state of knowledge strongly suggests that long-term physical activity, whether in work or play, affords some degree of protection from coronary artery disease.

REFERENCES

1 Bevegård, B. S., and Shepherd, J. T.: Regulation of the Circulation during Exercise in Man, *Physiol. Rev.*, 47:178, 1967.

2 Rowell, L. B.: Human Cardiovascular Adjustments to Exercise and Thermal Stress, *Physiol. Rev.*, 54:75, 1974.

3 Vatner, S. F., and Pagani, M.: Cardiovascular Adjustments to Exercise: Hemodynamics and Mechanisms, *Prog. Cardiovasc. Dis.*, 19:91, 1976.

4 Smith, E. E., Guyton, A. C., Manning, R. D., and White, R. J.: Integrated Mechanisms of Cardiovascular Response and Control during Exercise in the Normal Human, *Prog. Cardiovasc. Dis.*, 18:421, 1976.

5 Clausen, J. P.: Circulatory Adjustments to Dynamic Exercise and Effect of Physical Training in Normal Subjects and in Patients with Coronary Artery Disease, *Prog. Cardiovasc. Dis.*, 18:459, 1976.

6 Scheuer, J., and Tipton, C. M.: Cardiovascular Adaptations to Physical Training, *Annu. Rev. Physiol.*, 39:221, 1977.

7 Saltin, B., Hendriksson, J., Nygaard, E., Andersen, P., and Tansson, E.: Fiber Types and Metabolic Potentials of Skeletal Muscles in Sedentary Man and Endurance Runners, *Ann. N. Y. Acad. Sci.*, 301:3, 1977.

8 Committee on Exercise, American Heart Association: "Exercise Testing and Training of Apparently Healthy Individuals: A Handbook for Physicians," American Heart Association, New York, 1972.

9 Bruce, R. A.: Methods of Exercise Testing. Step Test, Bicycle, Treadmill, Isometrics, *Am. J. Cardiol.*, 33:715, 1974.

10 Gilbert, C. A.: Exercise Testing of Cardiac Function, in J. W. Hurst (ed.), "The Heart," 4th ed., McGraw-Hill Book Company, New York, 1978, p. 516.

11 Donald, K. W., Lind, A. R., McNicol, G. W., Humphreys, P. W., et al.: Cardiovascular Responses to Sustained (Static) Contractions, *Circ. Res.*, 20(suppl. 1):15, 1967.

12 Nutter, D. O., Schlant, R. C., and Hurst, J. W.: Isometric Exercise and the Cardiovascular System, *Mod. Concepts Cardiovasc. Dis.*, 41:11, 1972.

13 Åstrand, P. O., and Rodahl, K.: Physical Work Capacity, in "Textbook of Work Physiology," 2d ed., McGraw-Hill Book Company, New York, 1977, p. 289.

14 Felig, P., and Wahren, J.: Fuel Homeostasis in Exercise, *N. Engl. J. Med.*, 293:1078, 1975.

15 Gollnick, P. D.: Free Fatty Acid Turnover and the Availability of Substrates as a Limiting Factor in Prolonged Exercise, *Ann. N. Y. Acad. Sci.*, 301:64, 1977.

16 Galbo, H., Richter, E. A., Hilsted, J., et al.: Hormonal Regulation during Prolonged Exercise, *Ann. N. Y. Acad. Sci.*, 301:72, 1977.

17 Ekelund, L. G., and Holmgren, A.: Central Hemodynamics during Exercise, *Circ. Res.*, 20(suppl. 1):33, 1967.

18 Bevegård, S., Holmgren, A., and Jonsson, B.: The Effect of Body Position on the Circulation at Rest and during Exercise, with Special Reference to the Influence on the Stroke Volume, *Acta Physiol. Scand.*, 49:279, 1960.

19 Clausen, J. P., Klausen, K., Rasmussen, B., et al.: Central and Peripheral Circulatory Changes after Training of the Arms or Legs, *Am. J. Physiol.*, 225:675, 1973.

20 Horwitz, L. D., Atkins, J. M., and Leshin, S. J.: Role of the Frank-Starling Mechanism in Exercise, *Circ. Res.*, 31:868, 1972.

21 Vatner, S. F., Franklin, D., Higgins, C. B., et al.: Left Ventricular Response to Severe Exertion in Untethered Dogs, *J. Clin. Invest.*, 51:3052, 1972.

22 Ikkos, D., and Hanson, J. S.: Response to Exercise in Congenital Complete Atrioventricular Block, *Circulation*, 22:583, 1960.

23 Åstrand, P-O., and Saltin, B.: Maximal Oxygen Uptake and Heart Rate in Various Types of Muscular Activity, *J. Appl. Physiol.*, 16:977, 1961.

24 Hermansen, L., Ekblom, B., and Saltin, B.: Cardiac Output during Submaximal and Maximal Treadmill and Bicycle Exercise, *J. Appl. Physiol.*, 29:82, 1970.

25 Lock, J. D., Einzig, S., and Moller, J. H.: Hemodynamic Responses to Exercise in Normal Children, *Am. J. Cardiol.*, 41:1278, 1978.

26 Hartley, H. L.: Central Circulatory Function during Prolonged Exercise, *Ann. N. Y. Acad. Sci.*, 301:189, 1977.

27 Wilmore, H. H.: Acute and Chronic Physiological Responses to Exercise, in E. A. Amsterdam, J. H. Wilmore, and A. N. DeMaria (eds.), "Exercise in Cardiovascular Health and Disease," Yorke Medical Books, New York, 1977, p. 53.

28 Åstrand, P.-O., and Rodahl, K.: Respiration, in "Textbook of Work Physiology," 2d ed., McGraw-Hill Book Company, New York, 1977.

29 Clement, D. L., and Shepherd, J. T.: Regulation of Peripheral Circulation during Muscular Exercise, *Prog. Cardiovasc. Dis.*, 19:23, 1976.

30 Hultén, B., Thorstensson, A., Sjödin, B., et al.: Relationship between Isometric Endurance and Fibre Types in Human Leg Muscles, *Acta Physiol. Scand.*, 93:135, 1975.

31 Fisher, M. L., Nutter, D. O., Jacobs, W., et al.: Haemodynamic Responses to Isometric Exercise (Handgrip) in Patients with Heart Disease, *Br. Heart J.*, 35:422, 1973.

32 Lind, A. R., Taylor, S. H., Humphreys, P. W., et al.: Circulatory Effects of Sustained Voluntary Muscle Contraction, *Clin. Sci.*, 27:229, 1964.

254

33 Lind, A. R., and McNicol, G. W.: Circulatory Responses to Sustained Handgrip Contractions Performed during Other Exercise, Both Rhythmic and Static, *J. Physiol.*, 192:595, 1967.

34 Coote, H. H., Hilton, S. M., and Perez-Gonzalez, J. F.: The Reflex Nature of the Pressor Response to Muscular Exercise, *J. Physiol.*, 215:789, 1971.

35 McCloskey, O. I., and Mitchell, J. H.: Reflex Cardiovascular and Respiratory Responses Originating in Exercising Muscle, *J. Physiol.*, 224:173, 1972.

36 Fisher, M. L., and Nutter, D. O.: Cardiovascular Reflex Adjustments to Static Muscular Contractions in the Canine Hindlimb, *Am. J. Physiol.*, 226:648, 1974.

37 Sonnenblick, E. H., Braunwald, E., Williams, J. F., Jr., et al.: Effects of Exercise on Myocardial Force-Velocity Relations in Intact Unanesthetized Man: Relative Roles of Changes in Heart Rate, Sympathetic Activity, and Ventricular Dimensions, *J. Clin. Invest.*, 44:2051, 1965.

38 Stein, R. A., Michielli, D., Fox, E. L., et al.: Continuous Ventricular Dimensions in Man during Supine Exercise and Recovery. An Echocardiographic Study, *Am. J. Cardiol.*, 41:655, 1978.

39 Braunwald, E., Sonnenblick, E. H., Ross, J., Jr., et al.: An Analysis of the Cardiac Response to Exercise, *Circ. Res.*, 20(suppl. 1):44, 1967.

40 Horwitz, L. O., Atkins, J. M., and Dunbar, S. A.: Left Ventricular Dynamics during Recovery from Exercise, *J. Appl. Physiol.*, 39:449, 1975.

41 Ludbrook, P., Karliner, J. S., and O'Rourke, R. A.: Effects of Submaximal Isometric Handgrip on Left Ventricular Size and Wall Motion, *Am. J. Cardiol.*, 33:30, 1974.

42 Flessas, A. P., Connelly, G. P., Handa, S., et al.: Effects of Isometric Exercise on the End-Diastolic Pressure, Volumes, and Function of the Left Ventricle in Man, *Circulation*, 53:839, 1976.

43 Stefadouros, M. A., Grossman, W., ElShahawy, M., et al.: The Effect of Isometric Exercise on the Left Ventricular Volume in Normal Man, *Circulation*, 49:1185, 1974.

44 Kivowitz, C., Parmley, W. W., Donoso, R., et al.: Effect of Isometric Exercise on Cardiac Performance. The Grip Test, *Circulation*, 44:994, 1971.

45 Amende, I., Krayenbuehl, H. P., Rutishauser, W., et al.: Left Ventricular Dynamics during Handgrip, *Br. Heart J.*, 34:688, 1972.

46 Grossman, W., McLaurin, L. P., Saltz, S. B., et al.: Changes in the Inotropic State of the Left Ventricle during Isometric Exercise, *Br. Heart J.*, 35:697, 1973.

47 Shepherd, J. T.: Behavior of Resistance and Capacity Vessels in Human Limbs during Exercise, *Circ. Res.*, 20(suppl. 1):70, 1967.

48 Donald, D. E., Rowlands, D. J., and Ferguson, D. A.: Similarity of Blood Flow in the Normal and the Sym-

pathectomized Dog Hind Limb during Graded Exercise, *Circ. Res.*, 26:185, 1970.

49 Costin, J. C., and Skinner, N. S., Jr.: Competition between Vasoconstrictor and Vasodilator Mechanisms in Skeletal Muscle, *Am. J. Physiol.*, 220:462, 1971.

50 Donald, D. E.: Myocardial Performance after Excision of the Extrinsic Cardiac Nerves in the Dog, *Circ. Res.*, 34:417, 1974.

51 Martin, C. E., Shaver, J. A., Leon, D. F., et al.: Autonomic Mechanisms in Hemodynamic Responses to Isometric Exercise, *J. Clin. Invest.*, 54:104, 1974.

52 Blair, D. A., Glover, W. E., and Roddie, I. C.: Vasomotor Responses in the Human Arm during Leg Exercise, *Circ. Res.*, 9:264, 1961.

53 Zelis, R., Mason, D. T., and Braunwald, E.: Partition of Flood Flow to the Cutaneous and Muscular Beds of the Forearm at Rest and during Exercise in Normal Subjects and in Patients with Heart Failure, *Circ. Res.*, 24:799, 1969.

54 Rowell, L. B.: Regulation of Splanchnic Blood Flow in Man, *Physiologist*, 16:127, 1973.

55 Chapman, C. B., Henschel, A., Minckler, J., et al.: The Effect of Exercise on Renal Plasma Flow in Normal Male Subjects, *J. Clin. Invest.*, 27:639, 1948.

56 Wade, O. L., and Bishop, J. M.: The Distribution of Cardiac Output in Normal Subjects during Exercise, in "Cardiac Output and Regional Blood Flow," Blackwell Scientific Publications, Ltd., Oxford, 1962, p. 95.

57 Rushmer, R. F., Franklin, D. L., Van Citters, R. L., et al.: Changes in Peripheral Blood Flow Distribution in Healthy Dogs, *Circ. Res.*, 9:675, 1961.

58 Van Citters, R. L., and Franklin, D. L.: Cardiovascular Performance of Alaska Sled Dogs during Exercise, *Circ. Res.*, 24:33, 1969.

59 Vatner, S. F., Higgins, C. B., White, S., et al.: The Peripheral Vascular Response to Severe Exercise in Untethered Dogs before and after Complete Heart Block, *J. Clin. Invest.*, 50:1950, 1971.

60 Fixler, D. E., Atkins, J. M., Mitchell, J. E., et al.: Blood Flow to Respiratory, Cardiac and Limb Muscles in Dogs during Graded Exercise, *Am. J. Physiol.*, 231:1515, 1976.

61 Elkins, R. C., and Milnor, W. R.: Pulmonary Vascular Response to Exercise in the Dog, *Circ. Res.*, 29:591, 1971.

62 Hedlund, S., Nylin, G., and Regnstrom,: The Behavior of the Cerebral Circulation during Muscular Exercise, *Acta Physiol. Scand.*, 54:316, 1962.

63 Zobl, E. G., Talmers, F. N., Christensen, R. C., et al.: Effects of Exercise on the Cerebral Circulation and Metabolism, *J. Appl. Physiol.*, 20:1289, 1965.

64 Foreman, D. L., Sanders, M., and Bloor, C. M.: Total and Regional Cerebral Blood Flow during Moderate and

Severe Exercise in Miniature Swine, *J. Appl. Physiol.*, 40:191, 1976.

65 Khouri, E. M., Gregg, D. E., and Rayford, C. R.: Effect of Exercise on Cardiac Output, Left Coronary Flow and Myocardial Metabolism in the Unanesthetized Dog, *Circ. Res.*, 17:427, 1965.

66 Vatner, S. F., Higgins, C. B., Franklin, D., et al.: Role of Tachycardia in Mediating the Coronary Hemodynamic Response to Severe Exercise, *J. Appl. Physiol.*, 32:380, 1972.

67 Jorgensen, C. R., Gobel, F. L., Taylor, H. L., et al.: Myocardial Blood Flow and Oxygen Consumption during Exercise, *Ann. N. Y. Acad. Sci.*, 301:213, 1977.

68 Ball, R. M., Bache, R. J., Cobb, F. R., et al.: Regional Myocardial Blood Flow during Graded Treadmill Exercise in the Dog, *J. Clin. Invest.*, 55:43, 1975.

69 Barnard, J. R., Duncan, H. W., Livesay, J. J., et al.: Coronary Vasodilator Reserve and Flow Distribution during Near-Maximal Exercise in Dogs, *J. Appl. Physiol.*, 43:988, 1977.

70 Johnson, J. M.: Regulation of Skin Circulation during Prolonged Exercise, *Ann. N. Y. Acad. Sci.*, 301:195, 1977.

71 Eklund, B., Kaijser, L., and Knutsson, E.: Blood Flow in Resting (Contralateral) Arm and Leg during Isometric Contraction, *J. Physiol.*, 240:111, 1974.

72 Clement, D. L., and Shepherd, J. T.: Influence of Muscle Afferents on Cutaneous and Muscle Vessels in the Dog, *Circ. Res.*, 35:177, 1974.

73 Wickliffe, C., Nutter, D. O., and Crumly, H.: Regional Vascular Responses to the Somatopressor Reflex, *Physiologist*, 18:448, 1975.

74 Nordenfelt, I.: Haemodynamic Response to Exercise after Combined Sympathetic and Parasympathetic Blockade of the Heart, *Cardiovasc. Res.*, 5:215, 1971.

75 Horwitz, L. D., Atkins, J. M., and Leshin, S. J.: Effect of Beta-Adrenergic Blockade on Left Ventricular Function in Exercise, *Am. J. Physiol.*, 227:839, 1974.

76 Taylor, S. H., and Donald, K. W.: Circulatory Effects of Bretylium Tosylate and Guanethidine, *Lancet*, 2:389, 1960.

77 Bevegård, S., Jonsson, B., and Karlof, I.: Circulatory Response to Recumbent Exercise and Head-up Tilting in Patients with Disturbed Sympathetic Cardiovascular Control (Postural Hypotension): Observations on the Effect of Norepinephrine Infusion and Anti-gravity Suit Inflation in the Head-up Tilted Position, *Acta Med. Scand.*, 172:623, 1962.

78 Rushmer, R. F., Smith, O., and Franklin, D.: Mechanisms of Cardiac Control in Exercise, *Circ. Res.*, 7:602, 1959.

79 Goodwin, G. M., McCloskey, D. I., and Mitchell, J. H.: Cardiovascular and Respiratory Responses to Changes in Control Command during Isometric Exercise at Constant Muscle Tension, *J. Physiol.*, 226:173, 1972.

80 Mitchell, J. H., Reardon, W. C., McCloskey, D. I., et al.: Possible Role of Muscle Receptors in the Cardiovascular Response to Exercise, *Ann. N. Y. Acad. Sci.*, 301:232, 1977.

81 Korner, P. I.: Integrative Neural Cardiovascular Control, *Physiol. Rev.*, 51:312, 1971.

82 Alam, M., and Smirk, F. H.: Observations in Man upon a Blood Pressure Raising Reflex Arising from the Voluntary Muscles, *J. Physiol.*, 89:372, 1937.

83 Staunton, H. P., Taylor, S. H., and Donald, K. W.: The Effect of Vascular Occlusion on the Pressor Response to Static Muscular Work, *Clin. Sci.*, 27:283, 1964.

84 Hollander, A. P., and Bouman, L. N.: Cardiac Acceleration in Man Elicited by a Muscle-Heart Reflex, *J. Appl. Physiol.*, 38:272, 1975.

85 Liang, C. S., and Hood, W. B., Jr.: Afferent Neural Pathway in the Regulation of Cardiopulmonary Responses to Tissue Hypermetabolism, *Circ. Res.*, 38:209, 1976.

86 Tibes, U.: Reflex Inputs to the Cardiovascular and Respiratory Centers from Dynamically Working Canine Muscles. Some Evidence for Involvement of Group III or IV Nerve Fibers, *Circ. Res.*, 41:332, 1977.

87 Bristow, J. D., Brown, E. B., Jr., Cunningham, D. J. C., et al.: Effect of Bicycling on the Baroreflex Regulation of Pulse Interval, *Circ. Res.*, 28:582, 1971.

88 Cunningham, D. J. C., Petersen, E. S., Peto, R., et al.: Comparison of the Effect of Different Types of Exercise on the Baroreflex Regulation of Heart Rate, *Acta Physiol. Scand.*, 86:444, 1972.

89 McRitchie, R. J., Vatner, S. F., Boettcher, D., et al.: Role of Arterial Baroreceptors in Mediating Cardiovascular Response to Exercise, *Am. J. Physiol.*, 230:85, 1976.

90 Malliani, A., Recordati, G., and Schwartz, P. J.: Nervous Activity of Afferent Cardiac Sympathetic Fibers with Atrial and Ventricular Endings, *J. Physiol.*, 229:457, 1973.

91 Malliani, A., Lombardi, F., Pagani, M., et al.: Spinal Cardiovascular Reflexes, *Brain Res.*, 87:239, 1975.

92 Gupta, P. D.: Spinal Autonomic Afferents in Elicitation of Tachycardia in Volume Infusion in the Dog, *Am. J. Physiol.*, 229:303, 1975.

93 Åstrand, I.: Aerobic Work Capacity in Men and Women with Special Reference to Age, *Acta Physiol. Scand.*, 49(suppl. 169):1, 1960.

94 Saltin, B., Åstrand, P.-O.: Maximum Oxygen Uptake in Athletes, *J. Appl. Physiol.*, 23:353, 1967.

95 Daniels, J., Krahenbuhl, G., Foster, C., et al.: Aerobic Responses of Female Distance Runners to Submaximal

and Maximal Exercise, *Ann. N. Y. Acad. Sci.*, 301:726, 1977.

96 Strandell, T.: Circulatory Studies on Healthy Old Men, *Acta Med. Scand.*, 175(suppl. 414):1, 1964.

97 Julius, S., Antoon, A., Whitlock, L. S., et al.: Influence of Age on the Hemodynamic Response to Exercise, *Circulation*, 36:222, 1967.

98 Gerstenblith, G., Lakatta, E. G., and Weisfeldt, M. L.: Age Changes in Myocardial Function and Exercise Response, *Prog. Cardiovasc. Dis.*, 19:1, 1976.

99 Higgins, C. B., Vatner, S. F., Franklin, D., et al.: Effects of Experimentally Produced Heart Failure on the Peripheral Vascular Response to Severe Exercise in Conscious Dogs, *Circ. Res.*, 31:186, 1972.

100 Millard, R. W., Higgins, C. B., Franklin, D., et al.: Regulation of the Renal Circulation during Severe Exercise in Normal Dogs and Dogs with Experimental Heart Failure, *Circ. Res.*, 31:881, 1972.

101 Holloszy, J. O.: Adaptations of Muscular Tissue to Training, *Prog. Cardiovascular Dis.*, 18:445, 1976.

102 Gibbons, L. W., Cooper, K. H., Martin, R. P., et al.: Medical Examination and Electrocardiographic Analysis of Elite Distance Runners, *Ann. N. Y. Acad. Sci.*, 301:283, 1977.

103 Saltin, B., Blomqvist, G., Mitchell, J. H., et al.: Response to Exercise after Bed Rest and after Training, *Circulation*, 38(suppl. 7):1, 1968.

104 Gollnick, P. D., and Sembrowich, W. L.: Adaptations in Human Skeletal Muscle as a Result of Training, in E. A. Amsterdam, J. H. Wilmore, and A. N. DeMaria (eds.), "Exercise in Cardiovascular Health and Disease," Yorke Medical Books, New York, 1977, p. 70.

105 Brodal, P., Ingjer, F., and Hermansen, L.: Capillary Supply of Skeletal Muscle Fibers in Untrained and Endurance Trained Men, *Am. J. Physiol.*, 232:705, 1977.

106 Baldwin, K. M., Winder, W. W., Terjung, R. L., et al.: Glycolytic Enzymes in Different Types of Skeletal Muscle: Adaptation to Exercise, *Am. J. Physiol.*, 225:962, 1973.

107 Gollnick, P. D., Armstrong, R. B., Saltin, B., et al.: Effect of Training on Enzyme Activity and Fiber Composition of Human Skeletal Muscle, *J. Appl. Physiol.*, 34:107, 1973.

108 Badeer, H. S.: Resting Bradycardia of Exercise Training: A Concept Based on Currently Available Data, in P. E. Roy and G. Rona (eds.), "Recent Advances in Studies on Cardiac Structure and Metabolism," Vol. 20, University Park Press, Baltimore, 1975, p. 553.

109 Barnard, R. J., Corre, K., and Cho, H.: Effect of Training on the Resting Heart Rate of Rats, *Eur. J. Appl. Physiol.*, 35:285, 1976.

110 Ekblom, B., Åstrand, P.-O., Saltin, B., et al.: Effect of Training on Circulatory Response to Exercise, *J. Appl. Physiol.*, 24:518, 1968.

111 Saltin, B., and Grimby, G.: Physiological Analysis of Middle-aged and Old Former Athletes. Comparison with Still Active Athletes of the Same Ages, *Circulation*, 38:1104, 1968.

112 Boyer, J. L., and Kasch, F. W.: Exercise Therapy in Hypertensive Men, *J.A.M.A.*, 211:1668, 1970.

113 Clausen, J. P., and Trap-Jensen, T.: Effects of Training on the Distribution of Cardiac Output in Patients with Coronary Artery Disease, *Circulation*, 42:611, 1970.

114 Rousseau, M. F., Brasseur, L. A., and Detry, J. M. R.: Hemodynamic Determinants of Maximal Oxygen Uptake in Patients with Healed Myocardial Infarction: Influence of Physical Training, *Circulation*, 48:943, 1973.

115 Redwood, D. R., Rosing, D. R., and Epstein, S. E.: Circulatory and Symptomatic Effects of Physical Training in Patients with Coronary Artery Disease and Angina Pectoris, *N. Engl. J. Med.*, 286:459, 1972.

116 Holmgren, A., and Strandell, T.: The Relationship between Heart Volume, Total Hemoglobin and Physical Working Capacity in Former Athletes, *Acta Med. Scand.*, 163:149, 1959.

117 Morganroth, J., Maron, B. J., Henry, W. L., et al.: Comparative Left Ventricular Dimensions in Trained Athletes, *Ann. Intern. Med.*, 82:521, 1975.

118 Roeske, W. R., O'Rourke, R. A., Klein, A., et al.: Noninvasive Evaluation of Ventricular Hypertrophy in Professional Athletes, *Circulation*, 53:286, 1976.

119 Gilbert, C. A., Nutter, D. O., Felner, J. M., et al.: Echocardiographic Study of Cardiac Dimensions and Functions in the Endurance-trained Athlete, *Am. J. Cardiol.*, 40:528, 1977.

120 Underwood, R. H., and Schwade, J. L.: Noninvasive Analysis of Cardiac Function of Elite Distance Runners: Echocardiography, Vectorcardiography and Cardiac Intervals, *Ann. N. Y. Acad. Sci.*, 301:297, 1977.

121 DeMaria, A. N., Neumann, A., Leo, G., et al.: Alterations in Ventricular Mass and Performance Induced by Exercise Training in Man Evaluated by Echocardiography, *Circulation*, 57:237, 1978.

122 Ehsani, A. A., Hagberg, J. M., and Hickson, R. C.: Rapid Changes in Left Ventricular Dimensions and Mass in Response to Physical Conditioning and Deconditioning, *Am. J. Cardiol.*, 42:52, 1978.

123 Oscai, L. B., Molé, P. A., Brei, B., et al.: Cardiac Growth and Respiratory Enzyme Levels in Male Rats Subjected to a Running Program, *Am. J. Physiol.*, 220:1238, 1971.

124 Carew, T. E., and Covell, J. W.: Left Ventricular Function in Exercise-induced Hypertrophy in Dogs, *Am. J. Cardiol.*, 42:82, 1978.

125 Wyatt, H. L., and Mitchell, J. H.: Influences of Physical Training on the Heart of Dogs, *Circ. Res.*, 35:883, 1974.

126 Segel, L. D.: Myocardial Adaptation to Physical Con-

ditioning, in E. A. Amsterdam, J. H. Wilmore, and A. N. DeMaria (eds.), "Exercise in Cardiovascular Health and Disease," Yorke Medical Books, New York, 1977, pp. 95-107.

127 Stevenson, J. A. F., Feleki, V., Rechnitzer, P., et al.: Effect of Exercise on Coronary Tree Size in the Rats, *Circ. Res.*, 15:265, 1964.

128 Leon, A. S., and Bloor, C. M.: Effects of Exercise and Its Cessation on the Heart and Its Blood Supply, *J. Appl. Physiol.*, 24:485, 1968.

129 Tomanek, R. J.: Effects of Age and Exercise on the Extent of the Myocardial Capillary Bed, *Anat. Rec.*, 167:55, 1969.

130 Scheure, J., Kapner, L., Stringfellow, C. A., et al.: Glycogen, Lipid and High Energy Phosphate Stores in Hearts from Conditional Rats, *J. Lab Clin. Med.*, 75:924, 1970.

131 DeSchryver, C., Mertens-Strythagen, T., Becesi, I., et al.: Effect of Training on Heart and Skeletal Muscle Catecholamine Concentration in Rats, *Am. J. Physiol.*, 217:1589, 1969.

132 Salzman, S. H., Hirsch, E. Z., Hellerstein, H. K., et al.: Adaptation to Muscular Exercise: Myocardial Epinephrine-H^3 Uptake, *J. Appl. Physiol.*, 29:92, 1970.

133 Dowell, R. T., Stone, H. L., Sordahl, L., et al.: Contractile Function and Myofibrillar ATPase Activity in the Exercise-trained Dog Heart, *J. Appl. Physiol.*, 43:977, 1977.

134 Crews, J., and Aldinger, E. E.: Effect of Chronic Exercise on Myocardial Function, *Am. Heart J.*, 74:536, 1967.

135 Happ, A., Hansis, M., Gülch, R., et al.: Left Ventricular Isovolumetric Pressure-Volume Relations, Diastolic Tone, and Contractility in the Rat Heart after Physical Training, *Basic Res. Cardiol.*, 69:516, 1974.

136 Dowell, R. T., Cutilletta, A. F., Ruduik, M. A., et al.: Heart Functional Responses to Pressure Overload in Exercised and Sedentary Rats, *Am. J. Physiol.*, 230:199, 1976.

137 Penpargkul, S., and Scheuer, J.: The Effect of Physical Training upon the Mechanical and Metabolic Performance of the Rat Heart, *J. Clin. Invest.*, 49:1859, 1970.

138 Scheuer, J., and Stezoski, S. W.: Effect of Physical Training on the Mechanical and Metabolic Response of the Rat Heart to Hypoxia, *Circ. Res.*, 30:418, 1972.

139 Bersohn, M. M., and Scheuer, J.: Effects of Physical Training on End-Diastolic Volume and Myocardial Performance of Isolated Rat Hearts, *Circ. Res.*, 40:510, 1977.

140 Bhan, A. K., and Scheuer, J.: Effects of Physical Training on Cardiac Myosin ATPase Activity, *Am. J. Physiol.*, 228:1178, 1975.

141 Wilkerson, J. E., and Evonuk, E.: Changes in Cardiac and Skeletal Muscle Myosin ATPase Activities after Exercise, *J. Appl. Physiol.*, 30:328, 1971.

142 Penpargkul, S., Repke, D. I., Katz, A. M., et al.: Effect of Physical Training on Calcium Transport by Rat Cardiac Sarcoplasmic Reticulum, *Circ. Res.*, 40:134, 1977.

143 Baldwin, K. M., Winder, W. W., and Holoszy, J. O.: Adaptation of Actomyosin ATPase in Different Types of Muscle to Endurance Exercise, *Am. J. Physiol.*, 229:422, 1975.

144 Grimm, A. F., Kubota, R., and Whitehorn, W. V.: Properties of Myocardium in Cardiomegaly, *Circ. Res.*, 12:118, 1963.

145 Williams, J. F., Jr., and Potter, R. D.: Effect of Exercise Conditioning on the Intrinsic Contractile State of Cat Myocardium, *Circ. Res.*, 39:425, 1976.

146 Mole, P. A.: Increased Contractile Potential of Papillary Muscles from Exercise-trained Rat Hearts, *Am. J. Physiol.*, 234:H421, 1978.

147 Adams, W. C., McHenry, M. M., and Bernauer, E. M.: Long-term Physiologic Adaptations to Exercise with Special Reference to Performance and Cardiorespiratory Function in Health and Disease, in E. A. Amsterdam, J. H. Wilmore, and A. N. DeMaria (eds.), "Exercise in Cardiovascular Health and Disease," Yorke Medical Books, New York, 1977, p. 322.

148 Mitchell, J. H.: Exercise Training in the Treatment of Coronary Heart Disease, *Adv. Intern. Med.*, 20:249, 1975.

149 Committee on Exercise, American Heart Association: "Exercise Testing and Training of Individuals with Heart Disease or at High Risk for its Development: A Handbook for Physicians," American Heart Association, New York, 1972.

150 Hellerstein, H. K.: Anatomical Factors Influencing Effects of Exercise Therapy of ASHD Subjects, in H. Rosskamm and H. Reindell (eds.), "Das Chronisch Kranke Herz," Schaltauer, Stuttgart, 1973. p. 513.

151 Clausen, J. P., Larsen, O. A., and Trap Jensen, J.: Physical Training in the Management of Coronary Artery Disease, *Circulation*, 40:143, 1969.

152 Frick, M. H., and Katila, M.: Hemodynamic Consequences of Physical Training after Myocardial Infarction, *Circulation*, 37:192, 1968.

153 Sim, D. N., and Neill, W. A.: Investigation of the Physiological Basis for Increased Exercise Threshold for Angina Pectoris after Physical Conditioning, *J. Clin. Invest.*, 54:763, 1974.

154 Eckstein, R. W.: Effect of Exercise and Coronary Artery Narrowing on Coronary Collateral Circulation, *Circ. Res.*, 5:230, 1957.

155 Heaton, W. H., Marr, K. C., Capurro, N. L., et al.: Beneficial Effect of Physical Training on Blood Flow to Myocardium Perfused by Chronic Collaterals in the Exercising Dog, *Circulation*, 57:575, 1978.

156 McElroy, C. L., Gissen, S. A., and Fishbein, M. C.: Exercise-induced Reduction in Myocardial Infarct Size after Coronary Artery Occlusion in the Rat, *Circulation,* 57:958, 1978.

157 Selvester, R., Camp, J., and Sanmarcos, M.: Effects of Exercise Training on Progression of Documented Coronary Arteriosclerosis in Men, *Ann. N. Y. Acad. Sci.,* 301:495, 1977.

158 Mann, G. V., Garrett, H. L., Farhi, A., et al.: Exercise to Prevent Coronary Heart Disease. An Experimental Study of the Effects of Training on Risk Factors for Coronary Disease in Men, *Am. J. Med.,* 46:12, 1969.

159 Bonanno, J. A., and Lies, J. A.: Effects of Physical Training on Coronary Risk Factors, *Am. J. Cardiol.,* 33:760, 1974.

160 Enger, S. C., Herbjornsen, K., Erikssen, J., et al.: High Density Lipoproteins (HDL) and Physical Activity: The Influence of Physical Exercise, Age and Smoking on HDL-Cholesterol and the HDL-/Total Cholesterol Ratio, *Scand. J. Clin. Lab. Invest.,* 37:251, 1977.

161 Wood, P. D., Haskell, W., Klein, H., et al.: The Distribution of Plasma Lipoproteins in Middle-aged Male Runners, *Metabolism,* 25:1249, 1976.

162 Milvy, P., Forbes, W. F., and Brown, K. S.: A Critical Review of Epidemiological Studies of Physical Activity, *Ann. N. Y. Acad. Sci.,* 301:519, 1977.

163 Paffenburger, R. S., Jr., and Hale, W. E.: Work Activity and Coronary Heart Mortality, *N. Engl. J. Med.,* 292:545, 1975.

Alcohol and the Heart*

TIMOTHY J. REGAN, M.D. and PHILIP O. ETTINGER, M.D.

Alcohol is capable of producing a subacute myocarditis, often misdiagnosed because of the slowness of its evolution, and the coexistence, in the terminal period of cardiac murmurs.

H. VAQUEZ[1]

The toxic properties of ethyl alcohol during acute or chronic usage have long been recognized in terms of cerebral and hepatic function, but it has been traditionally thought that the heart was not similarly affected in the absence of complicating factors. As a specific disease entity, however, the concept of alcoholic cardiomyopathy has from time to time had some measure of acceptance. In Europe during the last century, there were repeated reports of diffuse disease of heart muscle in chronic alcoholic individuals, who apparently had low output heart failure.[1] Periods of economic distress with attendant nutritional deprivation have resulted in a different clinical presentation—the high output state of beriberi as a result of thiamine deficiency. Some concluded that this was the only cardiovascular effect of chronic alcoholism. In recent decades, however, when the industrialized countries have had a generally sufficient food supply, there have been numerous reports of low output heart failure in alcoholics, without clinical evidence of nutritional deficiency in the majority.[2–4]

Diagnostic difficulties persist, however, so that the appearance of heart disease in an alcoholic individual is frequently attributed to underlying cardiac pathology of rheumatic, hypertensive, or coronary etiology, often without adequate supporting evidence. Congestive cardiomyopathy may also be readily classified as idiopathic, particularly in a geographic setting where alcoholism is not epidemic. Even in many inner-city or Veterans Administration hospitals, where substantial numbers of alcoholic individuals are observed and congestive cardiomyopathy is common, admitting physicians not infrequently accept an initial negative history for alcoholism that is subsequently shown to be erroneous.

CARDIAC EPIDEMIOLOGY

A number of recent observations have indicated that ethanol alcohol may have chronic toxic effects on the cardiovascular system. An epidemiologic survey of industrial workers in Chicago revealed that problem drinkers had a significantly higher 15-year mortality from cardiovascular diseases and sudden death than did nonaddicted individuals. This difference was not attributable to the traditional cardiac risk factors.[5] Of interest here is the finding in a prospective epidemiologic study that intemperance itself is a risk factor; heavy alcohol consumption appeared to enhance the risk of developing heart disease,[6] but the pathologic nature of the process was not defined.

Response to Acute Ethanol Use

Several investigations have indicated that ethyl alcohol may simultaneously affect the function of many organs. In contrast to the popular view that ethanol has beneficial effects on the heart acutely, doses that are mildly intoxicating have been shown to adversely affect left ventricular function in some circumstances. This effect is in part dependent on prior experience with alcohol; that is, larger doses are required to demonstrate impaired pumping action of the heart in the chronic alcoholic subject without clinical evidence of heart disease.[7–9] For instance, 6 oz of scotch fed to normal individuals over a 2-h period has been found to diminish the force of heart muscle contraction at a mildly intoxicating blood level of 75 mg/100 ml[8] without affecting cardiac function in alcoholics who have no clinical evidence of heart disease. This effect progresses as blood levels rise and usually dissipates within a few hours after drinking ceases. Supporting the view that ethanol is acutely depressant to myocardium is the fact that ventricular dysfunction is rapidly reversed after 15 to 30 min of hemodialysis.[10]

In contrast to these findings in alcoholics without clinical evidence of heart disease, the patient who has already had at least one episode of heart failure may exhibit a greater sensitivity to the 6-oz dose of scotch,[11] with substantial elevation of filling pressure (Fig. 1). The response in such subjects who are not alcoholics may be qualitatively similar.[12] An important variation of the acute response to ethanol occurs when combined with other pharmacologic agents. Accidental or

* From the College of Medicine and Dentistry of New Jersey, New Jersey Medical School, Newark. The authors' research was supported by research grant AA00242 from the National Institute of Alcohol Abuse and Alcoholism.

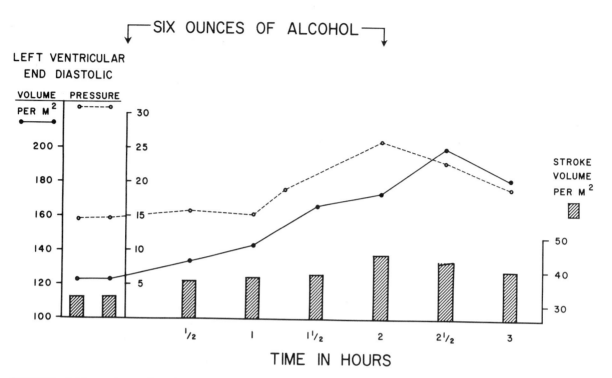

SIX OUNCES OF ALCOHOL

LEFT VENTRICULAR
END DIASTOLIC

VOLUME   PRESSURE
PER M^2

STROKE
VOLUME
PER M^2

TIME IN HOURS

FIGURE 1 These observations during the ingestion of 6 oz of scotch in an alcoholic patient with cardiac decompensation reveal a depressant effect on the left ventricle at a dose that has no effect in the noncardiac alcoholic. (*From T. J. Regan, Ethyl Alcohol and the Heart, Circulation, 44:957, 1971. Used by permission of the American Heart Association.*)

suicidal deaths have resulted from combining ethanol with barbiturates. Potentiation of the myocardial depressant effect has been observed experimentally with such a combination,[13] which is concurrent with respiratory depression.

The sympathetic nervous system presumably has an important role in modifying the cardiac response. Thus, blockade of this system has been shown to produce greater depression of left ventricular function during ethanol administration.[14] Intensification of the cardiovascular response to ethanol in animals treated with disulfiram,[15] an inhibitor of beta-hydroxylation which lowers levels of endogenous norepinephrine,[16] may well be on a similar basis. Since disulfiram is often used therapeutically, it is noteworthy that the interaction with recurrent alcohol use in human beings is characterized by hypotension, tachycardia, and hypokalemia. This reaction is quite variable and not solely explicable on the basis of blood acetaldehyde levels or the sympathetic nervous system.[17] It is noteworthy that the adrenal gland appears to respond with greater secretion of epinephrine, at least in response to a bolus infusion of ethanol,[18] and may participate with cardiac catecholamine stores to modulate the acute depressant effects of ethanol.

In considering the direct influence of ethanol on cardiac cells when administered acutely, changes of salts in the muscle are of major importance. The action in reducing force of contraction may well entail altered transcellular calcium movement[19] or fluxes at the microsomal level.[20] It is known that potassium and phosphate transiently leak out of the muscle cells after a large dose,[7] an effect that is not attributable to coronary blood flow reduction. The loss of cations may be related to an inhibitory effect of ethanol on active transport of potassium and sodium across cell membranes, which has been suggested as a basic mechanism of action of ethanol upon most cells.[21]

Another metabolic change is represented by alteration of lipid transport in the myocardium; the intake of larger doses of ethanol reduces the uptake of free fatty acid by the left ventricle, while increasing triglyceride uptake results in the accumulation of lipid in myocardium.[22] This response may contribute to pathologic changes observed in human myocardium at postmortem examination. Substantial increases in lipids, presumably triglycerides, have been observed in the alcoholic heart.[23]

It is noteworthy that noncardiac striated muscle, including uterine[24] and skeletal muscle,[25] are also depressed acutely by ethanol, although in the diaphragm this follows a period of enhanced contractility. With chronic use, the asymptomatic alcoholic may exhibit modest reduction of lactic dehydrogenase, as well as a small reduction in fast-twitch glycolytic fibers and volume of mitochondria.[26] The conditions required for acute myopathy and rhabdomyolysis are not well defined, but malnutrition and hypophosphatemia are frequently associated.[27]

Chronic Ethanol Use in Animal Models

While histologic abnormalities have been observed in 90 percent of unselected alcoholics in one postmortem series,[28] uncertainty as to the quantity of ethanol intake and the nutritional status of the patient, including electrolyte deficits and the possibility of heart disease from other causes, has obscured the relationship of excessive ethanol use and cardiomyopathy. Previous experiments with chronic ethanol use have yielded conflicting data in terms of the production of a functional deficit,[29,30] but the negative study used smaller quantities and was conducted for a relatively short period. Even in animal models with metabolic or morphologic abnormalities, the fact that heart failure has not been produced has raised a question as to whether the cardiomyopathy observed in human alcoholics is solely attributable to ethanol intake. It should be noted that the long ingestion period of at least 10 years that is apparently required in human beings, may be crucial to the development of clinical disease.

To eliminate some of the above variables, a group of young adult male dogs was maintained in a relatively normal nutritional state while receiving up to 36 percent of calories as ethanol, approximating the quantity reported in a population of human alcoholics.[31] To determine whether left ventricular functional and metabolic alterations in chronic ethanolism are time-dependent, a study was undertaken in young healthy mongrel dogs. Eight controls were compared to 8 experimental animals. Up to 36 percent of total daily calories was given as ethanol for an average of 18 months or 52 months. The short- and long-term groups were fed the same diet with vitamin supplements.[32]

Left ventricular function was assessed in the intact anesthetized dog using thermodilution for end-diastolic volume and stroke volume determinations. During preload increments with saline infusion, a significantly higher rise of end-diastolic pressure was observed in the ethanol group as compared to the controls, associated with reduced end-diastolic and stroke volumes. However, the responses were similar in short- and long-term alcoholic animals. Estimation of collagen in the left ventricle revealed significantly increased collagen accumulation in the myocardium of alcoholic animals, which is a basis for the compliance abnormality. Collagen was located in the interstitium by morphologic study and did not vary with duration.

Since elasticity of muscles has been attributed predominantly to extracellular structures,[33] increments of extracellular fibrous protein can diminish diastolic compliance. This view is supported by the observation that in the early stages of amyloid heart disease, amyloid accumulation, largely limited to the intercellular space, ultimately limits diastolic filling.[34,35] The presence of Alcian-positive staining material, as previously reported,[36] may represent an associated alteration in glycoprotein metabolism or may reflect carbohydrate molecules associated with collagen fibrils. Since left ventricular and septal weights did not differ from controls in the alcoholic groups, hypertrophy did not appear to contribute to the functional abnormality.

An index of left ventricular contractility, dp/dt normalized for preload and afterload, was significantly reduced, as was V_{ce}, only in the long-term animals. Myocardial water and cation distribution were assessed, using ^{51}Cr-EDTA to measure extracellular space. Cell accumulation of water and sodium was observed only in the long-term alcoholic group, without a reduction of cell potassium. In view of the dilatation of sarcoplasmic reticulum and subsarcolemmal regions observed by electron microscopy, it was postulated that edema of cardiac cells may limit the rate of calcium availability to contractile protein and thus affect contractile function in long-term alcoholism.

A prior study of a canine alcohol model concluded from analysis of glycerinated heart muscle preparations that the force-velocity relationship (V_{max} was significantly reduced.[37] The duration of ethanol feeding was approximately one-half of that in our long-term animals, which may explain the absence of changes in maximal developed tension, maximum rate of tension rise, and time to peak tension.

The pathogenesis of altered contractility in the long-term alcoholic animals is not clear. High-energy phosphate levels do not appear to be diminished,[37] and total calcium concentrations were not reduced in the long-term animals,[32] although an intracellular redistribution is not excluded.[27] While changes in the interstitium may limit the rate of calcium transport into myocardial cells, collagen accumulation was not different from that observed in the short-term animals. The report of enhanced sarcolemmal-myofibril distance observed in experimental alcoholism[38] may well be related to accumulation of sodium and water and may limit the rate of calcium movement to the myofibril. If this structural alteration affects a sufficient number of cardiac cells, then a basis for impaired contractility may exist. A direct effect of long-term ethanol use on contractile protein and its regulatory enzymes, present only in long-term animals, was not excluded.

Inhibition of sodium-potassium ATPase has been

LEFT VENTRICULAR CONTRACTILITY INDEX

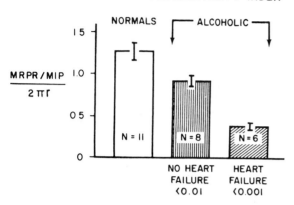

FIGURE 2 MRPR, maximum rate of pressure rise in the left ventricle; MIP, maximum isometric pressure; $2\pi r$, circumferential fiber lengths. (*From T.J. Regan, G.E. Levinson, H.A. Oldewurtel et al., Ventricular Function in Noncardiacs with Alcoholic Fatty Liver: Role of Ethanol in the Production of Cardiomyopathy, J. Clin. Invest., 48:397, 1969.*)

described in several organs as a result of chronic ethanol feeding.[39] However, the gain of sodium by the myocardium in long-term animals was not associated with potassium loss, in contrast to the situation when myocardial ATPase is inhibited by digitalis.[40] In addition, accumulation of water differs from the typical response to inhibition of this enzyme. Previous observations have indicated an altered fatty acid incorporation,[36] as well as composition of phospholipid,[41] in chronic ethanol models. Thus, one of the membrane properties limiting the entrance of sodium and water to the cell may be affected by altered phospholipid. It is noteworthy that even the long-term animals were able to maintain normal cell potassium concentrations.

These experiments support the view that chronic use of ethanol in substantial quantities can produce myocardial alterations that may be considered as antecedant to heart failure, analogous to the preclinical cardiomyopathy of human alcoholics (Fig. 2).[7] Whether development of heart failure in the animal model depends upon a longer period of ethanol ingestion or upon other factors, such as cigarette use, common to alcoholism in human beings remains to be elucidated. Intensification of interstitial collagen accumulation and intracellular cation abnormalities thought to be related to diminished contractility may be critical to progression of cardiac decompensation.

Preclinical Malfunction in Human Beings

That there is an equivalent functional abnormality in human beings is suggested by studies of alcoholic sub-jects with no symptoms or clinical evidence of heart disease or malnutrition.[7] Documentation of 10 to 15 years of alcoholism and the type of ethanol use was obtained from the patients' histories or from close relatives. Whiskey was the predominant alcoholic beverage consumed several times a week in amounts ranging from 0.5 to 2 pints per day. Liver biopsy revealed fatty liver without fibrosis. Left ventricular performance was studied by increasing afterload with angiotensin. The noncardiac alcoholic exhibited a significantly greater rise of ventricular end-diastolic pressure with a minimal increment of stroke volume as compared to nonalcoholic controls, confirmed in a subsequent study.[42] Diminished ventricular performance has also been observed during exercise in cirrhotic patients without clear evidence of cardiac disease.[43] Noninvasive studies that measure systolic time intervals have also confirmed that many asymptomatic subjects have modest depression of left ventricular function.[44,45] It is noteworthy that alcoholics with no clinical evidence of heart disease have been shown to accumulate alcian-blue-positive material in the myocardial interstitium (Fig. 3),[36,46] which may be a basis for the functional abnormality. Some degree of interstitial fibrosis may be present at this stage, as suggested by postmortem studies of alcoholics who succumb without clinical evidence of cardiac disease.[47]

Cardiac Failure

To test the thesis that cumulative effects of ethanol over a period of time may result in cardiac abnormality despite adequate nutrition, a well-compensated patient was fed scotch whiskey for a period of 5½ months at a daily dose of 12 to 16 oz.[7] After an interval of 6 weeks (Fig. 4), resting heart rate began to rise, and there was a prolonged circulation time and elevation of venous pressure without evidence of malnutrition. After 4 months, a ventricular diastolic gallop appeared, which persisted until ethanol was interrupted. Subsequently, without specific cardiac therapy, there was spontaneous restoration to normal. A major role of ethanol in the production of left-sided heart failure in this subject was substantiated by the gradual reversion of the cardiocirculatory abnormality after alcohol ingestion was interrupted. This observation supports the thesis that the myocardial disease is reversible at certain stages if intake of ethanol is discontinued.

In circumstances marked by progression of cardiac dysfunction in alcoholics, pulmonary congestion may lead to exertional or nocturnal dyspnea. If long sustained, or after repeated episodes, pulmonary hypertension and right-sided heart failure may become evident. Unless there is complicating papillary muscle insufficiency giving rise to mitral regurgitation, cardiomegaly may be moderate in extent and heart size may revert to near normal after central congestion is corrected during the initial episode of decompensation. In some patients, systemic or pulmonary emboli from mural thrombi may adversely affect the patient's course. These clinical events frequently seem to be precipitated by intensified drinking, but recurrent illness may apparently occur after a period of abstinence in some individuals.

In addition to the usual lack of specificity of the clinical signs and symptoms, high diastolic arterial blood pressure is not infrequently found during periods of severe congestive heart failure, which may lead to the false diagnosis of hypertensive heart disease. The blood pressure usually returns to normal following response to therapy. Hepatic cirrhosis and clear evidence of peripheral neuritis are not frequently present in patients with alcoholic cardiomyopathy.

HISTORY AND QUANTITATION

Several reports of cardiomyopathy have emphasized the difficulty in obtaining a history of alcoholism.[2–4]

There is a male predominance, and suggestive diagnosis aspects include social disruption, accident proneness, and a family history of chronic alcohol abuse. The major positive diagnostic feature is the history of ethanol ingestion in intoxicating amounts for many years, frequently marked by periods of spree drinking. This information may often be obtained only through persistent questioning over many visits with the patient or by communication with relatives. Negative aspects in the diagnosis include the exclusion of other causes of heart disease, namely hypertension, coronary artery disease, cor pulmonale, and congenital or valvular disease. Other forms of cardiomyopathy (viral, infiltrative, metabolic, etc.) must also be considered.

Not only are quantity, frequency, and duration of ethanol intake difficult to assess, but their relationship to organ pathology is not straightforward. It is probable that these factors have a similar importance for the varied chronic diseases secondary to alcohol abuse, so that information in relation to liver disease, for which there is more complete data, may in a general way be applicable to the heart. Alcoholic hepatitis

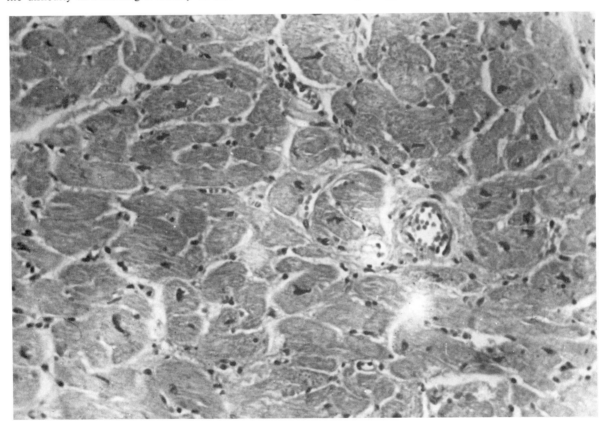

FIGURE 3 Myocardium from a patient with alcoholism without heart failure or infarction demonstrates significant accumulation of alcian blue material in the interstitium, a finding in the myocardium. (*From T. J. Regan, C. F. Wu, A. B. Weisse et al., Acute Myocardial Infarction in Toxic Cardiomyopathy without Coronary Obstruction, Circulation, 51:453, 1975. Used by permission of the American Heart Association.*)

usually develops after years of excessive drinking, although in a few patients it appears within a few years, while it may not develop in many even after several decades of drinking.[48] Over 80 percent were drinking for 5 years or longer before developing symptoms. The probability of developing alcoholic hepatitis is small in those who drink less than 80 g/day of ethanol (approximately 8 oz of 86-proof whiskey or 1 liter of wine)[49-51] or in those in whom ethanol provides less than 20 percent of total calories.[52] As the daily ethanol consumption increases to 80 to 160 g/day and the duration of drinking becomes longer, the risk of developing alcoholic liver disease increases.[53,54] The probability of alcoholic hepatitis or cirrhosis is great if the daily ethanol consumption exceeds 160 g (e.g., two-thirds of a bottle of whiskey, the approximately daily metabolic capacity of an average nondrinking person), and if the drinking, either steadily or in sprees, persists for 10 to 15 years or longer.[52-55]

Although five drinks of an alcohol beverage a day for many years has been suggested to increase cardiovascular mortality in an epidemiologic survey,[5] alcoholic patients with congestive cardiomyopathy usually give histories of heavier consumption. A somewhat higher threshold dose has been suggested by Koide.[56] In considering the incidence of heart disease in alcoholics, the widely held assumption that extracardiac disease such as cirrhosis is not usually associated with clinically evident heart disease, as well as the converse relationship, needs to be recognized. Whether this represents differential organ sensitivity or a protective effect of impaired hepatic function on development of cardiac disease is unknown. Germane to this issue are two studies of patients admitted for psychiatric disturbance, excluding those with evident cardiopulmonary problems. One group, described as predominantly periodic drinkers, had a 73 percent incidence of palpitation and almost half had dyspnea.[57] In the second study, nearly 40 percent had palpitation and one-third had dyspnea, but their coexistence in the same patient was not indicated.[58] These symptoms often appeared in subjects with an alcoholic history of less than 10 years and frequently disappeared on abstinence. It would appear that cardiac arrhythmias in alcoholics occur more frequently than overt cardiac decompensation.

OTHER CLINICAL CONSIDERATIONS

Hypertension

Although problem drinkers as a group may have higher blood pressures than do controls on random measurement,[1] these are usually within the range of normal. Intoxication itself may contribute to blood pressure rise, and the withdrawal state is not infrequently associated with transient elevation of arterial pressure. Ethanol administration produces vasoconstriction of skeletal muscle vessels associated with dilatation of vessels to the skin.[59] Predominance of the former may account for transient hypertension, but there is no clear evidence that chronic hypertension is produced.

A recent report of a large sample of subjects screened in a medical care program indicated that those reporting consumption of three or more drinks per day had a higher prevalence of arterial pressures above 160/95 mm Hg.[60] These findings were based on single measurements without information on the interval from the last drinking episode. Several reports have noted that after a short period of abstinence in subjects with no clinical evidence of heart disease, arterial pressure does not appear to differ from that of a control group[7,45,58,61] and usually declines spontaneously in those in whom it had been initially elevated.[58] Despite the fact that it appears unlikely that ethyl alcohol is an important factor in chronic hypertension, the role of transient blood pressure elevations needs to be considered in the pathogenesis of the cardiac syndromes associated with alcoholism.

Coronary Atherosclerosis

In an important study relating ethanol intake to the status of the coronary arteries, over 900 subjects presenting with chest pain or prior myocardial infarction had quantitative angiographic studies.[62] Significantly less atherosclerotic occlusive disease was found in subjects consuming larger amounts of ethanol, most evident in those over 60 years of age, with no effect in those under 40. These findings fit with the hypothesis that ethanol enhances the levels of high-density lipoproteins, which can facilitate the removal of cholesterol from the arterial wall.[63] That ethanol does affect the particular species of high-density lipoprotein that has such action remains to be demonstrated.

The angiographic study, however, revealed no effect of alcohol on the incidence of myocardial infarction. It should be recalled that earlier studies of coronary atherosclerosis at postmortem suggested that the cirrhotic had less vascular disease than noncirrhotic alcoholics, perhaps related to malnutrition in the former.[64] However, even this association has been challenged.[65-67]

Of interest, in view of the traditional belief that alcohol has a coronary vasodilator effect, are recent observations on the influence of ethanol in nonalcoholic individuals with classic stable pectoris angina and proved coronary artery disease.[67] Ten minutes after consuming an alcohol-containing beverage or a

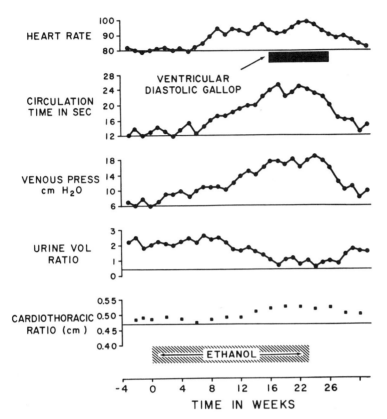

FIGURE 4 These are observations in a single, well-nourished patient receiving daily scotch, which resulted in evidence of heart failure. The failure regressed without medical treatment after interrupting alcohol intake. (*From T. J. Regan, G. E. Levinson, H. A. Oldewurtel, et al.: Ventricular Function in Noncardiacs with Alcoholic Fatty Liver: Role of Ethanol in the Production of Cardiomyopathy, J. Clin. Invest., 48:397, 1969.*)

noncaloric control, the patients underwent exercise stress testing. Ingestion of either 2 or 5 oz of ethanol was associated with a decreased duration of exercise required to precipitate angina and a significant increase in ischemic ST-segment depression. It had been previously observed that among male twin pairs discordant for heavy drinking, angina was significantly more prevalent in the alcohol user.[68] These observations suggest that even in the nonalcoholic individual, ethanol is not appropriate for the management of cardiac pain.

Atypical Myocardial Infarction

Precordial pain is often observed in myopathies of varied etiology; however, the association of alcoholism with the clinical syndrome of acute myocardial infarction has not previously been observed. Transmural myocardial scar has been found at postmortem examination in subjects with alcoholism and without significant coronary atherosclerosis. To elucidate this relationship, alcoholic subjects admitted to a coronary

care unit (CCU) with unequivocal evidence of acute transmural myocardial infarction were investigated.[46] Ten of 12 were without traditional coronary risk factors. Those with prior electrocardiograms frequently exhibited absent Q waves in leads I, V_5, and V_6, which, however, became manifest as the infarction evolved (Fig. 5). Examination of the coronary arteries at postmortem or by angiography showed no significant occlusive lesions.

Morphologic examination of the myocardium revealed concentric periarterial fibrosis, which was postulated to restrict coronary flow increments during periods of high blood flow requirements. This phenomenon is considered analogous to cardiac muscle necrosis associated with the periarterial lesions of constrictive pericarditis,[69] perhaps conditioned by the abnormal metabolism of cardiac cells in chronic alcoholism.

A thromboembolic process was deemed unlikely in this study on the basis of several observations. The patients without previous infarction did not have prior heart failure, cardiomegaly, evidence of arrhythmias, or valvular disease, which appear to be prerequisites for embolization from the left heart chambers.[70] Thrombocytosis and drugs affecting platelets were also not present. These patients were considered to have a preclinical form of toxic heart muscle disease prior to infarction, and mural thrombi have not been described at this stage.

Crucial to the thromboembolic postulate is the demonstration in such patients that emboli emanating from the left side of the heart are distributed to the systemic circulation in an incidence approximating that of proven mural thrombi. As a clinical model for the distribution of emboli in the arterial circulation, patients with prosthetic valves and a relatively high incidence of embolization show a striking noncoronary preponderance.[71] None of the total 12 patients in this series, representing 20 percent of CCU admissions for the given period, had evidence of embolization to any organ. Since angiography was not feasible during acute infarction, the presence of thromboembolism was assessed indirectly by serial determinations of circulating platelet levels, which are known to be altered during systemic thromboembolic phenomena.[72,73] The absence of a change in platelet count during the first day suggested that accelerated platelet turnover as a reflection of arterial thromboembolism was unlikely in these patients.

Although the pathogenesis of this entity is not known with certainty, an interaction with other consumable substances must be considered. Most ethanol users smoke cigarettes, which have been associated with infarction without significant coronary artery disease.[74,75] Also caffeine-containing beverages may interact with ethanol use and smoking and be significantly associated with myocardial infarction.[76]

Arrhythmias and the ECG

An association between alcohol use and cardiac arrhythmias, particularly atrial fibrillation, has long been suspected. However, the specific etiologic role of alcohol is difficult to establish, and indeed, doubt has existed as to the presence of any heart disease when overt cardiomyopathy is not present. Recent observations in our laboratory have indicated that chronic alcohol ingestion leads to cardiac conduction abnormalities and morphologic changes in an animal model.[40]

In an emergency room setting 32 separate dysrhythmic episodes requiring hospitalization were seen in 24 patients who drank heavily and habitually with superimposition of especially heavy ingestion prior to the arrhythmia.[78] Overt alcoholic cardiomyopathy was not present; the group was selected only insofar as all patients drank heavily, had arrhythmias, and had normal or borderline heart size (by x-ray) and normal or borderline ECGs after return to sinus rhythm. Cardiac arrhythmias developing in these circumstances probably are often misdiagnosed as "idiopathic," since little or no clinical evidence of heart disease remains after resolution of the rhythm problem and the extent of alcohol use may be unrecognized. Because of a rather typical weekend or holiday presentation, we have called this the "holiday heart syndrome," which we define as an acute cardiac rhythm and/or conduction disturbance associated with heavy ethanol consumption in a person without other clinical evidence of heart disease and disappearing, without evident residual, with abstinence. This report details numerous atrial and ventricular arrhythmias and one instance of transitory atrioventricular block (Fig. 6). The unusual season peak at year-end and early in the New Year

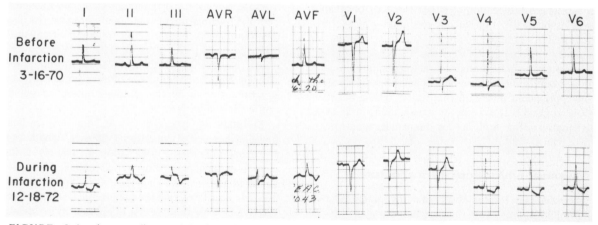

FIGURE 5 An electrocardiogram (*A*) taken prior to the episode of acute infarction illustrating absent Q waves in left ventricular leads. ECG (*B*) was taken during the admission for acute infarction. The recordings in the top tracings are from leads I to III, aV$_R$, aV$_L$, and aV$_F$; in the lower tracings, V$_{1-6}$ are shown. The absence of R in V$_1$ and V$_2$ corresponded to an anterior ventricular scar at postmortem examination. (*From T. J. Regan, C. F. Wu, A. B. Weisse, et al.: Acute Myocardial Infarction in Toxic Cardiomyopathy without Coronary Obstruction, Circulation, 51:453, 1975. Used by permission of the American Heart Association.*)

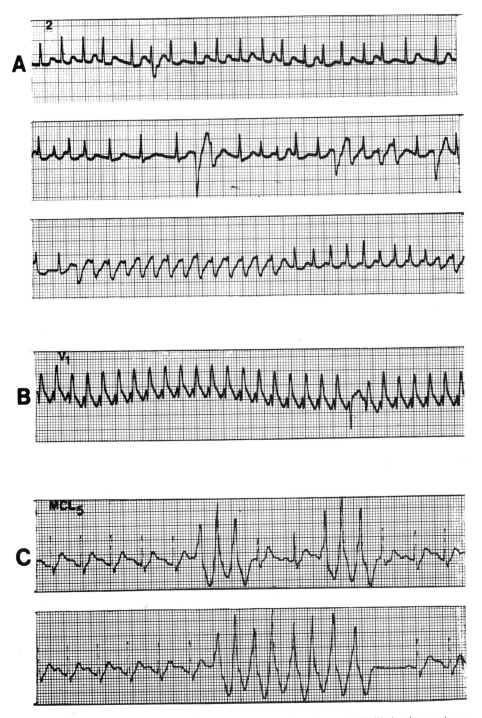

FIGURE 6 Electrocardiograms of illustrative cases. *A*. Case 2—atrial fibrillation is seen in top strip with one aberrant (Ashman) beat (the sixth). Within 10 min (next two strips), the rate accelerated with runs of wide complexes (? abberation or ventricular tachycardia) at a rate of 240 per minute. *B*. Case 3—atrial flutter with 1:1 conduction (verified later by carotid massage) at a rate of 250 per minute with RBBB aberration. A single normally conducted beat is seen. *C*. Case 4—runs of ventricular tachycardia 1 min following the end of a treadmill stress test (both strips). (*From T. J. Regan, et al., Ethyl Alcohol as a Cardiac Risk Factor, in W. P. Harvey et al. (eds.), Current Problems in Cardiology Copyright © 1977 by Year Book Medical Publishers, Inc., Chicago. Used by permission.*)

corresponds to the known peak of liquor sales at that time.

The mechanism by which these arrhythmias occur is not yet clear. In recent investigations from our laboratory, mild chronic conduction abnormalities, including H-V and QRS prolongation, were induced in otherwise healthy and well-nourished dogs that were fed ethyl alcohol in quantity for longer than 1 year.[40] In these animals, infiltration of the myocardial interstitium with alcian-blue-positive material and electron-microscopic evidence of intercalated disk disruption were observed, either of which alteration could have been responsible for prolonged conduction.

Cardiac conduction delays are believed to play an important role in arrhythmia production by facilitating reentry. Although the P-R, QRS, and Q-T prolongations observed in the above series of patients were of minor degree, it is possible that more severe localized areas of delay are present. Indeed, histologic evaluation of the heart in human cardiomyopathy and after alcoholic ingestion by animals emphasizes a variable, patchy distribution of lesions.

Because of the evident ventricular dysfunction in most patients (Fig. 7), we believe this to be an indication of preclinical cardiomyopathy in the majority of these patients. A few had systolic time intervals

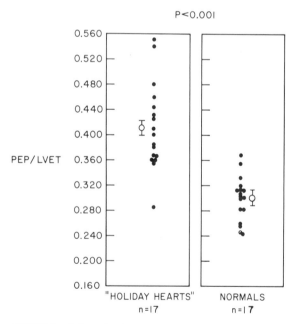

P<0.001

PEP/LVET

"HOLIDAY HEARTS"
n=17

NORMALS
n=17

FIGURE 7 Systolic time interval ratios (PEP/LVET) in patients with arrhythmias (left) and in normal subjects (right). Filled circles are individual data points, open circles are means, and standard errors are shown. (*From P. O. Ettinger, C. F. Wu, C. de la Cruz, et al.: Arrhythmias and the "Holiday Heart": Alcohol-associated Cardiac Rhythm Disorders, Am. Heart J., 95(5):555, 1978.*)

that were normal. Although we have not yet observed the transition to overt cardiomyopathy in any patient, perhaps because of the limited period of follow-up, this patient group includes at least 3 patients in whom a diagnosis of possible cardiomyopathy might be entertained because of borderline cardiomegaly.

To test the arrhythmogenic properties of ethanol, a study was undertaken to test the thesis that the electrical properties may be altered sufficiently in the chronic ethanolic animals to elicit arrhythmias in response to stimuli which evoked no ectopic beats in normal controls.[77] Both the basal state and the response to acute ethanol were examined. In the fasting state without ethanol in the bloodstream, these animals responded, as did normal animals, without a change in threshold to electrical stimulation.[78] This was also the case during isovolumic saline infusion given for the same time period as for animals infused with ethanol.

The chronic ethanolic animal responded within an hour with a reduced threshold to electrical stimulation, and the threshold progressively diminished as blood ethanol rose to levels still below that considered to be legally intoxicating. Ventricular fibrillation was observed in two animals at a 10-milliamp threshold which approximated the threshold seen in animals treated with acetylstrophanthidin at 60 percent of the toxic dose. This is in contrast to a separate group of animals who had been ingesting ethanol for a period of just 1 month. Acute administration of ethanol to these animals was not associated with change in the electrical threshold, so that recent short-term experience with ethanol is not a necessary condition for electrical instability of myocardium.

The animals exposed to chronic ethanol had normal levels of potassium, sodium, and magnesium, as well as normal levels of serum glucose and free fatty acids. During ethanol infusion the basal values did not change, so that there was no evident electrolyte or substrate alteration in extracellular fluids that contributed to this phenomenon.

While the underlying mechanism is not known, the animals which exhibited a reduced threshold to electrical stimulation had a progressive prolongation of QRS and Q-T$_c$ during ethanol which in certain circumstances could lead to ventricular tachycardia and fibrillation.[79] The suggestion of heterogeneity of conduction delays as judged from precordial leads implied that a reentry mechanism may give rise to tachycardia and fibrillation under these conditions.

Two previous studies of the myocardial conduction system during acute infusions of ethanol differed from our own in that conduction delays were seen in nonalcoholic animals in response to the infusion.[80,81] However, the ethanol infusate was substantially higher in concentration, and the blood levels were more rap-

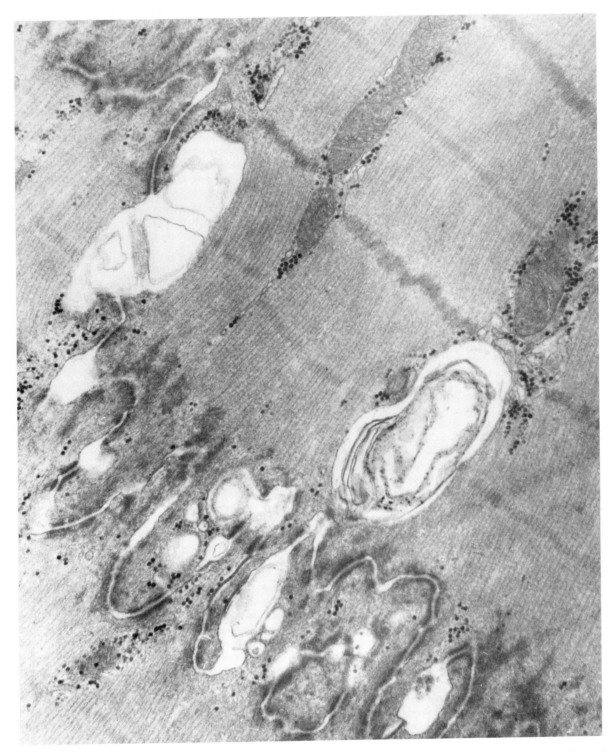

FIGURE 8 Intercalated disk of alcoholic dog. Cystic areas of dilatation of undifferentiated regions are apparent (curved arrows). A nexus (straight arrow) appears normal (× 9,500, × 47,500 final). (*From P. O. Ettinger, M. Lyons, H. A. Oldewurtel, and T. J. Regan: Cardiac Conduction Abnormalities Produced by Chronic Alcoholism, Am. Heart J., 91(1):66, 1976.*)

idly elevated. In one instance the ethanol was infused into the coronary artery.

Previous studies of the chronic canine model have indicated that after 2 years of ethanol ingestion there was dilatation of the specialized portion of the intercalated disk in ventricular muscle (Fig. 8) and Purkinje fibers as well as changes in the interstitium of the left ventricle marked by the accumulation of alcian-blue-positive material.[40] These may be the basis for the abnormalities of conduction in the basal state, which may be intensified by the myocardial loss of potassium during ethanol infusion.[22]

It is important to be aware that sudden unexpected death can apparently occur in alcoholics.[82] An earlier report had indicated that fatty liver was the principal pathologic finding, but there was no detailed histopathologic investigation of the heart.[83] In addition, in a series of 100 sudden deaths in which chronic alcoholism was apparently not known to be present, 18 percent, a significantly higher percentage than in the nonfatal myocardial infarction group, were associated with a large consumption of alcohol in the hours preceding death.[84] Some cardiac alcoholics who develop magnesium deficiency may encounter serious arrhythmias, apparently related to digitalis use, that are responsive to magnesium administration.[85] While these reports are circumstantial and other factors require consideration to establish a cause-and-effect relationship, the multiplicity of reports on arrhythmias in the alcohol[4,56,57,61,86] suggest that primary ventricular fibrillation related to chronic alcohol use probably occurs in some individuals.

SOCIAL USE IN PERSONS WITH CARDIAC DISEASE

Acute administration of 2 to 6 oz of spirits in nonaddicted as well as alcoholic individuals has been reported to transiently depress cardiac function.[8,9,11,12] It is not known if this dose will actually precipitate cardiac failure, as there has been no systematic study to examine this question. Prudence requires that alcoholics with cardiac disease be counseled to abstain from alcohol.[87] Nonalcoholics who are functionally class III or IV should be advised to restrict intake to perhaps one or at the most two drinks at a time, imbibed slowly over a 30- to 60-min period. This may be repeated, at most, once per day, after an approximate 6-h interval, if no untoward events occur. In view of the at least transient increase of blood pressure reported in individuals consuming a minimum of three drinks a day,[60] the same caution should be followed in patients with chronic hypertension.

PATHOLOGY

The gross anatomic features of the heart in human alcoholic cardiomyopathy are increase in cardiac weight; cardiac dilatation, including all chambers but particularly the ventricles; a high incidence of mural thrombi; and patent coronary arteries (<50 percent obstruction).[88] Histologically, these hearts are characterized by hypertrophy (increased diameters of the muscle cells), variable degrees of interstitial fibrosis, small foci of myocytolysis, and a variety of degenerative changes. Histochemical studies have demonstrated an increase in lipid droplets (triglyceride) and a decrease in the activity of a number of enzymes of oxidative metabolism. Ultrastructural studies have shown evidence of myofibrillar damage and lysis, dilatation of sarcoplasmic reticulum and T tubules, enlargement of nuclei, increased numbers of lipofuscin particles, irregularity of contour, and areas of partial separation of intercalated disks, as well as focal edema of capillary endothelial cells. Although intramyocardial coronary arteries have been reported to exhibit edema, fibrosis, and subendothelial humps,[89] significant occlusive disease does not appear to contribute to the myocardial pathology. None of the gross, histologic, histochemical, or electron-microscopic changes are sufficiently specific to allow a morphologic distinction to be made between alcoholic and nonalcoholic patients with congestive cardiomyopathy.

TREATMENT AND REVERSIBILITY

Management of alcoholic cardiomyopathy depends on the state of the disease when the addicted individual is first seen. Even in the absence of cardiac failure or enlargement, patients presenting with unexplained arrhythmias or absent septal Q waves should raise a high index of suspicion requiring verification of a negative history of alcoholism. The key to treatment at all stages involves complete abstinence. The alcoholic with cardiac abnormality may be approached effectively on an individual physician-patient relationship as well as in group therapy.

In the only available study of its kind, almost one-third of patients followed on an outpatient basis were found to have apparently maintained abstinence over a 3-year period.[87] The majority of these had an improved or unchanged cardiac status, similar to patients with hepatic cirrhosis who became abstinent.[90] Deaths occurred preponderantly in those who did not abstain. Some uncertainties exist, since the relative cardiac status on admission to the study was not described. It is noteworthy that more than 20 percent of those who allegedly were abstinent deteriorated in cardiac status. Presumably at certain stages of the disease, the pathogenetic mechanisms may continue unabated.

After the onset of clinical manifestations, traditional antiarrhythmic agents, dc countershock, digitalis, and diuretics may be used as needed. Electrolyte abnormalities may exist during the acute stage or can develop readily in patients with low salt intake or during diuresis. Since thromboembolism from endocardial thrombi is a prominent feature, occurring in as many as 80 percent of individuals in one series, anticoagulants are important when clinical evidence of heart disease is present.

REFERENCES

1 Ferrans, V. J., Rios, J. C., Gooch, A. S., Nutter, D., DeVita, V. T., and Datlow, D. W.: Alcoholic Cardiomyopathy, *Am. J. Med. Sci.*, 252:123, 1966.

2 Brigden, W., and Robinson, J.: Alcoholic Heart Disease, *Br. Med. J.*, 2:1283, 1964.

3 Burch, G. E., and Walsh, J. J.: Cardiac Insufficiency in Chronic Alcoholism, *Am. J. Cardiol.*, 6:864, 1960.

4 Fowler, N. O., Gueron, M., and Rowlands, D. T.: Primary Myocardial Disease, *Circulation*, 23:498, 1961.

5 Dyer, A. R., Stamler, J., Paul, O., Berkson, D. M., Lepper, M. H., McKean, H., Shekelle, R. B., Lindberg, H. A., and Garside, D.: Alcohol Consumption, Cardiovascular Risk Factors, and Mortality in Two Chicago Epidemiologic Studies, *Circulation*, 56:1067, 1977.

6 Wilhelmsen, L., Wedel, H., and Tibblin, G.: Multivariate Analysis of Risk Factors for Coronary Heart Disease, *Circulation*, 43:950, 1973.

7 Regan, T. J., Levinson, G. E., Oldewurtel, H. A., Frank, M. J., Weisse, A. B., and Moschos, C. B.: Ventricular Function in Noncardiacs with Alcoholic Fatty Liver: The Role of Ethanol in the Production of Cardiomyopathy, *J. Clin. Invest.*, 48:397, 1969.

8 Ahmed, S. S., Levinson, G. E., and Regan, T. J.: Depression of Myocardial Contractility with Low Doses of Ethanol in Normal Man, *Circulation*, 48:378, 1973.

9 Timmis, G. C., Ramos, R. G., Gorden, S., and Gangadharan, V.: The Basis for Differences in Ethanol-induced Myocardial Depression in Normal Subjects, *Circulation*, 51:1144, 1975.

10 Symbas, P. N., Tyras, D. H., Ware, R. E., and Baldwin, B. J.: Alteration of Cardiac Function by Hemodialysis during Experimental Alcohol Intoxication, *Circulation*, 45, 46(suppl. 2):227, 1972.

11 Regan, T. J.: Ethyl Alcohol and the Heart, *Circulation*, 44:957, 1971.

12 Conway, N.: Haemodynamic Effects of Ethyl Alcohol on Normal Human Volunteers, *Br. Heart J.*, 30:638, 1968.

13 Newman, W. H., and Valicenti, J. E., Jr.: Ventricular Function following Acute Alcohol Administration: A Strain-Gauge Analysis of Depressed Ventricular Dynamics, *Am. Heart J.*, 81:61, 1971.

14 Wong, M.: Depression of Cardiac Performance by Ethanol Unmasked during Autonomic Blockade, *Am. Heart J.*, 86:508, 1973.

15 Nokono, J., Holloway, J. E., and Schackford, J. S.: Effects of Disulfiram on the Cardiovascular Responses to Ethanol in Dogs and Guinea Pigs, *Toxicol. Appl. Pharmacol.*, 14:439, 1969.

16 Musacchio, J., Kopin, I. J., and Snuder, S.: Effects of Disulfiram on Tissue Norepinephrine Content and Subcellular Distribution of Dopamine, Tyramine and their β-hydroxylated Metabolites, *Life Sci.*, 3:769, 1964.

17 Sauter, A. M., Boss, D., and von Wartburg, J.-P.: Re-evaluation of the Disulfiram-Alcohol Reaction in Man, *J. Stud. Alcohol*, 38:1680, 1977.

18 Hirose, T., Higashi, R., Ikeda, H., Tamura, K., and Suzuki, T.: Effect of Ethanol on Adrenaline and Noradrenaline Secretion of the Adrenal Gland in the Dog, *Tohoku J. Exp. Med.*, 109:85, 1973.

19 Seeman, P., Chau, M., Goldberg, M., Sauks, T., and Sax, L.: The Binding of Ca^{2+} to Cell Membrane Increased by Volatile Anesthetics (Alcohols, Acetone, Ether) Which Induce Sensitization of Nerve or Muscle, *Biochem. Biophys. Acta.*, 225:185, 1971.

20 Retig, J. N., Kirchberger, M. A., Rubin, E., and Katz, A. M.: Effects of Ethanol on Calcium Transport by Microsomes Phosphorylated by Cyclic AMP-Dependent Protein Kinase, *Biochem. Pharmacol.*, 26:393, 1977.

21 Kalant, H., and Israel, Y.: Effects of Ethanol on Active Transport of Cations, in R. P. Mickel (ed.), "Biochemical Factors in Alcohol," 1967, pp. 25-37.

22 Regan, T. J., Koroxenidis, G. T., Moschos, C. B., Oldewurtel, H. A., Lehan, P. H., and Hellems, H. K.: The Acute Metabolic and Hemodynamic Responses of the Left Ventricular to Ethanol, *J. Clin. Invest.*, 45:270, 1966.

23 Ferrans, V. J., Hibbs, R. G., Weilbaecher, D. G., Black, W. C., Walsh, J. J., and Burch, G. E.: Alcoholic Cardiomyopathy: A Histochemical Study, *Am. Heart J.*, 69:748, 1965.

24 Gimeno, M. A. F., Benders, A. S., de Vastik, F. J., and Gimeno, A. L.: Effect of Ethanol on the Motility of Isolated Rat Myometrium, *Arch. Int. Pharmacodyn. Ther.*, 191:213, 1971.

25 Cooper, S. A., and Dretchen, K. L.: Biphasic Action of

Ethanol on Contraction of Skeletal Muscle, *Eur. J. Pharmacol.*, 31:232, 1975.

26 Kiessling, H.-H., Pilstrom, L., Bylund, A.-C., Piehl, K., and Saltin, B.: Effects of Chronic Ethanol Abuse on Structural and Enzyme Activities of Skeletal Muscle in Man, *Scand. J. Clin. Lab. Invest.*, 35:601, 1975.

27 Knochel, J. P., Bilbrey, G. L., Fuller, T. J., and Carter, N. W.: The Muscle Cell in Chronic Alcoholism: The Possible Role of Phosphate Depletion in Alcoholic Myopathy, *Ann. N.Y. Acad. Sci.*, 252:274, 1975.

28 Schenk, E. A., and Cohen, J.: The Heart in Chronic Alcoholism, *Pathol. Microbiol.*, 35:96, 1970.

29 Maines, J. E., and Aldinger, E. E.: Myocardial Depression Accompanying Chronic Consumption of Alcohol, *Am. Heart J.*, 73:55, 1967.

30 Lochner, A., Cowley, R., and Brink, A. J.: Effect of Ethanol on Metabolism and Function of Perfused Rat Heart, *Am. Heart J.*, 78:770, 1969.

31 Neville, J. N., Eagles, J. A., Sampson, G., and Olson, R. E.: The Nutritional Status of Alcoholics, *Am. J. Clin. Nutr.*, 21:1329, 1968.

32 Thomas, G., Haider, B., Oldewurtel, H. A., and Regan, T. J.: Progression of Myocardial Abnormalities in Chronic Alcoholism, submitted.

33 Brady, A. J.: Active State in Cardiac Muscle, *Physiol. Rev.*, 48:570, 1968.

34 Buja, L. M., Khoi, N. B., and Roberts, W. C.: Clinically Significant Cardiac Amyloidosis, *Am. J. Cardiol.*, 26:394, 1970.

35 Brigden, W.: Cardiac Amyloidosis, *Prog. Cardiovasc. Dis.*, 7:142, 1964.

36 Regan, T. J., Khan, M. I., Ettinger, P. O., Haider, B., Lyons, M. M., and Oldewurtel, H. A.: Myocardial Function and Lipid Metabolism in the Chronic Alcoholic Animal, *J. Clin. Invest.*, 54:740, 1974.

37 Sarma, J. S. M., Shigeaki, I., Fischer, R., Maruyama, Y., Weishaar, R., and Bing, R. J.: Biochemical and Contractile Properties of Heart Muscle after Prolonged Alcohol Administration, *J. Mol. Cell Cardiol.*, 8:951, 1967.

38 Alexander, C. S., Sekhri, K. K., and Nagasawa, H. T.: Alcoholic Cardiomyopathy in Mice. Electron Microscopic Observations, *J. Mol. Cell Cardiol.*, 9:247, 1977.

39 Israel, Y., Rosenmann, E., Hein, S., Colombo, G., and Canessa-Fischer, M.: Effects of Alcohol on the Nerve Cell, in Y. Israel and J. Mordones (eds.), "Biological Basis of Alcoholism," John Wiley & Sons, Inc., New York, 1971, p. 53.

40 Ettinger, P. O., Calabro, J., Regan, T. J., and Oldewurtel, H. A.: Origin of Acetylstrophanthidin-induced Ventricular Arrhythmias, *J. Clin. Invest.*, 59:193, 1977.

41 Reitz, R. C., Helsabeck, W., and Mason, D. P.: Effects of Chronic Alcohol Ingestion on the Fatty Acid Composition of the Heart, *Lipids*, 8:80, 1973.

42 Limas, C. J., Guiha, N. H., Lekagul, O., and Cohn, J. N.: Impaired Left Ventricular Function in Alcoholic Cirrhosis with Ascites. Ineffectiveness of Ouabain, *Circulation*, 49:755, 1974.

43 Gould, L., Shariff, M., and DiLieto, M.: Cardiac Hemodynamics in Alcoholic Patients with Chronic Liver Disease and Presystolic Gallop, *J. Clin. Invest.*, 48:860, 1969.

44 Spodick, D. H., Pigott, V. M., and Chirife, R.: Preclinical Cardiac Malfunction in Chronic Alcoholism. Comparison with Matched Normal Controls and with Alcoholic Cardiomyopathy, *N. Engl. J. Med.*, 287:677, 1972.

45 Wu, C. F., Sudhakar, M., Jaferi, G., Ahmed, S. S., and Regan, T. J.: Preclinical Cardiomyopathy in Chronic Alcoholics: A Sex Difference, *Am. Heart J.*, 91:281, 1976.

46 Regan, T. J., Wu, C. F., Weisse, A. B., Moschos, C. B., Ahmed, S. S., Lyons, M. M., and Haider, B.: Acute Myocardial Infarction in Toxic Cardiomyopathy without Coronary Obstruction, *Circulation*, 51:453, 1975.

47 Hognestad, J., and Teisberg, P.: Heart Pathology in Chronic Alcoholism, *Acta Pathol. Microbiol. Scand.*, 81:315, 1973.

48 Galambos, J. T.: Alcoholic Hepatitis, in F. Schaffner, S. Sherlock, and C. M. Leevy, (eds.), "The Liver and Its Diseases," Intercontinental Medical Book Corp., New York, 1974, p. 255.

49 Pequignor, G.: Die Rolle des Alkohols bei der Antiologies von Leberzirrhosen in Frankreich, *Munch. Med. Wochenschr.*, 103:1464, 1961.

50 Albot, G., Boisson, J., Chaput, J. C., and Rivjere, M.: Etude Comparative des Facteurs Toxiques et Nutritionnels dans les Hepatities Alcooliques Subaugues, *Rev. Int. Hepatol.*, 18:89, 1968.

51 Martini, G. A., and Bode, C.: The Epidemiology of Cirrhosis of the Liver, in A. Engle and T. Larsson (eds.), "Alcoholic Cirrhosis and Other Toxic Hepatopathies," Nord Bokhandelns Forlag, Stockholm, 1970, p. 315.

52 Ugarte, G., Iturriaga, H., and Insunza, I.: Some Effect of Ethanol on Normal and Pathologic Livers, in H. Popper and F. Schaffner (eds.), "Progress in Liver Diseases," Grune & Stratton, Inc., New York, 1970, p. 335.

53 Caroli, J., and Pequignot, G.: Enquete sur les Circonstances Dietetiques de la Cirrhose Alcoolique en France, *Proc. World Congr. Gastroenterol.*, 1:661, 1958.

54 Mackay, I. R., and Langford, L.: Blood Alcohol Estimation in Patients Attending an Outpatient Clinic, *Med. J. Aust.*, 1:778, 1963.

55 Lelback, W. K.: Leberschaden bei Chronischem Alkoholismus, *Acta Hepatosplenol.*, 13:321, 1966.

56 Hartel, G., Louhija, A., and Konttinen, A.: Cardiovascular Study of 100 Chronic Alcoholics, *Acta Med. Scand.*, 185:507, 1969.

57 Koide, T., Machida, K., Nakanishi, A., Ozeki, K., Mashima, S., and Kono, H.: Cardiac Abnormalities in Chronic Alcoholism. Evidence Suggesting an Association of Myocardial Abnormality with Chronic Alcoholism in 107 Japanese Patients Admitted to a Psychiatric Ward, *Jpn. Heart J.,* 13:418, 1972.

58 Koide, T., and Ozeki, K.: The Incidence of Myocardial Abnormalities in Man Related to the Level of Ethanol Consumption, *Jpn. Heart J.,* 15:337, 1974.

59 Fewings, J. D., Hanna, M. J. D., Walsh, J. A., and Whelan, R. H.: The Effects of Ethyl Alcohol on the Blood Vessels of the Hand and Forearm in Man, *Br. J. Pharmacol.,* 27:93, 1966.

60 Klatsky, A. L., Friedman, G. D., Siegelaub, A. B., and Gerard, M. J.: Alcohol Consumption and Blood Pressure, *N. Engl. J. Med.,* 296:1194, 1977.

61 Ettinger, P. O., Wu, C. F., de la Cruz, C., Jr., Weisse, A. B., Ahmed, S. S., and Regan, T. J.: Arrhythmias and the "Holiday Heart": Alcohol-associated Cardiac Rhythm Disorders, *Am. Heart J.,* 95:555, 1978.

62 Barboriak, J. J., Rimm, A. A., Anderson, A. J., Schmidhowser, M., and Tristani, F. E.: Coronary Artery Occlusion and Alcohol Intake, *Br. Heart J.,* 39:289, 1977.

63 Castelli, W. P., Gordon, T., Hjortland, M. C., Kagan, A., Doyle, J. T., Hames, C. G., Hulley, S. B., and Zukel, W. J.: Alcohol and Blood Lipids, *Lancet,* 8030:153, 1977.

64 Hirst, A. E., Hadley, G. G., and Gore, I.: The Effect of Chronic Alcoholism and Cirrhosis of the Liver on Atherosclerosis, *Am. J. Med. Sci.,* 249:143, 1965.

65 Wilens, S.: The Relationship of Chronic Alcoholism to Atherosclerosis. *J.A.M.A.,* 135:1136, 1947.

66 Parrish, H., and Eberly, A.: Negative Association of Coronary Atherosclerosis with Liver Cirrhosis and Chronic Alcoholism—a Statistical Fallacy, *J. Ind. Med. Assoc.,* 54:341, 1961.

67 Orlando, J., Aronow, W. S., Cassidy, J., and Prakash, R.: Effect of Ethanol on Angina Pectoris, *Ann. Intern. Med.,* 84:652, 1976.

68 Hrubec, Z., Cederlof, R., and Friberg, L.: Background of Angina Pectoris: Social and Environmental Factors in Relation to Smoking, *Am. J. Epidemiol.,* 103:16, 1976.

69 Levine, H. D.: Myocardial Fibrosis in Constrictive Pericarditis. Electrocardiographic and Pathologic Observations, *Circulation,* 48:1268, 1973.

70 Wenger, N. J., and Bauer, S.: Coronary Embolism, *Am. J. Med.,* 25:549, 1958.

71 Cleland, J., and Molloy, P. J.: Thromboembolic Complications of the Cloth-covered Starr-Edwards Prosthesis No. 2300 Aortic and No. 6300 Mitral, *Thorax,* 28:41, 1973.

72 Harker, L. A., and Slichter, S. J.: Platelet and Fibrogen Consumption in Man, *N. Engl. J. Med.,* 287:999, 1972.

73 Moschos, C. B., Lahiri, K., Manskopf, G., Oldewurtel, H. A., and Regan, T. J.: Effect of Experimental Coronary Thrombosis upon Platelet Kinetics, *Thromb. Diath. Haemorrh.,* 30:339, 1973.

74 Eliot, R. S., Baroldi, G., and Leone, A.: Necropsy Studies in Myocardial Infarction with Minimal or No Coronary Luminal Reduction Due to Atherosclerosis, *Circulation,* 44:1127, 1974.

75 Nixon, J. V., Lewis, H. R., Smitherman, T. C., and Shapiro, W.: Myocardial Infarction in Men in the Third Decade of Life, *Ann. Intern. Med.,* 85:759, 1976.

76 Wilhelmsen, L., Tibblin, G., Elmfeldt, D., Wedel, H., and Werko, L.: Coffee Consumption and Coronary Heart Disease in Middle-aged Swedish Men, *Acta Med. Scand.,* 201:547, 1977.

77 de la Cruz, C. L., Jr., Haider, B., Ettinger, P. O., and Regan, T. J.: Effects of Ethanol on Ventricular Electrical Stability in the Chronic Alcoholic Animal, *Alcoholism,* 1:158, 1977.

78 Matta, R. J., Verrier, R. L., and Lown, B.: Repetitive Extrasystole as an Index of Vulnerability to Ventricular Fibrillation, *Am J. Physiol.,* 230:1469, 1976.

79 Surawicz, B.: Ventricular Fibrillation, *Am. J. Cardiol.,* 28:268, 1971.

80 Kostis, J. B., Horstmann, E., Maurogeorgis, E., et al.: Effect of Alcohol on the Ventricular Fibrillation Threshold in Dogs, *Q. J. Stud. Alcohol,* 34:1315, 1973.

81 Goodkind, J. M., Gerber, N., Jr., Mellen, J., et al.: Altered Intracardiac Conduction after Acute Administration of Ethanol in the Dog, *J. Pharmacol. Exp. Ther.,* 194:633, 1975.

82 Sundby, P.: Alcoholism and Mortality, in "Universitetsforlaget" ("Alcohol Research in the Northern Countries"), Publ. 6, National Institute for Alcohol Research, Stockholm; University Center for Alcohol Study, New Brunswick, N.J., 1967.

83 Kramer, K., Kuller, L., and Fisher, R.: The Increasing Mortality Attributed to Cirrhosis and Fatty Liver, in Baltimore (1957–1966), *Ann. Intern. Med.,* 69:273, 1968.

84 Myers, A., and Dewar, H. A.: Circumstances Attending 100 Sudden Deaths from Coronary Artery Disease with Coroner's Necropsies, *Br. Heart. J.,* 37:1133, 1975.

85 Iseri, L. T., Freed, J., and Bures, A. R.: Magnesium Deficiency and Cardiac Disorders, *Am. J. Med.,* 58:837, 1975.

86 Singer, K., and Lundberg, W. B.: Ventricular Arrhythmias Associated with the Ingestion of Alcohol, *Ann. Intern. Med.,* 77:247, 1972.

87 Demarkis, J. G., Proskey, A., Rahimtoola, S. H., Jamil, M., Sutton, G. C., Rosen, K. M., Gummary, R. M., and Tobin, J. R.: The Natural Course of Alcoholic Cardiomyopathy, *Ann. Intern. Med.,* 80:293, 1974.

88 Ferrans, V. J., Buja, L. M., and Roberts, W. C.: Cardiac Morphologic Changes Produced by Ethanol, in M. A. Rothschild, M. Oratz, and S. S. Schreiber (eds.), "Alcohol and Abnormal Protein Biosynthesis, Biochemical and Clinical," Pergamon Press, Inc., New York, 1975, p. 139.

89 Factor, S. M.: Intramyocardial Small-Vessel Disease in Chronic Alcoholism, *Am. Heart J.,* 92:561, 1976.

90 Powell, W. J., Jr., and Klatskin, G.: Duration of Survival in Patients with Laennec's Cirrhosis, *Am. J. Med.,* 44:406, 1968.

Surgical Treatment of Wolff-Parkinson-White Syndrome*

WILL C. SEALY, M.D., EDWARD L. C. PRITCHETT, M.D., JACKIE KASELL, and JOHN J. GALLAGHER, M.D.

In the long vacation of 1906, Flack and I turned my study at Bredgar into a laboratory—microtome, oven, microscopes; we had a vast store of human hearts and were trapping moles, rats, mice, and hedgehogs with the intention of verifying and extending Tawara's discoveries on their hearts. I remember well one very hot day, late in the summer of 1906, my wife and I going out on our bicycles leaving Martin running serial sections of a mole's heart. On returning he bade me look through a microscope at a strange structure he had found at the junction of the superior cava with the right auricle. The structure was muscular but quite different from the musculature round about. I remembered the body I had seen in the MacKenzie hearts; we set to work and found it at the same site in all the mammalian hearts at our disposal. In structure it resembled the node of Tawara; hence we inferred it to be the site at which the cardiac rhythm was normally initiated.

ARTHUR KEITH[1]

The first successful interruption of a Kent bundle for the arrhythmias associated with the Wolff-Parkinson-White syndrome was carried out in 1968 on a man with intractable supraventricular tachycardia (SVT).[2] Since that time, 108 patients, selected from over 200 referred for evaluation of this problem, have been operated upon at Duke University Medical Center.[3] On the basis of this experience, the surgical treatment of the arrhythmias caused by the Kent bundle has improved to the point that the operation can now be confidently offered to patients with SVT that is refractory to drug control, to patients who have a pathway that can cause a life-threatening malignant ventricular arrhythmia, to young patients for whom a lifelong dependency on drugs constitutes an unacceptable burden, and to others who have either associated congenital or acquired heart disease that makes the arrhythmias poorly tolerated and difficult to control.

Until recently the classification of the Kent bundles

* From the Divisions of Thoracic Surgery and Cardiology, Duke University Medical Center, Durham, North Carolina. Supported in Part by N.I.H. Grant RR-30, from the General Clinical Research Center Branch, Division of Research Resources; and by N.I.H. Grants USPHS HL 15190, HL 17670, HL 13920, from the National Institutes of Health, Bethesda, Maryland. This work was done under Dr. Gallagher's tenure as an Established Investigator for the American Heart Association. Dr. Pritchett is the recipient of the NHLBI Young Investigator Research Award IR23 21347-01.

employed by us was based on Rosenbaum's analysis[4] of the electrocardiogram. After further experience it was found preferable to use an anatomic classification derived from our surgical findings. The pathways in this discussion are classified as follows: right free wall, right anterior septal, left free wall, and posterior septal (Figs. 1 and 2).

BACKGROUND

In 1930 Wolff, Parkinson, and White reported a group of young patients from Dr. White's clinic in Boston and Dr. Parkinson's in London whose electrocardiograms showed a short P-R interval and "functional"

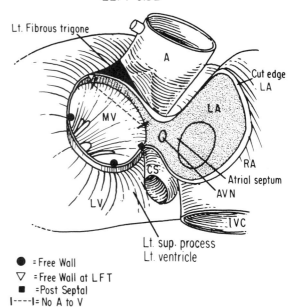

CLASSIFICATION KENT BUNDLES LEFT SIDE

● = Free Wall
▽ = Free Wall at LFT
■ = Post Septal
I----I = No A to V

FIGURE 1 This drawing shows the classification of Kent bundles on the left side based on our surgical findings. MV, mitral valve. A, aorta. LA, left atrium. RA, right atrium. AVN, atrioventricular node. CS, coronary sinus. RCA, right coronary artery. (*After W. A. McAlpine, "Heart and Coronary Arteries," Springer-Verlag New York, Inc., New York, 1975.*)

CLASSIFICATION KENT BUNDLES
RIGHT SIDE

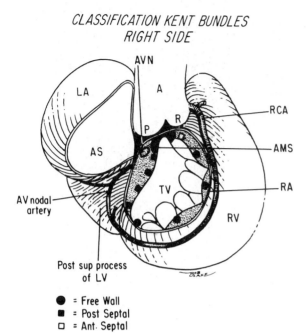

● = Free Wall
■ = Post Septal
□ = Ant. Septal

FIGURE 2 This drawing shows the pathways on the right side. AMS, atrial extension of the membranous septum. P and R, the sinuses of Valsalva, posterior and right. RV, right ventricle. AS, atrial septum. TV, tricuspid valve. (*After W. A. McAlpine, "Heart and Coronary Arteries," Springer-Verlag New York Inc., New York, 1975.*)

bundle branch block and whose histories included attacks of tachycardia.[5] In 1944 Ohnell used the term "pre-excitation" to describe the ECG changes.[6] The electrocardiographic changes have been noted fairly frequently on routine recordings (0.95 per thousand).[7] Although Holzman and Sherf[8] in 1932 and Wolferth and Wood[9] in 1933 suggested that the syndrome resulted from an anomalous connection between the atrium and the ventricle, it was not until 1943 that Wood, Wolferth, and Geckeler[10] described a Kent bundle in the heart of a young man known to have Wolff-Parkinson-White (W-P-W) syndrome who had died suddenly. The anomalous pathway was demonstrated in the right lateral free wall of the ventricle at a site where Kent,[11,12] in 1914, thought normal pathways existed. Following these observations there have been many elaborate electrophysiologic studies but very few additional anatomic ones, a fact that has greatly impeded the development of the surgical treatment of this disorder.

A REVIEW OF ANATOMIC DESCRIPTIONS

Persistence of the anomalous muscle connections between the atrium and the ventricle can be explained on both an embryologic and a phylogenetic basis, for muscle connections are found between the atria and the ventricles in the early stages of human development and are present in some adult lower animals. Truez[13] and Lunel[14] have discussed this problem and attribute the obliteration of all the connections except the atrioventricular (AV) node and His bundle in man, in the early embryonic stages, to the development of the annulus fibrosus. Their explanation, however, implies that the pathways are caught within the annulus and thus obliterated. This is not borne out by a review of the location of Kent pathways in anatomic studies nor by our surgical observations. The pathways can be at a distance from the annulus in the coronary sulcus fat.

A summary of the descriptions of Kent pathways reviewed for this chapter is shown in Table 1.[15–32] The tedious nature of the anatomic studies needed to find a Kent pathway explains, to some degree, why there is a paucity of information about them available for review. Literally hundreds of sections have to be done to find them, since the Kent bundles can be located anywhere around the annulus fibrosus. The pathways cannot be identified by sight or palpation. Their average size is 1.4 mm at their widest diameter, but some are less than 1 mm. The pathways, with three exceptions,[14,27,28] were all composed of working myocardium, and some contained multiple strands of fibers. More than one pathway has been described, Dreifus et al.[25] noting three in one patent. The pathways are usually just outside or immediately adjacent to the annulus fibrosus but do not perforate it in the manner that the His bundle perforates the right fibrous trigone. Only one Kent bundle reported by Mann,[23] three by Becker et al,[28] and one by Hackel[32] were in the fat in the coronary sulcus at a distance from the annulus. This turned out to be an important point. Pathways in the posterior septal region have been found in only 3 patients. In the 2 patients in which the anatomic studies were done by Truex,[13,25] the pathways were adjacent to the His bundle. A more recent example described by Becker was in the septum posterior to the His.[28] A right anterior septal pathway has been described by Becker et al.[28] As our experience increased,[3,33–35] we found that the pathways could be located in places other than those described in the

TABLE 1
Anatomic findings in 27 examples of Kent bundles

Width of Kent bundle	Average 1.3 mm (range, 0.1 to 7 mm)
Multiple strands in one bundle	9 patients
Multiple bundles	4 patients
Right free wall	9 patients
Left free wall	14 patients
Posterior septal	3 patients
Anterior septal	1 patient

above reports. Our deductions, derived from our surgical observations concerning the other locations of the Kent bundles, are included in the description of the surgical approach.

ELECTROPHYSIOLOGIC CONSIDERATIONS

The evaluation of the physiologic characteristics, as well as the location of Kent pathways, by preoperative electrophysiologic study is now accurate and dependable. The methods used were made possible by the His bundle studies devised by Sherlag[36] and the extrastimulus technique devised by Durrer[37] and Coumel.[38] From these examinations, the presence of pre-excitation can be confirmed, a search can be made for multiple pathways, and proof can be obtained that the pathway participates in the arrhythmia. The life-

threatening potential of a pathway can be measured, using as indicators the length of the effective refractory period of the pathway and the ventricular response to atrial fibrillation and flutter.[39–47]

Among the variations in the properties of a Kent pathway that can be shown by preoperative electrophysiologic study is the demonstration that the pathway has the capability to conduct only retrograde, that is, from ventricle to atrium.[48–56] Such a pathway can support an SVT, but obviously there would be no pre-excitation. In the strict sense of definition, such a patient would not have W-P-W syndrome.

The type of SVT found associated with W-P-W syndrome is almost always a "narrow QRS" one, for the anterograde conduction to the ventricle from the atrium is by the normal pathay. Retrograde conduction is by the Kent bundle. The SVT is usually triggered by a premature atrial impulse (Fig. 3). Rarely the impulse may enter the ventricle from the atrium

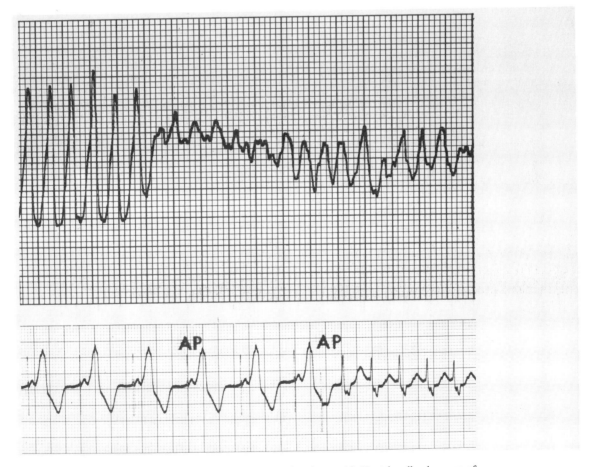

FIGURE 3 Surgery may be needed in the treatment of patients with Kent bundles because of recurrent episodes of SVT induced as shown in the lower rhythm strip by an induced atrial premature impulse (AP). The upper strip shows, beginning on the left, a fast ventricular rate resulting from atrial flutter conducted down the Kent bundle to the ventricle at a rate of 1:1. Ventricular fibrillation then ensued. This occurred during a study and was reverted easily.

via the Kent bundle, causing pre-excitation and a "wide QRS" tachycardia. In patients with more than one Kent bundle "wide QRS" tachycardia may occur as a result of the involvement of two Kent pathways in the reentrant circuit. In some patients during atrial fibrillation-flutter, because of short effective refractory period of the Kent bundle, the atrial and ventricular rates may be 1:1, causing the electrocardiogram to have the appearance of a ventricular tachycardia.[57-62] When this response occurs, it is, in fact, a malignant ventricular arrhythmia and can lead to ventricular fibrillation (Fig. 3).

CLINICAL EXPERIENCE

The evolution of the surgical procedure for interruption of a Kent bundle described in this section is based on our experience with 108 patients with this disorder.[3] About 40 percent of the patients had pathways that had the capacity to cause sudden death, as judged by history and electrophysiologic study. Sixty percent of the patients had pathways that caused SVT alone. They were deemed surgical candidates because of their poor response or intolerance to medication, the need of the young patient to avoid a lifelong dependency on medication, or the presence of an associated cardiac disorder that made the SVT poorly tolerated. The variety of cardiac problems presented by these patients is summarized in Table 2. There were 10 patients with only retrograde functioning pathways. There were 9 with multiple pathways, 1 patient having three Kent bundles.

SURGICAL TREATMENT

The control of SVT by surgery in patients with a Kent bundle is possible because the reentry circuit travels over two identifiable and accessible pathways. Divi-

TABLE 2
Other cardiac disorders (108 patients)

	Number of patients
Two Kent bundles	9
Three Kent bundles	1
Mahaim fibers	4
Retrograde function only	10
Ebstein's anomaly	10
Coronary artery disease	3
Mitral valve disease	3
Aortic valve disease	1
Cardiomyopathy	5
Ventricular septal defect	1

sion of one pathway, either the His bundle or the Kent bundle, will interrupt the reentry circuit. For control of the malignant ventricular arrhythmias only Kent division will be effective for obvious reasons. Surgery for division of either the Kent bundle or the His bundle has been carried out in the past by several surgeons with varying results. Lillehei[63] and Cartwright[64] interrupted the Kent bundle in 2 patients with Ebstein's anomaly with sutures used for tricuspid valve replacement. Burchell et al. identified at surgery a right free wall pathway in a patient with W-P-W syndrome undergoing surgery for an atrial septal defect.[65] Function of the Kent was obtunded temporarily by procaine injection. Although a variety of approaches to the pathway have been employed, most now divide the pathway on the atrial side after complete epicardial mapping.[66-74] Others have divided the His bundle electively rather than search for the Kent.[75-78] Based on the few anatomic descriptions available to guide us, we first interrupted the Kent bundle at the point it entered the ventricle at the latter's insertion into the annulus fibrosus.[2] Later the division point was changed to the atrial side of the pathway. Using this approach there was less chance of injury to the AV valves and coronary vessels, thus avoiding troublesome bleeding from the posterior surface of the heart when the left free wall pathways were divided.

The surgical procedure as developed in our hospital consists of two steps. The first is the epicardial mapping of the activation sequences of the atrium and the ventricle for location of the Kent bundle (Fig. 4). The second step is its division. Mapping of the activation sequences of the epicardial surface of the heart in man in the operating room was done first by Barker, Macleod, and Alexander in 1930,[79] using methods first described by Lewis.[80] In 1967 Durrer and Roos[81] and then Burchell et al.[65] did epicardial maps on patients with W-P-W syndrome. A similar technique was reported from Duke University in 1969 in the first patient successfully treated by surgery.[2] Boineau and Moore have also determined epicardial activation sequences in a dog[82] and in a squirrel monkey[83] with Kent bundles causing pre-excitation. Our current technique, recently described in detail, consists of both atrial and ventricular mapping.[84] Electrodes are attached to each of the two heart chambers on the side where the pathway is thought to be, as determined by the preoperative studies. Each electrode has both recording and pacing capabilities. The ventricular one is the reference electrode. The heart is divided by an arbitrary grid into 53 squares. A hand-held electrode that can record in the unipolar and bipolar modes is used to record the surface electrogram over each square on the grid. This is timed against the reference during pacing of the atrium and is read out on a special digital timer. The earliest area of activation on the

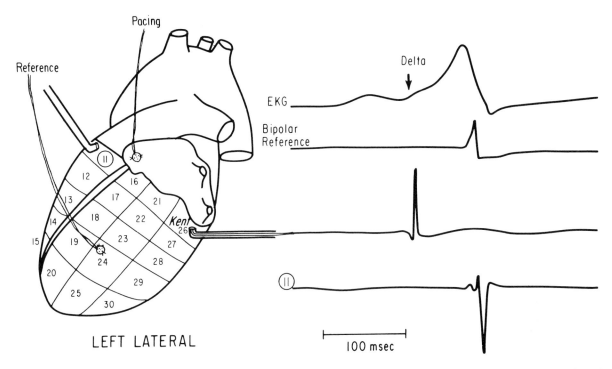

FIGURE 4 This is an illustration of the method used for measurements of the epicardial activation sequences of the atria and ventricles. An electrode is sutured to the atrium for pacing and to the ventricle for reference and pacing on the side of the heart where the pathway is located. A hand-held electrode is used to determine the activation time in relationship to the reference at sites on an arbitrary grid. The atrial activation times are also obtained at points just above the coronary sulcus during either SVT or ventricular pacing. The location of the Kent bundle in this illustration is at square number 26. It occurs simultaneously with the delta wave and much in advance of the activation at square 26 at some distance from the Kent bundle.

ventricle and atrium denotes the location of the pathway. This is always adjacent to the annulus fibrosus at the site where the pathway crosses the annulus. In the posterior septal group, however, the earliest area may be on either side of the crux and frequently shows a ''time lag'' between the onset of the delta on the surface electrocardiogram and the earliest epicardial electrogram. This means that pathways in this area can be located at some distance from this point, a finding consistent with distribution of septal pathways over a wide area. Right anterior septal pathways activate the right ventricle over the infundibulum, which is at a great distance from the pathway's location, but on retrograde pacing the early atrial site is close to the pathway's site. Other problems with precise localization occur because of the varying depths of the coronary sulcus caused by the angle made between the atria and ventricles at the annulus fibrosus. For atrial mapping, SVT is induced. However, the retrograde mapping can be troublesome if ventricular pacing is needed, for cardiac output may be so reduced that partial support with cardiopulmonary bypass may be required. This may also occasionally have to be done in some patients during SVT. As shown in Fig. 5, an isochronous map can be constructed from the activation sequences.

Once the pathway has been found, the surgeon prepares to open the heart for its interruption. The only exceptions to the open heart approach have been 2 patients who had very superficial left free wall pathways that were interrupted by the cryothermia probe applied to the epicardial surface of the heart.[85] These 2 patients had a sharp negative deflection on the surface electrogram obtained at the pathway site. All other patients have had either Kent or His bundle interruption attempts. In some of the latter, the His bundle was electively interrupted, while in others it was divided after failure to find the Kent. His bundle interruption has been achieved usng cryothermia in most patients.[35,86] When the latter fails, the surgical division may require complete separation of the atrial septum from the right fibrous trigone.

The methods for Kent bundle interruption will be described according to their location, starting first with an analysis of the operative observation made on the patients on whom it was missed, followed by the conclusions we have drawn from this analysis. The current technique will then be described.

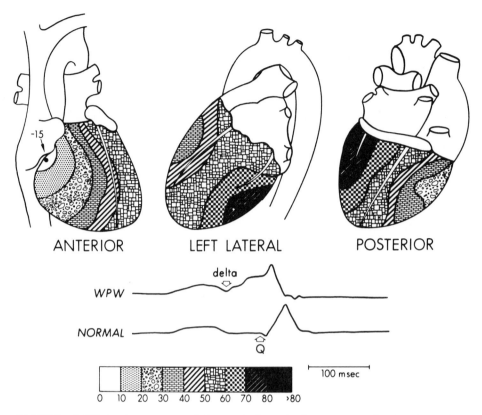

ANTERIOR   LEFT LATERAL   POSTERIOR

WPW

NORMAL

100 msec

0 10 20 30 40 50 60 70 80 ›80

FIGURE 5 This isochronous map of the ventricular activation sequence of a right free wall pathway can be prepared from the data obtained from the mapping just described. The upper tracing, showing pre-excitation, was obtained before division. The lower, normal tracing was obtained after interruption.

The published reports describing the Kent bundles and the speculation concerning their origin led us to assume that the pathways were either adjacent to or even entered the ventricles by perforations in the annulus fibrosus. It was for this reason that early in our experience the dissection for interruption included only the myocardium and not the fat in the coronary sulcus. Continued experience taught us that the location of the pathways at the crossing points was more complicated than this (Fig. 6).

Right Free Wall Pathways

Experience with 2 patients made us realize that the pathways on the right free wall can be at some distance from the annulus fibrosus, coursing in the fat in the coronary sulcus. The first patient had a right free wall pathway that was easily found on epicardial mapping. The atrial endocardium was divided just above the annulus fibrosus, and the fat pad separated from the ventricular muscle for a short distance. Pre-excitation was obliterated, a Weckenbach phenomenon occurred on atrial and ventricular pacing, and the post-interruption epicardial mapping was normal. Five days

after surgery the patient developed SVT again. Another electrophysiologic study showed that the pathway was present but would only conduct retrograde and yet support SVT. At the second operation the epicardial attachment to the atrium just above the fat in the coronary sulcus was incised, and the fat in the sulcus was completely separated from the atrium, exposing the annulus. The more extensive separation of the fat from the ventricle was then done, and finally the atrial incision from the previous operation was opened. Another patient operated upon early in our experience with a mild Ebstein's anomaly had a pathway that still retained its retrograde conduction capability after division of just the atrial wall.[87] A third patient was reoperated upon because pre-excitation was again apparent 5h after the operation. This pathway, prior to surgery, had caused an episode of ventricular fibrillation and severe brain damage. Eight other patients with right free wall pathways had only the atrial myocardium divided above the annulus but without extensive separation of the fat from the ventricle. Their pathways must have been close to the annulus. This led us to devise the operation for right free wall pathways shown in Figs. 7 and 8. The epicardium is first divided at its attachment to the atrium above the fat pad in the coronary sulcus. The fat in the coronary sulcus, along with the right coronary artery, and vein, is then separated from the atrium and the external surface of the annulus fibrosus. The superior aspect of the ventricle is freed of fat inferiorly to the epicardial attachment to the ventricle. Then through a right atriotomy the endocardial incision is made in the right atrium just above the annulus fibrosus at a point corresponding to the epicardial site of the pathway. The entire thickness of the atrial wall is divided, and fibers along the external surface of the annulus are gently pulled apart. As long as the myocardium is kept in view the coronary vessels will be protected during the operation. Intermittent cross-clamping of the aorta and induced fibrillation may be required for the precise incision through the endocardium. In the final step the endocardial site is closed, then the right atriotomy, and finally the epicardium.

Right Anterior Septal Pathways

The early point of activation on the ventricle in this group is at a distance from the pathway over the infundibulum. However, the early atrial point is close to it. The second and eighth patients in our series of 108 patients had pathways in this location. Attempts to divide the pathways on the ventricular side failed

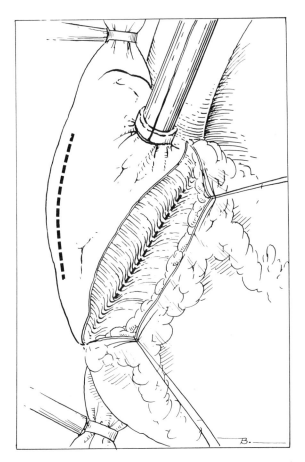

FIGURE 7 This is a drawing of the operation now used for right free wall pathways. The epicardium is incised just above the fat pad in the coronary sulcus. The coronary fat is then separated from the atrial wall, exposing the external aspect of the annulus. The separation is continued down the ventricular wall almost to the epicardial attachment to the ventricle. The dotted line shows the incision that will be made in the endocardium after the atriotomy. (*From W. C. Sealy, J. J. Gallagher, and E. L. C. Pritchett, The Surgical Anatomy of Kent Bundles Based on Electrophysiologic Mapping and Surgical Exploration, J. Thorac. Cardiovasc. Surg., in press. Used by permission of Journal of Thoracic and Cardiovascular Surgery.*)

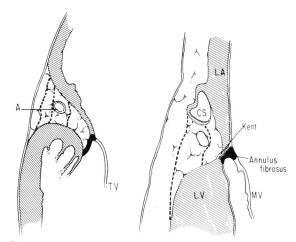

Right Lat. Free Wall

FIGURE 6 The panel on the left shows a drawing of a vertical section through the right heart wall made at right angles to the annulus fibrosus. This shows where we believe pathways to be, judged from our surgical experience. Note the angle between the atrium and the ventricle and the depth of the coronary sulcus caused by this. In the panel on the right, a copy has been made of a microscopic section reported by Brechenmacher.[26] A left free wall Kent pathway is shown immediately adjacent to the annulus fibrosus. The dashed line indicates where pathways could be, based on our surgical experience.

for reasons that are obvious. A clearer definition of the anatomic and electrophysiologic relationships in this area led to success in the other 6 patients. The pathway is approached by a right atriotomy. The most important step is to identify the atrial extension of the membranous ventricular septum which protects the His bundle. The His bundle can be found with the mapping probe if the surgeon is uncertain about its location. The incision for division of the Kent bundle is begun on the right atrial endocardium just anterior to the membranous ventricular septum. The myocardium is divided, and the fat on the summit of the muscular ventricular septum is separated from the under-

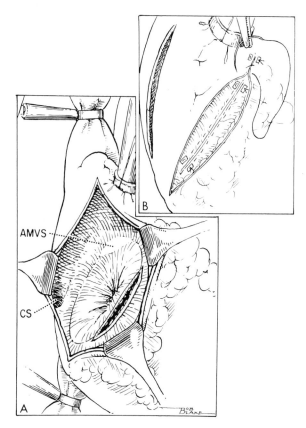

FIGURE 8 This is a drawing of the inside of the right atrium exposed by an atriotomy. An incision is then made above the annulus through the entire thickness of the atrial wall. In the upper block at B, the incision through the annulus is shown, having been closed with a running stitch, and the epicardium is next sutured to the atrial wall. (*From W. C. Sealy, J. J. Gallagher, and E. L. C. Pritchett, The Surgical Anatomy of Kent Bundles Based on Electrophysiologic Mapping and Surgical Exploration, J. Thorac. Cardiovasc. Surg., in press. Used by permission of Journal of Thoracic and Cardiovascular Surgery.*)

lying muscle. It is then carried anteriorly for 1.5 to 2.0 cm out onto the free wall of the right atrium. The epicardial attachment to the free wall of the atrium is then divided at this point and deflected downward, just as is done for the free wall pathways. This carries the right coronary artery downward with the coronary sulcus fat. The epicardium in the sulcus between the aorta and the right atrium can be left intact. The incision above the annulus is closed from the endocardial side, and the epicardium is then reattached.

Left Free Wall Pathways

The technique for the division of left free wall pathways is similar to that for the right free wall, except that the epicardial attachments to the atrium and ventricle are not divided. Our current technique evolved from experiences with 4 patients in whom pre-excitation persisted, but whose pathways would no longer support an SVT, possibly an example of a partially interrupted Kent bundle. There were 2 more patients in whom the pre-excitation was corrected, but their pathways would still support SVT because of retained retrograde function. One additional patient, operated upon the first time at another hospital, had her pathway divided at a second operation at our hospital, using the technique of extensive separation of the fat from the atrial and ventricular myocardium. Left free wall pathways can be located adjacent to the left fibrous trigone. Two were missed in this location because the incision did not extend to this point. Two additional patients had pathways on the free wall that were missed because of failure to do the extensive separation of the fat from the myocardium. Two patients had their pathways divided by the cryothermic probe applied to the epicardium indicating their superficial location.[85] Thus the pathways on the left free wall are not unlike those on the right. They can be located underneath the epicardium, adjacent to the annulus fibrosus, or in between (Fig. 2). Based on an experience of Baird,[74] they may originate in the atrial muscle that surrounds the coronary sinus on the free wall, dropping down through the coronary sulcus fat to the ventricular myocardium.

The left free wall pathways are approached by a left atriotomy made through the interatrial groove (Fig. 9). The heart is put in arrest with cold cardioplegia. Deep hypothermia of 26°C is used. The point is found on the annulus corresponding to the epicardial location of the pathway. The atrium just above the annulus fibrosus is next incised for 1 to 1.5 cm on each side of this point, followed by extensive separation of the fat in the coronary sulcus from both the atria and the ventricle. The epicardium is kept intact because of possible troublesome bleeding that can occur in this area of the heart.

Posterior Septal Pathways

Posterior septal pathways have been the most troublesome to interrupt because of the difficulty in determining their exact localization by mapping, their location in areas where the anatomy is complicated, and the possibility that they may be adjacent to the His bundle. Our experience has proved that entry into the ventricle from the atrium can occur over the wide span between the atrial extension of the membranous ventricular septum to the epicardium over the crux. These observations are based on the following clinical experiences. Two patients had the His and Kent bundles interrupted by the same incision, while in 2 other patients, interruption of the His bundle was not accompanied by interruption of the Kent bundle. In 6 patients, in our recent experience, pathways between the membranous ventricular septum and the crux were successfully interrupted. One other patient had a pathway underneath the epicardium that probably originated in the atrial muscle that surrounds the coronary sinus. The Kent bundle was divided when the epicardium was separated from the inferior aspect of the coronary sinus.

A series of steps have been designed for posterior septal pathways to cover all the variations (Figs. 10 and 11). In the first step the right atrium is opened, the His bundle is identified by the mapping probe, and the location of the atrial extension of the membranous ventricular septum is determined. A 2- to 2.5-cm incision in the septal portion of the right atrium is then made above the annulus fibrosus, beginning just back of the membranous ventricular and atrial septum but anterior to the ostium of the coronary sinus. This opens a large triangular space on the summit of the muscular ventricular septum. The fat is separated from the top of this structure, exposing the left atrial wall, and is then extended to the epicardium over the crux. The inferior surface of the coronary sinus is also freed of fat. Then the incision is extended posteriorly and laterally to the free wall. The epicardium is then separated from the atrium as described for right free wall pathways. If this step does not result in interruption of the pathway, the left atrium is opened in the manner just described for left free wall pathways. The left atrium just above the mitral valve annulus is then incised at a point posterior to the right fibrous trigone. This allows entry to the triangular supraventricular space and right atrial cavity. If the left atrial approach fails, then the attachment of the atrial septum is separated from the right fibrous trigone. This last maneuver would, of course, interrupt the His bundle and would only be done when the Kent pathway has the potential to cause a malignant ventricular arrhythmia.

Two procedures are carried out after division of the pathway to prove that the operation has been successful. When the heart's rhythm is regular, but while still on bypass, the atrium is paced at increasing rates to check for a Wenckebach phenomenon. This may be repeated from the ventricular side and would be done for all retrograde functioning pathways. The presence of a Wenckebach phenomenon indicates that the bypass pathways have been interrupted. After re-

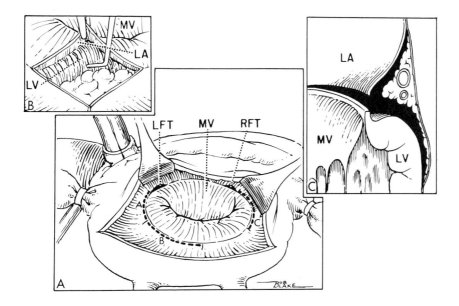

FIGURE 9 This drawing shows the approach to pathways on the left side. In the bottom panel, the left atrial cavity is shown after exposure through the interatrial groove. The dotted line beginning at the left fibrous trigone (LFT) and marked A is the incision used for a left free wall pathway that enters the ventricle from the atrium adjacent to the left fibrous trigone. Dotted line B shows the type of incision used for the usual left free wall pathway. In dotted line C is an incision that will be referred to later but is one that may be used as a second stage for the division of a septal pathway. In the upper left panel the fat is shown being separated from the left ventricle with a nerve hook. This is the key to the operative success. The right-hand panel shows the extent of the dissection of the fat that has to be done in order to be certain that the pathways are divided. RFT, right fibrous trigone. (*From W. C. Sealy, J. J. Gallagher, and E. L. C. Pritchett, The Surgical Anatomy of Kent Bundles Based on Electrophysiologic Mapping and Surgical Exploration, J. Thorac. Cardiovasc. Surg., in press. Used by permission of Journal of Thoracic and Cardiovascular Surgery.*)

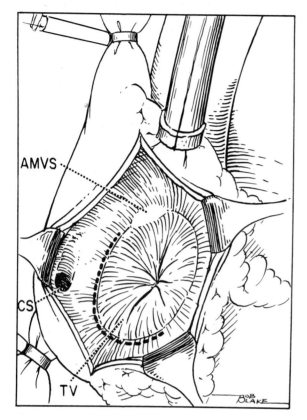

FIGURE 10 This drawing shows the approach to a posterior septal pathway which may show earliest ventricular activation on either side of the crux. A right atriotomy is done first, and an incision is then begun as shown in the dotted line just posterior to the atrial extension of the membranous ventricular septum (AMVS). It is carried posteriorly to the free wall. CS, coronary sinus. (*From W. C. Sealy, J. J. Gallagher, and E. L. C. Pritchett, The Surgical Anatomy of Kent Bundles Based on Electrophysiologic Mapping and Surgical Exploration, J. Thorac. Cardiovasc. Surg., in press. Used by permission of Journal of Thoracic and Cardiovascular Surgery.*)

warming and closure of the heart and while on partial bypass, another complete map of the atrial and ventricular activation sequences is done to be certain that there are no other pathways present, as well as to provide further assurance that the Kent has been divided.

In some patients, either by election or because of failure to divide the Kent, the His bundle may be divided to correct the SVT. This procedure has been described elsewhere.[35]

SUMMARY OF CLINICAL EXPERIENCE

Our clinical experience is divided into the first 40 and the last 68 patients (Tables 3 and 4). This division

point in the series was selected because at this time we began to do extensive separation of the fat in the coronary sulcus from the ventricular and atrial myocardium. The wide expanse of the septum that could harbor posterior septal pathways was also appreciated, and the systematic approach to them was developed during this period. In Tables 3 and 4, both right and left free wall and anterior septal pathways have been combined, since the procedures for their interruption are similar. In the last part of the series we have not missed a pathway on the right, being suc-

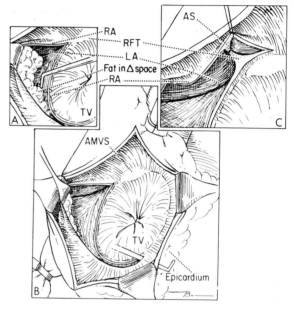

FIGURE 11 As shown in panel A in posterior septal pathways, the fat is cleared from the superior aspect of the muscular ventricular septum and from the left atrial wall. The separation is carried posteriorly beneath the coronary sinus to the epicardium over the crux. As shown in panel B, the incision is extended posteriorly and laterally to the free wall. When it reaches the free wall the epicardium is separated from the atrium, and the incision is made through and through, as shown by the nerve hook passing from the endocardium through the epicardium. If this maneuver does not successfully divide the pathway, then the left atrium is opened just as shown in Fig. 8. An incision is made beginning at the right fibrous trigone, extending to the free wall and going through the thickness of the left atrium, opening into the right atrium, and exposing the superior aspect of the muscular septum. If this maneuver fails, then as shown in the upper right panel, the atrial septum is completely separated from the right fibrous trigone, thereby interrupting the Kent bundle as well as the His bundle. (*From W. C. Sealy, J. J. Gallagher, and E. L. C. Pritchett, The Surgical Anatomy of Kent Bundles Based on Electrophysiologic Mapping and Surgical Exploration, J. Thorac. Cardiovasc. Surg., in press. Used by permission of Journal of Thoracic and Cardiovascular Surgery.*)

cessful in the 14 on this side. However, 2 patients with right free wall pathways did require a second operation. Three patients had His bundle interruption because of failure to interrupt their left free wall pathways. Since the three pathways were adjacent to the left fibrous trigone, the awareness of this possibility should prevent it from happening in other patients. The results in the posterior septal group are still not as good as in the others, having missed 3 of 14. With techniques now being developed, it may be possible to decide when a posterior septal pathway courses with the AV node-His bundle.

There have been no deaths and only one complication in the last 68 patients. One patient developed constrictive pericarditis 8 months after the operation secondary to the postpericardiotomy syndrome. This was successfully corrected.

Special problems have arisen in the group with other cardiac complications. In 2 patients who had posterior septal pathways with other significant cardiac disease, but who only had SVT, a His bundle interruption has been done electively, since this entails only a right atriotomy. Forced His bundle interruption was done because of failure to interrupt the Kent bundle in 5 of the first 40 patients and in 3 of the last 68.

In 7 patients, most of whom were seen early in our experience, radio-frequency pacemakers have been attached to the atrium on the side of the pathway, and no attempt was made to interrupt the Kent bundle.

An Ebstein's anomaly was present in 10 of the patients. The details of the surgery have been reported elsewhere.[87] The overlap of the ventricle over the

TABLE 3

Results in first 40 patients with Wolff-Parkinson-White syndrome

	Free wall and anterior septal	Posterior septal	Total
Number of patients	27	13	40
Kent divided	19	3	22
Kent obtunded	4	4	8
Kent missed	1	5	6
His divided, elective	0	1	1
His divided, forced	1	4	5
Deaths	3	0	3
No SVT by surgery	20	8	28
No SVT by surgery + drugs	3	4	7

TABLE 4

Results in last 68 patients with Wolff-Parkinson-White syndrome

	Free wall and anterior septal	Posterior septal	Total
Number of patients	53	15	68
Kent divided	49	11	60
Kent obtunded	0	0	0
Kent missed	4	3	7
His divided, elective	0	1	1
His divided, forced	3	0	3
Deaths	0	0	0
No SVT by surgery	52	12	64
No SVT by surgery + drugs	0	0	0

atrium may occur and will have to be separated before the pathway can be successfully interrupted.

Surgery to correct the tachyarrhythmias caused by a Kent bundle is now developed to the point that an operation can be safely and successfully performed. Thus, logically, the question of the expansion of the indications for surgery arises. The presence of pre-excitation on the electrocardiogram is not an indication for surgery. However, since W-P-W syndrome, which includes the tachycardia, is a congenital heart disorder, should not the indications for surgical treatment be as liberal as those for other congenital heart diseases? In some of the latter the presence of the anomaly may be the indication for surgery. Although such an indication is too loose for application to patients with W-P-W syndrome, the association of troublesome SVT in a young person with W-P-W syndrome ought to be an indication for surgery, irrespective of whether or not drugs are effective in controlling it. In addition to the prevention of SVT, should not the role of surgery be expanded in order to prevent sudden death from malignant ventricular arrhythmias that occur in W-P-W syndrome? This event is likely to occur in the young. Thus, electrophysiologic evaluation is needed for more young people with W-P-W syndrome in order to identify this group of patients.

The success of the surgical treatment of W-P-W syndrome could be the opening wedge to the application of surgery in the definitive treatment of other arrhythmias. This expansion will depend upon the further refinements of clinical electrophysiologic studies.

REFERENCES

1 Keith, A.: The Sino-Auricular Node: A Historical Note, *Br. Heart J.,* 4:77, 1942.

2 Sealy, W. C., Hattler, B. G., Jr., Blumenschein, S. D., and Cobb, F. R.: Surgical Treatment of Wolff-Parkinson-White Syndrome, *Ann. Thor. Surg.,* 8:1, 1969.

3 Sealy, W. C., Gallagher, J. J., and Pritchett, E. L. C.: The Surgical Anatomy of Kent Bundles Based on Electrophysiologic Mapping and Surgical Exploration, *J. Thorac. Cardiovasc. Surg.,* in press.

4 Rosenbaum, F. F., Hecht, H. H., Wilson, F. N., and Johnston, F. D.: The Potential Variations of the Thorax and the Esophagus in Anomalous Atrioventricular Excitation (Wolff-Parkinson-White Syndrome), *Am. Heart J.,* 29:281, 1945.

5 Wolff, L., Parkinson, J., and White, P. D.: Bundle Branch Block with Short P-R Interval in Healthy Young People Prone to Proxysmal Tachycardia, *Am. Heart J.,* 5:685, 1930.

6 Ohnell, R. F.: Preexcitation, a Cardiac Abnormality, *Acta Med. Scand.* [suppl.], 152:1, 1944.

7 Smith, R. F.: The Wolff-Parkinson-White Syndrome as an Aviation Risk, *Circulation,* 29:272, 1964.

8 Holzman, M., and Scherf, D.: Uber Elektrokardiogramme mit Verkurzter Vorhof-Kramer-Distanz und Positiven P-Zacken, *Z. Klin. Med.,* 121:404, 1932.

9 Wolferth, C. C., and Wood, F. C.: The Mechanism of Production of Short P-R Intervals and Prolonged QRS Complexes in Patients with Presumably Undamaged Hearts: Hypothesis of an Accessory Pathway of Auriculo-Ventricular Conduction (Bundle of Kent), *Am. Heart J.,* 8:297, 1933.

10 Wood, F. C., Wolferth, C. C., and Geckeler, G. D.: Histologic Demonstration of Accessory Muscular Connections between Auricle and Ventricle in a Case of Short P-R Interval and Prolonged QRS Complex, *Am. Heart J.,* 25:454, 1943.

11 Kent, A. F. S.: A Conducting Path between the Right Auricle and the External Wall of the Right Ventricle in the Heart of the Mammal, *J. Physiol.,* 48:57, 1914.

12 Kent, A. F. S.: Illustrations of the Right Lateral Auriculo-Ventricular Junction in the Heart, *J. Physiol.,* 48:63, 1914.

13 Truex, R. C., Bishof, J. K., and Hoffman, E. L.: Accessory Atrio-Ventricular Bundles of the Devloping Human Heart, *Anat. Rec.,* 131:45, 1958.

14 Lunel, A. A. V.: Significance of Annulus Fibrosus of Heart in Relation to AV Conduction and Ventricular Activiation in Cases of Wolff-Parkinson-White Syndrome, *Br. Heart J.,* 34:1263, 1972.

15 Kimball, J. L., and Burch, G.: The Prognosis of the Wolff-Parkinson-White Syndrome, *Ann. Intern. Med.,* 27:239, 1947.

16 Levine, H. D., and Burge, J. C., Jr.: Septal Infarction with Complete Heart Block and Intermittent Anomalous Atrioventricular Excitation (Wolff-Parkinson-White Syndrome): Histologic Demonstration of a Right Lateral Bundle, *Am. Heart J.,* 36:431, 1968.

17 Lev, N., Gibson, S., and Miller, R. A.: Ebstein's Disease with Wolff-Parkinson-White Syndrome. Report of a Case with a Histopathologic Study of Possible Conduction Pathways, *Am. Heart J.,* 49:724, 1955.

18 Truex, R. C., Bishof, J. K., and Downing, D. F.: Accessory Atrioventricular Muscle Bundles. II. Cardiac Conduction System in a Human Specimen with Wolff-Parkinson-White Syndrome, *Anat. Rec.,* 137:417, 1960.

19 Lev, M., Kennamer, R., Prinzmetal, M., and Mesquita, Q. H.: A Histopatholoic Study of the Atrioventricular Communications in Two Hearts with the Wolff-Parkinson-White Syndrome, *Circulation,* 24:41, 1961.

20 Lev, M., Sodi-Pallares, D., and Friedland, C.: A Histopathologic Study of the Atrioventricular Communications in a Case of WPW with Incomplete Left Bundle Branch Block, *Am. Heart J.,* 66:399, 1963.

21 Rosenberg, H. S., Klima, T., McNamara, D. G., and Leachman, R. D.: Atrioventricular Communication in the Wolff-Parkinson-White Syndrome, *Am J. Clin. Pathol.,* 56:79, 1971.

22 Lunel, A. A. V.: Significance of Annulus Fibrosus of Heart in Relation to AV Conduction and Ventricular Activation Cases of Wolff-Parkinson-White Syndrome, *Br. Heart J.,* 34:1263, 1972.

23 Mann, R. B., Fisher, R. S., Scherlis, S., and Hutchins, G. M.: Accessory Left Atrioventricular Connection in Type A Wolff-Parkinson-White Syndrome, *Johns Hopkins Med. J.,* 132:242, 1973.

24 James T. N., and Puech, P.: De Subitaneis Mortibus. IX. Type A Wolff-Parkinson-White Syndrome, *Circulation,* 50:1264, 1974.

25 Dreifus, L. S., Wellens, H. J. J., Watanabe, Y., Kimbiris, D., and Truex, R.: Sinus Bradycardia and Atrial Fibrillation Associated with the Wolff-Parkinson-White Syndrome, *Am. J. Cardiol.,* 38:149, 1976.

26 Brechenmacher, C., Laham, J., Iris, L., Gerbaux, A., and Lenegre, J.: Etude Histologique des Voies Anormales de Conduction dans un Syndrome de Wolff-Parkinson-White et dans un Syndrome Lown-Ganong-Levine, *Arch. Mal. Coeur,* 67:507, 1974.

27 Brechenmacher, C., Coumel, P., Fauchier, J. P., Cachera, J. P., and James, T. N.: De Subitaneis Mortibus. XXII. Intractable Paroxysmal Tachycardia Which Proved Fatal in Type A Wolff-Parkinson-White Syndrome, *Circulation,* 55:408, 1977.

28 Becker, A. E., Anderson, R. H., Durrer, D. and Wellens, H. J. J.: The Anatomical Substrates of Wolff-Parkinson-White Syndrome, *Circulation,* 57:870, 1978.

286

29 Davies, M. J.: "Pathology of the Conducting Tissue of the Heart," Butterworth and Co. (Publishers), Ltd., London, 1971, p. 150.

30 Segers, M., Sanabria, T., Lequime, J., and Denolin, H.: Le Syndrome de Wolff-Parkinson-White. Mise en Evidence d'une Connexion A-V Septale Directe, *Acta Cardiol.,* 2:21, 1947.

31 Schumann, G., Janson, H. H., and Anschutz, F.: Zur Pathogenese des WPW Syndroms, *Virchows Arch. [Pathol. Anat.],* 349:48, 1970.

32 Hackel, D. B.: Personal Communication.

33 Sealy, W. C., Wallace, A. G., Ramming, K. P., Gallagher, A. G., and Svenson, R. H.: An Improved Operation for the Definitive Treatment of the Wolff-Parkinson-White Syndrome, *Ann. Thorac. Surg.,* 17:107, 1974.

34 Sealy, W. C., and Wallace, A. G.: Surgical Treatment of Wolff-Parkinson-White Syndrome, *J. Thorac. Cardiovasc. Surg.,* 68:757, 1974.

35 Sealy, W. C., Anderson, R. W., and Gallagher, J. J.: Surgical Treatment of Supraventricular Tachyarrhythmias, *J. Thorac. Cardiovasc. Surg.,* 73:511, 1977.

36 Sherlag, B. J., Lau, S. H., and Helfant, R. H.: Catheter Technique for Recording His Bundle Activity in Man, *Circulation,* 39:13, 1969.

37 Durrer, D., Schoo, L., Schuilenburg, R. M., and Wellens, H. J. J.: The Role of Premature Beats in the Initiation and Termination of Supraventricular Tachycardia in the Wolff-Parkinson-White Syndrome, *Circulation,* 36:644, 1967.

38 Coumel, P. H., Cabrol, C., Fabiato, A., Gourgon, R., and Slama, R.: Tachycardia Permanente par Rhythme Reciproque, *Arch. Mal Coeur,* 60:1830, 1967.

39 Gallagher, J. J., Gilbert, M., Svenson, R. H., Sealy, W. C., Wallace, A. G., and Kasel, J.: Wolff-Parkinson-White Syndrome: The Problems, Evaluation and Surgical Correction, *Circulation,* 51:767, 1975.

40 Gallagher, J. J., Svenson, R. H., Sealy, W. C., and Wallace, A. G.: The Wolff-Parkinson-White Syndrome and the Pre-excitation Dysrhythmias: Medical and Surgical Management, *Med. Clin. North Am.,* 60:101, 1976.

41 Wellens, H. J. J.: The Electrophysiologic Properties of the Accessory Pathways in the Wolff-Parkinson-White Syndrome, in H. J. J. Wellens, K. I., Lie and M. J. Janse (eds.), "The Conduction System of the Heart," H. E. Stenfert Kroese B. V., Leiden, 1976, p. 567.

42 Gallagher, J. J., Sealy, W. C., Kasell, J., and Wallace, A. G.: Multiple Accessory Pathways in Patients with the Pre-excitation Syndrome, *Circulation,* 54:571, 1976.

43 Gallagher, J. J., Sealy, W. C., Wallace, A. G., and Kasel, J.: Correlation between Catheter Electrophysiologic Studies and Findings on Mapping of Ventricular Excitation in the WPW Syndrome, in H. J. J. Wellens, H. Lie, M. J. Janse (eds.), "The Conduction System of the

Heart," H. E. Stenfert Kroese B. V., Amsterdam, 1976, p. 588.

44 Tonkin, A. M., Miller, H. C., Svenson, R. H., et al.: Refractory Periods of the Accessory Pathway in the Wolff-Parkinson-White Syndrome, *Circulation,* 52:563, 1975.

45 Svenson, R. H., Miller, H., Gallagher, J. J., et al.: Electrophysiological Evaluation of the Wolff-Parkinson-White Syndrome: Problems in Assessing Antegrade and Retrograde Conduction over the Accessory Pathways, *Circulation,* 52:552, 1975.

46 Wellens, J. J., Durrer, D.: Wolff-Parkinson-White Syndrome and Atrial Fibrillation: Relation between Refractory Period of the Accessory Pathway and Ventricular Rate during Atrial Fibrillation, *Am. J. Cardiol.,* 34:777, 1974.

47 Gallagher, J. J., Kasell, J., Sealy, W. C., Pritchett, E. L. C., and Wallace, A. G.: Epicardial Mapping in the Wolff-Parkinson-White Syndrome, *Circulation,* 57:854, 1978.

48 Sung, R. J., Gelband, H., Castellanos, A., Aranda, J. M., and Myerburg, R. J.: Clinical and Electrophysiologic Observations in Patients with Concealed Accessory Atrioventricular Bypass Tracts, *Am. J. Cardiol.,* 40:839, 1977.

49 Gillette, P. C.: Concealed Anomalous Cardiac Conduction Pathways: A Frequent Cause of Supraventricular Tachycardia, *Am. J. Cardiol.,* 40:848, 1977.

50 Barold, S. S., and Coumel, P.: Mechanisms of Atrioventricular Junctional Tachycardia: Role of Re-entry and Concealed Accessory Bypass Tracts, *Am. J. Cardiol.,* 39:97, 1977.

51 Coumel, P., Attuel, P., and Flammang, D.: "The Role of the Conduction System in Supraventricular Tachycardia," in H. J. J. Wellens, H. Lie, and M. J. Janse (eds.), "The Conduction System of the Heart," H. E. Stenfert Kroese, B. V., Amsterdam, 1976, p. 424.

52 Zipes, D. P., DeJoseph, R. L., and Rothbaum, D. A.: Unusual Properties of Accessory Pathways, *Circulation,* 49:1200, 1974.

53 Neuss, H., Schlepper, M., and Thormann, J.: Analysis of Re-entry Mechanisms in Three Patients with Concealed Wolff-Parkinson-White Syndrome, *Circulation,* 51:75, 1975.

54 Tonkin, A. M., Gallagher, J. J., Svenson, R. H., et al.: Anterograde Block in Accessory Pathways with Retrograde Conduction in Reciprocating Tachycardia, *Eur. J. Cardiol.,* 3:143, 1975.

55 Sung, R. J., Castellanos, A., Gelband, H., et al.: Mechanism of Reciprocating Tachycardia during Sinus Rhythm in Concealed Wolff-Parkinson-White Syndrome, *Circulation,* 54:338, 1976.

56 Pritchett, E. L. C., Gallagher, J. J., Sealy, W. C., Anderson, R. W., Campbell, R. W. F., Sellers, T. D. J.,

and Wallace, A. G.: Supraventricular Tachycardia Dependent upon Accessory Pathways in the Absence of Ventricular Pre-excitation, *Am. J. Med.,* 64:214, 1978.

57 Dreifus, L. S., Haiat, R., and Watanabe, Y.: Ventricular Fibrillation: A Possible Mechanism of Sudden Death in Patients with Wolff-Parkinson-White Syndrome, *Circulation,* 43:520, 1971.

58 Bashore, T. M., Sellers, T. D., Jr., Gallagher, J. J., et al.: Ventricular Fibrillation in the Wolff-Parkinson-White Syndrome, *Circulation,* 54 (suppl. 4):186, 1976. (Abstract.).

59 Dreifus, L. S., Wellens, H. J. J., Watanabe, Y., et al.: Sinus Bradycardia and Atrial Fibrillation Associated with the Wolff-Parkinson-White Syndrome, *Am. J. Cardiol.,* 38:149, 1976.

60 Lem, C. H., Toh, C. C. S., and Chia, B. L.: Ventricular Fibrillation in Type B Wolff-Parkinson-White Syndrome, *Aust. N.Z.J. Med.,* 4:515, 1974.

61 Kaplan, M. A., and Cohen, K. L.: Ventricular Fibrillation in the Wolff-Parkinson-White Syndrome, *Am. J. Cardiol.,* 24:259, 1969.

62 Okel, B. B.: The Wolff-Parkinson-White Syndrome: Report of a Case with Fatal Arrhythmia and Autopsy Findings of Myocarditis, Interatrial Lipomatous Hypertrophy and Prominent Right Moderator Band, *Am. Heart J.,* 75:673, 1968.

63 Lillehei, C. W., Kalke, B. R., and Carlson, R. G.: Evolution of Corrective Surgery for Ebstein's Anomaly, *Circulation,* 35(Suppl. 1):111, 1967.

64 Cartwright, R. S., Smeloff, E. A., Cayler, G. G., Fong, W. Y., Huntley, A. C., Blake, J. R., and McFall, R. A.: Total Correction for Ebstein's Anomaly by Means of Tricuspid Replacement, *J. Thorac. Cardiovasc. Surg.,* 47:755, 1964.

65 Burchell, H. B., Frye, R. L., Anderson, M. W., and McGoon, D. C.: Atrioventricular and Ventriculoatrial Excitation in Wolff-Parkinson-White Syndrome. (Type B). Temporary Ablation at Surgery, *Circulation,* 36:663, 1967.

66 Cole, J. S., Wills, R. E., Winterscheid, L. C., Reichenbach, D. D., and Blackmon, J. R.: The Wolff-Parkinson-White Syndrome. Problems in Evaluation and Surgical Therapy, *Circulation,* 42:111, 1970.

67 Lindsay, A. E., Nelson, R. M., Abildskov, J. A., and Wyatt, R.: Attempted Surgical Division of the Preexcitation Pathway in Wolff-Parkinson-White Syndrome, *Am. J. Cardiol.,* 28:581, 1971.

68 Fontaine, G., Guiraudon, G., Bonnet, M., Bruhat, M., Grosgogeat, Y., and Cabrol, C.: Section d'un faisceau de Kent dans un cas de Syndrome de Wolff-Parkinson-White de Type A-B, *Arch. Mal. Coeur,* 65:925, 1971.

69 Iwa, T.: Surgical Experiences with the Wolff-Parkinson-White Syndrome, *J. Cardiovasc. Surg.,* 17:549, 1976.

70 Iwa, T.: Surgical Management of Wolff-Parkinson-White

Syndrome, in O. S. Narula (ed.) "His Bundle Electrocardiography and Clinical Electrophysiology," F. A. Davis Company, Philadelphia, 1975, p. 387.

71 McFaul, R. C., Davis, Z., Giuliani, E. R., Ritter, D. G., and Danielson, G. K.: Ebstein's Malformation. Surgical Experience at the Mayo Clinic, *J. Thorac. Cardiovasc. Surg.,* 72:910, 1976.

72 Kugler, J. D., Gillette, P. C., Duff, D. F., Cooley, D. A., and McNamara, D. G.: Elective Mapping and Surgical Division of the Bundle of Kent in a Patient with Ebstein's Anomaly Who Required Tricuspid Valve Replacement, *Am. J. Cardiol.,* 41:602, 1978.

73 Cabrol, C., and Guiraudon, G. Discussion of paper entitled The Surgical Problems with the Identification and Interruption of the Bundle of Kent (presented at Annual Meeting of the American Association for Thoracic Surgery, New Orleans, Louisiana, May 1978), *J. Thorac. Cardiovasc. Surg.,* in press.

74 Baird, D.: Discussion of paper entitled The Surgical Problems with the Identification and Interruption of the Bundle of Kent (presented at the Annual Meeting of the American Association or Thoracic Surgery, New Orleans, Louisiana, May 1978), *J. Thorac. Cardiovasc. Surg.,* in press.

75 Dreifus, L. S., Nichols, H., Morse, D., Watanabe, Y., and Truex, R.: Control of Recurrent Tachycardia of Wolff-Parkinson-White Syndrome by Surgical Ligature of the A-V Bundle, *Circulation,* 38:1030, 1968.

76 Edmonds, J. H., Jr., Ellison, R. G., and Crews, T. L.: Surgically Induced Atrioventricular Block as Treatment for Recurrent Atrial Tachycardia in Wolff-Parkinson-White Syndrome, *Circulation,* 39, 40(suppl. 1):105, 1969.

77 Latour, H., Peuch, P., Grocleau, R., Craptal, P. A., and Dufoix, R.: Le Traitement Chirurgical des Acces de Tachycardie Paroxystique Graves du Syndrome de Wolff-Parkinson-White et ses Limites, *Arch. Mal. Coeur,* 63:977, 1970.

78 Coumel, P., Waynberger, M., Fabiato, A., Slama, R., Aigueperse, J., and Bouvrain, Y.: Wolff-Parkinson-White Syndrome. Problems in Evaluation of Multiple Accessory Pathways and Surgical Therapy, *Circulation,* 45:1216, 1972.

79 Barker, P. S., MacLeod, A. G., and Alexander, J.: The Excitatory Process Observed in the Exposed Human Heart, *Am. Heart J.,* 5:720, 1930.

80 Lewis, T., and Rothschild, M. A.: The Excitatory Process in the Dog's heart. II The Ventricles, *Philos. Trans. R. Soc. Lond.,* 206:181, 1915.

81 Durrer, D., and Roos, J. P.: Epicardial Excitation of the Ventricles in a Patient with Wolff-Parkinson-White Syndrome (Type B), *Circulation,* 35:15, 1967.

82 Boineau, J. P., Moore, E. N., Spear, J. F., and Sealy, W. C.: Basis of Static and Dynamic ECG Variations in WPW. Anatomic and Electrophysiologic Observations in Right and Left Ventricular Pre-excitation, *Am. J. Cardiol.,* 32:32, 1973.

83 Boineau, J. P., and Moore, E. N.: Evidence for Propagation of Activation Across an Accessory Atrioventricular Connection in Types A and B Pre-excitation, *Circulation*, 41:375, 1970.

84 Gallagher, J. J., Kasell, J., Sealy, W. C., Pritchett, E. L. C., and Wallace, A. G.: Epicardial Mapping in the Wolff-Parkinson-White Syndrome, *Circulation*, 57:854, 1978.

85 Gallagher, J. J., Sealy, W. C., Kasell, J., Anderson, R. W., Millar, R., Campbell, R. W. F., Harrison, L., Pritchett, E. L. C., and Wallace, A. G.: Cryoablation of Accessory Atrioventricular Connections: A New Technique for Correction of the Pre-excitation Syndrome, *Circulation*, 55:471, 1977.

86 Harrison, L., Gallagher, J. J., Kasell, J., Anderson, R. W., Mikat, E., Hackel, D. B., and Wallace, A. G.: Cryosurgical Ablation of the AV Node-His Bundle: A New Method for Producing A-V Block, *Circulation*, 55:463, 1977.

87 Sealy, W. C., Gallagher, J. J., Pritchett, E. L. C., and Wallace, A. G.: Surgical Treatment of Tachyarrhythmias in Patients with Both an Ebstein's Anomaly and a Kent Bundle, *J. Thora. Cardiovasc. Surg.*, 75:847, 1978.

88 McAlpine, W. A.: "Heart and Coronary Arteries," Springer-Verlag New York Inc., New York, 1975.

Antiplatelet Medication and Cardiovascular Disease*

SIDNEY F. STEIN, M.D. and BRUCE L. EVATT, M.D.

Grayish-granulous looking plugs, composed, apparently, of colourless corpuscles and coagulated fibrin, are sometimes seen to block up an artery.

THOMAS WARTON JONES[1]

INTRODUCTION

Over 125 years have passed since Thomas Warton Jones first observed the formation of a white thrombus, and during that time we have made remarkable progress in understanding how platelets function. After a vessel is injured, platelets adhere to areas not protected by an endothelial surface and form a platelet plug which terminates blood loss. Those properties of platelets which allow them to prevent hemorrhage, however, also allow them to form thrombi which may obstruct critical vessels. Over the past few years, with increasing recognition of the fundamental role of the platelet in the genesis of arterial thrombi and atherosclerosis, enthusiasm for the use of drugs which might inhibit platelet function has increased. The ability of drugs to inhibit platelet function has generally been inferred from a series of in vitro tests that bear little resemblance to in vivo conditions. It has therefore become necessary to assess the antithrombotic properties of putative platelet function inhibitors in large clinical trials. The growing body of evidence suggesting that platelet function inhibitors may be useful in the treatment of arterial thrombosis and atherosclerosis is reviewed below and, where possible, well-designed double-blind clinical studies are stressed.[2–18]

RATIONALE FOR ANTIPLATELET THERAPY

Thrombogenesis

The four major factors affecting the mechanism of thrombus formation in vivo are the rate of blood flow, the condition of the vessel wall, changes in platelet function, and changes in the circulating coagulation

* From the Department of Medicine, Emory University School of Medicine (Dr. Stein) and Center for Disease Control, Atlanta.

factors.[16] During the past decade the role of these factors in the initiation of the clotting mechanism has been under intense investigation. One of the results of this effort has been the discovery that arterial and venous thrombi are formed under different conditions.[19] Since arterial thrombi are most likely to produce a sudden catastrophic event in the patient, new therapeutic approaches aimed at preventing arterial thrombi had to be considered.

The first step in the formation of an arterial thrombus is the adhesion of platelets to collagen or other substances found beneath abnormal or disrupted endothelial surfaces such as a rheumatic heart valve or an atherosclerotic plaque.[20–23] These platelets are thought to be recruited from platelet-rich zones near the vessel walls of the arteries. Since most of the platelets do not come in contact with the vessel wall, other platelets have to be recruited to form the subsequent platelet plug. When platelets adhere to the vessel wall, they change in shape and secrete certain constituents of their granules. This secretory process is similar to secretory reactions in other cells. When performed by platelets, this process is called the "release reaction" and is probably mediated by prostaglandin $H_2(G_2)$ or thromboxane A_2 (Fig. 1).[24,25] The materials secreted by the platelets include vasoconstrictors, coagulation factors, and most importantly, other substances such as adenosine diphosphate (ADP) which promote platelet aggregation, thrombus formation, and hemostasis.

ADP initiates the "aggregation" which recruits platelets into the platelet plug. When exposed to ADP, platelets in the vicinity of the platelets adhering to the vessel wall aggregate and are added to the expanding platelet mass. Small amounts of thrombin which are formed just before the fibrin clot is generated may also initially stimulate platelet function in hemostasis.[21] This concept is highly speculative, however, and its importance in vivo is not clear. Later, fibrin formation, probably initiated at sites on the platelet membrane, helps stabilize the platelet mass.

Although it is apparent that arterial thrombi are very dependent upon platelet function, initiation of venous thrombi may be more dependent upon the rate of blood flow[16] and activation of the clotting cascade. Rather than forming a white platelet plug at the head

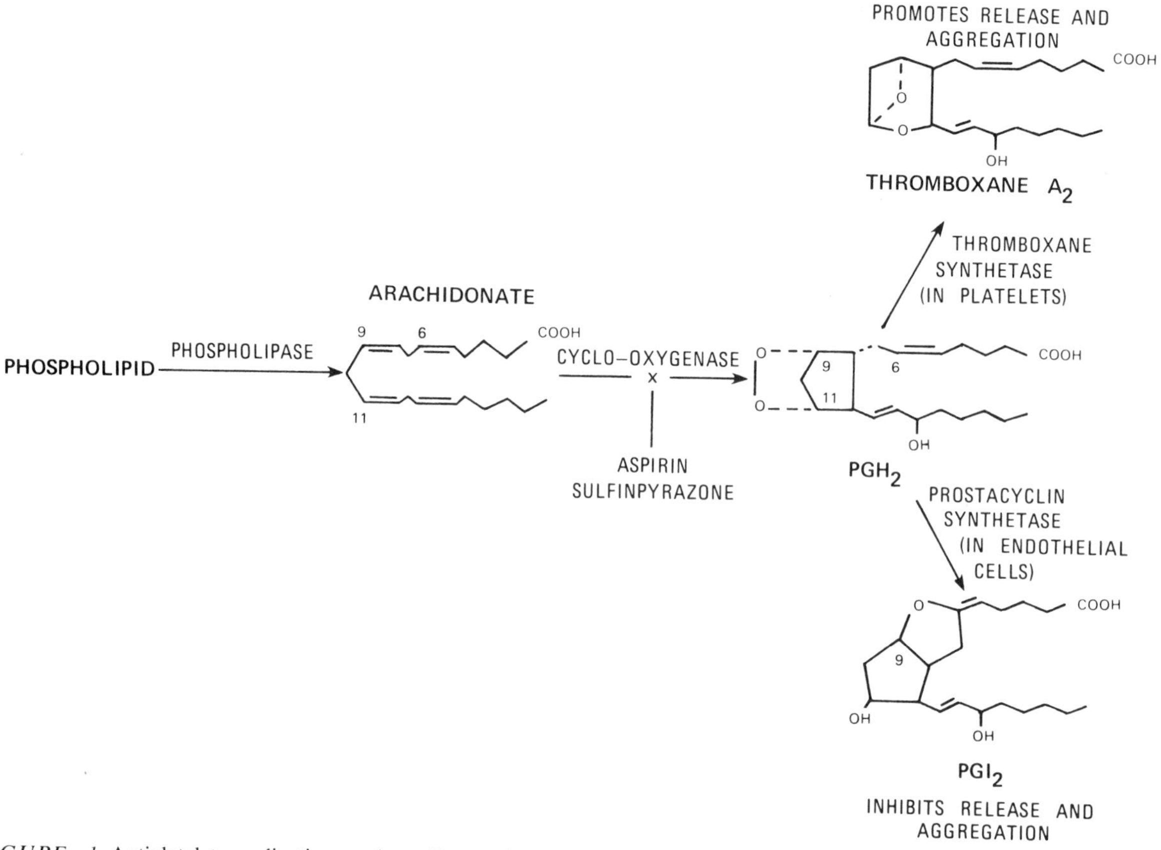

FIGURE 1 Antiplatelet medication and cardiovascular disease.

of an arterial thrombus, platelets are more uniformly distributed in venous thrombi, and a fibrin lattice forms the major component. It would be expected, then, that conventional anticoagulants (i.e., heparin or coumadin), which exert their influence upon clotting factors and are very effective in the management of venous thrombi, would be less effective in preventing thrombi from developing in arteries.[26]

It thus becomes apparent that the clinician who is interested in preventing or treating diseases produced by arterial thrombi would consider platelet suppressive agents. Since platelets have many functions related to the development of arterial thrombi, i.e., adhesion, the release reaction, and aggregation, a number of agents which affect these functions will have to be considered.

Accelerated platelet destruction or excessive or abnormal platelet function may constitute a major risk to patients, and treating them with platelet suppressive agents may reduce the chance of their developing catastrophic arterial thrombi. Patients with such conditions include those with older prosthetic mitral valves[27]

in whom a shortened platelet survival has been found. Also, spontaneous platelet aggregation has been reported in the blood of patients with arterial insufficiency and deep-vein thrombosis.[28,29] Increased sensitivity of platelets to aggregation of ADP and epinephrine has been reported in patients with diabetes mellitus, and increased platelet coagulant activity has been observed in patients with transient cerebral ischemia.[31] Although these latter observations have not been critically assessed, they point to areas in which antiplatelet therapy may potentially be of benefit.

Other cellular elements of the blood, such as red blood cells and white blood cells, may play passive roles in thrombus formation, but the extent to which these are important is as yet unclear.[16] Certainly, red blood cells contain large amounts of ADP which can be released in the presence of hemolysis and induce platelet aggregation. Likewise, the blood viscosity is predominantly dependent on the hematocrit levels and deviation of viscosity from normal which can greatly affect the rate of blood flow in the microcirculatory system, thus aggravating problems with stasis. However, except in the treatment of the rare patient with polycythemia rubra vera or promyelocytic leukemia, no rational therapeutic approach to the prevention of arterial thrombi has been aimed at either red blood cells or white blood cells.

Atherogenesis

The pathogenetic role of the platelet in arterial thrombus formation has been characterized for quite some time, but only in the past 5 years has evidence been found that the platelet plays an important role in the formation of atherosclerotic lesions. As far back as 1856, Virchow hypothesized that atherosclerotic plaques developed at sites of endothelial injury.[32] Immediately after injury occurs, platelets adhere to the connective tissue beneath the lost endothelium and proceed to aggregate and degranulate. Within days, smooth muscle cells begin migrating through the internal elastic lamina into the intima, where they proliferate and form an atherosclerotic plaque. Thus, smooth muscle cell proliferation is the *sine qua non* of atherosclerosis.[32,33] Apparently, a basic, heat-stable, nondialyzable macromolecule is released from the platelets adhering to the exposed subendothelium, and smooth muscle cell proliferation is subsequently promoted.[33,34] The hypothesis that smooth muscle cell proliferation is dependent upon secretion of a platelet factor is supported by the fact that smooth muscle cells in culture will proliferate only when mixed with serum prepared in the presence of platelets; if platelets are removed from plasma before it is converted to serum, the serum will be ineffective in promoting smooth muscle cell proliferation in vitro.[33-35] The hypothesis that a platelet secretory product stimulates proliferation of smooth muscle cells which form the atherosclerotic lesion is further supported by observations made in chronically homocystinemic baboons. These animals suffer chronic chemical endothelial cell injury associated with a decreased platelet survival and smooth muscle cell proliferation. Animals so treated with homocystine develop classical atherosclerotic lesions over a 3-month period. However, if the animals are treated with the platelet function inhibitor dipyridamole, the platelet survival returns to normal and no atherosclerotic lesions develop, even though endothelial desquamation continues.[14,15,36]

Two other lines of evidence implicate adequate platelet function as a necessary condition for the development of atherosclerosis:

1 Severe thrombocytopenia (platelet counts of approximately 5,000 per microliter) suppresses atherogenesis in rabbits whose aortic endothelium has been removed by a balloon catheter.[37]

2 The incidence of atherosclerosis is lower in pigs with von Willebrand's disease, a disorder of platelet function, than in normal pigs fed the same high cholesterol diet.[16,38]

PHARMACOLOGY AND METHODS OF ACTION OF ANTIPLATELET DRUGS

As Weiss has pointed out,[12] the word "antiplatelet" is a term without precise meaning. It has been used to describe drugs with various properties, including the ability to (1) inhibit in vitro the adhesion, retention, or aggregation of platelets, perhaps at drug concentrations that are unattainable in man; (2) inhibit platelet-induced thrombus formation; and (3) prolong in vivo platelet survival in clinical conditions associated with a shortened survival either by diminishing platelet reactivity or by suppressing the pathologic event which resulted in platelet activation (i.e., endothelial cell loss).

The characteristics of an ideal platelet function inhibitor have been well described.[14,16,18] Such a drug should be nontoxic, be effective when taken orally, have a reasonable duration of action, and have in vivo antithrombotic properties while carrying little risk of causing hemorrhage. Although many drugs have been noted to interfere with platelet function in vitro, only a few have been shown to have in vivo antithrombotic effects, and of these, only aspirin, sulfinpyrazone, and dipyridamole appear to have the potential for widespread clinical use in the next few years.

Aspirin

The use of aspirin in the prevention of myocardial infarction and other diseases caused by arterial occlusions has been stimulated by recent studies of the pharmacology of aspirin and its interrelationship with the prostaglandin pathway. The hypothesis that platelet function is very important in the initiation and development of arterial thrombi provides the rationale for using drugs which affect the prostaglandin pathway to prevent occlusive venous and arterial disease.

The prostaglandins (PG) are found virtually everywhere within the body.[39] There is little evidence that they are stored in any appreciable amounts, and thus they appear to be locally synthesized and released by various stimuli, depending upon the particular tissue.[40-45] They do not circulate to any extent and thus appear to act as local hormones, profoundly affecting the function of cells and tissues in their immediate area. The immediate prostaglandin precursor, arachidonic acid, is probably bound to phospholipids and triglycerides. Its release must be preceded by the activation of lipases, i.e., phospholipase A_2 and possibly triglyceridelipase (Fig. 1).[21,46]

In platelets, arachidonic acid is esterified to the two positions of glycerol and the phospholipids. When platelets are stimulated by contact with collagen, release of the acid is thought to be secondary to a specific lipase, phospholipase A_2. When released, the arachidonic acid serves as a substrate for another enzyme, cyclo-oxygenase, which then catalyzes the formation of a cyclic endoperoxide, prostaglandin H_2.[25] Availability of the substrate, arachidonic acid, regulates the reaction. The cyclic endoperoxide profoundly affects platelet function by causing aggregation with other platelets and the release reaction. Further metabolism[47] yields an even more potent vasoconstrictor and platelet aggregating agent, thromboxane A_2, by the interaction of PGH_2 and thromboxane synthetase.[24] This material is extremely labile and has a half-life of about 30 s.[21]

Aspirin is thought to block the conversion of arachidonic acid to the pharmacologically active intermediates by acetylating the enzyme cyclo-oxygenase.[25,48-51] This acetylation reaction parallels other aspirin effects upon the platelet and is permanent, that is, it persists throughout the life-span of the aspirin-treated platelet.[48] Physiologically, the effect blocks the platelet release reaction induced by ADP and collagen as measured in vitro[52-54] but does not affect adhesion. Clinically, it is manifest as a minimally prolonged bleeding time in normal subjects and a markedly prolonged one in patients who have congenital defects of their coagulation system.[54-56] The effect can be achieved in vivo with doses of no more than 300 to 600 mg/day.[57]

On a theoretical basis, however, the blockage of arachidonic acid by aspirin may not be the most efficient site of action for an antiplatelet drug. This is because there are other metabolic pathways for PGH_2 besides the synthesis of thromboxane. For instance, another enzyme, PGI_2 synthetase, which is present in the endothelial cells of arteries and veins, catalyzes the synthesis of PGI_2 (prostacyclin) from PGH_2.[58,59] Prostacyclin is a potent inhibitor of platelet aggregation and the release reaction. Thus, agents such as aspirin, which block prostaglandin synthesis at an early stage, both inhibit and prevent the inhibition of platelet function. These agents could be less effective than antiplatelet drugs which act at a later step, blocking thromboxane synthesis, while leaving intact the PGI_2 pathway. However, the amount of aspirin necessary to inhibit the cyclo-oxygenase in endothelial cells is much greater than that necessary to inhibit cyclo-oxygenase in platelets.[60] Thus the pathway for formation of products that inhibit platelet aggregation should remain intact at dosage levels of aspirin which

will inhibit the formation of products that stimulate platelet aggregation.

Sulfinpyrazone

Sulfinpyrazone (Anturane) belongs to the category of nonsteroidal anti-inflammatory agents, although it has minimal anti-inflammatory activity. It is a pyrazole compound related to phenylbutazone and has been used in the past as a uricosuric agent for treating gout. At concentrations higher than those attained clinically, sulfinpyrazone inhibits the platelet release reaction and thus the secondary phase of ADP or epinephrine-induced aggregation.[3,6,9,12,13,23,61,62] It has no effect on primary ADP aggregation and does not elevate platelet cyclic AMP.[63,64] Like aspirin, sulfinpyrazone appears to inhibit platelet cyclo-oxygenase; unlike aspirin, its effect is only transient.[65,66] Interestingly, blood levels of sulfinpyrazone that prolong a shortened platelet survival in vivo are inadequate to demonstrate an abnormality of in vitro platelet function (aggregation) and will not lead to prolongation of the bleeding time.[67-70] Thus, while it has been speculated that sulfinpyrazone may act on the vessel wall,[16,17] there was little evidence to support this hypothesis until recent studies demonstrated that high concentrations of sulfinpyrazone prevent homocysteine-induced endothelial cell injury.[71] At the present time the mechanism by which sulfinpyrazone manifests its antithrombotic properties in vivo remains uncertain.

Dipyridamole

Dipyridamole (Persantine) is a pyrimido-pyrimidine compound and has been used as a vasodilator for the treatment of angina pectoris for over 15 years. At concentrations higher than those clinically attainable, dipyridamole inhibits aggregation of platelets by thrombin and collagen, primary and secondary aggregation of platelets by ADP and epinephrine, and the platelet release reaction.[19,53,72-75] At similar concentrations, it has sometimes been reported to reduce the retention of platelets on glass-bead filters.[62] Interestingly, none of the in vitro abnormalities are observed in platelets which have been exposed to clinically attainable concentrations of the drug. At these same concentrations, however, dipyridamole has a demonstrable effect in reducing thrombus formation, prolonging platelet survival in conditions associated with an accelerated rate of platelet consumption, and preventing the development of atherosclerosis in experimental homocystinemia.[4-6,13-15,26,36,76] Dipyridamole increases the platelet cyclic AMP concentrations by inhibiting phosphodiesterase activity.[2,77] Exactly how dipyridamole exerts its antithrombotic effect is not certain. Analogous pyrimido-pyrimidine compounds, which are more potent inhibitors of phosphodiesterase and platelet aggregation than dipyridamole, seem to have somewhat reduced antithrombotic properties.[72,78-80]

ISCHEMIC HEART DISEASE

The rationale for using platelet function inhibitors in treating patients with ischemic heart disease has been well explained by Harker et al.[14] Platelets may form a thrombus in a major coronary artery, embolize from a proximal coronary artery lesion to the microcirculation of the heart,[81] or circulate as aggregates with the potential of obstructing the microcirculation.[82] In addition, platelets play a pathogenetic role in atherogenesis and produce thromboxane A_2, which may initiate intense coronary artery spasm. Thrombosis of a major coronary artery is often found after myocardial infarction,[83] but inasmuch as the thrombi are not always found in patients who die suddenly after a myocardial infarction and are more often found in patients who die several days after their infarct, it is not certain whether thrombosis is a cause or a consequence of myocardial infarction.[84,85] Platelet aggregates have been found in the microcirculation of the heart of rats that were subjected to stress, and they have been found in greater numbers in the cardiac microcirculation of patients who die suddenly after a myocardial infarction than in those of patients whose death may be attributed to another cause.[82,86] Furthermore, it has been shown that when dogs are pretreated with a variety of antiplatelet agents, they are protected against myocardial infarction while receiving an infusion of epinephrine.[87] In addition, as Weiss has noted,[13] increased in vitro platelet aggregation has been associated with hypercholesterolemia, smoking, stress, and diabetes. In platelet survival studies performed in patients with angiographically proved coronary artery disease, over half the patients had a shortened platelet survival which could be improved with the use of sulfinpyrazone[88] or dipyridamole.[89] It is thus apparent that there is adequate rationale for clinical trials of platelet function inhibitors in patients with a proved history of ischemic heart disease.

Several uncontrolled and largely retrospective studies suggest that aspirin may diminish the risk of myocardial infarction. The Boston Collaborative Drug Surveillance Group reported two studies done on over 14,000 patients, some of whom had been hospitalized with myocardial infarction.[90] In both studies they found that patients hospitalized for heart attack were much less likely to be users of aspirin than patients hospitalized for other reasons. One group of 8,000 middle-aged men had been treated with one or two aspirins a day for a period of 7 years, and it was asserted that none of these patients had ever had a myocardial infarction.[91] An autopsy series on patients with rheumatoid arthritis revealed an incidence of acute myocardial infarction of 4 percent, a figure much lower than the expected rate of 31 percent.[92] However, in another study involving over 1 million men and women, the negative correlation between incidence of myocardial infarction and use of aspirin was less apparent.[93] A multicenter randomized prospective double-blind study of aspirin use in men who had suffered a recent myocardial infarction was conducted in Wales. Patients received either placebo or 300 mg of aspirin once a day. Total mortality was reduced 12 percent in 6 months, 25 percent in 12 months, and 34 percent in 24 months for those patients receiving aspirin. While this trend was favorable, it was not statistically significant.[94] A closer analysis of the data, however, revealed that those patients who entered the study less than 6 weeks after suffering myocardial infarction had an overall mortality of 7.8 percent in the aspirin-treated group and 13.2 percent in the placebo-treated group—a difference which is statistically significant. Those men who entered the study after having had infarcts more than 6 months earlier had a mortality rate of 8.8 percent in the aspirin-treated group and 8.3 percent in the placebo-treated group.[18] It is possible, then, that aspirin may have its greatest effect on those patients whose myocardial infarction is most recent. It is unfortunate, therefore, that the Coronary Drug Project Aspirin Study was conducted on a group of men whose qualifying myocardial infarction had occurred several years before the study was initiated. No patient had his qualifying myocardial infarction less than 2 years before entering the study, and 75 percent of the patients had had their infarct 5 years or more before beginning the study. Over 1,500 men were randomized to receive either placebo or aspirin, 324 mg three times a day. After 28 months, overall mortality was 5.8 percent in the aspirin-treated group and 8.3 percent in the placebo-treated group—a difference of 30 percent.[95] While this is a favorable trend, it does not reach statistical significance. At the present time, one large double-blind study using aspirin alone is in progress in this country. The Aspirin Myocardial Infarction Study (AMIS) includes 4,200 men and women with a history of a myocardial infarction occurring between 2 months and 3 years before entry. Patients have been randomized to receive either placebo or 500 ng of aspirin twice a day. The end points for this study are recurrent myocardial infarction or death, and the follow-up period is 3 years.[96]

Thirteen studies have been reported in which dipyridamole was administered to patients with coronary artery disease.[16,18] In none of these studies can the end point of myocardial infarction and death be adequately evaluated because either the number of patients entered was too few, the drug dose was too small, or the duration of the study was too short. One study involving the use of dipyridamole and aspirin is in progress. The Persantine-Aspirin Re-infarction Study (PARIS) includes 2,000 men and women with a history of myocardial infarction occurring between 2 months and 3 years before they entered the study. The end points for this study are recurrent myocardial infarction or death, and the follow-up period is 2 years. Four hundred patients will receive placebo, 800 patients will receive 324 mg of aspirin three times a day, and 800 patients will receive a combination of 75 mg of dipyridamole and 324 mg of aspirin, both taken three times a day.[96] The results of this study are awaited with interest.

A group of 96 elderly men with a history of either myocardial infarction alone or myocardial infarction and stroke were treated with placebo or sulfinpyrazone, 200 mg three times a day. The patients were followed for 4 years or less, and deaths from vascular causes were significantly lower in the group receiving sulfinpyrazone. Overall, 18 percent of the patients receiving sulfinpyrazone died, and 53 percent of those receiving placebo died.[97] It is possible, however, that the improved mortality could merely reflect a drug effect on the course of cerebrovascular disease. Recently, a preliminary report on Anturane Reinfarction Trial (ART) was published.[98] In the study, 1,475 men and women were enrolled between 25 and 35 days after a myocardial infarction. They were randomized to receive either placebo or sulfinpyrazone, 200 mg four times a day. To date the average follow-up time has been 8.4 months and for cardiac deaths, the annual death rate was 9.5 percent in the placebo group and 4.9 percent in the sulfinpyrazone group. The annual sudden cardiac death rate was 6.3 percent in the placebo group and 2.7 percent in the sulfinpyrazone group, with sudden deaths making up 61 percent of the total cardiac mortality. Both of these differences are highly statistically significant. Why sulfinpyrazone was so effective in diminishing the rate of sudden cardiac deaths remains uncertain. Perhaps it inhibits the dissemination of platelet microemboli into the microcirculation of the heart where they may cause fatal arrhythmias, or perhaps it has some unknown direct action upon the myocardium. This study is still in progress and final results are awaited.

While we are awaiting definitive results on the value of antiplatelet drugs from the AMIS, PARIS, and ART studies, how should we treat our patients with recent myocardial infarction? Neither aspirin nor sulfinpyrazone is a benign drug; each has its serious complications. Still, with the high mortality in the first year after myocardial infarction, it would not seem unreasonable to treat patients who can tolerate the therapy with sulfinpyrazone, 200 mg four times a day for a period of 1 year, with adequate precautions being observed. Once the efficacy of antiplatelet drugs is firmly established, we will be able to approach the treatment of patients more rationally. One should not be surprised if antiplatelet therapy is not shown to significantly improve the survival of patients after a myocardial infarction. After all, coronary artery disease becomes clinically manifest only late in its course, and it might be that platelet function inhibitors would be more effective if started earlier in the course of the disease.

CEREBRAL VASCULAR DISEASE

Although the clinical effectiveness of antiplatelet agents in cerebral vascular disease remains controversial,[16,99] recent studies have indicated that such agents are potentially useful. One area of major emphasis has been that of patients who have experienced transient ischemic attacks (TIA). Between 4 and 10 percent of these patients will develop strokes each year, and a total of 25 to 40 percent of patients who have experienced TIAs will develop a stroke within 5 years of the initial TIA.[16] It has been shown that TIAs are frequently associated with atherosclerotic lesions of the extracranial portions of the internal carotid and basilar arteries[13] and that they may result from microembolization of platelet thrombi developing on these lesions. This theory has been given credence by the observation of passage of microemboli in retinal arterioles during attacks of monocular vision loss, amaurosis fugax.[100–102] Also, autopsy material on patients with histories of vascular and cerebral ischemia have shown microemboli composed of platelet aggregates.[103] In 1972, Evans reported the results of a double-blind randomized study performed on 20 patients who had had recurrent attacks of amaurosis fugax and who were treated with sulfinpyrazone.[104] Each patient received either a placebo or 200 mg of sulfinpyrazone four times a day for 6 weeks and then was treated with the alternative therapy for an additional 6 weeks. The incidence of the amaurosis attacks was significantly lowered by sulfinpyrazone treatment. A year later, Deykin et al. reported a retrospective study of 26 patients with TIAs, 15 of whom had been treated with 300 mg of aspirin twice daily.[105] Although there were no differences between the ultimate occurrence of cerebral infarction or death, 82 percent who had received no aspirin had additional TIAs, whereas only 13 percent of those who had received aspirin reported additional TIAs. In 1975, results of another study supported the use of antiplatelet therapy in cerebral vascular disease. A double-blind study was performed by

Blakely and Gent on 99 institutionalized males over a 4-year period.[97] These subjects had previously had a stroke, either singly or in combination with a myocardial infarction. Each of two groups received either placebo or sulfinpyrazone, 200 mg three times a day. The results showed a clear statistically significant benefit in terms of overall survival for the sulfinpyrazone-treated group.

Findings of several recent studies support results of these previous studies. In a group of 25 patients with TIAs and shortened platelet survival, Steele et al. showed that sulfinpyrazone was effective in returning platelet survival to normal and reducing the number of TIAs experienced by these patients.[106] The study was interesting in that it suggested a relationship between TIA frequency and the platelet survival.

Another double-blind randomized study was performed at 10 cooperating U.S. centers on a group of 178 patients who had had TIAs.[107] These patients were randomly allocated to either aspirin or placebo therapy and were followed to determine the incidence of subsequent TIAs, death, cerebral infarction, or retinal infarction. Although no significant difference was found between aspirin and the placebo treatments as determined by the absolute end points of death, cerebral infarction, or retinal infarction, significant benefits were shown in particular subgroups. There was a statistical difference favoring aspirin therapy in patients with a history of multiple TIAs and in those with carotid lesions appropriate to their symptoms. In addition, when patients having at least as many TIAs in the first 6 months after randomization as they had had in the 3 months prior to study entry were included with those having an absolute end point, there was a significant difference in favor of aspirin. Therefore, it appeared that certain subgroups of patients with cerebral ischemia were more likely to benefit from aspirin therapy. In addition, a recent study has been reported by the Canadian Cooperative Trial of Platelet Suppressive Drugs and Transient Cerebral Ischemia. This multicenter double-blind placebo control study of 585 patients who have had at least one TIA has shown some surprising results.[108] Aspirin in the dosage of 325 mg four times a day reduced the risk of stroke and death by approximately one-half in males but had no effect in females. Sulfinpyrazone in a dose of 800 mg/day was without effect, in contrast to previous findings.

Presently, there is no evidence that dipyridamole is useful in the prophylaxis of TIAs or other types of cerebral ischemia.[109] In light of the recent studies, it seems reasonable to recommend that 1200 to 1300 mg of aspirin per day be used as a prophylaxis against TIAs in symptomatic males who can tolerate the therapy.

ARTIFICIAL SURFACES

Thromboembolism remains a major problem for patients with prosthetic heart valves. With the older, more thrombogenic valves, as many as 50 percent of the patients would experience a thromboembolic episode. Even with newer valves, 5 to 10 percent of the patients still experience such an episode.[27,110–113] Platelet survival studies in patients with prosthetic heart valves have repeatedly demonstrated shortened platelet survivals,[27,76,114,115] presumably because platelet material is deposited on and subsequently embolized from the valve surface. Indeed, one study shows that the rate of platelet consumption is proportional to the surface area of the prosthetic valve.[76] However, a shortened platelet survival has been demonstrated in patients with mitral valve disease before surgery, and this has correlated with the risk of subsequent thromboembolic episodes after valve implantation.[116] Conducting postoperative platelet survival studies, Weily showed that 62 percent of the patients with a shortened platelet survival experienced a thromboembolic episode, whereas the same fate awaited only 9 percent of those with a normal platelet survival.[27] Thus there was a close correlation between platelet survival and the incidence of thromboembolism. Furthermore, a history of thromboembolic episodes before surgery correlated with shortening of the platelet survival after surgery. In one study, the platelet half-life in patients without a previous history of an embolic episode was 3.4 days after valve insertion, while it was only 2.5 days postoperatively in those patients with a previous history of an embolic event.[27,68] Both dipyridamole[76] and sulfinpyrazone[67] have been shown to increase the platelet survival in patients with prosthetic heart valves, which indicates that they can decrease platelet consumption. In the dipyridamole study, 400 mg/day of dipyridamole was required to normalize the platelet survival. However, if 1 g of aspirin were taken concomitantly with 100 mg of dipyridamole once a day, the platelet survival could also be normalized. Aspirin by itself did not normalize the platelet survival, and how it potentiates the action of dipyridamole remains unknown. Based on such studies, a regimen of 75 mg of dipyridamole and 330 mg of aspirin taken together three times a day has the capability of normalizing a shortened survival without subjecting the patient to the side effects produced by high doses of dipyridamole.[26] The sulfinpyrazone study showed that 800 mg of sulfinpyrazone a day, but not 400 mg per day, would normalize the platelet survival in patients with mitral valve prostheses. One well-controlled study has shown the utility of platelet function inhibitors in controlling thromboembolic episodes in patients with prosthetic heart valves.[117,118] One hundred and sixty-three patients with thrombogenic prosthetic mitral and aortic valves were treated with oral anticoagulants and randomized to receive either a placebo or dipyridamole, 100 mg four times a day. Fourteen percent of the patients receiving placebo experienced emboli, while only 1.3 percent of the patients receiving dipyridamole did. The death rate in both groups was unaffected by the therapy; however, no patients in the dipyridamole group died of an embolic event, whereas 2 of 10 patients in the placebo group did. Arrants treated 39 patients with prosthetic valves with oral anticoagulation and dipyridamole.[119,120] He reported a lower incidence of embolic episodes in these patients than in 20 historical controls. The results of this study, however, are probably biased in favor of dipyridamole because the historical controls had more thrombogenic valves implanted. In another report, 11 patients experiencing embolic phenomenon while on oral anticoagulants alone stopped having these episodes when dipyridamole was added to the regimen.[121] Two other studies showed a decreased incidence of embolic phenomena after a platelet function inhibitor was added to the regimen of prosthetic valve patients taking an oral anticoagulant; in one study, ½ g of aspirin per day was added,[122] while in the other study, 1 g of aspirin daily was added.[123] The evidence suggests that patients should now be treated with an oral anticoagulant as well as with platelet function inhibitors, and the regimen recommended by Harker of 75 mg of dipyridamole taken together with 330 mg of aspirin three times a day seems most reasonable.[26]

Thrombus formation continues to be a frequent problem in the management of arteriovenous shunts used for hemodialysis.[124] Animal studies have shown that thrombosis of arteriovenous shunts can be reduced by the use of aspirin,[125] sulfinpyrazone,[126] dipyridamole,[127,128] and its analogues.[71] One study has shown that the shortened platelet survival observed in hemodialysis patients with arteriovenous shunts could be restored toward normal with the use of dipyridamole.[5] The most informative studies in the area were those performed by Kaegi.[129,130] His group showed that sulfinpyrazone, 200 mg three times a day, significantly reduced the number of patients developing thrombi (50 percent versus 80 percent) and reduced the rate of thrombus formation by a factor of 4. This study represents a definitive example of the efficacy of platelet function inhibitors in the reduction of thrombus formation associated with arteriovenous shunts.

VENOUS THROMBOSIS

The use of antiplatelet drugs for the prevention of venous thrombosis remains much more controversial than their use in the prevention of arterial thrombosis.[13,17,131] Certainly from the theoretical point of view, platelets play a more prominent role in the initiation of arterial thrombi, for the high flow rates in arteries favor a platelet-rich zone near the wall of the blood vessel, and in addition, many of the activated clotting factors are swept away. On the other hand, venous thrombosis is much more dominated by the presence of stasis. Furthermore, unlike arterial thrombi, which are easily detected because of their catastrophic clinical effects, venous thrombi can frequently escape detection. Thus, results of clinical trials must be judged on the basis of the methods used in detecting venous thrombi.[18] This is because studies which rely solely on fibrinogen-scanning techniques may be relatively insensitive to thrombi of the iliac and high femoral veins, whereas studies based upon phlebography run extra risks of side effects and are not easily repeated.[12]

Because of the large number of studies performed in this field and the number of recent reviews, most individual studies will not be reviewed here. The reader is referred to several good reviews on the subject.[13,14,18]

The drug which has been studied most often is aspirin. Although these studies do not conclusively show that aspirin, either alone or in combination with dipyridamole, can prevent venous thrombosis, certain trends are developing. Although aspirin has not proved to be of benefit in some studies,[132,133] at least 10 studies dealing primarily with prophylaxis for hip operations suggest that aspirin may reduce the incidence of postoperative venous thrombosis.[14,134] These studies have been criticized because of the methodology used in performing them.[18] However, Harris et al. recently reported on a well-controlled study in which phlebography was used as the diagnostic end point.[134] They reported that 600 mg. of aspirin administered twice daily significantly reduced the incidence of thrombosis after hip replacement. This study, like the one performed by the Canadian Cooperative Trial on transient cerebral ischemias, demonstrated that the protective effect was limited to men.[108] Another study performed by Zechert also suggested that aspirin in the dosage of 500 mg three times a day may also reduce the incidence of pulmonary emboli in patients undergoing hip operations.[135] Although heparin and oral anticoagulants currently remain the recommended therapy for the prevention of venous thrombosis, these studies point out the possibility that aspirin may be useful in preventing venous thrombosis in selected high-risk patients.[12] However, it is only fair to point out that studies in which aspirin was found to be beneficial in preventing venous thrombosis have been conducted primarily with patients in the setting of surgery, a situation in which vascular injury may accentuate the role of the platelet in the initiation of a venous thrombus.

PERIPHERAL VASCULAR DISEASE

Little data are available on the use of antiplatelet agents in the treatment of patients with peripheral vascular disease. Patients with stable peripheral vascular disease generally have normal platelet survivals,[5,26] and thus a therapeutic role for antiplatelet agents may be limited. There are a few anecdotal reports, mainly in the British literature, on the treatment of patients with intermittent peripheral arterial ischemia. Ten patients with painful and cyanotic fingers and/or toes associated with thrombocytosis responded favorably to treatment with 300 to 1,000 mg of aspirin per day;[136-138] 1 of these patients did not benefit from 150 mg of di-

pyridamole per day. Another patient with Raynaud's disease apparently benefited from the use of aspirin,[139] and 2 patients with postembolic upper extremity ischemia may have benefited from dipyridamole.[140]

FUTURE TRENDS

The platelet function inhibitors that are currently available are not particularly powerful or specific and have been discovered largely by accident. In the future we can look forward to the development of analogues of PGI_2, more potent and specific anti-inflammatory and pyrimido-pyrimidine compounds, drugs that may prevent endothelial cell loss, and drugs that negate the effect of platelet mitogenic factor. With these drugs, antiplatelet therapy will undoubtedly play a more important role in the prevention of thrombosis and atherosclerosis.

REFERENCES

1 Jones, T. W.: Guys Hosp. Rep. (2nd series), 7 (part 1):35, 1850.

2 Mustard, J. F., and Packham, M. A.: Factors Influencing Platelet Function: Adhesion, Release, and Aggregation, *Pharmacol. Rev.,* 22:97, 1970.

3 Mustard, J. F., Kinlough-Rathbone, R. L., and Packham, M. A.: Recent Status of Research in the Pathogenesis of Thrombosis, *Thromb. Diath. Haemorrh.,* 59:(Supplement)157, 1974.

4 Harker, L. A., Slichter, S. J.: Arterial and Venous Thromboembolism: Kinetic Characterization and Evaluation of Therapy, *Thromb. Diath. Haemorrh.,* 31:188, 1974.

5 Harker, L. A., and Slichter, S. J.: Platelet and Fibrinogen Consumption in Man, *N. Engl. J. Med.,* 287:999, 1972.

6 Sherry, S., Brinkhous, K. M., Genton, E., and Stengle, J. M. (eds.): "Thrombosis," National Academy of Science, Washington, D.C., 1969.

7 Weiss, H. J. (ed.): Platelets and Their Role in Hemostasis, *Ann. N. Y. Acad. Sci.,* 201:1, 1972.

8 Didisheim, P. T., Shimamoto, T., and Yamazaki, H.: Platelets, Thrombosis and Inhibitor, *Thromb. Diath. Haemorrh.,* 60:(suppl.)1, 1974.

9 Hirsh, J., Cade, J. F., Gallus, A. S., and Schombaum, E. (eds.): "Platelets, Drugs and Thrombosis," Karger, Basel, 1974.

10 Jensen, K. G., and Killman, S. A. (eds.): Antiplatelet Drugs and Thrombosis, *Ser. Haematol.,* 8(3):50, 1976.

11 Spaet, T. H.: Optimism in the Control of Atherosclerosis, *N. Engl. J. Med.,* 291:576, 1974.

12 Weiss, H. J.: Antiplatelet Therapy, *N. Engl. J. Med.,* 298:1344, 1403, 1978.

13 Weiss, H. J.: Antiplatelet Drugs—a New Pharmacologic Approach to the Prevention of Thrombosis, *Am. Heart J.,* 92:86, 1976.

14 Harker, L. A., Hirsh, J., Gent, M., et al.: Critical Evaluation of Platelet Inhibiting Drugs in Thrombotic Disease, *Prog. Hematol.,* 9:229, 1975.

15 Harker, L. A., Ross, R., Slichter, S. J., et al.: Homocystine-induced Arteriosclerosis: The Role of Endothelial Cell Injury and Platelet Response in Its Genesis, *J. Clin. Invest.,* 58:731, 1976.

16 Didisheim, P., and Fuster, V.: Actions and Clinical Status of Platelet Suppressive Agents, *Sem. Hematol.,* 15:55, 1978.

17 Verstraete, M.: Are Agents Effecting Platelet Functions Clinically Useful?, *Am. J. Med.,* 61:897, 1976.

18 Genton, E., Gent, M., Hirsh, J., et al.: Platelet Inhibiting Drugs in the Prevention of Clinical Thrombotic Disease, *N. Engl. J. Med.,* 293:1174, 1236, 1296, 1975.

19 Mustard, J. F., and Packham, M. A.: Platelets, Thrombosis and Drugs, *Drugs,* 9:19, 1975.

20 Weiss, H. J.: Platelets: Physiology and Abnormalities of Function, *N. Engl. J. Med.,* 293:531, 1975.

21 Majerus, P. W.: Why Aspirin?, *Circulation,* 54:357, 1976.

22 Caen, J. P., Bronberg, S., and Kubisz, P.: "Platelets: Physiology and Pathology," Stratton Intercontinental, New York, 1977.

23 Packham, M. A., and Mustard, J. F.: Clinical Pharmacology of Platelets, *Blood,* 50:555, 1977.

24 Hamberg, M., Svensson, J., and Samuelsson, B.: Thromboxanes: A New Group of Biologically Active Compounds Derived from Prostaglandin Endoperoxides, *Proc. Natl. Acad. Sci. USA,* 72:2994, 1975.

25 Hamberg, M., Svensson, J., Wakabayashi, T., and Samuelsson, B.: Prostaglandin Endoperoxides. Novel Transformations of Arachidonic Acid in Human Platelets, *Proc. Natl. Acad. Sci. USA,* 71:3400, 1974.

26 Harker, L. A.: In Vivo Evaluation of Antithrombotic Therapy in Man, *Thromb. Diath. Haemorrh.,* 60 (suppl.):481, 1974.

27 Weily, H. S., Steele, P. P., Davis, H., et al.: Platelet Survival in Patients with Substitute Heart Valves, *N. Engl. J. Med.,* 290:534, 1974.

28 Wu, K. K., Barnes, R. W., and Hoak, J. C.: Platelet Hyperaggregability in Idiopathic Recurrent Deep Vein Thrombosis, *Circulation,* 53:687, 1976.

29 Wu, K. K., Hoak, J. C.: Spontaneous Platelet Aggregation in Arterial Insufficiency: Mechanisms and Implications, *Blood,* 44:934, 1974.

30 Kwaan, H. C., Colwell, J. A., Cruz, S., et al.: Increased Platelet Aggregation in Diabetes Mellitus, *J. Lab. Clin. Med.,* 80:236, 1972.

31 Walsh, P. N., Pareti, F. I., and Corbett, J. J.: Platelet Coagulant Activities and Serum Lipids in Transient Cerebral Ischemia, *N. Engl. J. Med.,* 295:854, 1976.

32 Ross, R., and Glomset, J. A.: Atherosclerosis and the Arterial Smooth Muscle Cell, *Science,* 180:1332, 1973.

33 Ross, R., and Glomset, J. A.: The Pathogenesis of Atherosclerosis, *N. Engl. J. Med.,* 295:369, 420, 1976.

34 Ross, R., Glomset, J., Kariya, B., et al.: A Platelet Dependant Serum Factor That Stimulates the Proliferation of Arterial Smooth Muscle Cells In Vitro, *Proc. Natl. Acad. Sci. USA,* 71:1207, 1974.

35 Ross, R., Glomset, J., and Harker, L.: Response to Injury and Atherogenesis, *Am. J. Pathol.,* 86:675, 1977.

36 Harker, L. A., Slichter, S. J., Scott, C. R., et al.: Homocystinemia, *N. Engl. J. Med.,* 291:537, 1974.

37 Friedman, R. J., Stemerman, M. D., Wenz, B., et al.: The Effect of Thrombocytopenia on Experimental Arteriosclerotic Lesion Formation in Rabbits, *J. Clin. Invest.,* 60:1191, 1977.

38 Fuster, V., Byrne, J. M., Fass, D. N., et al.: Arterial Lesions in Normal and von Willebrand Pigs Receiving a High Chloresterol Diet, *Circulation,* 54:137, 1976.

39 Christ, E. J., and Van Dorp, D. A.: Comparative Aspects of Prostaglandin Biosynthesis in Animal Tissues, in G. Raspe (ed.), "Advances in the Biosciences," Vol. 9, Pergamon Press, New York, 1972, p. 35.

40 Aiken, J. W., and Vane, J. R.: Intrarenal Prostaglandin Release Attentuates the Renal Vasoconstrictor Activity of Angiotensin, *J. Pharmacol. Exp. Ther.,* 184:678, 1973.

41 Ferreira, S. H., and Vane, J. R.: Prostaglandins: Their Disappearance from and Release into the Circulation, *Nature,* 216:868, 1976.

42 McGiff, J. C., Terrangno, N. A., Colina, J., et al.: Prostaglandins and Their Relationships to the Kallekrein-Kinin Systems, in J. J. Pisano and K. F. Austen (eds.), "Chemistry and Biology of the Kallikrein-Kinin System in Health and Disease" [DHEW Publication No. (NIH) 76–791], U.S. Government Printing Office, Washington, D.C., 1971, p. 267.

43 Needleman, P., Marshall, G. R., and Sobel, B. E.: Hormone Interactions in the Isolated Rabbit Heart: Synthesis and Coronary Vasomotor Effects of Prostaglandins, Angiotensin, and Bradykinin, *Circ. Res.,* 37:802, 1975.

44 Needleman, P.: The Synthesis and Function of Prostaglandins in the Heart, *Fed. Proc.,* 35:2376, 1976.

45 Piper, P., and Vane, J.: The Release of Prostaglandins from Lung and Other Tissues, *Ann. N.Y. Acad. Sci.,* 180:363, 1971.

46 Needleman, P., and Daley, G.: Cardiac and Coronary Prostaglandin Synthesis and Function, *N. Engl. J. Med.,* 298:1122, 1978.

47 Hamberg, M., Svensson, J., and Samuelsson, B.: Prostaglandin Endoperoxides. A New Concept Concerning the Mode of Action and Release of Prostaglandins, *Proc. Natl. Acad. Sci. USA,* 71:3824, 1974.

48 Smith, J. B., and Willis, A. L.: Aspirin Selectively Inhibits Prostaglandin Production in Human Platelets, *Nature [New Biol.],* 231:235, 1971.

49 Roth, G. J., and Majerus, P. W.: The Mechanism of the Effect of Aspirin on Human Platelets. I. Acetylation of a Particulate Fraction Protein, *J. Clin. Invest.,* 56:624, 1974.

50 Roth, G. J., Stanford, N., and Majerus, P. W.: The Acetylation of Prostaglandin Synthase by Aspirin, *Proc. Natl. Acad. Sci. USA,* 72:3073, 1975.

51 Rome, L. H., Lands, W. E. M., Roth, G. J., and Majerus, P. W.: Aspirin as an Acetylating Agent for Prostaglandin Synthetase, *Prostaglandins,* 11:23, 1976.

52 O'Brien, J. R.: Effects of Salicylates on Human Platelets, *Lancet,* 1:779, 1968.

53 Zucker, M. B., and Peterson, J.: Effect of Acetyl-salicylic Acid, and Other Non-steroidal Anti-inflammatory Agents, and Dipyridamole on Human Blood Platelets, *J. Lab. Clin. Med.,* 76:66, 1970.

54 Weiss, H. J., Aledort, L. M., and Kochwa, S.: The Effects of Salicylates on the Hemostatic Properties of Platelets in Man, *J. Clin. Invest.,* 47:2169, 1968.

55 Mielke, C. H., Daneshiro, M. M., Maher, I. A., Weiner, J. M., and Rapaport, S. I.: The Standardized Normal Ivy Bleeding Time and its Prolongation by Aspirin, *Blood,* 34:204, 1969.

56 Kaneshiro, M. M., Mielke, C. H., Kasper, C. K., and Rapaport, S. I.: Bleeding Time after Aspirin in Disorders of Intrinsic Clotting, *N. Engl. J. Med.*, 281:1039, 1969.

57 Vane, J. R.: Inhibition of Prostaglandin Synthesis as a Mechanism of Action for Aspirin-like Drugs, *Nature [New Biol.]*, 231:232, 1971.

58 Moncada, S., Gryglewski, R., Bunting, S., et al.: An Enzyme Isolated from Arteries Transforms Prostaglandin Endoperoxides to an Unstable Substance That Inhibits Platelet Aggregation, *Nature,* 263:663, 1976.

59 Moncada, S., Higgs, E. A., and Vane, J. R.: Human Arterial and Venous Tissues Generate Prostacyclin (Prostaglandin X), a Potent Inhibitor of Platelet Aggregation, *Lancet,* 1:18, 1977.

60 Ketton, J., Carter, C., Buchanan, M. R., et al.: Thrombogenic Effect of High Dose Aspirin in Injury Induced Experimental Venous Thrombosis, *Clin. Res.,* 26:350, 1978.

61 Biochemistry and Pharmacology of Platelets, *Ciba Found. Symp.,* 35:1, 1975.

62 Weiss, H. J.: Pharmacology of Platelet Inhibition, *Prog. Hemostasis Thromb.,* 1:199, 1972.

63 Packham, M. A., Warrior, E. S., Glynn, M. F., et al.: Alteration of the Response of Platelets to Surface Stimule by Pyrazole Compounds, *J. Exp. Med.,* 126:171, 1967.

64 Packham, M. A., and Mustard, J. F.: The Effect of Pyrazole Compounds on Thrombin Induced Platelet Aggregation, *Proc. Soc. Exp. Biol. Med.,* 130:72, 1968.

65 Ali, M., and McDonald, J. W. D.: Effect of Sulfinpyrazone on Platelet Prostaglandin Synthesis and Platelet Release of Seritonin, *J. Lab. Clin. Med.,* 89:868, 1977.

66 McDonald, J. W. D., Ali, M., Nagi, G. R., et al.: Inhibition of Platelet Prostaglandin Synthetase and Platelet Release Reaction by Sulfinpyrazone, *Blood,* 46:10, 1975.

67 Steele, P. P., Weily, H. S., Davies, H., et al.: Platelet Function Studies in Coronary Artery Disease, *Circulation,* 48:1194, 1973.

68 Weily, H. S., and Genton, E.: Altered Platelet Function in Patients with Prosthetic Mitral Valves. Effects of Sulfinpyrazone Therapy, *Circulation,* 42:967, 1970.

69 Genton, E., and Steele, P. P.: Platelet, Drugs and Heart Disease, in J. Hirsh, J. F. Cade, A. S. Gallus, et al. (eds): "Platelets, Drugs and Thrombosis," Karger, Basel, 1975, p. 263.

70 Smythe, H. A., Ogryzlo, M. A., Murphy, E. A., et al.: The Effects of Sulfinpyrazone (Anturane) on Platelet Economy and Blood Coagulation in Man, *Can. Med. Assoc. J.,* 93:818, 1965.

71 Harker, L. A., Wall, R. T., Harlan, J. M., et al.: Sulfinpyrazone Prevention of Homocysteine-induced En-

dothelial Cell Injury in Arteriosclerosis, *Clin. Res.,* 26:544A, 1978.

72 Cucuianu, M. P., Nishizawa, E. E., and Mustard, J. F.: Effect of Pyrimido-Pyrimidine Compounds on Platelet Function, *J. Lab. Clin. Med.,* 77:958, 1971.

73 Eliasson, R., and Bygdeman, S.: Effect of Dipyridamole and Two Pyrimido-Pyrimidine Derivatives on the Kinetics of Human Platelet Aggregation and on Platelet Adhesiveness, *Scand. J. Lab. Invest.,* 24:145, 1969.

74 Emmons, T. R., Harrison, M. J. G., Honour, A. J., et al.: Effect of Dipyridamole on Human Platelet Behavior, *Lancet,* 2:603, 1965.

75 Kinlough-Rathbone, R. L.: The Effects of Other Drugs on Platelet Function, in J. Hirsh, J. F. Cade, A. S. Gallus, et al. (eds): "Platelets, Drugs and Thrombosis," Karger, Basel, 1975, p. 124.

76 Harker, L. A., and Slichter, S. J.: Studies of Platelet and Fibrinogen Kinetics in Patients with Prosthetic Heart Valves, *N. Engl. J. Med.,* 283:1302, 1970.

77 Mills, D. C. D., and Smith, J. B.: The Influence on Platelet Aggregation of Drugs That Affect the Accumulation of Adenosine 3', 5'-cyclic Monophosphate in Platelets, *Biochem. J.,* 121:185, 1971.

78 Rifkin, T. L., and Zucker, M. B.: The Effect of Dipyridamole and RA 233 on Human Platelet Function in Vitro, *Thromb. Diath. Haemorrh.,* 29:694, 1973.

79 Hassanein, A. A., Turpil, A. G. G., McNicol, G. P., et al.: Effect of RA 233 on Platelet Function in Vivo, *Br. Med. J.,* 2:83, 1970.

80 Elkeles, R. S., and Hampton, J. R.: Effect of a Pyrimido-Pyrimidine Compound on Platelet Behaviour in Vitro and in Vivo, *Lancet,* 2:751, 1968.

81 Haerem, J. W.: Mural Platelet Microthrombi and Major Acute Lesions of Main Epicardial Arteries in Sudden Coronary Death, *Atherosclerosis,* 19:529, 1974.

82 Haft, J. I., and Fani, K.: Platelet Aggregation in the Heart Induced by Stress, *Circulation,* 47:353, 1973.

83 Constantinides, P.: Placque Fissures in Human Coronary Thrombosis, *J. Atheroscl. Res.,* 6:1, 1966.

84 Spain, D. M., and Bradess, V. A.: The Relationship of Coronary Thrombosis to Coronary Atherosclerosis and Ischemic Heart Disease, *Am. J. Med. Sci.,* 240:701, 1960.

85 Roberts, W. C., and Buja, L. M.: The Frequency and Significance of Arterial Thrombi in Other Observations in Fatal Acute Myocardial Infarction, *Am. J. Med.,* 52:425, 1972.

86 Haerem, J. W.: Platelet Aggregates in Intramyocardial Vessels of Patients Dying Suddenly and Unexpectedly of Coronary Artery Disease, *Atherosclerosis,* 15:199, 1972.

87 Haft, J. I., Gershengorn, K., Krang, P. D., et al.: Protection Against Epinephrine Induced Myocardial Ne-

crosis by Drugs That Inhibit Platelet Aggregation, *Am. J. Cardiol.,* 30:838, 1972.

88 Steele, P., Battock, P., and Genton, E.: Effects of Clofibrate and Sulfinpyrazone on Platelet Survival Time in Coronary Artery Disease, *Circulation,* 52:473, 1975.

89 Ritchie, J. L., and Harker, L. A.: Platelet and Fibrinogen Survival in Coronary Atherosclerosis: Response to Medical and Surgical Therapy, *Am. J. Cardiol.,* 39:595, 1977.

90 Boston Collaborative Drug Surveillance Group: Regular Aspirin Intake and Acute Myocardial Infarction, *Br. Med. J.,* 1:440, 1974.

91 Craven, L. L.: Experiences with Aspirin (Acetylsalicylic Acid) in the Non-specific Prophylaxis of Coronary Thrombosis, *Miss. Valley Med. J.,* 75:38, 1953.

92 Cobb, S., Anderson, F., and Bauler, W.: Length of Life and Cause of Death in Rheumatoid Arthritis, *N. Engl. J. Med.,* 249:553, 1953.

93 Hammond, E. C., and Garfinkel, L.: Aspirin and Coronary Heart Disease: Findings of a Prospective Study, *Br. Med. J.,* 1:269, 1975.

94 Elwood, P. C., Cochrane, A. L., Burr, M. L., et al.: A Randomized Control Trial of Acetylsalicylic Acid in the Secondary Prevention of Mortality from Myocardial Infarction, *Br. Med. J.,* 1:436, 1974.

95 The Coronary Drug Project Research Group: Aspirin and Coronary Heart Disease, *J. Chronic Dis.,* 29:625, 1976.

96 Klimt, C. R., Doub, P. H., and Doub N. H.: Clinical Trials in Thrombosis: Secondary Prevention of Myocardial Infarction, *Thromb. Haemostasis (Stuttg),* 35:49, 1976.

97 Blakely, J. A., and Gent, M.: Platelet Drugs and Longevity in a Geriatric Population, in J. Hirsh, J. F. Cade, A. S. Gallus, et al. (eds.), "Platelets, Drugs and Thrombosis," Karger, Basel, 1975, p. 284.

98 Anturane Reinfarction Trial Research Group: Sulfinpyrazone in the Prevention of Cardiac Death after Myocardial Infarction, *N. Engl. J. Med.,* 298:289, 1978.

99 Genton, E., Barnett, H. J. M., Fields, W. S., et al.: XIV. Cerebral Ischemia: The Role of Thrombosis and Antithrombotic Therapy, *Stroke,* 8:150, 1977.

100 Fisher, C. M.: Observations of the Fundus Oculi in Transient Monocular Blindness, *Neurology (Minneap)* 9:333, 1959.

101 Russell, R. W. R.: Observations on the Retinal Blood Vessels in Monocular Blindness, *Lancet,* 2:1422, 1961.

102 Ashby, M., Oakley, N., Lorentz, I., et al.: Recurrent Transient Monocular Blindness, *Br. Med. J.,* 2:894, 1963.

103 Gunning, A. J., Pickering, G. W., Robb-Smith, A. H. T., et al.: Mural Thrombosis of the Internal Carotid Artery and Subsequent Embolism, *Q. J. Med.,* 33:155, 1964.

104 Evans, G.: Effect of Drugs That Suppress Platelet Surface Interaction on Incidence of Amaurosis Fulga and Transient Cerebral Ischemia, *Surg. Forum,* 23:239, 1972.

105 Dyken, M. L., Kolar, O. J., and Jones, F. H.: Differences in the Occurrence of Carotid Transient Ischemic Attacks Associated with Antiplatelet Aggregation Therapy, *Stroke,* 4:732, 1973.

106 Steele, P. P., Weily, H. S., Davies, H., et al.: Effect of Sulfinpyrazone on Platelet Survival Time in Patients with Transient Cerebral Ischemic Attacks, *Stroke,* 8:396, 1977.

107 Fields, W. S., Lemak, N. A., Frankowski, R. F., et al.: Controlled Trial of Aspirin in Cerebral Ischemia, *Stroke,* 8:301, 1977.

108 The Canadian Cooperative Study Group: A Randomized Trial of Aspirin and Sulfinpyrazone in Threatened Stroke, *N. Engl. J. Med.,* 299:53, 1978.

109 Acheson, J., Danta, G., and Hutchinson, E. C.: Controlled Trial of Dipyridamole in Cerebral Vascular Disease, *Br. Med. J.,* 1:614, 1969.

110 Genton, E.: Cardiac Embolic Disease, in S. Sherry, K. M. Brinkhous, E. Genton, et al. (eds.), "Thrombosis," National Academy of Sciences, Washington, D.C., 1969, p. 184.

111 Barnhorst, D. A., Oxman, H. A., Connolly, D. C., et al.: Isolated Replacement of the Mitral Valve with the Starr-Edwards Prosthesis, *J. Thorac. Cardiovasc. Surg.,* 71:230, 1976.

112 Duvoisin, G. E., Brandenburg, R. O., and McGoon, D. C.: Factors Affecting Thromboembolism Associated with Prosthetic Heart Valves. *Circulation,* 35 (suppl. 1):70, 1967.

113 Gadboys, H. L., Litwak, R. S., Niemetz, J., et al.: Role of Anticoagulants in Preventing Embolization from Prosthetic Heart Valves, *J.A.M.A.,* 202:134, 1967.

114 Lander, H., Kinlough, R. L., and Robson, H. N.: Reduced Platelet Survival in Patients with Starr-Edwards Prostheses, *Br. Med. J.,* 1:688, 1965.

115 Steele, T. P., Weily, H. S., Davies, H., et al.: Platelet Survival Time Following Aortic Valve Replacement, *Circulation,* 51:358, 1975.

116 Steele, T. P., Weily, H. S., Davies, H., et al.: Platelet Survival in Patients with Rheumatic Heart Disease, *N. Engl. J. Med.,* 290:537, 1974.

117 Sullivan, J. M., Harken, D. E., and Gorlin, R.: Pharmacologic Control of Thromboembolic Complications of Cardiac Valve Replacement. A Preliminary Report. *N. Engl. J. Med.,* 279:576, 1968.

118 Sullivan, J. M., Harken, D. E., and Gorlin, R.: Pharmacologic Control of Thromboembolism Complications of Cardiac Valve Replacement, *N. Engl. J. Med.,* 284:1391, 1971.

119 Arrants, J. E., and Hairston, T.: Use of Persantin in Preventing Thromboembolism Following Valve Replacement, *Am. Surg.,* 38:432, 1972.

120 Arrants, J. E., Hairston, T., and Lee, W. H., Jr.: Use of Dipyridamole (Persantine) in Preventing Thromboembolisms Following Valve Replacement, *Chest*, 58:275, 1970.

121 Meyer, J. S., Charney, J. Z., Rivera, V. M., et al.: Cerebral Embolization: Prospective Clinical Analysis of 42 Cases, *Stroke*, 2:541, 1971.

122 Altman, R., Boullon, F., Rouvier, J., et al.: Aspirin and Prophylaxis of Thromboembolic Complications in Patients with Substitute Heart Valves, *J. Thorac. Cardiovasc. Surg.*, 72:127, 1976.

123 Dale, J.: Prevention of Arterial Thromboembolism with Acetylsalicylic Acids in Patients with Prosthetic Heart Valves, *Thromb. Haemostasis*, 38:66, 1977.

124 Berger, S., and Salzman, E. D.: Thromboembolic Complications of Prosthetic Devices, *Prog. Hemostasis Thromb.*, 2:273, 1974.

125 Zucker, M. B., and Peterson, J.: Inhibition of Adenosine Diphosphate Induced Secondary Aggregation and Other Platelet Functions by Acetylsalicylic Acid Ingestion, *Proc. Soc. Exp. Biol. Med.*, 127:547, 1968.

126 Mustard, J. F., Roswell, H. C., Smythe, H. A., et al.: The Effect of Sulfinpyrazone on Platelet Economy and Thrombus Formation in Rabbits, *Blood*, 29:859, 1967.

127 Didisheim, P., and Owen, C. A.: Effect of Dipyridamole (Persantin) and Its Derivatives on Thrombosis and Platelet Function, *Thromb. Diath. Haemorrh.*, 42 (suppl):267, 1970.

128 Didisheim, P.: Inhibition by Dipyridamole of Arterial Thrombosis in Rats, *Thromb. Diath. Haemorrh.*, 20:257, 1968.

129 Kaegi, A., Pineo, G. F., Shimizu, A., et al.: Arterial Venous Shunt Thrombosis: Prevention by Sulfinpyrazone, *N. Engl. J. Med.*, 290:304, 1974.

130 Kaegi, A., Pineo, G. F., Shimizu, A., et al.: The Role of Sulfinpyrazone in the Prevention of Arterial Venous Shunt Thrombosis, *Circulation*, 52:497, 1975.

131 Heiden, D., Mielke, C. H., Jr., Rodvien, R.: Impairment by Heparin of Primary Hemostasis and Platelet (^{14}C)5-Hydroxytryptamine Release, *Br. J. Haematol.*, 36:427, 1977.

132 O'Brien, J. R., Tulevski, V., and Etherington, M.: Two in Vivo Studies Comparing High and Low Aspirin Dosage, *Lancet*, 1:399, 1971.

133 Effect of Aspirin on Post-operative Venous Thrombosis: Report of the Steering Committee of a Trial Sponsored by the Medical Research Council, *Lancet*, 2:441, 1972.

134 Harris, W. H., Salzman, E. W., Athanasoulis, C. A., et al.: Aspirin Prophylaxis of Venous Thromboembolism after Total Hip Replacement, *N. Engl. J. Med.*, 297:1246, 1977.

135 Zeckert, F.: "Thrombosen, Embolien and Aggregation-shemmer in der Chirugie," F. J. Schattauer, Stuttgart, 1975.

136 Vreeken, J., and van Aken, W. G.: Spontaneous Aggregation of Blood Platelets as a Cause of Idiopathic Thrombosis in Recurrent Painful Toes and Fingers, *Lancet*, 2:1394, 1971.

137 Biermé, R., Boneu, B., Guiraud, B., et al.: Aspirin and Recurrent Painful Toes and Fingers in Thrombocythaemia, *Lancet*, 1:432, 1972.

138 Preston, F. E., Emmanuel, I. G., Winfield, D. A., et al.: Essential Thrombocythaemia and Peripheral Gangrene, *Br. Med. J.*, 3:548, 1974.

139 Fitzgerald, D. E., and Butterfield, W. J. H.: A Case of Increased Platelet Antiheparin Factor in a Patient with Raynaud's Phenomena and Gangrene Treated by Aspirin, *Angiology*, 20:317, 1969.

140 Wilding, R. P., and Flute, R. T.: Dipyridamole in Peripheral Upper Limb Ischemia, *Lancet*, 1:999, 1974.

Arrhythmias Related to Abnormal Repolarization[*]

PAUL F. WALTER, M.D.

The chance of sudden death in someone relatively well has to be carefully weighed against the probable advantage—precisely as when advising an operation. . . . Death has occurred not only after large doses, but almost at once after small or moderate doses, whether normal rhythm has been restored or not.

J. PARKINSON and M. CAMPBELL[1]

INTRODUCTION

The Q-T interval in the scalar electrocardiogram is a clinically useful indirect measure of recovery of ventricular excitability. Prolongation of the Q-T interval has diagnostic value in a number of clinical circumstances. The purpose of this chapter is to review those disorders in which prolongation of ventricular recovery may be associated with serious ventricular tachyarrhythmias (Table 1).

These disorders form a heterogeneous group and may seem totally unrelated. Common to all, however, is prolongation of ventricular recovery time as measured by the Q-T interval, the occurrence of ventricular arrhythmias, and a risk of sudden death. Clinical and experimental observations suggest that delayed repolarization is not just a coincidental finding but is related causally to the ventricular arrhythmias. Another common feature is the marked variability in any individual's susceptibility to ventricular tachyarrhythmias. Our clinical experience and several reports in the literature suggest that a combination of factors known to prolong ventricular recovery is more likely to produce ventricular arrhythmia than a single predisposing circumstance or drug.[1a,2]

Although knowledge of the pathogenesis of these disorders is incomplete, obvious differences do exist. Dysfunction of the cardiac sympathetic nerves, whether related to disease of the central nervous system or to abnormalities of intracardiac neural elements, may be the major factor in some cases. Alteration in cardiac cell membrane function induced by drugs or electrolyte abnormalities may be the decisive factor in other cases.

* From the Department of Medicine, Emory University School of Medicine and the Veterans Administration Hospital, Atlanta.

THE T WAVE

The T wave represents the electrical forces resulting from recovery of activated muscle fibers to their resting state. The morphology of the T wave depends on the sequence of ventricular repolarization. This sequence is determined by the shape and duration of ventricular action potentials. The normal sequence of ventricular repolarization has been studied most extensively in the dog heart. Measurements of local functional refractory periods of monophasic action potentials have produced similar findings.[3,4] In normal ventricles the activation sequence proceeds from endocardium to epicardium and from apex to base. Recovery properties are inversely related to the activation sequence: areas of the ventricles that are activated early have long recovery and areas of the ventricles that are activated late have short recovery properties. Therefore, local refractory periods and monophasic action potentials are longest in the endocardium and apex and shortest in the epicardium and base.[3,4] The normal sequence of repolarization may be disturbed by a change in recovery properties in various areas of the ventricle. The temporal and spatial patterns of this change will alter the magnitude and form of the T wave.[5]

The mechanisms responsible for a long Q-T interval are incompletely understood. Certain drugs or electrolyte disturbances which lengthen action poten-

TABLE 1
Prolonged repolarization arrhythmias

1 "Congenital syndromes"
    Jervell and Lange-Nielsen syndrome
    Romano-Ward syndrome
2 Quinidine syncope
3 Psychotropic drugs
    Phenothiazines
    Tricyclic antidepressants
4 Bradycardia
5 Electrolyte abnormalities
    Hypokalemia
    Hypomagnesemia
6 Central nervous system disorders
7 Coronary atherosclerotic heart disease
8 Mitral valve prolapse syndrome
9 Fasting and liquid protein diets

tial duration may also prolong the Q-T interval. Alteration of recovery properties in selected areas of the ventricle may produce inhomogeneity of recovery and thereby prolong ventricular repolarization. Whatever the mechanism, the result is a prolonged recovery sequence, as indicated by a long Q-T interval, a broad T wave, or a T-U wave.

THE U WAVE

The origin of the U wave in the electrocardiogram remains controversial. The major theories of U wave formation are (1) delayed repolarization of certain portions of the ventricles, (2) negative afterpotentials in the ventricular myocardium, and (3) repolarization in the Purkinje system.[6] Direct evidence for any of these hypotheses has not been presented. The clinical importance of a large U wave that merges with or overshadows the T wave is more settled. Clinical studies confirm that a large U wave is one of the electrocardiographic abnormalities commonly seen in patients in whom delayed repolarization is complicated by serious ventricular arrhythmias.[7]

PHYSIOLOGY OF VENTRICULAR ARRHYTHMIAS

The electrophysiologic explanation for the ventricular tachyarrhythmias which complicate the delayed repolarization syndrome is not known. The most widely accepted hypothesis is that a long Q-T-U interval is correlated with nonuniform recovery, a requisite of reentry.[8] Experimental observations suggest that with lengthening of the Q-T interval comes prolongation of the ventricular vulnerable period and a greater susceptibility to ventricular arrhythmias.[9] It should be noted that the vulnerable period and the duration of refractoriness in different portions of the ventricle

cannot be determined from the surface ECG. However, it is clinically useful to consider the interval between the apex of the T wave and the end of repolarization as an estimate of the duration of the relative refractory period in at least some parts of the ventricle.[10] The basis for ventricular vulnerability appears in part related to inhomogeneous excitability of the ventricle during its relative refractory period.[9] Because of nonuniform rates of repolarization at various segments of ventricular myocardium, an impulse generated during the vulnerable period may find some segments responsive and others refractory. The impulse may be forced to propagate along a tortuous and irregular wave front, creating the setting for reentry.

VENTRICULAR TACHYCARDIA

The ventricular tachycardias associated with prolonged ventricular repolarization have several distinctive features (Fig. 1). The premature contractions which initiate ventricular tachycardia may originate from the atria or AV junction as well as from the ventricles. These premature contractions have a long coupling interval and interrupt the U wave or late portion of the T wave to incite ventricular arrhythmias. The ventricular tachycardia that follows is commonly of the *torsade de pointes* type.[8,11,12]

Torsade de pointes was first described in detail in the French literature.[12] It is now recognized as a distinct ventricular arrhythmia, intermediate in its morphology between classical ventricular tachycardia and ventricular fibrillation.[11,12] The main features of the tachycardia are as follows: (1) the Q-T interval is usually quite prolonged (0.60 s or more) with enlarged and prolonged T or T-U waves; (2) the premature contraction which incites the ventricular tachycardia has a long coupling interval but, because of the delay in repolarization, falls on the T or U wave; (3) the QRS complexes are bizarre in appearance and during the

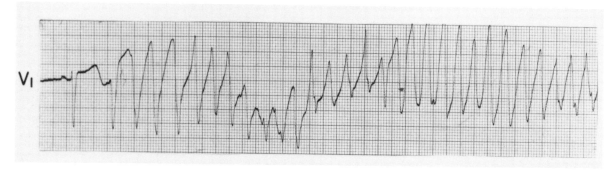

V_1

FIGURE 1 Torsade de pointes ventricular tachycardia. Rhythm strip of a 52-year-old man who abused alcohol and had hypokalemia (3.0 mEq/liter) and hypomagnesemia (1.1 mg/dl). The premature contraction which incites the tachycardia has a long coupling interval, and the QRS axis indulates during the tachycardia. Q-T$_c$ interval normalized, and the tachycardia ceased after correction of the electrolyte abnormalities.

fast phase have a frequency of 200 to 250 beats per minute; (4) the QRS axis undulates over runs of 5 to 20 beats, with definite changes in direction, producing a picture of torsion around an imaginary line—hence the French designation *torsade de pointes;* (5) the tachycardia stops spontaneously but may recur quickly or degenerate into ventricular fibrillation.[11,12] *Torsade de pointes* occurs in the context of chronic atrioventricular block or sinoatrial block or in conditions that produce a long Q-T interval.[11,12] It has been seen with a variety of disorders characterized by delayed ventricular repolarization, including the Jervell and Lange-Nielsen syndrome,[13] the Romano-Ward syndrome,[8] hypokalemia,[14] hypomagnesemia,[11] subarachnoid hemorrhage,[15] or during treatment with quinidine,[8] phenothiazines,[11] or tricyclic antidepressants.[11] *Torsade de pointes* is a rare complication of myocardial

infarction[16] and myocarditis.[17] Electrical stimulation of the right ventricle may induce it on rare occasions.[18] The treatment of *torsade de pointes* varies greatly because of the different inciting causes; however, quinidine and similar agents are contraindicated because they may cause further slowing of intraventricular conduction and prolongation of ventricular repolarization, thereby aggravating the arrhythmias.[11,12]

CONGENITAL SYNDROMES

In 1957 Jervell and Lange-Nielsen described a syndrome characterized by congenital deafness, bizarre prolongation of the Q-T interval, recurring syncope, and sudden and unexpected death[19] (Fig. 2). In the

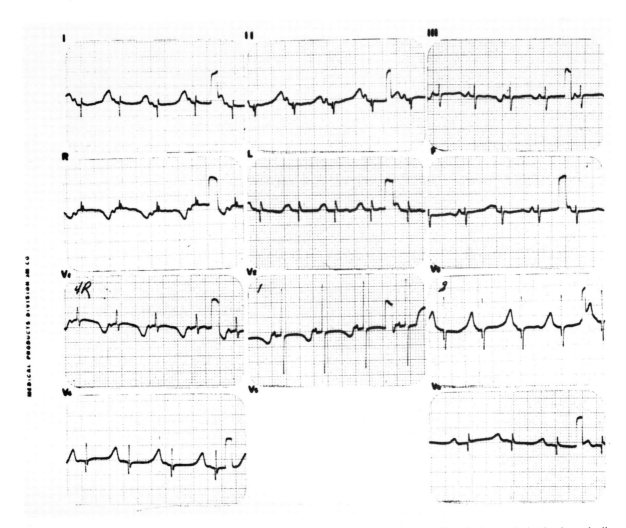

FIGURE 2 The electrocardiogram of a 2-day-old infant with Romano-Ward syndrome. Ventricular repolarization is markedly delayed, the Q-T interval is 0.44 s., and the Q-T$_c$ interval is 0.61 s. The child died at age 3 weeks from refractory ventricular tachyarrhythmias despite treatment with propranolol. At autopsy, the heart and great vessels were within normal limits. The specialized conduction tissue and neural elements were not studied. (Courtesy of Dr. William Plauth, Jr.)

Norwegian family described, 4 of 6 siblings developed syncopal episodes in the first years of life, and 3 of those affected died suddenly at the ages of 4, 5, and 9 years. A syndrome with all the features of the Jervell and Lange-Nielsen syndrome except congenital deafness was reported by Romano and his colleagues in 1963[20] and by Ward in 1964.[21] Both reports documented ventricular arrhythmias coinciding with the syncopal episodes in these children. Since the original description of these syndromes, several hundred clinical reports have appeared in the literature. It is apparent that patients with these syndromes who hear normally (Romano-Ward) outnumber those who are deaf (Jervell and Lange-Nielsen).[22] Since the clinical presentation and the cardiac manifestations are identical, the following discussion applies to both syndromes.

Clinical Manifestations, Long Q-T Syndromes

The major clinical feature of the syndromes is repeated syncope. Loss of consciousness may occur without warning or be preceded by palpitations or an aura. Seizure activity has been noted with severe episodes, and urinary incontinence is frequent even in the absence of seizures. These episodes are frequently mistaken for atypical epilepsy, although the electroencephalogram is normal.[13] A clinical picture consisting of atypical seizures with a normal electroencephalogram and of premature ventricular contractions on the ECG may be the first clues to the presence of a long Q-T syndrome. Minor attacks without loss of consciousness may be mistaken for hysterical behavior.

The syncopal episodes usually begin early in life, commonly in infancy, although the onset has been as late as the second or third decade. The frequency of attacks is variable, from several times a day to one every several years. The close relationship of syncope to physical or emotional stress has been emphasized in many reports.[22–24] Loud noises, febrile illnesses, menstruation, and pregnancy are less common precipitating factors.[23,25] No metabolic or electrolyte abnormalities can be detected at the time of the attacks.

The prevailing view is that there is heritable transmission of the long Q-T syndrome. The syndrome with deafness is thought to be transmitted as an autosomal recessive trait; without deafness, it is transmitted as an autosomal dominant trait with variable penetrance of the gene. Doubt about the validity of this hypothesis has been raised,[26] based in part on the discovery of several families with Q-T prolongation in whom some affected siblings were deaf and others had normal hearing, on the documentation of many cases

with no known afflicted family members, and on the wide variability in clinical and electrocardiographic severity.

The most consistent electrocardiographic abnormality is prolongation of the Q-T interval. While generally greatly prolonged, the Q-T interval may vary spontaneously or in response to fright or excitement. A few patients may have normal or minimally prolonged Q-T intervals at rest which lengthen considerably as the heart rate accelerates with exercise.[27,28] Increased sympathetic tone is probably responsible for this effect, since atrial pacing to the same heart rate in these patients is accompanied by normal shortening of the Q-T interval, and atrial pacing does not enhance sympathetic activity.[24]

The T waves are typically large, broad, and generally bizarre. T wave alternans, or T wave alternation in amplitude and polarity without a concomitant change in the QRS complex is another important feature.[29] This is best detected if multiple ECG leads are recorded. T wave alternans may appear during any activity that causes an abrupt increase in sympathetic nervous system discharge. In some cases it bodes ill, for it may be followed by ventricular arrhythmias.[22,24,27] The ventricular arrhythmias that produce syncope are either a uniform ventricular flutter (250 to 300 beats per minute) or the *torsade de pointes* type of ventricular tachycardia.[30] Many episodes of ventricular arrhythmias stop spontaneously, but some degenerate into ventricular fibrillation and sudden death. Abnormal sinus node function may be present in some patients as evidenced by a slow resting sinus rate and an inappropriately modest increase in heart rate with exercise.[27] Atrioventricular block with a narrow QRS complex has been recorded in a few patients.[24]

Pathogenesis

The pathogenesis of the long Q-T syndromes has not been fully clarified. A disturbance in myocardial metabolism, focal degeneration within the sinus node, and dysfunction of the autonomic nervous system are the major hypotheses put forward.[22] The first two hypotheses have little supportive data. However, there is strong evidence that an abnormality in adrenergic neural control is a fundamental problem in patients with long Q-T syndromes. The following discussion summarizes the experimental and clinical evidence that favors this hypothesis.

EXPERIMENTAL

In experimental animals, removal of the right stellate ganglion or stimulation of the left stellate ganglion lengthens the Q-T interval and increases the amplitude of the T wave.[31] Electrical stimulation of the left stellate ganglion may also produce T wave alternans.[29] Although the innervation of the left and right stellate ganglia overlap, the left predominates over the posterior wall of the left ventricle, while the right prevails over the anterior portion. Stimulation of either stellate ganglion shortens the duration of myocardial action potentials and shortens the recovery time in the area of the myocadium innervated by the ganglion. It is not surprising that surgical ablation of the right stellate ganglion should lengthen the Q-T interval, since removal of sympathetic activity would be expected to prolong recovery time. It is less obvious how left stellate stimulation, known to shorten the refractory period of the posterior aspect of the dog ventricle, can prolong the Q-T interval. Shorter duration of repolarization on the posterior wall may possibly unmask previously cancelled electrical forces from the anterior wall, resulting in a net prolongation of the Q-T interval.[31] The observation worthy of emphasis is that either an increase or decrease in sympathetic tone in a discrete area of the ventricle may result in Q-T interval prolongation.[31] In dogs, ablation of the left stellate ganglion increases the threshold for ventricular fibrillation, while ablation of the right stellate decreases the fibrillation threshold.[32]

CLINICAL

There is substantial experimental and clinical data in support of the view that nonhomogeneous cardiac sympathetic activity is involved in the pathogenesis of the long Q-T syndromes.[29,31–33] This imbalance could originate in the brain, in the sympathetic chain, in the adrenergic terminals in the myocardium, or in any combination of these sites. Although there is individual variability, dominance of left sympathetic activity seems to occur most frequently. Left dominance could result from increasd activity of the left sympathetic nerves or decreased activity of the right sympathetic nerves.

Schwartz et al., in 1975, stated that a local myocardial abnormality might also be involved in the pathogenesis, and if such were the case, the sympathetic activity might only serve as a triggering mechanism.[22] This was somewhat prophetic in light of the recent and important study by James et al., who studied the hearts from 8 patients who suffered a long Q-T syndrome, syncopal attacks, and sudden death.[26] Focal neuritis and neural degeneration were present in all 8 hearts. The neuropathology was found most often in and near the sinus node and atrioventricular node and adjacent to the arterial branches within the ventricles and in the epicardium. These degenerative neural lesions were invariably associated with inflammation.

The cause for the neuritis could not be determined. Chronic infection, noninfectious toxins, or some degenerative process are possibilities.

The asymmetrical focal distribution of the neural lesions might explain some of the cardiac abnormalities. Sinus bradycardia may be related to the disease of the nerves in and around the sinus node. Focal destruction of nerves found in the ventricular myocardium could contribute to the abnormal ventricular repolarization.

Ventricular Arrhythmias

Catecholamines shorten the action potential duration of ventricular muscle fibers. With uneven distribution or activity of ventricular sympathetic nerve endings, stronger stimulation may result in a nonuniform decrease in refractory periods. According to Han et al., a nonuniform decrease in refractoriness predisposes to reentry.[34] This view is widely accepted as the explanation for the ventricular arrhythmias in the Q-T syndrome; however, it is uncertain whether the small differences in refractoriness in separate regions of the ventricle are sufficient to permit reentry.[35]

Only a few patients with Q-T syndrome have been studied with programed electrical stimulation of the heart. In 7 patients suffering from repeated episodes of ventricular tachycardia and ventricular fibrillation, Wellens was unable to initiate the ventricular arrhythmias with stimulation of the heart.[36] The inability to precipitate ventricular tachycardia by this technique might be a point against a reentrant mechanism. A more likely explanation for the failure to produce tachycardia is that augmented sympathetic activity, an essential requirement, was not present at the time of study.

Prognosis

Symptomatic patients with a prolonged Q-T syndrome have a poor prognosis. Without treatment the mortality is distressingly high, especially in childhood and adolescence.[22] Syncopal episodes may continue for years, but in those patients who survive long enough the frequency of attacks tends to diminish. However, adulthood confers no absolute protection from sudden death, and fatalities have occurred in patients in the fifth decade of life.[24]

Treatment

All symptomatic patients suffering from the Jervell and Lange-Nielsen or Romano-Ward syndrome should be treated. Asymptomatic patients with a long Q-T interval but no ventricular arrhythmias or syncope do not require treatment, but should be observed closely. In asymptomatic patients, it may be useful to perform an exercise test as part of the follow-up examinations, since exercise-induced Q-T interval lengthening, T-U wave alternans, or ventricular arrhythmias provide indication for treatment. The electrocardiographic response to exercise in asymptomatic patients has not been studied, but prudence would dictate such a recommendation until more information is available.

Symptomatic patients should be instructed to avoid strenuous physical and mental stresses, since these may provoke attacks. Any stressful diagnostic or surgical procedure should be carried out under continuous electrocardiographic monitoring.

Because of the extraordinarily high incidence of sudden death in these syndromes, the effectiveness of therapy in suppressing ventricular arrhythmias must be known.[37] This can be accomplished with exercise testing, with ambulatory electrocardiographic monitoring, and in select cases, with electrocardiographic monitoring during psychological stress testing.

The treatment of these syndromes remains empirical. Many medications have been tried along with cardiac pacing and stellate ganglionectomy. Treatment failures have occurred with all forms of therapy. The determination of a therapeutic success is hampered by the inexplicable waxing and waning of the clinical manifestations.

The most favorable therapeutic results have been obtained by antagonizing the effects of sympathetic activity on the heart with beta-adrenergic blocking drugs or by surgical removal of the left stellate and first thoracic ganglion. James et al. have expressed some reservations about this approach.[26] They emphasize that the problem is an imbalance in cardiac sympathetic neural activity and not one of a generalized sympathetic overactivity. The erratic distribution of the neural disease could make the pharmacologic actions of beta-adrenergic blocking agents unpredictable.

Despite these reservations, the superiority of beta-adrenergic blocking agents over any other medication has been amply demonstrated.[22] In most patients, propranolol is effective in abolishing syncopal attacks or reducing their frequency, although the Q-T interval on the ECG remains unchanged.[24,27] Some supposed propranolol failures have been caused by an inadequate dose.[30] Propranolol is surprisingly well tolerated by most patients despite the presence of sinus bradycardia.[22]

Both diphenylhydantoin and phenobarbital have been given for an erroneous diagnosis of epilepsy. Diphenylhydantoin may shorten the Q-T interval and has been effective in some patients.[38] Digitalis may shorten the Q-T interval but has had little effect in

suppressing attacks.[39] Quinidine, procainamide, and disopyramide prolong ventricular repolarization and are contraindicated in these syndromes. Epinephrine and phenylephrine have induced ventricular fibrillation in these patients.

Implantation of an artificial pacemaker may be required if propranolol causes symptomatic bradycardia or if there is associated atrioventricular block.[24] A demand ventricular pacemaker should deliver a stimulus only after an asystolic interval of 850 ms is exceeded, so that the pacing stimulus will not interrupt the repolarization phase of the preceding ventricular beat. If atrioventricular conduction is normal, atrial pacing is preferred because it is known, at least acutely, to shorten the Q-T interval.

Moss and McDonald in 1971 reported the first dramatic success with left stellate ganglionectomy for the treatment of the long Q-T syndrome.[33] The surgery resulted in a shortening of the Q-T interval and in the disappearance of syncopal attacks. Subsequently, stellate ganglion blockade and/or surgical removal has been attempted by others with no uniform result. The change in the Q-T interval following pharmacologic blockade of the stellate ganglia is unpredictable.[22] This may be related to the erratic distribution of the cardiac neural disease (see above) or to the unreliability of the procedure itself. The appearance of Horner's syndrome does not prove effective blockade of sympathetic fibers to the heart.[22] The needle could induce a mechanical stimulation of the stellate ganglion and increase sympathetic discharge to the heart. Stellate ganglion blockade, performed under local anesthesia, does not predict accurately the results of stellectomy.

Surgical ablation of a stellate ganglion along with the first thoracic ganglion should not be considered unless medical treatment fails. Medical failure is not declared until the patient has received high doses of propranolol and a trial of diphenylhydantoin, alone or in combination. Ordinarily the left stellate ganglion is removed. Removal of the right stellate alone is not done unless the Q-T interval shortens with blockade of the right and does not change or lengthens with blockade of the left. Only a small number of patients have had surgical removal of a stellate ganglion. In the largest series, Schwartz reported that left stellectomy suppressed syncopal attacks refractory to medical therapy in all 11 patients in the series.[40]

ACQUIRED Q-T SYNDROMES

There are several important differences between this group of acquired forms of Q-T prolongation and the Jervell and Lange-Nielsen or Romano-Ward syndrome. Victims of the acquired forms are usually adults. Syncope occurs independent of emotional or physical stress. The Q-T prolongation is usually a transient phenomenon and may be abolished by withdrawal of a drug, correction of an electrolyte abnormality, insertion of a pacemaker, or healing of a stroke.

Acquired Q-T Syndrome: Drug Related

QUINIDINE

"Quinidine syncope" is characterized by a loss of consciousness as a result of ventricular arrhythmias in patients receiving therapeutic but nontoxic doses of quinidine (Figs. 3 and 4). The relationship of syncope and sudden death to the administration of quinidine was recognized before the mechanism of syncope was known to be ventricular arrhythmia. Quinidine-induced syncope is characterized by recurrent short paroxysms of ventricular tachycardia or, less frequently, ventricular fibrillation. The syncopal attacks usually occur without premonitory symptoms and persist for a few seconds to several minutes.[41] Most episodes of ventricular tachycardia terminate spontaneously, but ventricular fibrillation may supervene. In a recent study of hospitalized patients, this complication of quinidine therapy was found in 0.6 percent of patients receiving the drug.[42]

A review of the reported cases of quinidine syncope reveals two interesting findings. Ninety percent of patients received quinidine to terminate or prevent recurrence of atrial fibrillation or atrial flutter.[8] Most patients were also taking digitalis. Is this combination

of atrial fibrillation/flutter and digitalis of importance in the genesis of quinidine-induced ventricular tachycardia or is the association simply fortuitous? There is no definitive answer to this question, but clearly, quinidine-induced ventricular tachycardia can also occur when the drug is given to suppress ventricular arrhythmias in patients not taking digitalis.[43]

There are several reasons to be concerned about the combined use of digitalis and quinidine. Although digitalis shortens the Q-T interval, the combination of digitalis and quinidine produces an electrocardiogram with a depressed ST segment, low T wave, and a prominent U wave.[44] While it is not known if these electrocardiographic changes reflect increased susceptibility to ventricular arrhythmias, ventricular tachycardia is induced more readily in the hearts of dogs receiving both drugs.[45] Also, the plasma digoxin concentration increases when quinidine is given.[46] The clinical importance of these observations will only be resolved by further investigations.

Quinidine syncope should not be confused with quinidine toxicity. Quinidine toxicity is characterized by cinchonism, systemic hypotension, and electrocardiographic evidence of impaired atrioventricular and intraventricular conduction. Quinidine plasma levels are in the toxic range in patients with quinidine toxicity, whereas quinidine syncope occurs with small or usual doses and the plasma concentration may be above, within, or below the therapeutic range. There is a remarkable absence of the manifestations of toxicity in patients with quinidine-induced ventricular arrhythmias.[41–43,78] The QRS duration is usually normal in patients with quinidine syncope. Delay in repolarization which may accompany quinidine can be ex-

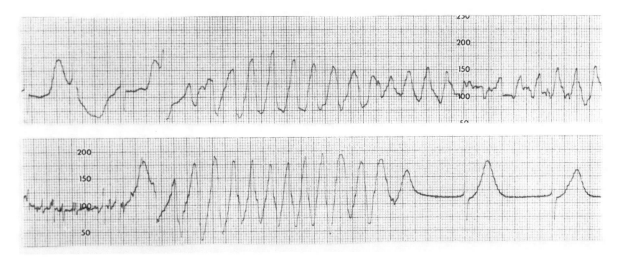

FIGURE 3 Quinidine-induced syncope in an elderly woman taking quinidine sulfate, 800 mg/day, and digoxin, 0.25 mg/day. Top: *torsade de pointes* ventricular tachycardia. Bottom: spontaneous termination of tachycardia. The Q-T interval prior to tachycardia was 0.72 s, and in the beat immediately following, it was 0.60 s. (Courtesy of Dr. Felix Rogers.)

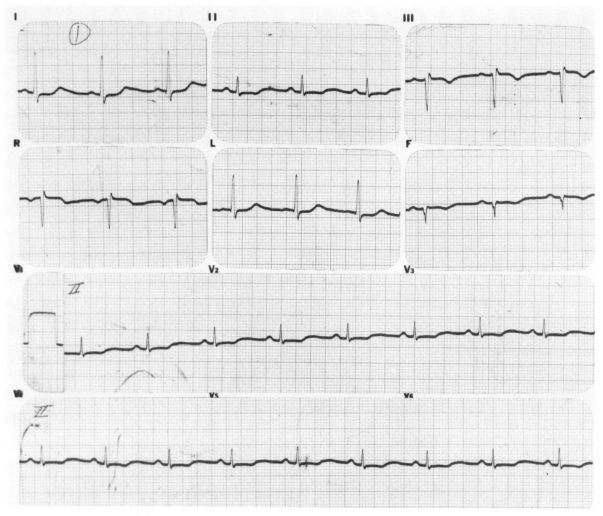

FIGURE 4 The electrocardiogram was recorded 15 min before the appearance of ventricular fibrillation. A 31-year-old man was taking quinidine sulfate, 800 mg/day, plus digoxin, 0.25 mg/day, for the prevention of atrial fibrillation. Quinidine had been tolerated previously, but ventricular arrhythmias appeared when hypokalemia (3.1 mEq/liter) developed. The Q-T$_c$ interval was 0.55 s. Prolonged repolarization most apparent in lead II.

plained by changes in the ventricular action potentials.[48] Q-T-U interval prolongation can be attributed to an increase in the action potential duration. The wide, low-amplitude T wave relates to the prolongation and decreased slope of phase 3. Lengthening of the action potential duration is more marked at lower serum potassium levels and at slower heart rates.[7,48] A marked increase in the Q-T-U interval is the usual electrocardiographic abnormality recorded when ventricular arrhythmias complicate quinidine therapy. T-U wave alternans suggests a severe repolarization abnormality and should serve as a warning of impending ventricular tachyarrhythmias.[7] Many of the published electrocardiograms show the *torsade de pointes* variety of ventricular tachycardia.[7,8,41,43,47]

Treatment of quinidine syncope The goal of therapy is to support the patient until the quinidine effects on ventricular repolarization have dissipated. Therapy should be planned with the expectation that repeated episodes of ventricular tachycardia or ventricular fibrillation are likely to occur over the ensuing 12 to 18 h. Multiple electrical countershocks have been required in some instances.[8] Numerous drugs have been tried, but no clear preference has emerged. Drugs with pharmacologic effects similar to quinidine-procainamide and disopyramide should not be given. Worsening of the ventricular arrhythmias following the administration of procainamide is documented.[43] Sodium bicarbonate and sodium lactate are useful in the treatment of quinidine toxicity but probably have little beneficial effect when the ventricular arrhythmias are associated with a narrow QRS complex, which is the usual finding. Success has been reported with the use of lidocaine and diphenylhydantoin in some patients.[8,43] An intravenous infusion of isoproterenol beginning at 0.5 to 1.0 μg/min may warrant a trial. The fact that beta-adrenergic amines shorten the action potential duration of ventricular muscle provides a theoretical justification for their use in ventricular arrhythmias associated with delayed repolarization and prolonged Q-T.[48] Successful therapy with intravenous administration of bretylium tosylate has been reported.[43,49] Bretylium is an adrenergic nerve blocking drug.[50] In the laboratory, it will reverse the quinidine-induced increase in ventricular action potential duration.[51] Potassium administration may be effective therapy if quinidine syncope is associated with hypokalemia. We have encountered 1 patient, and a similar patient has been reported in whom potassium therapy was successful.[52] There is a rational basis for this treatment, since the effect of quinidine on the action potential duration is known to be increased at lower serum potassium concentrations.[48] It should be emphasized that potassium is contraindicated when the QRS complex is wide (quinidine toxicity) because it may further slow intraventricular conduction.

Many of the episodes of ventricular arrhythmia appear within the first week of quinidine therapy; therefore, patients should be observed carefully during this period. No reliable method of predicting patients at risk for quinidine-induced arrhythmia is known.

A patient who has had quinidine syncope should not receive the drug again because ventricular arrhythmias tend to recur with subsequent doses.[41] If the Q-T interval is prolonged before therapy and there are premature ventricular contractions, the administration of quinidine may be associated with an increased risk owing to the production of the R-on-T phenomenon.[53] Patients who develop marked Q-T interval prolongation during quinidine therapy may have a high risk for the development of ventricular arrhythmias.[42,43] The duration of marked Q-T interval lengthening prior to the onset of ventricular arrhythmias and the sensitivity of this warning sign have not been studied. However, if marked repolarization delay is detected, it is certainly advisable to stop the drug.

Although the electrophysiologic effects of procainamide and quinidine are similar, there are many fewer reports of ventricular arrhythmias following procainamide therapy.[54] The reasons for this discrepancy are not known. A lesser degree of Q-T interval prolongation at comparable therapeutic serum levels may be an important factor.[48] Disopyramide, a quinidine-like drug, has recently been approved for general clinical use. A single oral dose of disopyramide may produce minimal Q-T interval lengthening.[55] Ventricular fibril-

lation, associated with a prolonged Q-T interval during disopyramide therapy, has been reported.[56,57] The frequency of this complication of disopyramide treatment will only become apparent with its more widespread use.

PSYCHOTROPIC DRUGS

The phenothiazines and the tricyclic antidepressants are clearly associated with electrocardiographic changes, cardiac arrhythmias, and even sudden death. It is disturbing that serious ventricular arrhythmias can occur in young adults with antecedent heart disease who are receiving therapeutic doses of these psychotropic drugs.[58] This discussion focuses on one cardiac complication of psychotropic drug therapy, that of delayed ventricular repolarization with ventricular arrhythmias. Other cardiovascular complications do occur with these drugs, such as systemic arterial hypotension, atrioventricular and intraventricular conduction defects, atrial tachyarrhythmias, and bradycardia.

Phenothiazines The effects of phenothiazines (Figs. 5 and 6) on ventricular repolarization are similar to those of quinidine. Also, thioridazine (Mellaril) has, in the dog, been shown to reverse atrial flutter and ventricular tachycardia as effectively as quinidine.[59] Phenothiazines prolong the duration of phase 3 in Purkinje fibers and ventricular muscle and may shorten the duration of phase 2.[60,61] These effects explain the repolarization abnormalities in the electrocardiogram induced by phenothiazines in usual therapeutic doses. The earliest electrocardiographic changes are lengthening of the Q-T interval, widening and blunting of the T wave, and increased U wave amplitude.[58,62] These changes are present in the electrocardiograms of approximately 50 percent of patients receiving 100 to 300 mg of thioridazine daily and are predictable at daily doses exceeding 800 mg.[44,62,63] A delay in ventricular repolarization is less likely to occur with the administration of therapeutic doses of chlorpromazine (Thorazine) and is infrequent with trifluoperazine (Stelazine). Toxic doses of phenothiazines produce the additional change of QRS widening, since higher concentrations of the drugs slow the upstroke velocity of the action potential.[60]

There is a definite although apparently low risk of ventricular arrhythmias or sudden death with phenothiazine therapy in usual doses. The earlier reports dealt primarily with the risk of ventricular arrhythmias or sudden death in patients who received a toxic drug overdose or who had underlying heart disease. More recent studies demonstrate a greater problem. Ventricular arrhythmias can occur in patients without pre-

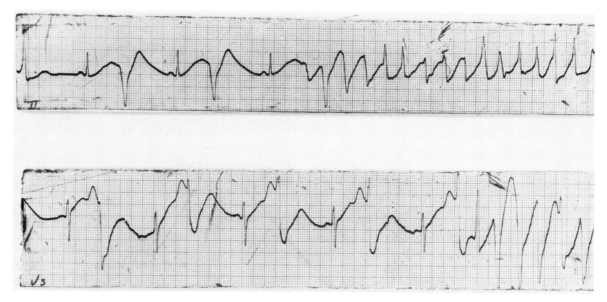

FIGURE 5 Recurrent ventricular tachyarrhythmias resulting from thioridazine administration, 300 mg/day, and hypomagnesemia (0.9 mg/dl). There is marked prolongation of ventricular repolarization. This patient, a 34-year-old man, had no history of heart disease.

vious heart disease who are receiving usual therapeutic doses of phenothiazines.[58,64] As could be predicted by the frequency of electrocardiographic changes, the arrhythmogenic potential of thioridazine far exceeds that of any other phenothiazine derivative. The maximum dose of thioridazine recommended by the manufacturer and some authorities in psychopharmacology is 800 mg/day.[65] A number of patients with

thioridazine-related ventricular tachycardia have received an excessive daily dose (800 to 3600 mg).[58,66] Over 50 percent of these patients have, in addition to ventricular tachyarrhythmias, either bundle branch block or complete atrioventricular block.[66]

Review of the small number of patients with ventricular tachyarrhythmias induced by therapeutic doses of thioridazine reveals that some patients had severe

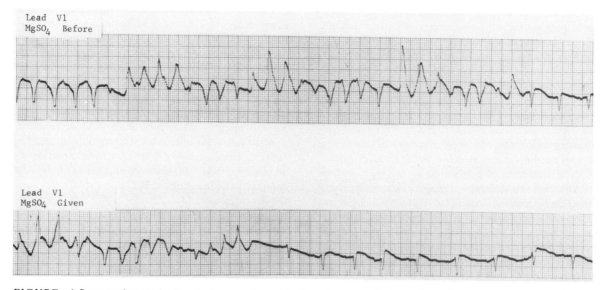

FIGURE 6 Same patient as in Fig. 5. Recurrent *torsade de pointes* ventricular tachycardia was refractory to lidocaine, diphenylhydantoin, propranolol, potassium infusion, and overdrive pacing. It was abolished by the administration of magnesium sulfate.

hypokalemia which may have potentiated the occurrence of ventricular arrhythmias, leading to the suggestion that the use of thioridazine may be dangerous when hypokalemia exists.[67] Thioridazine, 300 mg/day, plus hypomagnesemia produced refractory ventricular tachyarrhythmias in a patient seen at our institution. The arrhythmias stopped when magnesium sulfate was given. Magnesium is a cofactor in the sodium- and potassium-dependent adenosine triphosphatase enzyme system. Phenothiazines exert an inhibitory effect on this enzyme system in muscle membranes.[60,63] These factors provide a theoretical basis for magnesium replacement in this clinical situation. The combination of thioridazine and tricyclic antidepressant has produced troublesome ventricular arrhythmias.[1] It appears that tricyclic antidepressants, hypokalemia, or hypomagnesemia may, in combination with phenothiazine, produce an additive effect on prolongation of ventricular repolarization. There are additional reasons why the concurrent use of a tricyclic antidepressant with a phenothiazine may increase the risk of ventricular arrhythmias. Studies in human beings suggest that each drug inhibits the metabolism of the other, resulting in higher serum concentrations.[2,68]

Postmortem examination of the hearts of victims of phenothiazine-related sudden cardiac death has not provided an explanation for these events. There may be no demonstrable morphologic changes.[69] Intramyocardial arteriolar lesions with some surrounding myofibrillar degeneration has been noted in some fatal cases.[70,71] Detailed studies of the cardiac conduction system and neural elements have not been reported.

Treatment There is no specific treatment for the cardiovascular toxicity of the phenothiazines. Therapy must be directed toward control of the cardiovascular complications until the tissue levels of the drug reach a nontoxic range. Suppression of ventricular tachyarrhythmias consequent to phenothiazine therapy is often difficult. The ventricular arrhythmias may persist for as long as 48 h.[1,67] Repeated dc electrocardioversion may be required. Quinidine, procainamide, and disopyramide are contraindicated because their electrophysiologic actions are similar to those of the phenothiazines, as discussed above. The quinidine actions of slowing intraventricular conduction and prolonging ventricular repolarization aggravate the preexisting electrophysiologic abnormalities. Lidocaine can be given safely to these patients because, at therapeutic concentrations, it has little effect on intraventricular conduction and does not prolong ventricular repolarization.[50] Unfortunately, the success of lidocaine therapy has been, at best, modest.[1,58,67,70] Potassium should be given if hypokalemia is present.[1,67] If the ventricular arrhythmias are associated with some electrocardiographic evidence of conduction impairment

(atrioventricular block or a wide QRS complex), it is prudent to withhold potassium replacement until a temporary transvenous pacemaker has been inserted, as potassium may increase AV block. Propranolol may be tried in refractory cases but should be used in conjunction with a temporary pacemaker in case resulting bradycardia is severe. Temporary overdrive pacing may suppress the ventricular arrhythmias and warrants a trial when drug therapy fails.[58,64]

The use of caution may prevent many future complications from these drugs. Phenothiazines should not be given at doses exceeding the manufacturer's recommendation. Concomitant therapy with phenothiazines, tricyclic antidepressants, and quinidine should be avoided. The serum potassium and magnesium levels should be maintained in the normal range and should be monitored along with the ECG. As thioridazine is the most dangerous of the phenothiazines, it should probably be avoided in patients with heart disease, in favor of one of the phenothiazines less often associated with cardiac arrhythmias.

Tricyclic antidepressants Major cardiac arrhythmias associated with tricyclic antidepressant therapy occur almost exclusively in patients taking an excessive dose of these drugs (Fig. 7). The problem of tricyclic overdosage is not confined to adults, since these drugs are used in the treatment of enuresis in children. The majority of overdosages in children are accidental and occur in children under 4 years of age.[72]

The electrocardiographic effects of tricyclic antidepressants are similar to those produced by quinidine and the phenothiazines.[44,73] Tricyclic antidepressants prolong the Q-T interval, widen the QRS complex, and broaden and decrease the amplitude of the T wave. Reversible and generally minor electrocardiographic changes are found in approximately 20 percent of patients receiving therapeutic doses.[62] The electrocardiographic abnormalities are more pronounced when toxic doses are ingested. The QRS complex may exceed 0.15 s in duration.[74] A marked delay in ventricular repolarization with large bizarre T-U waves is common. However, isolated reports confirm that ventricular tachycardia may follow from usual therapeutic doses,[75] which is not surprising in view of the similarity of these drugs to quinidine and the phenothiazines.

The cardiac arrhythmias accompanying tricyclic antidepressant toxicity include sinus tachycardia, ventricular premature contractions, supraventricular tachycardia, ventricular tachycardia, and heart block.

Thorstrand studied 153 patients with tricyclic antidepressant poisoning.[74] Amitriptyline (Elavil) was the drug most often involved, and the average dose ingested was approximately 1,000 mg. The heart rate exceeded 90 beats per minute in 73 percent of the pa-

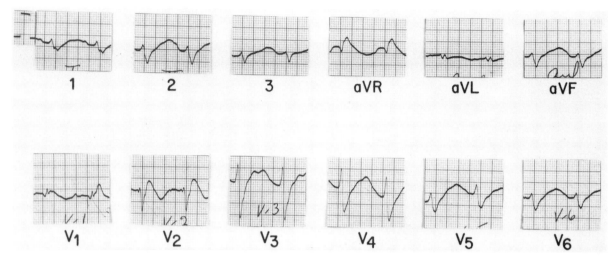

FIGURE 7 Amitriptyline overdose in a 19-year-old female. There was associated hypokalemia (2.4 mEq/liter) as a result of diuretic therapy. The QRS complex is wide (0.20 s), and the Q-T$_c$ interval is increased (0.61 s). (Courtesy of Dr. Laurence Lesser.)

tients. The mean of the QRS duration was 0.11 s, exceeding this in 42 percent of the cases. Q-T interval prolongation was found in half the patients, and the T waves were often broad or flat.

The pharmacologic effects of tricyclic antidepressants on the cardiovascular system are complex because these drugs possess anticholinergic and antiadrenergic as well as quinidine-like actions.[76] In experimental animals and possibly in human beings, imipramine (Tofranil) has antiarrhythmic properties similar to those of quinidine.[73,77,78] Tricyclic antidepressants increase the duration of the action potential and prolong phase 3 repolarization in rabbit atria.[44] At higher concentrations, the maximal rate of rise of phase 0 of the action potential is decreased. This finding correlates with the slowing of intraventricular conduction that occurs with an overdose of the agents. The H-V interval is consistently prolonged, sometimes markedly so, in patients overdosed with a tricyclic antidepressant,[79] whereas at therapeutic levels the H-V interval is normal or only minimally increased.[78,79]

Treatment The treatment for tricyclic antidepressant toxicity is difficult because of the complex pharmacologic actions of these drugs on multiple organ systems. Patients suffering from severe toxicity may present with coma, seizures, hypotension, cardiac arrhythmias, and metabolic and/or respiratory acidosis. Hypotension, hypothermia, severe acidosis, and a markedly prolonged QRS and Q-T interval are signs of severe toxicity and may portend a fatal outcome.[80,81] The mortality in a large series of patients with tricyclic antidepressant poisoning was 3 percent.[80]

Sodium bicarbonate is one of the most useful agents in the treatment of tricyclic poisoning. It is effective in the treatment of the accompanying metabolic acidosis and of the cardiac arrhythmias.[72] The administration of sodium bicarbonate reinstated normal sinus rhythm in 9 of 12 children.[72] Its beneficial effects derive from the sodium ion because alkalinization with tromefamol is ineffective.[82] The increased availability of sodium ions might increase the upstroke velocity of phase 0 of the action potential and thereby improve intraventricular conduction. A specific effect of sodium bicarbonate on ventricular repolarization other than to correct metabolic acidosis is unknown. The anticholinesterase agents physostigmine and neostigmine effectively combat the central nervous system toxicity of tricyclic antidepressants.[76,83] They also slow the marked sinus tachycardia that occasionally accompanies an overdose.[83,84] Anticholinesterase drugs have not been shown to improve intraventricular conduction or to shorten ventricular repolarization, which is understandable in view of the minimal cholinergic innervation of the ventricles.[85] Convulsions and cholinergic poisoning are the major side effects of anticholinesterase therapy.[86]

Heart block persisting after the administration of appropriate amounts of sodium bicarbonate is best treated with a transvenous pacemaker. Overdrive pacing warrants a trial in patients with refractory ventricular arrhythmias. Propranolol has abolished recurrent ventricular tachycardia in a few patients but may cause hypotension or bradycardia.[87]

Guidelines offered for the prevention of phenothiazine toxicity apply equally to the tricyclic antidepressants. Tricyclic antidepressants should not be used in patients receiving quinidine-like antiarrhythmic drugs or phenothiazines, as this combination increases the likelihood of cardiotoxicity. Preliminary evidence suggests that doxepin (Sinequan) may be the safest antidepressant drug for patients with cardiac disease or isolated bundle branch block.[76,79]

Bradycardia

Motte et al. found that chronic bradyarrhythmias were the most common cause of *torsade de pointes* ventricular tachycardia.[12] The most frequent cause of chronic bradyarrhythmia is chronic atrioventricular block.[17,88] Occasionally, *torsade de pointes* is a complication of advanced sinoatrial block or of second-degree atrioventricular block.[89]

Loss of consciousness in patients with complete atrioventricular block is the result either of standstill of the ventricular pacemaker or of paroxysms of ventricular tachycardia. When heart block is complicated by episodes of ventricular tachycardia, the electrocardiogram recorded between episodes may show abnormal ventricular repolarization. The Q-T interval may be as long as 0.80 s, and there may be marked inversion of a broad T wave in the right and midprecordial leads.[12]

The ventricular arrhythmias associated with heart block can usually be controlled by cardiac pacing. Increasing the heart rate with a cardiac pacemaker shortens ventricular repolarization and changes intraventricular conduction.[11] These effects probably play an important role in the suppression of ventricular arrhythmias. The optimal pacemaker rate for suppression of ventricular arrhythmias is not necessarily 70 to 72 beats per minute. The most effective pacing rate should be established by use of a temporary pacing catheter and an external pulse generator prior to the insertion of a permanent pacemaker, unless a permanent pacemaker with a variable pacing rate is used. Quinidine and other type I antiarrhythmic drugs are contraindicated in AV block because they aggravate both the conduction disturbance and the repolarization abnormality.

Electrolyte Abnormalities

The importance of any single electrolyte deficiency in the genesis of a cardiac arrhythmia is difficult to establish because electrolyte abnormalities rarely occur in isolation (see Figs. 1, 4, 5, 6, and 8). Cardiac elec-

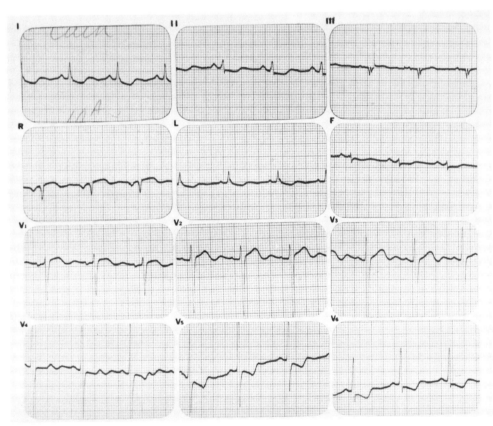

FIGURE 8 Prolonged ventricular repolarization in a 61-year-old man with severe arterial hypertension and a hypokalemic (3.0 mEq/liter) chloremic metabolic alkalosis. Prominent U waves are most apparent in lead V$_4$. Ventricular bigeminy and brief bursts of ventricular tachycardia were controlled by correction of the electrolyte abnormalities.

trical activity may be altered by the additional factors of organic heart disease, other electrolyte deficiencies, or the presence of cardioactive drugs. A recent case report illustrates the complexities of the problem.[90] This report describes a 45-year-old woman with primary prolongation of the Q-T interval of at least 5 years' duration. She had no cardiac symptoms until hypokalemia and a combination of amitriptyline and perphenazine (Triavil) therapy resulted in life-threatening ventricular arrhythmias. Despite reservations about cause and effect, it is clear that hypokalemia, hypomagnesemia, and possibly hypocalcemia play an important role in the production of some cardiac arrhythmias. The importance of an electrolyte deficiency is most apparent when it occurs in combination with other arrhythmogenic factors.

Hypokalemia is known to cause cardiac arrhythmias and to impair atrioventricular conduction, especially in patients receiving digitalis or suffering from heart disease. Atrial and ventricular ectopic contractions become frequent as the serum potassium level falls below 3.2 mEq/liter.[91] Hypokalemia as the sole cause of ventricular fibrillation or ventricular tachycardia must be rare. Some reports purporting to show this relationship are not convincing because the patients were seriously ill or were receiving quinidine.[92] However, 2 cases of life-threatening ventricular arrhythmia resulting from chronic hypokalemia caused by primary hyperaldosteronism and familial periodic paralysis have been described.[14] Neither patient received cardiac drugs prior to the onset of the arrhythmia. There was no clinical evidence of underlying organic heart disease, although the possibility of hypokalemia-related myocardial degenerative lesions could not be excluded.[91]

Hypomagnesemia has been implicated as a cause of delayed ventricular repolarization and ventricular tachyarrhythmias (see p. 315).[2] Hypomagnesemia is less common than hypokalemia and is less often sought. The clinical circumstances associated with magnesium deficiency include chronic alcoholism, diabetic acidosis, diuretic therapy, cirrhosis of the liver, and malabsorption syndromes. Patients with hypomagnesemia who develop ventricular tachycardia may abuse alcohol, take digitalis, and be potassium depleted.[93,94]

The effects of isolated hypomagnesemia on ventricular repolarization and the electrocardiogram are unsettled. A prevalent view is that repolarization is not prolonged unless there is associated hypokalemia.[91,95] In chronic experimental magnesium deficiency the electrocardiographic changes resemble those of hypokalemia.[93] The mechanism by which chronic hypomagnesemia alters ventricular repolarization is not known. A reduction in the activity of the magnesium-dependent sodium potassium ATPase enzyme

might result in the inability of cells to maintain the high intracellular potassium concentration.[93,96] Also, insufficient activation of this magnesium-dependent enzyme may impair the correction of intracellular potassium deficits.[96]

Although both hypokalemia and hypocalcemia prolong the Q-T interval, cardiac arrhythmias are commonly observed with hypokalemia but are rarely seen with isolated hypocalcemia. The dissimilar effects of hypokalemia and hypocalcemia on ventricular repolarization may partially explain this difference. Hypokalemia shortens the absolute refractory period but prolongs the relative refractory period.[91] Hypocalcemia prolongs the absolute refractory period but does not change the relative refractory period. A longer relative refractory period is generally associated with an increased propensity to reentrant arrhythmias.[9,10] These differences are also reflected in the electrocardiogram. With a decrease in extracellular potassium, there is progressive depression of the ST segment, a decrease in the amplitude of the T wave, and an increase in the amplitude of the U wave.[91,95] With hypocalcemia the onset of the T wave is delayed, the duration of the T wave is not altered or is only modestly increased, and the U wave is not recognizable.[91,95]

Only a few authors have reported ventricular tachyarrhythmias as a clinical manifestation of hypocalcemia.[97,98] In these patients the serum calcium was very low (3.0 and 4.2 mg/dl), and 1 patient had severe hypokalemia.[98] Recurrent ventricular fibrillation was abolished in both patients by an infusion of calcium. The ablation of ventricular arrhythmias by a pharmacologic dose of calcium or any other electrolyte does not confirm a causal relationship.

Repolarization alternans refers to alternation in amplitude or in polarity of the T wave, U wave, or T-U wave, unaccompanied by changes in the QRS complex. This phenomenon has been observed in association with a variety of disorders in which marked prolongation of ventricular repolarization is uniformly present. Repolarization alternans has been recognized in patients with idiopathic long Q-T interval syndromes,[29] combined hypokalemia and hypocalcemia,[98] chronic alcohol abuse with hypomagnesemia,[94,99] and a combination of quinidine use, hypomagnesemia, and hypocalcemia.[7] These episodes of T or U wave alternans often precede or follow those of ventricular tachyarrhythmias.[7,29,94,98]

TREATMENT—ELECTROLYTE DEFICIENCY

The treatment of ventricular tachycardia associated with hypokalemia or hypomagnesemia usually requires parenteral therapy as a result of the gravity of the clinical situation, even though potassium salts are safer when administered by mouth. An intravenous potassium infusion of 1 mEq/min may cause high-grade atrioventricular block.[91] The most rapid infusion rate generally considered safe is 20 mEq/h.

Magnesium must be given parenterally, either by vein or muscle. Small doses are given (10 mEq or 2.5 ml of a 50% solution of magnesium sulfate), using clinical response and serum levels to guide therapy.

A time lag of many hours may elapse between electrolyte replacement and suppression of the serious ventricular arrhythmia, during which additional therapy may be needed. Overdrive pacing is the treatment of choice.[11,12] Pacing from the right atrium will preserve properly timed atrial contraction and enhance cardiac output unless there is AV block. Only occasionally will pacing rates greater than 100 to 120 beats per minute be required.[14,90,93]

Antiarrhythmic drugs are rarely effective in serious ventricular arrhythmias related to electrolyte imbalance. Quinidine, procainamide, and disopyramide are contraindicated, as discussed earlier (see "Clinical Manifestations, Long Q-T Syndromes").[14] Lidocaine and diphenylhydantoin are only modestly helpful.[92–94] There are several reports of successful therapy with bretylium tosylate and mexiletine.[14,90,92]

Diseases of the Central Nervous System

In 1954, Burch et al. identified an electrocardiographic pattern peculiar to certain patients with cerebrovascular accidents.[100] The most consistent electrocardiographic finding is a prolonged Q-T-U interval.[101] Large upright or deeply inverted T waves and prominent U waves are commonly seen in the precordial leads. The electrocardiographic findings are not pathogenic of an intracranial lesion and may be caused by electrolyte imbalance, myocardial ischemia, quinidine, or complete heart block. A prolonged Q-T interval has also been found in patients with other intracranial disorders, i.e., trauma, infection, tumor, and idiopathic epilepsy[31,101,102] (Fig. 9). Similar electrocardiographic changes have occurred acutely during neurosurgical procedures.[101,103] We and others have observed patients with intracranial tumors who developed Q-T interval prolongation and large inverted T waves without any change in their neurologic status.[23]

The electrocardiographic changes are not caused by an increase in intracranial pressure, but appear to be related to injury of those areas of the brain which

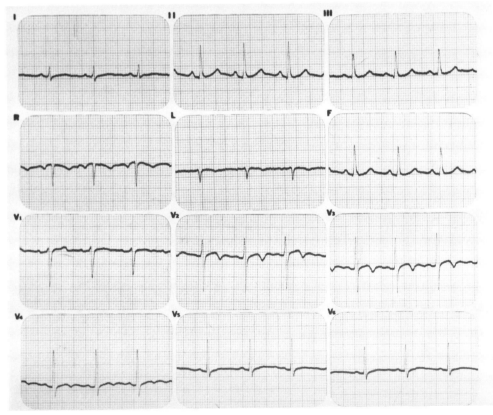

FIGURE 9 T wave change with U waves following repeated grand mal seizures. The electrocardiogram, 2 days later, was within normal limits. There was no clinical evidence of heart disease in this 42-year-old man.

contain the cortical representation of the autonomic nervous system.[101,103] In experimental animals, stimulation of the stellate ganglia or areas of the brain with known sympathetic connections can produce repolarization abnormalities resembling those observed in human beings.[31] Some observers attribute the electrocardiographic changes found in patients with central nervous system lesions to scattered subendocardial hemorrhages.[104] In the majority of patients, however, pathologic studies fail to reveal abnormalities of the heart or coronary arteries.[101,103]

That the central nervous system can induce delay in ventricular repolarization with the subsequent development of ventricular tachyarrhythmias is suggested by several reports. Recurrent ventricular fibrillation was observed in 2 patients with subarachnoid hemorrhage and in 1 patient with a transient hemiparesis.[8,105] Marked Q-T-U prolongation was observed on the electrocardiograms of these patients between episodes of fibrillation. Neurologic improvement in the 2 survivors resulted in return of the Q-T intervals to normal and cessation of recurrent ventricular fibrillation

The incidence of ventricular arrhythmias in patients with neurologic events is unknown. Continuous electrocardiographic monitoring is advisable for those patients with marked Q-T interval prolongation. Supportive care with drug therapy (lidocaine, diphenylhydantoin, or propranolol) or overdrive pacing should be given while hope for neurologic improvement exists.

Coronary Atherosclerotic Heart Disease

Marked prolongation of the Q-T interval is sufficiently uncommon after myocardial infarction that its presence, especially when associated with ventricular tachycardia of the *torsade de pointes* type* suggests another complication (Fig. 10). In one report, 4 of 5 acute infarction patients with prolonged Q-T intervals and ventricular tachycardia had other potential causes of delayed repolarization.[16] These included complete heart block, severe hypokalemia, and quinidine therapy. Suppression of the ventricular tachycardia is not easily achieved. Overdrive pacing should be tried and any associated electrolyte or metabolic abnormality corrected.[106] Quinidine, procainamide, and similar antiarrhythmic agents are contraindicated.

Although marked Q-T interval prolongation with attendant ventricular arrhythmias is an infrequent complication of acute myocardial infarction, a modest increase in the Q-T interval is quite common. Do-

roghazi and Childers found that the Q-T interval was transiently prolonged in 43 percent of patients with acute myocardial infarction.[107] During the first week after infarction, the rate corrected Q-T_c interval increased from a mean of 0.404 to 0.448 s in their patients. The important questions raised by these observations have not been answered. What is the cause of the increase in the Q-T interval and what influence does a modest prolongation of the Q-T interval have on the genesis of ventricular arrhythmias? Interest in the Q-T interval has been extended to a study of its value as a predictor of sudden death in patients with prior myocardial infarction. In a small postinfarction study group, the incidence of Q-T prolongation was greater in patients who suffered sudden death.[108]

Mitral Valve Prolapse Syndrome

The mitral valve prolapse syndrome is a common and usually benign condition, often associated with premature ventricular contractions and supraventricular tachyarrhythmias (Fig. 11). Progressive mitral regurgitation, bacterial endocarditis, and sudden death occur as rare complications.[109] The incidence of sudden death is low in this syndrome, even in patients with frequent premature ventricular contractions.[110,111] Sudden death may occur without warning or may be preceded by syncopal episodes.[109] It may occur with exercise, at rest, or during sleep.[110] Ventricular tachyarrhythmias are probably the major cause of sudden death.

Although infrequent, the occurrence of ventricular tachycardia and ventricular fibrillation in patients with mitral valve prolapse is well documented.[110,112–116] Mitral valve prolapse should be considered in all patients, especially women, presenting with drug-resistant ventricular arrhythmias.[113] The relationship between ventricular arrhythmias and repolarization abnormalities in the resting electrocardiogram in patients with mitral valve prolapse is controversial. Some observers have noted a high prevalence of inferolateral ST segment and T wave abnormalities and Q-T interval prolongation in the electrocardiogram of patients with ventricular arrhythmias.[110,113,115] Other observers have found no correlation.[112,116] This discrepancy suggests that factors other than delayed repolarization may be responsible for arrhythmias in patients with this syndrome. It is possible that ventricular arrhythmias may result from increased mechanical stress on the papillary muscles and their insertion sites.[117]

Antiarrhythmic treatment is not indicated for asymptomatic patients who have frequent ventricular premature contraction, pairs of ventricular ectopic beats, or even multiform ventricular ectopic contractions.[110] This conservative approach is defensible because sudden death is a rare complication of this syn-

---

* See p. 317 for discussion of *torsade de pointes* ventricular tachycardia.

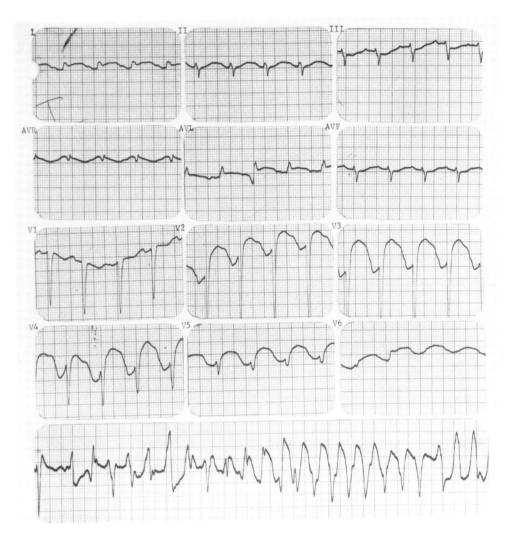

FIGURE 10 Acute anterior and lateral myocardial infarction with prolonged ventricular repolarization and ventricular tachycardia. No other factors known to lengthen ventricular repolarization were apparent. The Q-T$_c$ interval 0.55 s. (Courtesy of Dr. Laurence Lesser.)

drome despite the common occurrence of ectopic ventricular contractions. Patients having bothersome symptoms related to premature ventricular contractions and patients with runs of ventricular tachycardia should be treated. Propranolol has been recommended for the treatment of the mitral valve prolapse syndrome because of its antiarrhythmic properties. The response to propranolol is variable, and many therapeutic failures have been reported.[113,114,116,117] Combined propranolol/diphenylhydantoin therapy has suppressed ventricular arrhythmias in some patients but has failed in others.[113,117,118] Aprindine or mexiletine, new antiarrhythmic agents with local anesthetic effects, have been effective in abolishing refractory ventricular arrhythmias in a total of 21 patients with mitral valve prolapse.[57,113,115] These drugs have been approved for investigational studies in patients in the

United States. Overdrive pacing or mitral valve replacement may be considered when life-threatening ventricular arrhythmias persist despite an adequate trial of medical therapy.[116,117]

Fasting and Liquid Protein Diets

Sudden death has been reported in times of famine.[119] It has also been reported as a consequence of therapeutic starvation for obesity. In a well-documented case reported by Garnett et al., sudden death occurred in a 20-year-old woman with no history of heart disease.[120] Intractable ventricular arrhythmias developed on the seventh day of refeeding after a therapeutic fast. Her electrocardiogram after initial cardiac arrest showed low QRS voltage and a greatly prolonged Q-

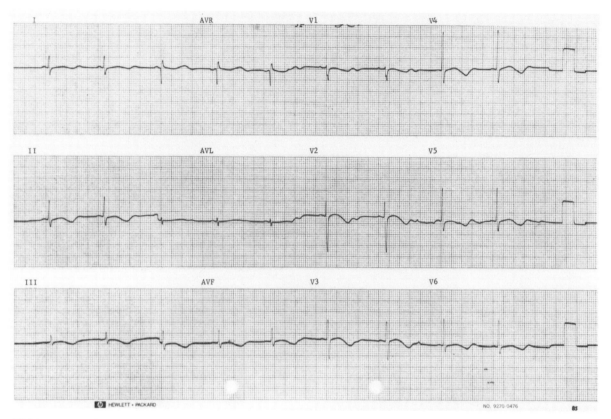

FIGURE 11 Mitral valve prolapse syndrome in an 18-year-old female with delayed ventricular repolarization and one documented episode of ventricular tachycardia. The patient was not receiving medication, and the serum electrolytes were normal when the electrocardiogram was recorded. (Courtesy of Dr. Candace Miklozek.)

T interval. Recently, sudden death has been reported in association with liquid protein diets.[121,122] By December 1977, 15 cases had been recorded.[122] All patients were obese women, ranging in age from 25 to 51 years. None had a history of heart disease or other underlying medical problems which could have caused death. Eleven patients died suddenly while on the diet, and 4 patients died during refeeding. Ventricular arrhythmias were documented in 9 patients. The electrocardiograms showed Q-T interval prolongation in 6 to 9 patients. In 1 patient, a prolonged Q-T interval had been demonstrated on an electrocardiogram taken 4 years prior to beginning of diet.[121] At autopsy, focal lymphocytic infiltration of the myocardium was observed in 7 of 13 patients. A reduction in myocardial fiber size with fragmentation of the myofibrils has been found with starvation and in 1 patient on a liquid protein diet.[120,121]

The pathogenesis of the cardiac arrhythmias and death is uncertain. Delayed ventricular repolarization appears to be an important factor in some patients. The mechanisms by which liquid protein diets and therapeutic starvation may prolong ventricular repo-

larization is unknown. Serum potassium levels in the fatal cases were low in some patients but normal in others.[122] Tissue depletion of magnesium is a recognized complication of prolonged fasting in human beings.[123] Available serum levels of calcium and magnesium were in the low normal range in the patients who died. In experimental animals, prolonged fasting causes suppression of the sympathetic nervous system.[124] Upon refeeding, sympathetic activity increases. Theoretically an abrupt increase in sympathetic activity to a heart that is deficient in magnesium and unaccustomed to a high level of sympathetic tone could have an adverse effect on ventricular repolarization.

There is no specific treatment for the ventricular arrhythmias that complicate prolonged starvation or liquid protein diets. Rapid atrial pacing and the administration of magnesium may be tried, but their effectiveness is not established. Patients taking a liquid protein diet should be carefully observed for symptoms suggestive of a cardiac arrhythmia and for a prolonged Q-T interval or premature ventricular contractions in the electrocardiogram.

Electrolytes, specifically potassium, calcium, phosphate, and magnesium, should be monitored. Refeeding after prolonged fasting should be gradual and closely supervised. As the liquid protein diet regimen for weight reduction is associated with an increased risk of sudden death in previously healthy individuals without known heart disease, it should not be generally recommended.

REFERENCES

1 Parkinson, J., and Campbell, M.: The Quinidine Treatment of Auricular Fibrillation, *Q. J. Med.*, 22:281, 1929.

1a Heiman, E. M.: Cardiac Toxicity with Thioridazine-Tricyclic Antidepressant Combination, *J. Nerv. Ment. Dis.*, 165:139, 1977.

2 Gram, L. E., and Overo, K. F.: Drug Interaction: Inhibitory Effect of Neuroleptics on Metabolism of Tricyclic Antidepressants in Man, *Br. Med. J.* 1:463, 1972.

3 Burgess, M. J., Green, L. S., Millar, K., Wyatt, R., and Abildskov, J. A.: The Sequence of Normal Ventricular Recovery, *Am. Heart J.*, 84:660, 1972.

4 Autenrieth, G., Surawicz, B., and Kuo, C. S.: Sequence of Repolarization on the Ventricular Surface in the Dog, *Am. Heart J.*, 89:463, 1975.

5 Surawicz, B.: The Pathogenesis and Clinical Significance of Primary T-Wave Abnormalities, in R. C. Schlauf and J. W. Hurst (eds.), "Advances in Electrocardiography," Grune & Stratton, Inc., New York, 1972, p. 377.

6 Watanabe, Y., and Toda, H.: The U Wave and Aberration Conduction. Further Evidence for the Purkinje Repolarization Theory on Genesis of the U Wave, *Am. J. Cardiol.*, 41:23, 1978.

7 Luca, C.: Right Ventricular Monophasic Action Potential during Quinidine-induced Marked T and U Wave Abnormalities, *Acta Cardiol.*, 32:305, 1977.

8 Reynolds, E. W., and Vander Ark, C. R.: Quinidine Syncope and the Delayed Repolarization Syndromes, *Mod. Concepts Cardiovasc. Dis.*, 45:117, 1976.

9 Han, J., and Goel, B. G.: Electrophysiologic Precursors of Ventricular Tachyarrhythmias, *Arch. Intern. Med.*, 129,749, 1972.

10 Surawicz, B.: The Input of Cellular Electrophysiology into the Practice of Clinical Electrocardiography, *Mod. Concepts Cardiovasc. Dis.*, 44:41, 1975.

11 Krikler, D. M., and Curry, P. V. L.: Torsade de Pointes, an Atypical Ventricular Tachycardia, *Br. Heart J.*, 38:117, 1976.

12 Motte, G., Coumel, P., Abitbol, G., Dessertenne, G., and Slama, R.: Le Syndrome QT Long et Syncopes par "Torsade de Pointes," *Arch. Mal. Coeur.*, 63:831, 1970.

13 Shelby, P. J., and Driver, M. V.: An Unusual Cause of Apparent Epilepsy: ECG and ECG Findings in a Case of Jervell Lange-Nielsen Syndrome, *J. Neurol. Neurosurg. Psychiatry*, 40:1102, 1977.

14 Curry, P., Stubbs, W., Fitchett, D., and Krikler, D.: Ventricular Arrhythmias and Hypokalemia, *Lancet*, 2:231, 1976.

15 Ranquin, R., and Parizel, G.: Ventricular Fibrillo-Flutter ("Torsade de Pointes"): An Established Electrocardiographic and Clinical Entity, *Angiology*, 28:115, 1977.

16 Dalle, X. S., Meltzer, E., and Kravitz, B.: A New Look at Ventricular Tachycardia, *Acta Cardiol.*, 22:519, 1967.

17 Finley, J. P., Radford, D. J., and Freedom, R. M.: Torsade de Pointes Ventricular Tachycardia in a Newborn Infant, *Br. Heart J.*, 40:421, 1978.

18 Evans, T. R., Curry, P. V. L., Fitchett, D. H., and Krikler, D. M.: "Torsade de Pointes" Initiated by Electrical Ventricular Stimulation, *J. Electrocardiol.*, 9:255, 1976.

19 Jervell, A., and Lange-Nielsen, F.: Congenital Deaf-Mutism, Functional Heart Disease with Prolongation of the QT Interval, and Sudden Death, *Am. Heart J.*, 54:59, 1957.

20 Romano, C., Gemme, G., and Pongiglione, R.: Aritmie Cardiache Rare Dell' eta' Pediatrica. II. Accessi Sincopali per Fibrillazione Ventricolane Parossistica, *Clin. Pediatr. (Phila.)*, 45:656, 1963.

21 Ward, O. C.: A New Familial Cardiac Syndrome in Children, *J. Irish Med. Assoc.*, 54:103, 1964.

22 Schwartz, P. J., Periti, M., and Malliani, A.: The Long Q-T Syndrome, *Am. Heart J.*, 89:378, 1975.

23 Vincent, G. M., Abildskov, J. A., Burgess: Q-T Interval Syndromes, *Prog. Cardiovasc. Dis.*, 16:523, 1974.

24 Roy, P. R., Emanuel, R., Ismail, S. A., Hassan, E. I., and Tayib, M.: Hereditary Prolongation of the Q-T Interval. Genetic Observations and Management in Three Families with Twelve Affected Members, *Am. J. Cardiol.*, 37:237, 1976.

25 Frank, J. P., and Friedberg, D. Z.: Syncope with Prolonged QT Interval, *Am. J. Dis. Child.*, 130:320, 1976.

26 James, T. N., Froggatt, P., Atkinson, W. J., Lurie, P. R., McNamara, D. G., Miller, W. W., Schloss, G. T., Carroll, J. F., and North, R. C.: De Subitaneis

Mortibus xxx. Observations on the Pathophysiology of the Long QT Syndromes with Special Reference to Neuropathology of the Heart, *Circulation,* 57:1221, 1978.

27 Von Bernuth, G., Belz, G. G., Evertz, W., and Stauch, M.: QTU-Abnormalities, Sinus Bradycardia and Adams-Stokes Attacks Due to Ventricular Tachyarrhythmia, *Acta Paediatr. Scand.,* 62:675, 1973.

28 Garza, L. A., Vick, R. L., Nora, J. J., and McNamara, D. C.: Heritable QT Prolongation without Deafness, *Circulation,* 41:39, 1970.

29 Schwartz, P. J., and Malliani, A.: Electrical Alternation of the T Wave: Clinical and Experimental Evidence of Its Relationship with the Sympathetic Nervous System and with the Long Q-T Syndrome, *Am. Heart J.,* 89:45, 1975.

30 Chaudron, J. N., Heller, F., Van den Berghe, H. B., and LeBacq, E. G.: Attacks of Ventricular Fibrillation and Unconsciousness in a Patient with Prolonged QT Interval. A Family Study, *Am. Heart J.,* 91:783, 1976.

31 Yanowitz, F., Preston, J. E., and Abildskov, J. A.: Functional Distribution of Right and Left Stellate Innervation to the Ventricles: Production of Neurogenic Electrocardiographic Changes by Unilateral Alteration of Sympathetic Tone, *Circ. Res.,* 18:416, 1966.

32 Schwartz, P. J., Snebold, N. G., and Brown, A. M.: Effects of Unilateral Cardiac Sympathetic Denervation on the Ventricular Fibrillation Threshold, *Am. J. Cardiol.,* 37:1034, 1976.

33 Moss, A. J., and McDonald, J.: Unilateral Cervicothoracic Sympathetic Ganglionectomy for the Treatment of Long QT Interval Syndrome, *N. Engl. J. Med.,* 285:903, 1971.

34 Han, J., Garcia de Jalon, P. D., and Moe, G. K.: Fibrillation Threshold of Premature Ventricular Responses, *Circ. Res.,* 18:18, 1966.

35 Wit, A. L., Hoffman, B. F., and Rosen, M.: Electrophysiology and Pharmacology of Cardiac Arrhythmias 1X. Cardiac Electrophysiologic Effects of Beta Adrenergic Receptor Stimulation and Blockade. Part A, *Am. Heart J.,* 90:521, 1975.

36 Wellens, H. J. J.: Value and Limitations of Programmed Electrical Stimulation of the Heart in the Study and Treatment of Tachycardias, *Circulation,* 57:845, 1978.

37 Radford, D. J., Izukawa, T., and Rowe, R. D.: Evaluation of Children with Ventricular Arrhythmias, *Arch. Dis. Child.,* 52:345, 1977.

38 Ratshin, R. A., Hunt, D., Russell, R. O., Jr., and Rackley, C. E.: QT Interval Prolongation, Paroxysmal Ventricular Arrhythmias, and Convulsive Syncope, *Ann. Intern. Med.,* 75:919, 1971.

39 Olley, P. M., and Fowler, R. S.: The Surdo-Cardiac Syndrome and Therapeutic Observations, *Br. Heart J.,* 32:467, 1970.

40 Schwartz, P. J.: Experimental Reproduction of the Long Q-T Syndrome, *Am. J. Cardiol.,* 41:374, 1978. (Abstract.)

41 Selzer, A., and Wray, H. W.: Quinidine Syncope. Paroxysmal Ventricular Fibrillation Occurring during Treatment of Chronic Atrial Arrhythmias, *Circulation,* 30:17, 1964.

42 Cohen, I. S., Jick, H., and Cohen, S. I.: Adverse Reactions to Quinidine in Hospitalized Patients: Findings Based on Data from the Boston Collaborative Drug Surveillance Program, *Prog. Cardiovasc. Dis.,* 20:151, 1977.

43 Koster, R. W., and Wellens, H. J. J.: Quinidine-induced Ventricular Flutter and Fibrillation without Digitalis Therapy, *Am. J. Cardiol.,* 38:519, 1976.

44 Surawicz, B., and Lasseter, K. C.: Effect of Drugs on the Electrocardiogram, *Prog. Cardiovasc. Dis.,* 13:26, 1970.

45 Kwit, N. T., and Gold, H.: Further Experimental Observations on the Combined Effects of Digitalis and Quinidine on the Heart, *J. Pharmacol. Exp. Ther.,* 50:180, 1934.

46 Ejuinsson, G.: Effect of Quinidine on Plasma Concentrations of Digoxin, *Br. Med. J.,* 1:279, 1978.

47 Jenzer, H. R., and Hagemeijer, F.: Quinidine Syncope: Torsade de Pointes with Low Quinidine Plasma Concentrations, *Eur. J. Cardiol.,* 4:447, 1976.

48 Hoffman, B. F., Rosen, M. R., and Wit, A. L.: Electrophysiology and Pharmacology of Cardiac Arrhythmias. VII. Cardiac Effects of Quinidine and Procaineamide B, *Am. Heart J.,* 90:117, 1975.

49 VanderArk, C. R., Reynolds, E. W., Kahn, D. R., and Tullett, G.: Quinidine Syncope. A Report of Successful Treatment with Bretylium Tosylate, *J. Thorac. Cardiovasc. Surg.,* 72:464, 1976.

50 Bassett, A. L., and Hoffman, B. F.: Antiarrhythmic Drugs: Electrophysiological Actions, *Annu. Rev. Pharmacol.,* 11:143, 1971.

51 DeAzavedo, I. M., Watanabe, Y., Dreifus, L. S.: Electrophysiologic Antagonism of Quinidine and Bretylium Tosylate, *Am. J. Cardiol.,* 33:633, 1974.

52 Oravetz, J., and Slodki, S. J.: Recurrent Ventricular Fibrillation Precipitated by Quinidine, *Arch. Intern. Med.,* 122:63, 1968.

53 Pick, A.: Manifestations of a Vulnerable Phase in the Human Heart, in B. Surawicz and E. D. Pellegrino (eds.), "Sudden Cardiac Death," Grune & Stratton, Inc., New York, 1964, p. 44.

54 Read, J. M.: Fatal Ventricular Fibrillation following Procaineamide Hydrochloride Therapy, *J.A.M.A.,* 149:1390, 1952.

55 Hulting, J., and Jansson, B.: Antiarrhythmic and Electrocardiographic Effects of Single Oral Doses of Disopyramide, *Eur. J. Clin. Pharmacol.,* 11:91, 1977.

56 Frieden, J.: Quinidine Effects Due to Disopyramide, *N. Engl. J. Med.,* 298:975, 1978.

57 Zipes, D. P., and Troup, P. J.: New Antiarrhythmic Agents. Amiodarone, Aprinidine, Disopyramide, Ethmozin, Mexiletine, Tocainide, Verapamil, *Am. J. Cardiol.,* 41:1005, 1978.

58 Fowler, N. O., McCall, D., Chou, T., et al.: Electrocardiographic Changes and Cardiac Arrhythmias in Patients Receiving Psychotropic Drugs, *Am. J. Cardiol.,* 37:223, 1976.

59 Madan, B. R., and Pendse, V. K.: Antiarrhythmic Activity of Thioridazine Hydrochloride (Mellaril), *Am. J. Cardiol.,* 11:78, 1963.

60 Arita, M., and Surawicz, B.: Electrophysiologic Effects of Phenothiazines on Human Atrial Fibers, *Jpn. Heart J.,* 14:398, 1973.

61 Arita, M., and Surawicz, B.: Electrophysiologic Effects of Phenothiazines on Canine Cardiac Fibers, *J. Pharmacol. Exp. Ther.,* 184:619, 1973.

62 Crane, G. E.: Cardiac Toxicity and Psychotropic Drugs, *Dis. Nerv. Syst.,* 31:534, 1970.

63 Leestma, J. E., and Koenig, K. L.: Sudden Death and Phenothiazines, *Arch. Gen. Psychiatr.,* 18:137, 1968.

64 Schoonmaker, F. W., Osteen, R. T., and Greenfield, J. C.: Thioridazine (Mellaril)-induced Ventricular Tachycardia Controlled with an Artificial Pacemaker, *Ann. Intern. Med.,* 65:1076, 1966.

65 Gelenberg, A. J.: Cardiac Arrhythmias after Psychotropic Drugs, *Am. J. Cardiol.,* 40:297, 1977.

66 Kelly, H. G., Fay, J. E., and Laverty, S. G.: Thioridazine Hydrochloride (Mellaril): Its Effect on the ECG and a Report of Two Fatalities with ECG Abnormalities, *Can. Med. Assoc. J.,* 89:546, 1963.

67 Sydney, M. A.: Ventricular Arrhythmias Associated with Use of Thioridazine Hydrochloride in Alcohol Withdrawal, *Br. Med. J.,* 4:467, 1973.

68 El-Yousef, M. K.: Tricyclic Antidepressants and Phenothiazides, *J.A.M.A.,* 229:1419, 1974.

69 Moore, M. T., and Book, M. H.: Sudden Death in Phenothiazine Therapy, *Psychiatr. Q.,* 44:389, 1970.

70 Giles, T. D., and Modlin, R. K.: Death Associated with Ventricular Arrythmia and Thioridazine Hydrochloride, *J.A.M.A.,* 205:108, 1968.

71 Richardson, H. L., Graupner, K. I., and Richardson, M. E.: Intramyocardial Lesions in Patients Dying Suddenly and Unexpectedly, *J.A.M.A.,* 195:254, 1966.

72 Brown, T. C.: Sodium Bicarbonate Treatment for Tricyclic Antidepressant Arrhythmias in Children, *Med. J. Aust.,* 2:380, 1976.

73 Bigger, J. T., Giardina, E. G. B., Perel, J. M., et al.: Cardiac Antiarrhythmic Effect of Imipramine Hydrochloride, *N. Engl. J. Med.,* 296:206, 1977.

74 Thorstrand, C.: Cardiovascular Effects of Poisoning with Tricyclic Antidepressants, *Acta Med. Scand.,* 195:505, 1974.

75 Scollins, M. J., Robinson, D. S., and Nies, A.: Cardiotoxicity of Amitriptyline, *Lancet,* 2:1202, 1972.

76 Jefferson, J. W.: A Review of the Cardiovascular Effects and Toxicity of Tricyclic Antidepressants, *Psychosom. Med.,* 37:160, 1975.

77 Schmitt, H., Cheymol, G., and Gilbert, J. C.: Effects Anti-arythmisants et Hemodynamiques de l'Imipramine et de la Chlorimipramine, *Arch. Int. Pharmacodyn. Ther.,* 184:158, 1970.

78 Brorson, L., and Wennerblom, B.: Electrophysiological Methods in Assessing Cardiac Effects of the Tricyclic Antidepressant Imipramine, *Acta Med. Scand.,* 203:429, 1978.

79 Burrows, G. D., Vohra, J., Hunt, D., Sloman, J. G., Scoggins, B. A., and Davies, B.: Cardiac Effects of Different Tricyclic Antidepressant Drugs, *Br. J. Psychiatry,* 129:335, 1976.

80 Thorstrand, C.: Clinical Features in Poisonings by Tricyclic Antidepressants with Special Reference to the ECG, *Acta Med. Scand.,* 199:337, 1976.

81 Spiker, D. G., Weiss, A. N., Chang, S. S., Ruwitch, J. F., and Biggs, J. T.: Tricyclic Antidepressant Overdose: Clinical Presentation and Plasma Levels, *Clin. Pharm. Ther.,* 18:539, 1975.

82 Gaultier, M.: Sodium Bicarbonate and Tricyclic Antidepressant Poisoning, *Lancet,* 2:1258, 1976.

83 Raymond, C. W.: Neostigmine Methylsulfate in the Treatment of Cardiac Arrhythmia Induced by Perphenazine-Amitriptyline, *Can. Med. Assoc. J.,* 114:102, 1976.

84 Tobis, J., Das, B. W.: Cardiac Complications in Amitriptyline Poisoning. Successful Treatment with Physostigmine, *J.A.M.A.,* 235:1474, 1976.

85 Bigger, J. T., Jr., Kantor, S. J., Glassman, A. H., and Perel, J. M.: Is Physostigmine Effective for Cardiac Toxicity of Tricyclic Antidepressant Drugs?, *J.A.M.A.,* 237:1311, 1977.

86 Newton, R. W.: Physostigmine Salicylate in the Treatment of Tricyclic Antidepressant Overdose, *J.A.M.A,* 231:941, 1975.

87 Roberts, R. J., Mueller, S., and Laver, R. M.: Propranolol in the Treatment of Cardiac Arrhythmias Associated with Amitriptyline Intoxication, *J. Pediatr.,* 82:65, 1973.

88 Krikler, D. M.: A Fresh Look at Cardiac Arrhythmias. Pathogenesis and Presentation, *Lancet,* 1:913, 1974.

89 Rossi, L., and Matturni, L.: Histopathological Findings in Two Cases of Torsade de Pointes with Conduction Disturbances, *Br. Heart. J.,* 38:1312, 1976.

326

90 Schneider, R. R., Bahler, A., Pincus, J., and Stimmel, B.: Asymptomatic Idiopathic Syndrome of Prolonged Q-T Interval in a 45-Year-Old Woman. Ventricular Tachyarrhythmias Precipitated by Hypokalemia and Therapy with Amitriptyline and Prephenazine, *Chest,* 71:210, 1977.

91 Surawicz, B.: Relationship between Electrocardiogram and Electrolytes, *Am. Heart J.,* 73:814, 1967.

92 Redleaf, P. D., and Lerner, I. J.: Thiazide-induced Hypokalemia with Associated Major Ventricular Arrhythmias, *J.A.M.A.,* 206:1302, 1968.

93 Loeb, H. S., Pietras, R. J., Gunnar, R. M., and Tobin, J. R. Jr.: Paroxysmal Ventricular Fibrillation in Two Patients with Hypomagnesemia, *Circulation,* 37:210, 1968.

94 Bashour, T., Rios, J. C., and Gorman, P.: U Wave Alternans and Increased Ventricular Irritability, *Chest,* 64:377, 1973.

95 Vander Ark, C. R., Ballantine, F., and Reynolds, E. W., Jr.: Electrolytes and the Electrocardiogram, *Cardiovasc. Clin. 5* (3. Complex Electrocardiography 1):270, 1973.

96 Dyckner, T., and Wester, P. O.: Intracellular Potassium after Magnesium Infusion, *Br. Med. J.,* 1:822, 1978.

97 Kambara, H., Iteld, B. J., and Phillips, J.: Hypocalcemia and Intractable Ventricular Fibrillation, *Ann. Intern. Med.,* 86:583, 1977.

98 Navarro-Lopez, F., Cinca, J., Sanz, G., Periz, A., Magrina, J., and Betriv, A.: Isolated T Wave Alternans, *Am. Heart J.,* 95:369, 1978.

99 Ricketts, H. H., Denison, E. K., and Haywood, L. J.: Unusual T Wave Abnormality. Repolarization Alternans Associated with Hypomagnesemia, Acute Alcoholism, and Cardiomyopathy, *J.A.M.A.,* 207:365, 1969.

100 Burch, G. E., Myers, R., and Abildskov, J. A.: A New Electrocardiographic Pattern Observed in Cerebrovascular Accidents, *Circulation,* 9:719, 1954.

101 Abildskov, J. A., Millar, K., Burgess, M. J., and Vincent, W.: The Electrocardiogram and the Central Nervous System, *Prog. Cardiovasc. Dis.,* 13:210, 1970.

102 Hugenholtz, P. G.: Electrocardiographic Abnormalities in Cerebral Disorders. Report of Six Cases and Review of the Literature, *Am. Heart J.,* 63:451, 1962.

103 Cropp, G. J., and Manning, G. W.: Electrocardiographic Changes Stimulating Myocardial Ischemia and Infarction Associated with Spontaneous Intracranial Hemorrhage, *Circulation,* 22:25, 1960.

104 Koskelo, P., Punsar, S., and Sipila, W.: Subendocardial Hemorrhage and ECG Changes in Intracranial Bleeding, *Br. Med. J.,* 1:1479, 1964.

105 Parizel, G.: Life-threatening Arrhythmias in Subarachnoid Hemorrhage, *Angiology,* 24:17 1973.

106 Lopez, L., and Sowton, E.: Overdriving by Pacing to Suppress Ventricular Ectopic Activity, *J. Electrocardiol.,* 5:65, 1972.

107 Doroghazi, R. M., and Childers, R.: Time-related Changes in the Q-T Interval in Acute Myocardial Infarction: Possible Relation to Local Hypocalcemia, *Am. J. Cardiol.,* 41:684, 1978.

108 Schwartz, P. J., and Wolf, S.: QT Interval Prolongation as Predictor of Sudden Death in Patients with Myocardial Infarction, *Circulation,* 57:1074, 1978.

109 Devereaux, R. B., Perloff, J. K., Reichek, N., and Josephson, M. E.: Mitral Valve Prolapse, *Circulation,* 54:3, 1976.

110 Winkle, R. A., Lopes, M. G., Popp, R. L., and Hancock, E. W.: Life-threatening Arrhythmias in the Mitral Valve Prolapse Syndrome, *Am. J. Med.,* 60:961, 1976.

111 Jeresaty, R. M.: Sudden Death in the Mitral Valve Prolapse-Click Syndrome, *Am. J. Cardiol.,* 37:317, 1976.

112 DeMaria, A. N., Amsterdam, E. A., Vismara, L. A., Neumann, A., and Mason, D. T.: Arrhythmias in the Mitral Valve Prolapse Syndrome, *Ann. Intern. Med.,* 84:656, 1976.

113 Wei, J. Y., Bulkey, B. H., Schaeffer, A. H., Greene, H. L., and Reid, P. R.: Mitral-Valve Prolapse Syndrome and Recurrent Ventricular Tachyarrhythmias, *Ann. Intern. Med.,* 89:6, 1978.

114 Shappell, S. D., Marshall, C. E., Brown, R. E., and Bruce, T. A.: Sudden Death and the Familial Occurrence of Mid-systolic Click, Late Systolic Murmur Syndrome, *Circulation,* 48:1128, 1973.

115 Campbell, R. W. F., Godman, M. G., Fiddler, G. I., Marquis, R. M., and Julian, D. G.: Ventricular Arrhythmias in Syndrome of Balloon Deformity of Mitral Valve. Definition of Possible High Risk Group, *Br. Heart J.,* 38:1053, 1976.

116 Ritchie, J. L., Hammermeister, K. E., and Kennedy, J. W.: Refractory Ventricular Tachycardia and Fibrillation in a Patient with the Prolapsing Mitral Leaflet Syndrome. Successful Control with Overdrive Pacing, *Am. J. Cardiol.,* 37:314, 1976.

117 Cobbs, B. W., and King, S. B., III: Ventricular Buckling: A Factor in the Abnormal Ventriculogram and Peculiar Hemodynamics Associated with Mitral Valve Prolapse, *Am. Heart J.,* 93:741, 1977.

118 Pocock, W. A., and Barlow, J. B.: Post-exercise Arrhythmias in the Billowing Posterior Mitral Leaflet Syndrome, *Am. Heart J.,* 80:740, 1970.

119 Zimmer, R., Weill, J., and Dubois, M.: The Nutritional Situation in the Camps of the Unoccupied Zone of France in 1941 and 1942 and Its Consequences, *N. Engl. J. Med.,* 230:303, 1944.

120 Garnett, E. S., Barnard, D. L., Ford, J., et al.: Gross Fragmentation of Cardiac Myofibrils after Therapeutic Starvation for Obesity, *Lancet,* 1:914, 1969.

121 Michiel, R. R., Sneider, J. S., Dickstein, R. A., et al.: Sudden Death in a Patient on a Liquid Protein Diet, *N. Engl. J. Med.,* 298:1005, 1978.

122 Food and Drug Administration: Protein Diets, *FDA Drug Bull.* 8:2, 1978.

123 Felig, P.: Four Questions about Protein Diets, *N. Engl. J. Med.,* 298:1025, 1978.

124 Landsberg, L., and Young, J. B.: Fasting, Feeding and Regulation of the Sympathetic Nervous System, *N. Engl. J. Med.,* 298:1295, 1978.

Cardiovascular Nuclear Medicine*

H. WILLIAM STRAUSS, M.D., KENNETH A. McKUSICK, M.D., and GERALD M. POHOST, M.D.

INTRODUCTION

The application of radioactive tracers to the evaluation of heart disease and cardiac physiology dates to the 1920s, when Blumgart and Weiss[1] and their associates applied the cloud chamber, developed by Wilson, to observe the arrival of intravenously administered tracer at a distant site in order to measure the circulation time noninvasively in intact human beings. This tracer application occurred at the time that DeBorglis and Schröedinger had published the wave mechanics theory (1924–1926), before Pavlov published his work in conditioned reflexes (1926), and long before the development of artificial radioactivity. Since this early application of radioactive tracers to the evaluation of physiology, radioactive tracers have been used to determine almost every aspect of cardiac structure and function, from the evaluation of protein and electrolyte turnover rates in cardiac muscle to the assessment of drug levels in blood and the evaluation of cardiac structure and function. Table 1 lists the important landmarks in the development of cardiovascular nuclear medicine.

TRACER DETERMINATION OF CARDIAC STRUCTURE

Static Blood Pool Scan

METHOD

The static cardiac blood pool scan is performed after the intravenous administration of a tracer that remains in the vascular compartment, such as technetium 99m-labeled albumin, red blood cells, or ionic indium 113m (which combines in vivo with the β_1-globulin in transferrin) (Table 2). The scan supplies information about overall cardiac size, relationship of the cardiac blood pool to that of the lungs and liver, and the relative thickness of the myocardium of the right and left ventricles (in the absence of pericardial disease). Scans which record 800 to 1000 counts per square centimeter are of sufficient quality to clearly define the cardiac

borders. The image represents the mean position of the heart during the several minute intervals of imaging. Since the heart spends the majority of time in diastole, the image is an approximation of the mid-diastolic heart size. The diaphragmatic excursion dur-

TABLE 1

Landmarks in cardiovascular nuclear medicine in human beings

Measurement of circulation time in man	1927
Development of radiocardiogram	1947
Cardiac blood pool scan for pericardial effusion	1958
Myocardial imaging for distribution of perfusion (intravenous tracer)	1962
Myocardial imaging for acute infarct	1962
Nuclear angiocardiography	1963
Digoxin assay	1967
Global left ventricular function by first pass	1968
Myocardial imaging for distribution of perfusion (particle injection)	1969
Regional left ventricular function by gated blood pool scan	1970
Regional myocardial perfusion reserve	
Noninvasively	1972
Invasively	1973
Global left ventricular function reserve	1977
Global right ventricular function	1978

TABLE 2

A Tracers for static blood pool imaging

Nuclide	Substrate
Technetium 99m	Albumin
Iodine 123	
Carbon 11 monoxide	Red blood cells
Technetium 99m	
Indium 113 m	Transferrin

B Indications for cardiac blood pool scan

1 Enlarging cardiac size.
2 Onset of congestive cardiac failure in a patient with viral syndrome or uremia.
3 Determine relative ventricular chamber size in patients with chronic lung disease and symptoms of increasing shortness of breath.
4 Determine the presence of a large clot or mass within a cardiac chamber in a patient manifesting unusual signs of systemic embolization.
5 Detection of ventricular aneurysm in a patient who experiences congestive failure following myocardial infarction.

* From the Departments of Radiology and Medicine, Massachusetts General Hospital, Boston.
    Supported by Cardiovascular Nuclear Medicine Training Grant USPHS HL07416-1 and Ischemic SCOR Grant NHLBI HL-17665-04.

ing quiet respiration is about 1.5 cm and does not significantly degrade the image. The examination should always be performed in at least two views: usually the anterior and the left anterior oblique. The left anterior oblique scan should clearly delineate the septum.

Although technetium pertechnetate can be used for the evaluation of the cardiac blood pool, it is not recommended, since the tracer rapidly diffuses out of the vasculature and enters effusion, decreasing the contrast between the cardiac blood pool of the heart and the surrounding structures.

Detection of Ventricular Aneurysms, Intracardiac Masses, and Left Ventricular Dilatation

The diagnosis of ventricular aneurysm can occasionally be suspected from these images if one sees an outpouching of the blood pool that breaks the usually gently curving convex border associated with the normal ventricular outline.

Occasionally, intracardiac masses, such as myxomata or clots[2] can be detected as focal regions of decreased tracer activity in the cardiac blood pool.

The diagnosis of pericardial effusion can be made by echocardiography with a sensitivity equal to or exceeding that of tracer methods if the effusion is freely moving.[3] If the effusion is loculated, however, the tracer method may be more sensitive. In many institutions where both techniques are available, the echo method has largely supplanted the tracer technique for initial evaluation for possible effusion.

Marked dilatation of the cardiac chambers can be detected on static blood pool scanning, as can marked enlargement of the great vessel, such as occurs in poststenotic dilation or aneurysm. However, the size of individual chambers and their anatomic relation to one another are easier to evaluate from a nuclear angiocardiogram.[4] Occasionally, ventricular septal defects can be seen on the static blood pool scan as a focal absence in the septum. However, these are also better visualized during the nuclear angiocardiogram.

NUCLEAR ANGIOCARDIOGRAM— INDICATIONS

Nuclear angiocardiography is the diagnostic procedure in which the course of the radionuclide is followed with a scintillation camera as it traverses the heart and great vessels following intravenous injection (Fig. 1). Since the first studies were performed by

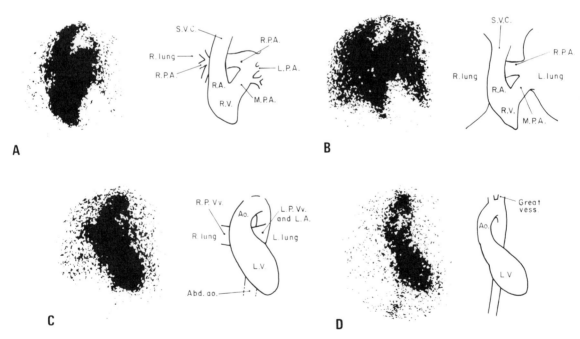

FIGURE 1 Radionuclide angiocardiogram performed in the anterior position following the intravenous administration of 20 mCi of 99m$_{Tc}$ pertechnetate. Frame A, recorded 5 s following intravenous injection, shows the superior vena cava, right atrium, right ventricle, pulmonary outflow tract. Frame B, recorded 2 s later, reveals pulmonary outflow tract and lungs with a space where the left ventricle will reside. Frame C, recorded 2 s later, reveals the left atrium, left ventricle, and aorta. Frame D, recorded 2 s later, reveals left ventricle and aorta. Should shunting be present, refilling of the right ventricle and promulgation of transit through the lungs will be observed.

Bender and Blau in 1963,[5] there has been steady improvement in the technique, so that the findings in various congenital and acquired cardiac conditions[4,6,7] have been defined.

Nuclear angiocardiography is particularly well suited to the evaluation of three groups of patients: (1) those for whom the catheterization procedure must be kept as short as possible (e.g., the patient with transposition of the great vessels in whom a septostomy is planned); the tracer procedure gives an indication of the presence and site of the disease; (2) those for whom a catheter procedure is not indicated but a definite diagnosis is sought by family or physician (e.g., a patient with a murmur suggestive of a ventricular septal defect but without significant clinical compromise); (3) those for whom a repeat evaluation of a known disease is indicated such as ventricular septal defect.

Methods

Three major components of the examination are important to obtain information of diagnostic quality: (1) intravenous bolus injection of nuclide; (2) collimation and count rate response of the scintillation camera; (3) method of data recording. The volume containing the tracer activity should be kept to a minimum to minimize the length of the bolus. A long bolus hinders interpretation, since tracer may be present in the right and left sides of the heart at the same time. Younger patients have shorter circulation times than do older individuals and consequently require shorter imaging intervals in order to obtain adequate separation of specific chambers and vessels. Adequate data can be obtained when a dose of 8 to 20 mCi/m^2 is administered intravenously (proportionally higher doses are required in children than adults) and images are recorded at 0.3-s intervals.

The choice of collimator depends on the age of the patient, size of the lesion, and the tracer used. The pinhole collimator magnifies the image on the face of the detector, thereby improving the approximately 1.5-cm resolution at the detector surface. The resolution is inversely related to the magnification factors. If the patient is a large child, then the gain in resolution using the pinhole collimator may be more than offset by the loss of sensitivity, and the high-resolution parallel hole collimator or converging multihole collimator may be preferable.

No preparation is required for patients who are cooperative. In a younger or uncooperative patient, sedation is useful because the patient must remain absolutely still during the imaging procedure. Crying and increased intrathoracic pressure may impede the bolus and reverse certain shunts.

The position selected for the examinations—ante-

rior, left anterior oblique (LAO), or left lateral—depends on the anatomy to be demonstrated. If shunting at the ventricular level is suspected, the LAO position is best; on the other hand, if the diagnosis of pulmonic stenosis is a serious consideration, an anterior position is preferred.

Several injection techniques have been suggested to produce a good bolus of tracer: (1) preloading a catheter with a dose and injecting a large flushing bolus (five to ten times the volume of isotonic or hypertonic solution); (2) a two-part syringe containing the dose in the forward compartment and a flushing solution in the rear compartment; and (3) the method of Oldendorf, using a blood pressure cuff inflated above systolic pressure to induce ischemic vasodilatation and injecting while the cuff is on, with rapid removal of the cuff to give a bolus. It is desirable, if possible, to inject the tracer in the upper extremity, in the basilic vein (since it has a more direct course to the heart) of the right arm, so that activity coming into the heart via the vena cava can be clearly differentiated from that leaving via the aorta.

The distribution of the nuclide can be recorded from the scintillation camera on (1) list mode into a computer; (2) computer frame mode into a computer; and (3) photographic film. The distinct advantage of the first two formats is the preservation of raw data, which can be replayed and integrated, viewed with adjustable contrast, and photographed as desired. In addition, early and late portions of the study can be superimposed to permit the ready appreciation of specific lesions.[8] The technique which records directly on film has a major advantage of low initial cost but has the liability of requiring a preset recording time and oscilloscopic intensity. The recording devices employed must be capable of handling the necessary framing rates with minimal dead time. The multi-image format devices have essentially no dead time and are more suitable for this type of examination. A minimal number of events must be contained in an image to provide a recognizable picture. If shorter recording intervals are used, the data from several intervals must be added together to provide an interpretable examination. After 1 min of rapid sequence recording, an image of 300,000 counts is recorded for delineation of the cardiac borders.

INTERPRETATION

It is useful to view the static high-count density image first to establish the relationship of cardiac to lung blood pools and the relationship of intracardiac blood pools to each other.[4] Examination of sequential images gives information about the temporal relationships of chamber filling. The duration of the bolus in the vena cava must be evaluated when seeking evidence of shunting. The major criteria for left-to-right shunting is the reentry of the bolus in the right heart, after the bolus has passed through the lungs to the left heart.

Once the quality of the bolus has been established, the anatomy of the chambers, pulmonary artery, and aorta can be evaluated and the sequence of chamber filling determined.

If the injection is satisfactory, slow passage of activity through all segments of the cardiopulmonary tree is an indication of heart failure. Delay confined to a particular segment suggests more localized impedance (e.g., as a result of incompetence of one or more valves, shunting, or possibly aneurysmal dilatation of a chamber).

Quantification of Shunts

Observing the path of tracer transit through the heart and great vessels permits the subjective assessment of the presence or absence of a shunt. The quality of blood shunted through an abnormal connection can be quantified if the quantity or transit of tracer through either the cardiac chambers, the lungs, or a systemic capillary bed is monitored at the time of tracer administration.

Right-to-Left Shunts

Tracers such as xenon or microspheres, when administered intravenously, should not traverse the lungs to arrive in the systemic circulation in the absence of a significant anatomic shunt for the microspheres or an anatomic or significant V/Q abnormality with xenon. Following intravenous administration of these tracers, no significant increase in activity should be seen over a systemic capillary bed unless a significant shunt is present. Precordial monitoring is less desirable for the detection of right-to-left shunts than that over a systemic capillary bed, since some activity will always appear under precordial detector owing to underlying lung.

A simple and safe method for shunt quantification utilizes the intravenous administration of microspheres and a scintillation detector placed over the head.[9] A small measured amount of blood pool tracer is administered intravenously, and the transit of tracer through the head is recorded using a digital rate meter. Immediately following the plateau of activity from this injection, a second measured dose of tracer tagged to microspheres is administered intravenously, and the increase in activity in the head is measured 60 s later. The curve resulting from the initial dose of tracer is plotted on semilog paper, and the initial downslope of tracer clearance is extrapolated to the abscissa. The area under the curve is integrated and the mean transit

time calculated. By multiplying the reciprocal of the mean transit time by the integrated area under the curve, the portion of the injected dose that was delivered to the vascular bed is determined. From the injection of the microspheres, any increase in counts results from particles that were not trapped by capillaries, which will be delivered in relation to cardiac output in a fashion similar to the non-microsphere-bound activity. Thus the increase in activity from the administration of microspheres, as a fraction of the injected dose, divided by the fraction of cardiac output arriving under the detector obtained from the initial injection provides a means of quantifying right-to-left shunts.

In patients without significant right-to-left shunts, there is no increase in activity following microsphere administration. With this technique less than 1 percent shunting was found in patients with chronic lung disease. However, when one patient was examined shortly after cardiac arrest, a shunt of 20 percent was found, which was not present on reevaluation several days later (possibly the result of transient shunting through a patent foramen ovale in this patient with altered pressures). Another potential use of this procedure is in the evaluation of patients with multiple pulmonary arteriovenous anastomoses. In our limited experience with this condition, the nuclear angiocardiogram appears normal in structure, but the transit time from the right to the left side of the heart is rapid. The shunt quantification revealed that 50 percent of administered particles reached the systemic circulation.

The lung scan can serve as an indicator of right-to-left shunting if the scan includes the kidneys. With the techniques employed to image the lungs, at least 15 percent of particles must pass to the systemic circulation before the kidneys will be seen.

Although the particle distribution for shunt detection has the potential hazard of embolizing to the arterial circulation, it appears to cause no damage when the number of particles is kept to a minimum (50,000) and they are administered slowly (over several seconds). A potential advantage of the particle method is the differentiation of shunting from nonventilated lung from that caused by anatomic connections. The xenon method would give an abnormal result when perfusion of nonventilated lung occurs, whereas the particle method would not.

Left-to-Right Shunts

The situation with left-to-right shunting is more difficult, since there are no tracers that only traverse left-to-right shunts. The techniques employed usually utilize the alteration in transit caused by the shunt. If a detector is placed over the lungs[10] or a region of interest set to record counts following intravenous administration of tracer, the alterations in the pulmonary transit curve induced by the shunt can serve as a qualitative or rough quantitative test. The time required for the initial upstroke of the curve from base line to apex is called T-1. After a second interval of time, equal to T-2, has elapsed, the activity should have decreased to 32 percent of that at T-1. If the activity concentration is greater than this, and the injection was a good bolus, the presence of a shunt is confirmed, the magnitude of which is related to the alteration in the curve.[11]

The magnitude of the shunt can be quantified by the method of Malte et al.[12] by integrating the peaks which occur in the lung. The area under the initial curve represents total flow through the lung and the area under the second early recirculation peak is caused by the shunt. To calculate the pulmonary systemic flow ratio, the difference between the two curves is calculated to determine the systemic flow, and the initial value from the first curve is divided by the calculated systemic flow. The measurement of the areas under the curves is best made with the aid of a computer, since the curves are complex and the first must be stripped from the second point by point (gamma variate fit program).[13]

In addition to shunt quantification, superior vena cava obstruction[14] and differentiation of vascular from nonvascular lesions in the thorax[15] can be determined with this technique.

The nuclear angiocardiogram may also be used to differentiate ventricular septal defect from papillary muscle rupture in patients recovering from acute myocardial infarction.[16] The sudden onset of a murmur and deterioration in the condition in these patients suggests that either the septum or a papillary muscle has ruptured. The intravenous administration of a very small volume of tracer and sequential images in the LAO position can clearly define the recirculation into the right ventricle. The bolus volume must be made as small as possible in these patients, since they are usually in congestive failure. The bolus will be prolonged even under the best of circumstances, and a large volume of tracer would lengthen the bolus so much that it may make evaluation of reentry of tracer into the right heart very difficult.

DETERMINATION OF CARDIAC FUNCTION (Table 3)

The radiocardiogram initially described by Prinzmetal in 1947[17] employed a Geiger tube placed over the precordial region at a strip chart recorder to define the initial tracer passage of sodium-24 following intravenous injection through the heart and lungs. From this

TABLE 3
Measurement of cardiac function

Indications		Findings
1 Acute infarction	a	Establish prognosis—inversely related to ejection fraction.
	b	Determine efficacy of acute interventions by changes in EF, end-diastolic volumes, and regional wall motion.
2 Congestive failure	a	Separate diffuse from focal ventricular dysfunction by correlating EF and regional wall motion abnormalities.
	b	Estimate foward and regurgitant flow in patients with valvular regurgitation.
	c	Differentiate right from left ventricular dysfunction by chamber volume and EF.
3 Suspected cor pulmonale	a	Measure right ventricular function; determine effect of therapy on function.
4 Left ventricular function reserve	a	Detect occult coronary disease by a fall in EF or new regional wall motion abnormality at stress.
	b	Detect incipient failure with aortic regurgitation by increase in pulmonary blood volume or fall in EF at stress.
	c	Monitor patients taking cardiotoxic drugs such as adriamycin for incipient failure.
5 Systemic embolization	a	Detect aneurysm of the left ventricle.
	b	Identify atrial myxoma as a zone of decreased activity in the atrium with appropriate motion.

measurement, the transit time from the right to the left side of the heart was defined, and measurements of shunting were possible. However, because of the rapid diffusion of ^{24}Na from the vasculature, it was impossible to make adequate measurements of cardiac output. In 1952, MacIntyre and his colleagues reported on a simple method for the noninvasive measurement of cardiac output using radioiodinated serum albumin.[18] These investigators recorded the precordial dilution curve and, after an interval of equilibration, drew a venous blood sample. From measurement of the activity in a known volume of blood and the precordial curve, cardiac output can be readily determined. It was not until 1969, however, the Mullins and his colleagues described a method for recording end-diastolic and end-systolic volumes of the heart.[19] These investigators recorded the initial passage of the nuclide through the heart in synchrony with the ECG, employing an Anger scintillation camera. The data were then replayed through a computer system, and several cycles were added together at their end-diastolic points and several in systole. The added images were then photographed, their outlines defined, and the volumes to the chambers determined. This technique was improved upon by Shelbert and his colleagues, who reported on methods of calculating the ejection fraction directly from the amount of radioactivity in the ventricular chambers.[20] This "counts approach" has the advantage of being relatively independent of geometric assumptions. This initial transit approach has been evaluated by Zaret and his colleagues as a means of serially studying patients with myocardial infarction,[21] chronic stable angina,[22] and cardiomyopathy.[23] Recent technical improvements in scintillation-imaging devices permit recording of high count rates during the initial passage of tracer through the heart so that definition of portions of walls of the ventricle is greatly improved. Thus the first transit technique has also been useful in identifying regional wall motion abnormalities. One of the difficulties with the initial transit approach, however, is that only one measurement is possible per tracer injection, and relatively large doses of tracer are needed to make these measurements because of the requirement of a high photon flux during the passage of tracer through the heart. Thus, because of the radiation burden, it is difficult to make multiple measurements over a short period of time, such as required to assess an intervention. The recent development by Holman and his colleagues of the 9 min half-life generator system, tungsten-tantalum-178,[24,25] makes it likely that, in the future, multiple measurements will be possible with the initial transit technique in a short interval of time.

An alternative approach to the measurement of ventricular function is following equilibration of a blood pool tracer in the vasculature. This technique relies on the assumption that a continuously moving object can be successfully imaged if images are recorded rapidly enough and synchronized through movement of the object. This is analogous to shining a strobe light on a moving object and matching the frequency of strobe flashes with the motion to be examined. In the case of equilibrium blood pool imaging, synchronization is obtained by observing the patient's ECG and using the R wave as an indicator for the commencement of another cardiac cycle.[26] Thereafter, the cardiac cycle is divided up into a fixed number of segments, and data from each segment are recorded into a computer system.[27-29] Data from consecutive beats are summed until a higher resolution is obtained. The technique has the advantage of providing ex-

tremely high resolution images of the heart, which permit excellent delineation of regional wall motion abnormalities (Fig. 2). Computers presently employed are capable of recording up to 127 segments in each cardiac cycle. The number of cycles employed to record data can be controlled by the operator and may be as short as 100 cycles under certain exercise circumstances or as long as several thousand cycles, depending on the quality of data required and the stability of the patient at the time of measurement. It is critically important for these multiple gated images to have a blood pool tracer which will remain totally within the vasculature. Most laboratories are presently employing in vivo labeled red blood cells.[30] The labeling is carried out by injecting patients with a mixture of stannous ions (usually in the form of stannous pyrophosphate). Following intravenous injection, this material appears to enter the red blood cell and cause a change to occur in the hemoglobin. The ^{99m} Tc pertechnetate is administered intravenously 20 min thereafter and appears to bind to the hemoglobin of the red blood cell. The efficiency of labeling is commonly over 90 percent, and the stability of the label over an interval of 4 h is excellent.

The imaging procedure is performed by placing electrodes on the patient and ascertaining that the gate is properly functioning. Thereafter, the radioactive pharmaceutical is injected, and images are recorded in the anterior, 45° left anterior oblique, and 60° left posterior oblique positions. Immediately following the recording of data, the information is available for replay as a cineangiographic study on a computer screen. The "average cardiac cycle" is replayed over and over again at a rate that is adjustable by the operator so that global and regional function of each of the cardiac chambers can be evaluated. Viewing these films allows definition of wall motion abnormalities by simple inspection. In addition, programs are presently being developed to define the borders of the ventricle automatically so that objective determinations of regional function will be possible without requiring operator interaction.[31] Through multiple gated data, both ejection fraction and volumes of the left ventricle can be defined, using highly reproducible computer programs.[28] The volume curve data have been correlated with contrast angiographic left ventricular volumes ($R = 0.94$). These studies have already proved to be of value in patients with acute myocardial infarction as an objective measurement of ventricular function,[32] to differentiate aneurysm from diffuse hypokinesis of the left ventricle[33] in patients presenting with congestive cardiac failure,[34,35] to determine whether right ventricular dysfunction is a cause of low cardiac output in patient with inferior wall infarction,[36] to detect the presence of intraatrial masses[2,37] (Figs. 3 to 7), and to define the alteration and configuration of the left ventricular chamber caused by hypertrophic cardiomy-

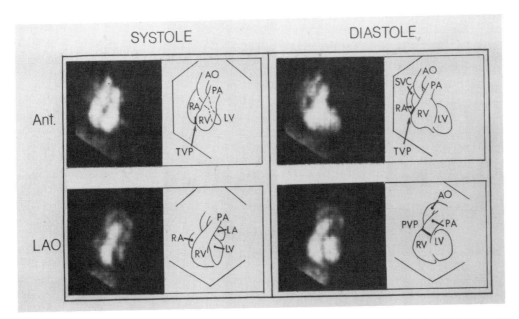

FIGURE 2 Gated blood pool scan recorded in the anterior position (top frames), in the 45° LAO position (bottom frames), at the end of systole (left-hand panels), and at the end of diastole (right-hand panels). In the anterior position, the tricuspid valve plane, right atrium, right ventricle, left ventricle, pulmonary outflow tract, and aorta are all defined. At end-systole, the right atrium is full, while at end-diastole, it is empty. The great vessels appear fuller at the end of systole than at the end of diastole. The left ventricle appears to move in all of its segments. The LAO position permits better separation of the right ventricle from the left than is possible in the anterior position. The septum is very well defined in this view (particularly helpful in evaluating patients with suspected hypertrophy).

opathies,[38] Since the tracer equilibrates in the blood pool following intravenous administration, multiple measurements are possible over the course of several hours. This means that the patients can be studied before and after interventions. Nichols et al. evaluated two groups of patients with the multiple gated acquisition study: a group with unstable angina, and a group with acute myocardial infarction, both with low cardiac output states requiring intraaortic balloon count to pulsation.[39] The data revealed that although hemodynamic improvement was found in all patients placed on the balloon pump, the extent of regional wall motion abnormality did not change in patients with infarction, while patients with unstable angina showed marked improvement.

Recent work by Borer et al. combines the use of multiple gated acquisition imaging with supine stress testing to identify patients with diminished left ventricular function reserve.[29] In normal patients, the ejection fraction increases with exercise by greater than 5 percent. In a group with coronary artery disease, ejection fraction fell and new regional wall motion abnormalities were seen in those with hemodynamically significant lesions. Comparison between the rest and exercise multiple gated examinations offers a very sensitive means of identifying occult coronary artery disease by the impact of hemodynamically significant lesions on ventricular function reserve at peak

stress. However, the results of this test are nonspecific, since other causes of compromised ventricular function, such as aortic insufficiency, cardiomyopathy, or extensive previous scar as a result of myocardial infarction without additional ischemia, may cause an abnormal response at peak stress.

Because of the observation that ventricular function is commonly altered by myocardial ischemia, with a resultant fall in ejection fraction and an increase in systolic volume, a question was raised about the possible change in pulmonary blood volume. Nichols et al. investigated a series of normal subjects with upright bicycle exercise and found that, normally, pulmonary blood volume diminishes at peak exercise.[40] In a group of patients with hemodynamically significant coronary artery lesions, however, an increase in regional pulmonary blood volume was observed. On inspection of the temporary relation of an increase in pulmonary blood volume to the alterations in cardiac volumes, it was observed that the pulmonary blood volume increased prior to the alteration in ejection fraction. To determine whether changes in pulmonary blood volume would offer a sensitive means of detecting occult coronary artery disease, studies were performed by Okada in a series of patients undergoing rest and stress multiple gated blood pool imaging.[41] Okada observed a fall in pulmonary blood volume in all subjects with hemodynamically insignificant coronary disease. In pa-

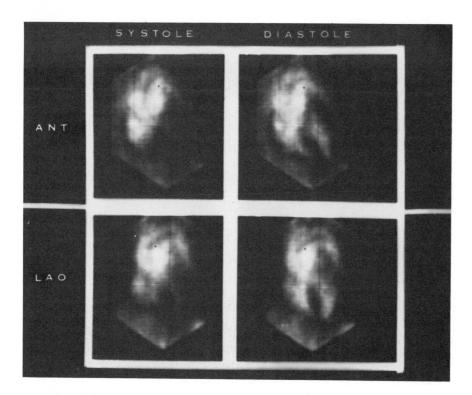

336

FIGURE 3 Gated scan performed at end-systole (left-hand panels) and at end-diastole (right-hand panels) in the anterior position (top panels) and at a 45° LAO position (bottom panels) in a patient with suspected hypertrophic cardiomyopathy. Since the gated scans evaluate the blood pool, an area where a blood pool is minimal shows up as a zone of decreased tracer concentration. The myocardium, pericardium, and associated fat pads are such areas. In the absence of pericardial effusion, an increased space between the left ventricular outline and the adjacent lung or between the left ventricular and right ventricular silhouettes in the LAO view suggests the possibility of myocardial hypertrophy. In this patient, the end-systolic volumes of the left ventricle are reduced, the ejection fraction is high, and the space between left and right ventricles suggests marked distortion of the normal septal architecture. This constellation of findings raises the possibility of hypertrophic cardiomyopathy. In particular, the unusual septal configuration is commonly encountered in this condition.

tients with hemodynamically significant coronary lesions involving the left coronary system, 85 percent of the patients developed an increase in pulmonary blood volume, while only 70 percent revealed a decrease in ejection fraction. In patients with right coronary disease, none of the patients developed an increase in pulmonary blood volume. The technique, then appears to offer a specific means of identifying occult left ventricular failure. It is unlikely, however, that the increase in pulmonary blood volume will be at all specific for coronary disease, since any circumstance which decreases left ventricular function in the face of normal right ventricular function should produce an increase in pulmonary blood volume.

One of the major clinical indications for the multiple gated blood pool scan at rest is the evaluation of left ventricular function in patients with increasing shortness of breath and known ischemic coronary disease. The investigation is commonly employed to screen patients for catheterization. If left ventricular function is relatively well preserved, then the patient is an excellent candidate for catheterization; but if left ventricular function is seriously impaired and the ejection fraction is reduced, the patients are unlikely to be good surgical candidates, in which case catheterization is often unnecessary.

NONIMAGING METHODS TO MEASURE VENTRICULAR FUNCTION

Two nonimaging approaches to the measurement of ventricular function have been described. The first

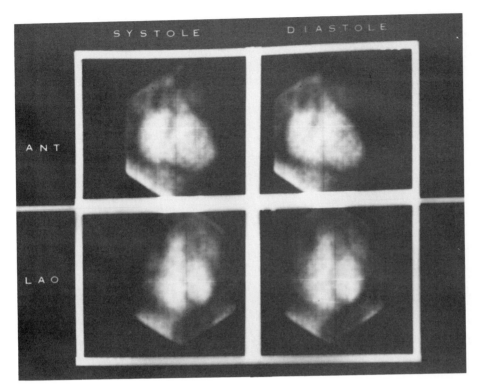

FIGURE 4 Gated blood pool scan at end-systole (left-hand panels), end-diastole (right-hand panels), in the anterior position (top panels), and in the 45° LAO position (bottom panels) in a patient with suspected cardiomyopathy. There is enlargement and poor motion of all four cardiac chambers. Although this syndrome agreed with the patient's clinical symptoms, it is important to ascertain that no technical artifact was responsible for this apparent poor function on scan. This can be done by determining that the gate was properly triggered and that the computer was properly functioning at the time of data recording.

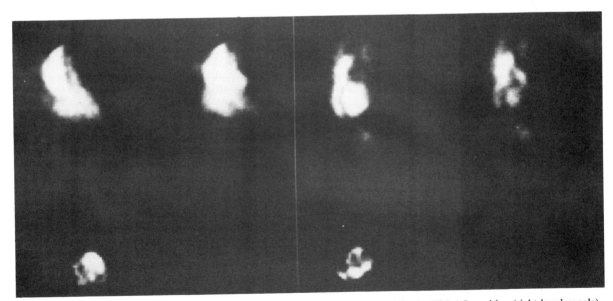

FIGURE 5 Gated scan performed in the anterior position (left-hand panels) and in the 45° LAO position (right-hand panels). The gated scan reveals excellent wall motion. This is ordinarily ascertained by comparing the outline of the end-diastolic images to that at end-systole. However, an alternative to this is to subtract the end-systolic image from the end-diastolic image to make a stroke volume image (bottom panels). This stroke volume image summarizes the data in a manner that can be directly comprehended by showing the change of wall motion from the end of diastole to the end of systole.

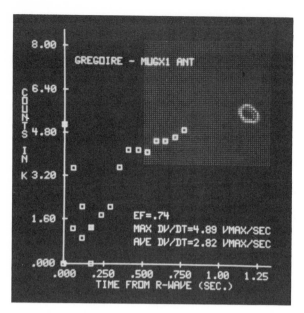

FIGURE 6 A left ventricular time-vs.-activity curve obtained from multiple gated acquisition imaging. Each point represents the net counts in the left ventricle and that portion of the cardiac cycle after the R wave. The ejection fraction is computed from the difference between end-diastolic counts and end-systolic counts, divided by the end-diastolic counts. These data require approximately 45 s to calculate using the nuclear medicine computer systems.

approach employs a simple scintillation probe detector with a high-fidelity analogue strip chart recorder to measure the initial passage of the tracer through the heart and great vessels.[42] This technique can be used to measure ejection fraction, cardiac output, and pulmonary blood volume at the bedside. A major disadvantage of this method is that the probe must be appropriately localized prior to tracer injection, a procedure which requires recording either a chest radiograph or an echocardiogram to localize the apex of the left ventricle.

The second approach employs a tracer which is equilibrated throughout the vasculature and a multi-scaler which records data in synchrony with the cardiac cycle (triggered by the patient's ECG).[43] This method has the advantage of providing an opportunity to make several "test measurements" to correctly localize the probe over the left ventricle. Thereafter, data are recorded from several hundred cardiac cycles to produce a time-vs.-activity curve, which is useful for the measurement of ejection fraction as well as ejection and filling rates. This technique is particularly useful because it permits definitive monitoring of patients over a prolonged period of time with relatively simple equipment. It may be possible in the future, with miniaturization of the components, to employ this technique for on-line continuous patient monitoring over a period of several hours or days.

MYOCARDIAL PERFUSION

Myocardial perfusion can be determined both invasively and noninvasively using radioactive tracers. Radioactive pharmaceuticals employed for the invasive determination of perfusion are usually xenon,[44] microspheres,[45] and more recently, krypton 81m.[46] Neither xenon nor microspheres can be administered intravenously for the study of myocardial perfusion, since particulates are larger than capillary size and hence could not traverse the lungs and most of the xenon administered intravenously would be lost in the passage through the alveolar capillaries prior to reaching the coronary circulation, because the air-blood partition coefficient is 8.75 to the other body temperatures.

Particles administered at the time of coronary arteriography will remain in place, obstructing a very small percentage of the precapillary arterioles until they are degraded in situ (approximate half-life 4 to 18 h depending on the particle preparation employed). The margin of safety in this procedure is great, even in patients with obliteration of a significant fraction of the coronary arterial tree. Jansen et al. have employed myocardial microsphere distribution techniques in several thousand patients without a mishap, which could be attributed to the intracoronary administration of particles.[45] However, it causes a potential problem in that it is important to keep the number of particles administered below 100,000. Images performed several hours following intracoronary administration will reflect conditions of perfusion at the time of tracer injection. Thus the scintillation camera can be located at a remote site from the catheterization laboratory. In the technique described by Jansen et al., tracer microspheres with one label were administered in the left coronary bed, and a second injection with a different label was administered in the right. The distribution of each tracer is determined by differential gamma spectometry at the time of imaging. One disadvantage of this tracer approach is that the relative distribution of blood flow between the two coronary beds investigated is not defined. Once the particles are administered into the proximal coronary artery, 100 percent of the dose will go into the distal coronary bed. This means that although a 99 percent stenosis may be present in the proximal vessel, the entire dose will be distributed distally. Therefore, the effect of proximal disease on distal flow distribution is not apparent with this technique.

To overcome this problem, the particles may be administered via the left ventricle or the left atrium at the time of catheterization. This approach has the advantage of showing the regional distribution of myocardial perfusion in the entire heart as a fraction of cardiac output, an important improvement over the direct intracoronary method. However, the direct intracoronary method is very useful to indicate where the flow arrives to a given zone via collaterals or only via the native circulation. The critical question that commonly arises at catheterization is whether a specific lesion is hemodynamically significant. This question is not clearly answered by the administration of particulate tracers under basal circumstances. The studies of Gould et al. in the dog demonstrated that the intracoronary administration of angiographic contrast material results in a considerable increase in coronary blood flow within 15 s of administration. Administration of microspheres at the time of maximal blood flow induced by injection of contrast media demonstrated alterations in the particle perfusion pattern caused by significant distal narrowings in the coronary vessels. Thus the hemodynamic significance of these distal lesions could be readily defined by combining

information from a rest and postcontrast hyperemia tracer procedure.

An alternative to the particulate approach uses an inert gas to evaluate regional coronary blood flow. Xenon gas (dissolved in saline solution) administered directly into the coronary arteries rapidly equilibrates with tissue.[44] After bolus injection, the rate of clearance of xenon from the tissue is related to blood flow and tissue, i.e., the blood partition coefficient. Regions of slow clearance have either lower flows or much greater solubility (such as fat) in normal myocardium. The determination of xenon clearance must be made immediately following tracer administration, which requires the presence of an imaging device in the catheterization laboratory. Ross, in his initial investigations of xenon clearance of global myocardium,

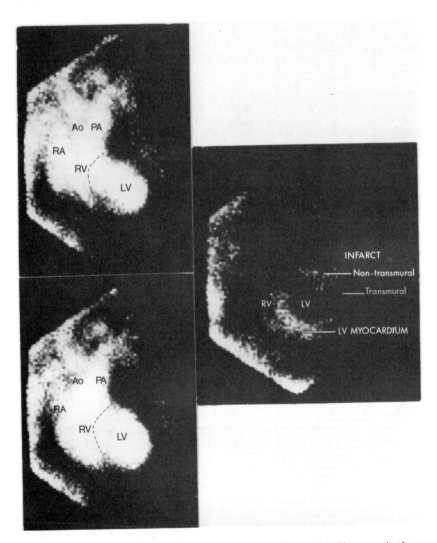

FIGURE 7 Gated blood pool scan in the anterior position and thallium scan in the same position performed on a patient with myocardial infarction. RA, right atrium; RV, right ventricle; AO, aorta; PA, pulmonary artery; — indicates the mitral and aortic valve planes, LV, left ventricle. The abnormality of regional wall motion is seen to correspond well with the zone of absent thallium concentration. (*From H. W. Strauss et al., "Atlas of Cardiovascular Medicine," The C. V. Mosby Company, St. Louis, 1978, with permission of the publisher.*)

found that it was difficult to separate normal subjects from those with abnormal myocardial perfusion, thus suggesting that global myocardial perfusion measurements were not satisfactory for the study of coronary artery disease.[48] The use of an imaging device with spatial resolution at least sufficient to divide the myocardium into 1-cm zones makes the determination of regional perfusion clinically useful. Cannon and his colleagues have found that patients with severe coronary artery narrowing may have a decrease in coronary artery blood flow, even in the absence of regional wall motion abnormalities.[49] In addition, the xenon approach permits repetitive measurement to be made over a short period of time so that the effects of nitroglycerin, pacing, and other interventions could be readily studied. Recently, Kaplan and his colleagues have reported using [81m] Kr as a means of measuring regional myocardial blood flow.[46] Krypton 81m is a radionuclide with a 13-s half-life, which, following direct intracoronary administration, rapidly equilibrates in myocardial tissue and clears with a half-time related to partition coefficient in blood flow. However, since the physical half-life of the radioactive pharmaceutical is short in comparison to the clearance half-time, the primary information gleaned from an image of the tracer during continuous infusion is the regional distribution of blood flow. Thus, moment-to-moment changes in the distribution of regional coronary blood flow can be recorded when the tracer is continuously infused in the coronary arteries and images are continuously recorded. This method offers the exciting prospect of being able to identify the onset of regional myocardial blood flow maldistribution and to relate this to global changes in ventricular function, such as increases in end-diastolic pressure.

MYOCARDIAL IMAGING WITH IONIC TRACERS (Table 4)

Imaging in the myocardium with intravenously administered nuclides was first accomplished by Carr and his colleagues in the early 1960s. Cesium-131, a low-energy x-ray radinuclide, was employed for the initial studies in both animals and patients.[50] Although it was possible to image anterior myocardial infarction, posterior and lateral infarcts were difficult to identify because of the physical properties of the tracer. These difficulties led Love and his colleagues to develop an improved collimator to image myocardial distribution of potassium 42,[51] a tracer with extremely high energy gamma. In Love's investigations, zones of myocardial infarction could be demonstrated, but areas supplied by narrowed coronary vessels appeared normal on the scan. This is not surprising, since according to the Sapirstein principle,[52] these tracers should be distrib-

TABLE 4
Clinical uses of thallium imaging

Indications		Findings
1 Suspected cardiomyopathy	a	Differentiate diffuse from focal myocardial disease.
2 Unstable angina	a	Define the zone of ischemia by comparing the areas of initial involvement to that found on redistribution imaging (in the absence of pain or ECG ischemia). Particularly useful in spasm.
3 Acute infarction	a	Identify the site and extent of damage, demonstration of periinfarction ischemia by serial imaging. Less useful for recurrent infarction.
4 Detect occult coronary disease	a	Identify focal areas of decreased thallium concentration which improve on serial imaging. More sensitive and specific than stress ECG alone. Particularly useful in patients with LBBB, in those taking digitalis, and in those who develop either silent ST-segment changes, or pain with no ECG abnormalities.
5 Evaluate significance of specific lesions in patients with known coronary artery disease	a	Low flow zones appear as decreased activity early which improves on serial images in the absence of chest pain and wall motion abnormalities.
	b	Define the zones of ischemia in patients with coronary disease.
6 Evaluation of patients after coronary bypass surgery	a	Define myocardial perfusion status to identify patency of grafts, and intraoperative infarction.

uted in relation to regional blood flow. Zones supplied by stenotic coronary vessels will usually have adequate blood flow at rest unless the stenoses are extreme. To detect regional myocardial malperfusion, an alteration in regional blood flow must be brought about by increasing myocardial demands. To achieve this, Zaret et al.[53] injected ionic potassium-43 at the time of peak exercise in patients with significant coronary artery disease and found, on scans performed immediately, alterations in the regional tracer distribution which were not apparent on repeat examination performed following tracer injection at rest. Subsequently, thallium-201 has been employed for detection of regional myocardial perfusion because of its physical properties.[54] As with the initial [43]K studies, injection of the tracer is commonly carried out at the time of peak stress, with imaging performed immediately thereafter. The type of stress used to induce the regional differences in myocardial blood flow does not appear to be a significant factor. Bicycle, treadmill, pacing, and pharmocologic stresses have all been utilized with success. The level of stress, however, is critically important. With a lesion of borderline hemodynamic significance, injection of tracer at a heart rate below that which produces maldistribution of myocardial perfusion will result in a normal-appearing image, while injection of tracer at the very peak effort that can be exerted by the patient may result in an abnormal study. It is important to note, however, that myocardial imaging offers information that is significantly different from that recorded with a coronary arteriogram: the arteriogram supplies detailed information about *structural abnormalities* of the coronary arteries, while the scan supplies information about the *perfusion* at the level of the muscle cell. The scan can be normal in the face of a totally obstructed coronary artery if collateral flow is sufficient; on the other hand, the scan may be abnormal in the face of a patent coronary vessel if recanalization of a vessel has occurred following an infarct. Recent clinical evidence from a number of centers has demonstrated that injection of thallium at the time of maximum exercise stress with immediate imaging, in comparison to a subsequent study performed at rest, was successful in identifying zones of myocardial ischemia as focal areas of decreased concentration on the stress-injected scan which were not present on the rest injected study (Figs. 8 to 11).[55] The scan data was more sensitive than stress ECGs performed simultaneously for the detection of myocardial ischemia. A comparison of the site and extent of abnormalities on scan to that appearing on the coronary arteriogram revealed a non-linear relationship between the two studies. One zone of the myocardium frequently became ischemic before the others and caused the patient to cease exercising, so that focal abnormalities might appear in only one zone, whereas anatomic examination reveals that the patient indeed has multivessel involvement. It appears that thallium imaging is most helpful in the evaluation of patients with suspected ischemic heart disease who have abnormal resting ECGs, since the stress ECG is difficult to interpret in these individuals. In addition, a thallium scan may be helpful in the evaluation of patients with suspected cardiomyopathy to differentiate focal from diffuse disease.

Studies by Maseri et al. in patients with coronary spasm[56] and by Pohost et al. in patients with myocardial ischemia induced by exercise[57] reveal that thallium "redistributes" into zones of myocardium which are viable but supplied by severely stenotic vessels. Therefore, most laboratories now perform serial im-

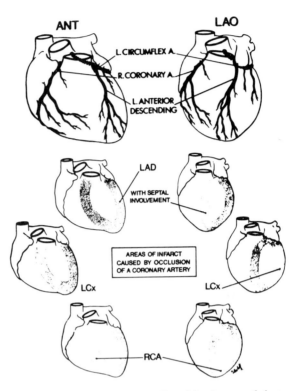

FIGURE 8 Diagrammatic outline of focal zones of abnormality encountered in myocardial infarction or ischemia on thallium image. The thallium scan in the anterior position (left-hand panels), 45° LAO position (center panels), and 70° LAO position (right-hand panels) in a patient examined with injection at rest (top) and at peak exercise (bottom). There is a normal distribution of thallium in the myocardium. (*From H. W. Strauss et al., "Atlas of Cardiovascular Nuclear Medicine," The C. V. Mosby Company, St. Louis, 1978, with permission of the publisher.*)

ages following a single injection of ^{201}Tl to differentiate areas of viable myocardium supplied by vessels with hemodynamically significant stenoses from areas of myocardial scar which show no change on serial images. Since these initial observations, it has become apparent that even at rest, patients with severe coronary stenosis may have malperfusion which can be detected by serial imaging.[58] This approach may be helpful in identifying the site and extent of myocardial ischemia in patients with unstable angina and the peri-infarction ischemic zone in patients with no acute myocardial infarction. In addition, the thallium scan will be particularly helpful in patients who have undergone coronary bypass surgery and who have recurrent chest discomfort. Recent work by Greenburg and his colleagues indicates that patients with patent grafts and no significant progression of disease in the native circulation have no evidence of ischemia on stress-injected thallium images.[59]

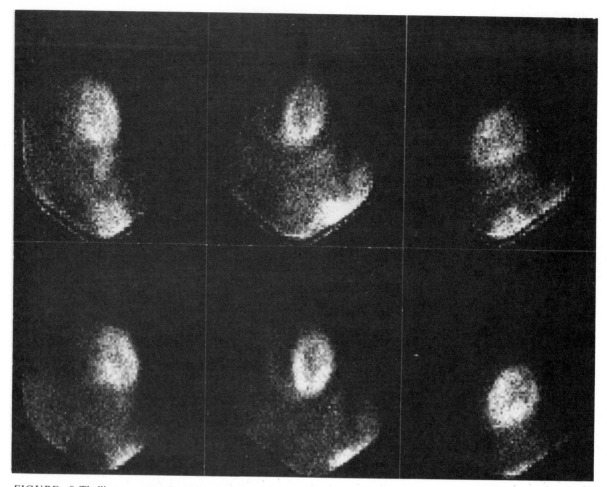

FIGURE 9 Thallium scans performed at peak exercise (bottom panels) and at rest (top panels) in the anterior position, 45° LAO position, and 70° LAO position in a normal subject.

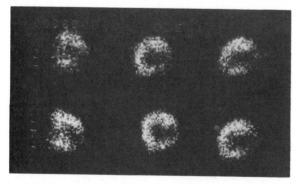

FIGURE 10 Thallium scans performed following injection at peak stress (top panels) and at redistribution (bottom panels) in the anterior position (left-hand panels), in the 45° LAO position (center panels), and in the 70° LAO position (right-hand panels). There is a focal zone of decreased tracer concentration involving the apex and posterior wall which is persistent. These abnormalities suggest the presence of myocardial scar in this individual with previous documented myocardial infarction and recurrent atypical chest pain. The ECG performed concurrently with the thallium scan revealed no new ischemic zones.

The myocardium represents an unusual problem for nuclear imaging since it is cone with activity in the periphery which is continuously moving during the relatively lengthy process of imaging. Gating of the scintillation camera can be useful in eliminating some of the blurring of cardiac motion, particularly if images are recorded through the entire diastolic interval. Even with gating techniques, however, the contrast between the myocardium and background is limited. Since the human eye works on a long scale for brightness, the viewer can be aided in the perception of alterations in myocardial perfusion by observing the thallium images from the screen of a computer which permits on-line contrast enhancement. Contrast enhancement, however, is a two-edged sword: (1) the myocardium normally has some heterogeneity of flow (as much as 15 percent in adjacent 1-cm regions); and (2) the statistical fluctuation of counts in an area of myocardium may vary up to 14 percent, depending on the count density of the scan. These two factors result in a scan that has a mottled appearance which may be very difficult to interpret. Smoothing the data, using digital averaging

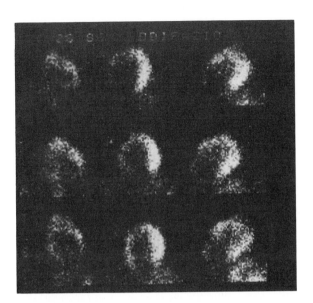

FIGURE 11 Thallium scan injected at peak stress (top panels) and imaged 30 min thereafter (center panels) and at 2½ h (bottom panels) in the anterior position (left panels), the 45° LAO position (center panels), and the 70° LAO position (right-hand panels) in a patient with documented myocardial infarction. The patient was evaluated at the time for recurrent chest pain with exercise. The thallium scan reveals a large zone of decreased tracer concentration involving the apex and inferior wall of the anterior and 70° LAO views and involving the septum and apical inferior segment on the 45° LAO view. There is a significant amount of "redistribution" involving the septum, while the apical inferior lesions remain unchanged. This combination of findings raises the likelihood of myocardial scar with associated septal ischemia.

techniques, or squinting at the image helps reduce some of these problems. Phantom studies performed by Cook demonstrated the lesions less than one-half the full thickness of the myocardium and smaller than 2.5 cm in diameter could not be delineated.[60] Subsequent work in animals by Markus et al. revealed that lesions smaller than 5 g of myocardium could not be detected. Because of the limitations of object contrast, a flow of maldistribution greater than 25 percent to an area of at least 2.5 cm in diameter is required for minimal visualization of a lesion on the thallium scan.

ACUTE INFARCT IMAGING (Table 5)

In this decade, successful localization of acute myocardial infarction in human beings has been achieved with a number of ^{99m}Tc radiopharmaceuticals including ^{99m}Tc glucoheptonate, ^{99m}Tc tetracycline, and ^{99m}Tc pyrophosphate. [99m]Tc tetracycline is limited for clinical use, because of slow clearance from blood, which results in a delay of at least 24 h following injection

before imaging can commence.[61] However, the concentration in acutely damaged myocardium is in direct proportion to the degree of tissue necrosis. [99m]Tc tetracycline, therefore, is a better indicator of the extent of necrosis than ^{99m}Tc pyrophosphate, the uptake of which is flow-limited in regions of poor perfusion.[62,63] [99m]Tc tetracycline accumulates in acutely infarcted myocardium but not in ischemic uninfarcted tissue, and there is a direct correlation between the reduction in blood flow and the relative increase in concentration of the radiopharmaceutical.[64] Furthermore, in animal studies a direct correlation has been demonstrated between ^{99m}Tc tetracycline concentration and the size of infarction. A sevenfold increase in concentration of ^{99m}Tc tetracycline over normal myocardium is found in damaged regions which are greater in extent than 40 percent of the myocardium, whereas only a twofold increase is found when the damaged zone is less than 15 percent of the myocardium. Such high levels of concentration have not been found in experimental work with ^{99m}Tc glucoheptonate, an infarctavid radiopharmaceutical which has some theoretical advantages:[65] the radiopharmaceutical concentrates in an infarcted myocardium as early as 5 h after the onset of chest pain in amounts sufficient for imaging and is not concentrated in the skeleton, as is ^{99m}Tc pyrophosphate. The low contrast between infarcted and noninfarcted myocardium 24 h after the onset of symptoms has limited the application of ^{99m}Tc glucoheptonate in clinical practice.[66]

The observations by Bonte that the bone-imaging radiopharmaceutical ^{99m}Tc pyrophosphate also accumulates in acutely damaged myocardium introduced infarct-avid imaging techniques into clinical cardiology.[67] The uptake of ^{99m}Tc pyrophosphate ([99m]Tc PyP) in necrotic myocardial tissue, unlike ^{99m}Tc tetracycline, which is thought to complex to denatured macromolecules, may be related to the presence of crystalline and precrystalline calcium mitochondria following myocardial infarction in cells that are irreversibly damaged, but also beyond the borders of the infarct in cells which are ischemic and only injured. Also, there

TABLE 5
Acute infarct imaging

Indications	Findings
Suspected acute infarction or extension	Identify zones of acute necrosis within 72 h of onset as areas of increased tracer concentration. Particularly useful following open heart surgery or to identify patients with sudden death syndrome who have sustained infarction.
Chest trauma	Zones of myocardial necrosis appear as areas of increased tracer localization.

is a temporal relationship between the uptake of ^{99m}Tc pyrophosphate following occurrence of myocardial necrosis and the curve of calcium deposition and resorption as infarction resolves.

Imaging may be performed 2 h after intravenous injection of ^{99m}Tc pyrophosphate, when the concentration in the cardiac blood pool has decreased to a level that will not obscure uptake in infarcted myocardium. Images are usually obtained in multiple projections with a high-resolution gamma scintillation camera. The resulting images are classified as to intensity and degree of localization,[68] with 2+ representing definite myocardial activity that is less than adjacent sternum, 3+ equal to adjacent sternum, and 4+ greater than sternal activity. ^{99m}Tc PyP infarct images may become positive as early as 12 h following myocardial necrosis, with peak accumulation usually at 2 to 3 days following injury. Positivity will usually subside by the seventh day but may persist in a small proportion of patients for months,[66] an occurrence which may be related to the development of ventricular aneurysm and dystrophic calcification or persistent myocardial necrosis. The overall incidence of false positive scanning, which is 8 to 20 percent, has also been reported secondary to regional wall dyssynergy, cardiomyopathy, recent high-energy cardioversion, calcification of the mitral annulus, pericardial calcification, diseases of the pleura, and tumor or fractures of the ribs.[69-71] Myocardial scintigraphy with ^{99m}Tc PyP is not specific for myocardial infarction but is a marker for muscle necrosis, including cardiac trauma and even metastatic tumor to the heart. The technique results in positive images in approximately one-third of patients with unstable angina pectoris.[72] Since there is a temporal correlation between ^{99m}Tc PyP myocardial imaging and the onset of resolution of infarction, sequential imaging over 2-week period provides a means of separating those patients with recent acute necrosis from those with positive uptake secondary to other causes.

^{99m}Tc pyrophosphate imaging is a sensitive test for detection of acute transmural infarction. In an analysis of 242 patients undergoing ^{99m}Tc PyP myocardial imaging, 108 of 115 patients with acute myocardial infarction had test results which were positive for the presence of myocardial necrosis. The 5 patients with infarction who had negative test results had been imaged more than 1 week after onset of chest pain and symptoms. Of the 129 patients without evidence of infarction, 117 had negative studies, whereas the remaining 12 who had moderately positive scans had unstable angina pectoris.[72] The persistent positivity following acute myocardial infarction that occurs in a variable percentage of patients appears to be related to the severity of disease as evidenced by congestive heart failure, persistent angina pectoris, and evidence of ventricular dyssynergy.[73] In 46 patients studied with ^{99m}Tc PyP scintigraphy, 41 percent retained low-grade intensity for up to 3 months after acute infarction. Significantly the most symptomatic postinfarction course, characterized by persistent severe angina pectoris and heart failure, was noted in those patients who had persistent activity. Myocardial tissue obtained at surgery or at necropsy from patients with persistently positive ^{99m}Tc PyP myocardial images has demonstrated significant myocardial degeneration and cytolosis or fibrosis of myocardial cells.[74] As might be expected, the intensity and extent of the myocardial uptake of ^{99m}Tc PyP may be correlated to the extent of acute myocardial infarction. A complication rate including cardiogenic shock, serious ventricular arrhythmias, extension of infarction in development of unstable angina pectoris, or death directly correlates to the myocardial image. The greatest complication rate occurs in those patients who have a massive increase in myocardial uptake with intensity equal to or greater than the sternum, as opposed to those patients in whom there is focal discrete uptake that is less intense than that in the sternum.[75] Although there is a general correlation between the extent of activity and the size of the myocardial infarction with ^{99m}Tc PyP, the ability to estimate the absolute size of a myocardial infarct by this radiopharmaceutical is limited because the concentration of the radiopharmaceutical is related to both the degree of tissue damage and the myocardial blood flow. A comparison of radiolabelled microspheres to ^{99m}Tc pyrophosphate in canine models of myocardial infarction demonstrates that uptake, of that ^{99m}Tc PyP is high when flow is reduced to 30 to 40 percent of normal but that the concentration falls as flow is further reduced. Regional myocardial perfusion is therefore an important determinant of the distribution within the myocardium of ^{99m}Tc PyP after coronary occlusion. It is improbable that infarcts weighing less than 3 g could be imaged with current nuclear medicine techniques. There is reasonable evidence that ^{99m}Tc PyP myocardial imaging is capable of sizing transmural acute anterior and anterior lateral myocardial infarctions but not inferior, nontransmural, or subendocardial myocardial infarctions. Possibly tomographic reconstructive techniques may provide a tool by which more accurate quantification of infarct size may be made. Accurate quantification may also become possible with the development of improved radiopharmaceuticals, such as was experimentally demonstrated with ^{131}I-labelled antibody to myosin, which concentrates with greatest activity within necrotic myocardium and which is not flow-limited, as is ^{99m}Tc PyP.[76.]

Improved myocardial infarct localization may be obtained by combining infarct-avid imaging with gated cardiac blood pool scanning, in which the extent of regional wall motion abnormality may be correlated with findings on ^{99m}Tc PyP scanning and comparison

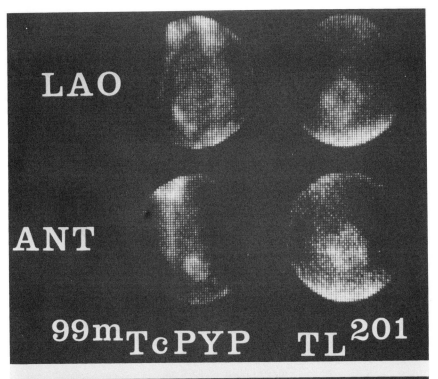

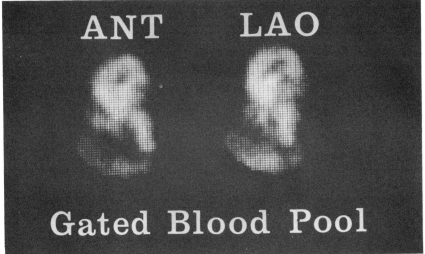

FIGURE 12 The patient is a 78 year-old woman with a previous history of congestive heart failure and chronic digitalization who complained of moderate chest pain 2 days prior to these studies. Upon admission, her ECG was unchanged from an ECG obtained 1 year prior to admission. Anterior and 50° LAO ^{99m}Tc pyrophosphate and ^{201}Tl chloride images were obtained sequentially without moving the gamma camera or the patient. There was 4+ concentration of the infarct-avid ^{99m}Tc Pyp in the septum and anterior wall, corresponding to perfusion defects on the ^{201}Tl images. The apical ^{201}Tl defect corresponds to an extensive apical aneurysm on the gated blood pool images, which also demonstrated severe hypokinesis of the septum and high anterior lateral wall. Repeat ^{99m}Tc Pyp images on day 10 and at 1 month became progressively negative, consistent with acute myocardial necrosis at the time of the initial study. Diagnosis: Acute septal and anterior infarction, previous apical infarction, with apical aneurysm. (Courtesy of Dr. Joseph D'Antonio, director, Division of Nuclear Medicine, St. Joseph's Hospital, Baltimore, Maryland.)

[201]Tl perfusion imaging. In one series of 80 patients with documented acute myocardial infarction, in whom 25 had nontransmural and 55 had transmural infarction, a combined ^{201}Tl perfusion and [99m]Tc PyP study was 100 percent sensitive for the detection of infarction, and there was close agreement as to infarct localization between the two techniques. Combined ^{201}Tl and [99m]Tc PyP imaging should permit differentiation of old from recent infarctions.

Currently, infarctavid imaging with [99m]Tc PyP provides a sensitive test for detection of acute myocardial infarction, provides a means for improved localization in size of infarction, and provides a practicing cardiologist with a prognostic indicator concerning the eventual course of a patient who has sustained a recent heart attack. It is primarily recommended for the detection of myocardial infarction (see Table) when the clinical diagnosis is obscured by limitations of the tests normally used for the diagnosis of acute myocardial infarction, such as creatine phosphokinase enzymes and electrocardiography.

PROSPECTS

The recent description of techniques to perform planar tomographic imaging and transverse section imaging using either gamma- or positron-emitting radionuclides opens up new vistas for study of the cardiovascular system with radionuclides. Tomographic imaging will permit far better quantification of lesion size and location than is presently possible with standard planar images. In addition, the ability to use "physiologic" tracers such as carbon-11, nitrogen-13, or oxygen-15 to measure substrate metabolism in the heart allows a better understanding of myocardial pathophysiology. Recent studies performed with glucose analogues and fatty acid analogues suggest that regional myocardial metabolism can be investigated and may offer new markers of regional myocardial ischemia or increased protein turnover which are not possible by other techniques. The development of short-lived radionuclide generator systems suitable for use in ventricular function measurements and the miniaturization of radiation detectors will permit on line moment-to-moment assessment of ventricular function in awake, alert, ambulatory individuals. Finally, the combined use of nuclear imaging techniques and hemodynamic measurements available routinely in the catheterization laboratory will offer improved understanding of cardiac function by allowing the ready generation of complex studies such as pressure-volume loops.

REFERENCES

1 Blumgart, H. C., and Weiss, S.: Studies on the Velocity of Blood. VII. The Pulmonary Circulation Time in Normal Resting Individuals, *J. Clin. Invest.,* 4:399, 1927.

2 Zaret, B. L., Hurley, P. J., and Pitt, B.: Non-invasive Scintiphotographic Diagnosis of Left Atrial Myxoma, *J. Nucl. Med.,* 13:81, 1972.

3 Christensen, E. E., and Bonte, F. J.: The Relative Accuracy of Echocardiography, Intravenous CO_2 Studies and Blood Pool Scanning in Detecting Pericardial Effusion in Dogs, *Radiology,* 91:265, 1968.

4 Hurley, P. J., Strauss, H. W., and Wagner, H. N.: Radionuclide Angiocardiography in Cyanotic Congenital Heart Disease, *Johns Hopkins Med. J.,* 127:46, 1970.

5 Bender, M., and Blau, M.: The Autofluoroscope, *Nucleonics,* 21:52, 1963.

6 Wesselhoeft, H., Hurley, P. J., Wagner, H. N., et al.: Nuclear Angiocardiography in the Diagnosis of Congenital Heart Disease in Infants, *Circulation,* 45:77, 1972.

7 Rosenthall, L.: Applications of the Gamma Ray Scintillation Camera to Dynamic Studies in Man, *Radiology,* 86:634, 1966.

8 Wagner, H. N.: The Heart and Circulation, in H. N. Wagner (ed.), "Nuclear Medicine," HP Publishing Company, New York, 1975, p. 113.

9 Strauss, H. W., Hurley, P. J., Rhodes, B. A., et al.: Quantification of Right to Left Transpulmonary Shunts in Man, *J. Lab. Clin. Med.,* 74:597, 1969.

10 Folse, R., and Braunwald, E.: Pulmonary Vascular Dilution Curves Recorded by External Detection in the Diagnosis of Left to Right Shunts, *Br. Heart J.,* 24:166, 1962.

11 Alazraki, N. P., Ashburn, W. L., Hagan, A., et al.: Detection of Left to Right Cardiac Shunts with the Scintillation Camera Pulmonary Dilution Curve, *J. Nucl. Med.,* 13:142, 1972.

12 Maltz, D. L., and Treves, S.: Quantitative Radionuclide Angiocardiography: Q_p:Q_s in Children, *Circulation,* 47:1049, 1973.

13 Parker, J. A., and Treves, S.: Radionuclide Detection, Localization and Quantification of Intracardiac Shunts and Shunts between the Great Arteries, in B. L. Holman, E. H. Sonnenblick, and M. Lesch (eds.), "Principles of Cardiovascular Nuclear Medicine," Grune & Stratton, Inc., New York, 1977, p. 189.

14 Rosenthall, L.: Measurement of Intrathoracic Circulation Times with the Gamma Ray Scintillation Camera, *Radiology,* 100:245, 1971.

15 Conway, J. J., and Sherman, J. O.: Evaluation of Chest Masses in Children with Early and Delayed Radionuclide Angiography, *Am. J. Roentgenol.,* 108:575, 1970.

16 Rigo, P.: Unpublished observations.

17 Prinzmetal, M., Corday, E., and Bergman, H. C.: Radiocardiography: A New Method for Studying the Blood Flow Through the Heart in Human Beings, *Science,* 108:340, 1948.

18 MacIntyre, W. J., Storassli, J. P., Krieger, H., et al.: ^{131}I-labeled Human Serum Albumin: Its Use in the Study of Cardiac Output and Peripheral Vascular Flow, *Radiology,* 59:849, 1952.

19 Mullins, C. B., Mason, D. T., Ashburn, W. L., et al.: Determination of Ventricular Volume by Radioisotope Angiography, *Am. J. Cardiol.,* 24:72, 1969.

20 Schelbert, H. R., Verba, J. W., Johnson, A. S., et al.: Non-traumatic Determination of Ejection Fraction by Radionuclide Angiocardiography, *Circulation,* 51:902, 1975.

21 Reduto, L. A., Berger, H. J., Cohen, L. S., et al.: Sequential Radionuclide Assessment of Left and Right Ventricular Performance following Acute Myocardial Infarction, *Circulation,* 55, 56(suppl. 3):65, 1977.

22 Marshall, R. C., Berger, H. J., Reduto, L. A., et al.: Effect of Oral Propranolol Therapy on Left Ventricular Performance in Coronary Artery Disease: Non-invasive Assessment by Sequential Radionuclide Angiocardiography, *Circulation,* 55, 56(suppl. 3):32, 1977.

23 Hellenbrans, W. E., Berger, H. J., O'Brien, R. T., et al.: Left Ventricular Performance in Thalassemia: Combined Radionuclide and Echocardiographic Assessment, *Circulation,* 55, 56(suppl. 3):49, 1977.

24 Holman, B. L., Harris, G. I., Neirinckx, R. D., et al.: Tantulum-178—a Short-lived Nuclide for Nuclear Medicine: Production of the Parent W-178, *J. Nucl. Med.,* 19:510, 1978.

25 Neirinckx, R. D., Jones, A. G., Davis, M. A., et al.: Tantulum-178: A Short-lived Nuclide for Nuclear Medicine: Development of a Potential Generator System, *J. Nucl. Med.,* 19:514, 1978.

26 Strauss, H. W., Zaret, B. L., Hurley, P. J., et al.: A Scintiphotographic Method for Measuring Left Ventricular Ejection Fraction in Man without Cardiac Catheterization, *Am. J. Cardiol.,* 28:575, 1971.

27 Green, M. V., Ostrow, H. G., Douglas, M. A., et al.: High Temporal Resolution ECG-gated Scintigraphic Angiocardiography, *J. Nucl. Med.,* 16:95, 1974.

28 Burow, R., Strauss, H. W., Singleton, R., et al.: Analysis of Left Ventricular Function from Multigated Acquisition (MUGA) Cardiac Blood Pool Imaging: Comparison to Contrast Angiography, *Circulation,* 56:1024, 1977.

29 Borer, J. S., Bachrach, S. L., Green, M. V., et al.: Real Time Radionuclide Cineangiography in the Non-invasive Evaluation of Global and Regional Left Ventricular Function at Rest and during Exercise in Patients with Coronary Artery Disease, *N. Engl. J. Med.,* 296:839, 1977.

30 Pavel, D. G., Zimmer, A. M., Patterson, V. N., et al.: In Vivo Labeling of Red Blood Cells with Tc-99m: A New Approach to Blood Pool Visualization, *J. Nucl. Med.,* 18:305, 1977.

31 Caldwell, J. H., Williams, D. L., Kennedy, J. W., et al.: Quantitative Semiautomated Radionuclide Technique for Determination of Regional Left Ventricular Function at Rest and during Exercise, *J. Nucl. Med.,* 19:710, 1978. (Abstract.)

32 Rigo, P., Murray, M., Strauss, H. W., et al.: Left Ventricular Function in Acute Myocardial Infarction Evaluated by Gated Scintiphotography, *Circulation,* 50:678, 1974.

33 Zaret, B. L., Strauss, H. W., Hurley, P. J., et al.: A Non-invasive Scintiphotographic Method for Detecting Regional Ventricular Dysfunction in Man, *N. Engl. J. Med.,* 284:1176, 1971.

34 Rigo, P., Murray, M., Strauss, H. W., et al.: Scintiphotographic Evaluation of Patients with Suspected Left Ventricular Aneurysm, *Circulation,* 50:895, 1974.

35 Nichols, A. B., McKusick, K. A., Dinsmore, R. E., et al.: Clinical Utility of Cardiac Blood Pool Imaging in the Assessment of Congestive Heart Failure, *Am. J. Med.,* in press.

36 Rigo, P., Murray, M., Taylor, D. R., et al.: Right Ventricular Dysfunction Detected by Gated Scintiphotography in Patients with Acute Inferior Myocardial Infarction, *Circulation,* 52:268, 1974.

37 Pohost, G. M., Pastore, J. O., McKusick, K. A., et al.: Detection of Left Atrial Myxoma by Gated Radionuclide Cardiac Imaging, *Circulation,* 55:88, 1977.

38 Pohost, G. M., Vignola, P. A., McKusick, K. A., et al.: Hypertrophic Cardiomyopathy: Evaluation by Gated Blood Pool Scanning, *Circulation,* 55:92, 1977.

39 Nichols, A. B., Pohost, G. M., Gold, H. K., et al.: Left Ventricular Function during Intra-aortic Balloon Pump Assessed by Multigated Cardiac Blood Pool Imaging, *Circulation,* in press.

40 Nichols, A. B., Cochavi, S., Strauss, H. W., et al.: Changes in Cardiopulmonary Blood Volume during Upright Exercise Testing in Patients with Coronary Artery Disease, *J. Nucl. Med.,* 19:711, 1978. (Abstract.)

41 Okada, R.: Personnel communication.

42 Steele, P., VanDyke, D., Trow, R. S., et al.: A Simple and Safe Bedside Method for Serial Measurement of Left Ventricular Ejection Fraction, Cardiac Output and Pulmonary Blood Volume, *Br. Heart J.,* 38:122, 1974.

43 Wexler, J. P., Strom, J., Sonnenblick, E. A., et al.: Validity of a Probe Technique for Ejection Fraction Determination, *J. Nucl. Med.,* 19:704, 1978.(Abstract.)

44 Maseria, A.: Myocardial Blood Flow in Man: Evaluation of Drugs, in H. W. Strauss, B. Pitt, and A. E. James (eds.), "Cardiovascular Nuclear Medicine," The C. V. Mosby Company, St. Louis, 1974, p. 163.

45 Jansen, C., Grames, G. M., and Judkins, M. P.: Myocardial Blood Flow in Man: Albumin Microsphere Tech-

nique, in H. W. Strauss, B. Pitt, and A. E. James (eds.), "Cardiovascular Nuclear Medicine," The C. V. Mosby Company, St. Louis, 1974, p. 211.

46 Kaplan, E., and Mayron, L. W.: Evaluation of Perfusion with the ^{81}Rb-^{81m}Kr Generator, *Sem. Nucl. Med.*, 6:163, 1976.

47 Gould, K. L., Lipscomb, K., and Hamilton, G. L.: Physiologic Basis for Assessing Critical Coronary Stenosis: Instantaneous Flow Response and Regional Distribution during Coronary Reactive Hyperemia as Measures of Coronary Flow Reserve, *Am. J. Cardiol.*, 33:87, 1974.

48 Ross, R. S.: Historical Perspective and Future Needs, in H. W. Strauss, B. Pitt, and A. E. James (eds.), "Cardiovascular Nuclear Medicine," The C. V. Mosby Company, St. Louis, 1974, p. 138.

49 Cannon, P. J., Dell, R. B., and Dwyer, E. M.: Measurement of Regional Myocardial Perfusion in Man with ^{133}Xenon and a Scintillation Camera, *J. Clin. Invest.*, 51:694, 1972.

50 Carr, E. A.: The Direct Diagnosis of Myocardial Infarction by Photoscanning after Administration of Cesium-131, *Am. Heart J.*, 68:627, 1964.

51 Love, W. D., and Smith, R. O.: Focusing Collimators for Use with the Hard Gamma Emitters of Rubidium-86 and Potassium-42, *J. Nucl. Med.*, 7:81, 1966.

52 Sapirstein, L. A., and Moses, L. E.: Cerebral and Cephalic Flow in Man: Basic Considerations of the Indicator Fractionation Technique, in R. M. Knisely, W. N. Tauxe, and E. B. Anderson (eds.), "Dynamic Clinical Studies with Radioisotopes," USEAC Technical Information Service, 1964.

53 Zaret, B. L., Strauss, H. W., Martin, N. D., et al.: Noninvasive Regional Myocardial Perfusion with Radioactive Potassium: Study of Patients at Rest and during Angina Pectoris, *N. Engl. J. Med.*, 288:809, 1973.

54 Strauss, H. W., Harrison, K., Langan, J. K., et al.: Thallium-201 for Myocardial Imaging: Relationship of Thallium-201 to Regional Myocardial Perfusion, *Circulation*, 51:641, 1975.

55 Trobaugh, G. B., Ritchie, J. L., and Hamilton, G. L.: Rest-Exercise Imaging in Coronary Artery Disease, in J. L. Ritchie, G. W. Hamilton, and F. J. Wackers (eds.), "Thallium-201 Myocardial Imaging," Raven Press, New York, 1978, p. 81.

56 Maseri, A., Parodi, O., Severi, S., et al.: Transient Transmural Reduction of Myocardial Blood Flow Demonstrated by Thallium-201 Scintigraphy as a Cause of Variant Angina, *Circulation*, 54:280, 1976.

57 Pohost, G. M., Zir, L. M., Morre, R. H., et al.: Differentiation of Transiently Ischemic from Infarcted Myocardium by Serial Imaging after a Single Dose of Thallium-201, *Circulation*, 55:294, 1976.

58 Gewirtz, H., Beller, G. A., Strauss, H. W., et al.: Transient Defects on Resting Thallium Scans in Patients with Coronary Artery Disease, *Circulation*, in press.

59 Greenberg, B. H., Hart, R., Botvinick, E. H., et al.: Thallium-201 Myocardial Perfusion Scintigraphy to Evaluate Patients after Coronary Bypass Surgery, *Am. J. Cardiol.*, 42:167, 1978.

60 Strauss, H. W., Pitt, B., Rouleau, J., et al.: Physiological and Technical Factors, in H. W. Strauss et al. (eds.), *Atlas of Cardiovascular Nuclear Medicine*, The C. V. Mosby Company, St. Louis, 1978, chap. 1.

61 Holman, B. L., Lesch, M., Zweiman, F. G., et al.: Detection and Sizing of Acute Myocardial Infarcts with ^{99m}Tc(Sn) Tetracycline, *N. Engl. J. Med.*, 291:159, 1974.

62 Zaret, B. L., Dicola, V. C., Donabedian, R. K., et al.: Dual Radionuclide Study of Myocardial Infarction: Relationships between Myocardial Uptake of Potassium-43, Technetium-99m Stannous Pyrophosphate, Regional Myocardial Blood Flow and Creatinine Phosphokinase Depletion, *Circulation*, 53:422-428, 1976.

63 Marcus, M. L., Tomanek, R. J., Ehrhardt, et al.: Relationships between Myocardial Perfusion, Myocardial Necrosis and Technetium-99m Pyrophosphate Uptake in Dogs Subjected to Sudden Coronary Occlusion, *Circulation*, 54:647, 1976.

64 Zweiman, F. G., Holman, B. L., O'Keefe, A., et al.: Selective Uptake of ^{99m}Tc Complexes and ^{67}Ga in Acutely Infarcted Myocardium, *J. Nucl. Med.*, 16:975, 1975.

65 Rossman, D. J., Strauss, H. W., Siegel, M. E., et al.: Accumulation of ^{99m}Tc-Glucoheptonate in Acutely Infarcted Myocardium, *J. Nucl. Med.*, 16:875-878, 1975.

66 Rossman, D. J., Rouleau, J., Strauss, H. W., et al.: Detection and Size Estimation of Acute Myocardial Infarction Using ^{99m}Tc-Glucoheptonate, *J. Nucl. Med.*, 16:980, 1975.

67 Bonte, F. J., Parkey, R. W., and Graham, K. D.: A New Method for Radionuclide Imaging of Myocardial Infarcts, *Radiology*, 110:473, 1974.

68 Parkey, R. W., Bonte, F. J., Meyer, S., et al.: A New Method for Radionuclide Imaging of Acute Myocardial Infarction in Humans, *Circulation*, 50:540, 1974.

69 Perez, L. A., Hayt, D. B., and Freeman, L. M.: Localization of Myocardial Disorders Other than Infarction with ^{99m}Tc-labeled Phosphate Agents, *J. Nucl. Med.*, 17:241, 1976.

70 Pugh, B. R., Buja, L. M., Parkey, R. W., et al.: Cardioversion and Its Potential Role in the Production of "False Positive" Technetium-99m Stannous Pyrophosphate Myocardial Scintigrams, *Circulation*, 54:399, 1976.

71 Wisneski, J. A., Rollo, F. D., and Gertz, E. W.: Tc-99m Pyrophosphate Myocardial Accumulation in the Absence of Acute Infarction: Correlation with Left Ventricular Wall Motion Abnormalities, *Circulation*, 53, 54(suppl. 2):81, 1976.

72 Parkey, R. W., Bonte, F. J., Stokely, G. M., et al.: Analysis of ^{99m}Tc(Sn) Pyrophosphate Myocardial Scintigrams in 242 Patients, *J. Nucl. Med.*, 16:556, 1975.

73 Olson, H. G., Lyons, K. P., Aronow, W. S., et al.: Fol-

low-up with ^{99m}Tc(Sn) Pyrophosphate Myocardial Scintigrams after Acute Myocardial Infarction, *Circulation,* 56:181, 1977.

74 Buja, N. M., Poliner, L. R., and Parkey, R. W., et al.: Clinical Pathological Study of Persistently Positive ^{99m}Tc Pyrophosphate Myocardial Scintigrams in Myocytolytic Degeneration after Myocardial Infarction, *Circulation,* 56:1016, 1977.

75 Holman, B. L., Chisolm, R. J., and Braunwald, E.: The Prognostic Complications of Acute Myocardial Infarct Scintigraphy with ^{99m}Tc Pyrophosphate, *Circulation,* 57:320, 1978.

76 Berger, H. J., Gottschalk, and Zaret, B. L.: Dual Radionuclide Study of Acute Myocardial Infarction, *Ann. Intern. Med.,* 88:145, 1978.